INSTRUMENTATION IN NUCLEAR MEDICINE

Volume I

CONTRIBUTORS TO THIS VOLUME

Ernest C. Anderson
Hal O. Anger
Saul Aronow
Fritz Berthold
Gordon L. Brownell
Ben C. Claunch
Stephen S. Friedland
Gerald J. Hine
John M. A. Lenihan
Robert Loevinger
Frank H. Low
William J. MacIntyre
Richard C. McCall
Johannes G. Mehl
John Myhill
Paul Numerof
Alan L. Orvis
Edward F. Polic
Edward Rapkin
Chester R. Richmond
Charles V. Robinson
Robert L. Schuch
Marvin A. Van Dilla
James A. Wall
Martin Wenzel
James B. Williams
Michael R. Zatzick

INSTRUMENTATION IN NUCLEAR MEDICINE

Edited by

GERALD J. HINE

Section of Medicine
Department of Research and Isotopes
International Atomic Energy Agency
Vienna, Austria
and
Radioisotope Service
Veterans Administration Hospital
Boston, Massachusetts

Volume I

1967

ACADEMIC PRESS New York San Francisco London

A Subsidiary of Harcourt Brace Jovanovich, Publishers

ACADEMIC PRESS INC.
111 Fifth Avenue, New York, New York 10003

United Kingdom Edition published by
ACADEMIC PRESS, INC. (LONDON) LTD.
24/28 Oval Road, London NW1

Library of Congress Catalog Card Number: 66-29674

PRINTED IN THE UNITED STATES OF AMERICA

LIST OF CONTRIBUTORS

Numbers in parentheses indicate the pages on which the authors' contributions begin.

Ernest C. Anderson (587), Los Alamos Scientific Laboratory, University of California, Los Alamos, New Mexico

Hal O. Anger (485), Donner Laboratory of Medical Physics and Biophysics, University of California, Berkeley, California

Saul Aronow (381, 461), Physics Research Laboratory, Massachusetts General Hospital, Boston, Massachusetts

Fritz Berthold (251), Laboratorium Professor Dr. Berthold, Wildbad (Schwarzwald), Federal Republic of Germany

Gordon L. Brownell (381), Physics Research Laboratory, Massachusetts General Hospital, Boston, Massachusetts

Ben C. Claunch (15), Radioisotope Service, Veterans Administration Hospital, Providence, Rhode Island

Stephen S. Friedland (73), Department of Physics, San Fernando Valley State College, Northridge, California, and Solid State Radiations, Inc., Los Angeles, California

Gerald J. Hine (95, 275, 327, 381, 429, 619), Section of Medicine, Department of Research and Isotopes, International Atomic Energy Agency, Vienna, Austria, and Radioisotope Service, Veterans Administration Hospital, Boston, Massachusetts*

John M. A. Lenihan (309), Regional Physics Department, Western Regional Hospital Board, Glasgow, Scotland

Robert Loevinger (619), Section of Medicine, Department of Research and Isotopes, International Atomic Energy Agency, Vienna, Austria

Frank H. Low (29), Picker Nuclear, White Plains, New York

William J. MacIntyre (351), Departments of Medicine and Psychiatry, Western Reserve University, Cleveland, Ohio

* Present address: Section of Medicine, International Atomic Energy Agency, Vienna, Austria.

Richard C. McCall (163), Controls for Radiation, Inc., Cambridge, Massachusetts†

Johannes G. Mehl (553), Division of Health, Safety, and Waste Disposal, International Atomic Energy Agency, Vienna, Austria‡

John Myhill (429), University of Sydney, and Institute of Medical Research, Royal North Shore Hospital of Sydney, Sydney, Australia

Paul Numerof (1), E. R. Squibb & Sons, New York, New York

Alan L. Orvis (119), Section of Biophysics, Mayo Clinic, Rochester, Minnesota

Edward F. Polic (227), Packard Instrument Company, Inc., Downers Grove, Illinois

Edward Rapkin (181), Consultant, Intertechnique, S. A., Plaisir (S. et O.), France

Chester R. Richmond (587), Los Alamos Scientific Laboratory, University of California, Los Alamos, New Mexico

Charles V. Robinson (57), Medical Physics Division, Medical Research Center, Brookhaven National Laboratory, Upton, New York

Robert L. Schuch (587), University of California at San Diego, La Jolla, California

Marvin A. Van Dilla (587), Los Alamos Scientific Laboratory, University of California, Los Alamos, New Mexico

James A. Wall (163), Controls for Radiation, Inc., Cambridge, Massachusetts

Martin Wenzel (251), Physiologisch-Chemisches Institut der Freien Universität, Berlin, Federal Republic of Germany

James B. Williams (327), Ames Atomium, Inc., Billerica, Massachusetts

Michael R. Zatzick (73), Solid State Radiations, Inc., Los Angeles, California

† Present address: Linear Accelerator Center, Stanford University, Stanford, California.

‡ Present address: Reactor Center Karlsruhe, Karlsruhe, Federal Republic of Germany.

FOREWORD

Nuclear medicine is slowly but steadily coming to be recognized as a medical discipline in its own right. Many of the spectacular developments in this field during the last two decades have been due to advances in instrumentation. Equipment for nuclear medicine has now not only reached a high degree of complexity but is offered by commercial manufacturers all over the world in such variety that it is difficult if not impossible for the average nuclear medicine specialist to select the equipment most suitable for his needs without outside advice. The present volume was written to provide such advice and, in addition, to discuss the physical principles of radiation measurement techniques so that the choice of equipment may be made with a proper regard to its practical applications.

Progress in nuclear medicine requires close collaboration between physician and medical physicist. Unfortunately, many nuclear medicine departments or smaller radioisotope laboratories cannot afford the services of a physicist. Therefore, this comprehensive treatise, the first to describe all aspects of instrumentation in nuclear medicine, is particularly recommended to the medically qualified specialist who would otherwise all too easily fall victim to the persuasion of some clever salesman.

The editor of this book is well known, not only as one of the editors of the "bible" of radiation dosimetry, but also as the author of numerous publications contributing to the advancement of techniques and instrumentation in nuclear medicine. He has enlisted the cooperation of an impressive group of authors, each an expert on the subject assigned to him. In addition, Dr. Hine has written a number of chapters himself.

Although an intergovernmental organization, the International Atomic Energy Agency is primarily science-oriented. It encourages its technical staff to undertake scientific work. This not only includes research in the Agency's laboratory but also the writing or editing of books, conference proceedings, and technical reports. The present volume is a splendid example of such work, and I am convinced that it will not only be consulted by all those responsible for the further development of instruments for nuclear medicine but will also find its place on the shelves of every nuclear medicine department.

HERBERT VETTER

Vienna, Austria
September, 1966

PREFACE

The application of nuclear radiation in medical diagnosis, research, and therapy—now classified as nuclear medicine—has advanced greatly during the past decade. This would not have been possible without the rapid growth in nuclear science and technology during the same period. Radiation detectors such as scintillation crystals and the liquid scintillation counting systems have become highly developed tools to which new types such as the semiconductor and thermoluminescence devices have been added recently. The associated electronic equipment has been greatly improved by switching from vacuum tubes to transistors and by developing new types of equipment such as multichannel analyzers and magnetic tape recorders. Last, but not least, a whole generation of equipment has evolved specifically for the needs of nuclear medicine. To these belong radioisotope scanners, scintillation cameras, and whole-body counters.

This treatise describes comprehensively both the fundamentals and recent developments of important instruments used in nuclear medicine. The theoretical as well as the experimental aspects are presented together with specific information on applications. For each topic as much detailed information is given as is presently available without including special features employed only by individual research workers or certain instrument manufacturers.

The treatise is divided into four parts. The first, which serves as an introduction, presents some of the fundamental concepts for the application of radioisotopes in medicine. In the second part, the various types of radiation detectors presently employed in nuclear medicine are discussed. In addition, the basic electronic components of counting and data-analysis equipment are explained for the nontechnical reader. The special instruments required for radiation safety monitoring are described in an additional chapter. The third part encompasses the various techniques for the measurement of biological samples. They are: liquid scintillation counting, radiochromatographic techniques, γ-ray sample counting, and nuclear activation analysis. The fourth and final part, covering radioisotope measurements *in vivo,* presents the various instruments and techniques specifically developed for nuclear medicine. Composed of eight chapters, it is the largest section of the book. The problems encountered in determining uptake and flow-rates of various compounds in organs by external γ-ray counting are discussed first. Then follows a detailed description of the various systems for delineating the radioisotope distribution within an organ: scanners with multihole collimators, positron scanning, and scintillation cameras. The final chapters deal with the different types of whole-body counters presently in use.

This work is not a description of the latest models of instruments available for nuclear medicine. It attempts rather to present something more important, basic knowledge concerning the purpose, performance, and limitations of each type of instrument and technique. This knowledge is required to make a rational selection of an instrument for a certain use and to achieve the best results with the instrument on hand. In order to enable the reader to obtain specific information about currently available instruments, the names, addresses, and a list of products of manufacturers in the United States and abroad are given in the Appendix of the book.

The reader is expected to be familiar with the physical properties of the radiation emitted by radioisotopes and the basic concepts of radiation detectors. Knowledge which has been available only from widely scattered sources of information is presented systematically for both the practicing physician and the specialist in nuclear medicine, including the hospital physicist. The researcher should also benefit from a study of this book because it contains technical details which only a group of specialists, such as the authors of the various chapters, could present. Most chapters contain a complete bibliography so the book may also serve as a useful reference source. Finally, the medical as well as the nonmedical student will find this book a needed guide through the rapidly growing field of instrumentation in nuclear medicine.

In an attempt to achieve a systematic and exhaustive presentation of all topics, numerous drafts of the various chapters were required. The authors as well as the editor were greatly aided by many people in the field to whom they are much indebted. In particular, the editor would like to express his thanks to Norman A. Baily, Belton A. Burrows, John A. Cardarelli, Arthur F. Dratz, Melvin H. Farmelant, Hobart W. Kraner, Robert Loevinger, Robert M. Parr, Herbert Vetter, and Richard E. Wainerdi.

GERALD J. HINE

Vienna, Austria
August, 1966

CONTENTS

Part II. Systems for Radiation Analysis

Part III. Measurements of Biological Samples

Chapter 9. PREPARATION OF SAMPLES FOR LIQUID SCINTILLATION COUNTING

EDWARD RAPKIN

Chapter 10. LIQUID SCINTILLATION COUNTING EQUIPMENT

EDWARD F. POLIC

Chapter 11. RADIOCHROMATOGRAPHIC COUNTING TECHNIQUES

FRITZ BERTHOLD AND MARTIN WENZEL

Chapter 12. γ-RAY SAMPLE COUNTING

GERALD J. HINE

Chapter 17. MULTIHOLE COLLIMATORS FOR SCANNING

JOHN MYHILL AND GERALD J. HINE

Chapter 18. POSITRON SCANNING

SAUL ARONOW

Chapter 19. RADIOISOTOPE CAMERAS

HAL O. ANGER

Chapter 20. SINGLE AND MULTIPLE DETECTOR SYSTEMS FOR WHOLE-BODY COUNTING

JOHANNES G. MEHL

Chapter 21. LARGE ORGANIC SCINTILLATION DETECTORS

MARVIN A. VAN DILLA, ERNEST C. ANDERSON, CHESTER R. RICHMOND, AND ROBERT L. SCHUCH

INSTRUMENTATION IN NUCLEAR MEDICINE

Volume I

PART I
FUNDAMENTAL CONCEPTS

CHAPTER 1

RADIOISOTOPES AND LABELED COMPOUNDS

PAUL NUMEROF
E. R. SQUIBB & SONS
NEW YORK, NEW YORK

I. RADIOPHARMACEUTICAL AGENTS IN NUCLEAR MEDICINE

Progress in clinical nuclear medicine and developments in instrumentation and radiopharmaceuticals are mutually dependent. The most advanced nuclear detection devices are useless if there is no labeled drug present in the tissue volume to be examined. Similarly, the most tissue-specific drug is of little value if suitable detection equipment is not available.

A labeled compound has one of its atoms substituted by a radioactive one, which may be an isotope of the same element (isotopic labeling), in the same position and without any other change in the molecule. In case a foreign radioisotope (such as ^{131}I) is used, the labeling is nonisotopic. A useful radiopharmaceutical agent must have a high tissue specificity to yield a good target-to-nontarget ratio. In addition it must possess the following characteristics:

(a) Radioisotope of suitable half-life.
(b) Isotope with suitable radiation characteristics.
(c) Ready incorporation into suitable agents by chemical or biological synthesis.
(d) Nontoxic in the concentrations to be administered.
(e) Moderate in cost.
(f) Available in convenient pharmaceutical dosage forms.

Radioisotopes of half-life sufficiently long to permit chemical processing, pharmaceutical formulation, and quality-control testing are essential for radioactive drugs to have any degree of widespread use. Although half-lives of seconds or minutes are not compatible with these requirements, isotopes of half-life as short as 12 hr can be employed for inorganic compounds.

The radiation characteristics of isotopes are also important. In diagnostic thyroid work, for example, one faces the anomalous situation where the γ-ray component of the isotope, ^{131}I, is essential for the measurement of radioiodine uptake and morphology. However, the radiation effects produced by ^{131}I are primarily caused by the β-ray component, which is not desired during diagnostic procedures. Conversely, for radiation therapy the β-ray component is the more important.

Facile synthesis of radiopharmaceutical agents is a matter of prime importance since difficulty in preparation must be associated with an increase in cost. Organic synthesis is preferable, since methods can usually be devised for incorporating the radioactive isotope at late stages of preparation, thus minimizing loss of radioactivity. In certain instances this method of approach is not feasible and biosynthetic methods are then employed. Good illustrations of biosynthetic preparations useful in clinical nuclear medicine are cyanocobalamin, which has not yielded to organic synthesis, and also selenomethionine.

The radiochemical purity of the labeled compound is that proportion of the radioisotope that is present in the stated chemical form. The requirement for radiochemical purity varies with the use for which the labeled compound is intended. Its radiochemical impurities are often the consequences of the conditions of synthesis or storage. Quality control depends not only on the examination or analysis of the product but also on the whole production process starting from the selection of the target material used for activation. There is only limited use for the traditional physical methods of purity testing in the analysis of radiopharmaceuticals.

For the materials in routine clinical use, exacting requirements apply in regard to freedom from toxic impurities, including pyrogens and microorganisms. Most of the labeled compounds can be sterilized by autoclaving. The most noteworthy exception is iodinated human serum albumin, which must be prepared aseptically in sterilized sealed glove boxes. Testing for sterility and pyrogens has its own problems, because of radioactive decay, and the small weights or volumes which are available. Standard pyrogen testing requires relatively large volumes of solutions to be injected into rabbits, which would involve large amounts of radioactivity.

An important feature of radiopharmaceuticals is the very small chemical level at which these agents are used. For thyroid uptake studies, a 25 μCi dose of ^{131}I weighs only 0.002 μg, which is a minor fraction of the normal daily iodine requirement of about 150 μg. In evaluation of kidney function the chemical level of the radioactive agent is generally a fraction of a milligram, much less than the amount of the same agent, unlabeled, where several grams are administered for radiological diagnostic purposes. In general, radiopharmaceuticals used at the diagnostic level employ agents well below the level at which pharmacological responses are observed.

II. IODINATED COMPOUNDS

A. Chemical Considerations

The ready availability of ^{131}I as a by-product of nuclear fission in reactor operation, the ease of its radiation measurement, and the unique requirement of the thyroid gland for iodine, served as potent stimuli for early widespread clinical application of this radioisotope. Subsequent experience disclosed a need for easily measured isotopically labeled compounds of potential usefulness in measurement of plasma volume, kidney function, and liver function. Fortunately, the chemical properties of iodine are amenable to incorporation into the variety of agents required for many different clinical applications (*13*). It is understandable why ^{131}I remains the most widely used radioisotope in clinical medicine, for no other element possesses such favorable radiation characteristics, chemical properties, ready availability, and moderate cost.

B. Iodide-Iodine

Most ^{131}I, in terms of both number of millicuries and number of patients studied, is used in diagnosis and treatment involving the thyroid gland. Production and distribution of this ^{131}I is generally as carrier-free iodide ion. Maintenance of ^{131}I as iodide ion is essential, since biochemical studies have shown thyroid accumulation of iodine to be chemically dependent (*6*). The ease with which iodide is oxidized to iodine by relatively mild oxidizing agents has presented a pharmaceutical problem, which has been met, in part, by the addition of reducing agents. However, the concentration of reducing agent in pharmaceutical preparations of iodide-^{131}I is limited, and noniodide chemical forms may develop in such samples retained for long periods of time.

In addition to the problem of chemical integrity in highly radioactive solutions of iodide-^{131}I, the problem of carrier-free concentrations must also be considered, since the weight of iodine per 1000 μCi of radioactivity is 8.1×10^{-12} gm. Solutions of even several millicuries per milliliter contain gravimetric concentrations of iodide far below those encountered in conventional chemical manipulations. Adsorption to glassware and chemical behavior contrary to that expected from the law of mass action are common phenomena.

These problems are of critical importance in the preparation of radioactive solutions for human use. Minimum standards of preparation have been established and appear in recent revisions of the *United States Pharmacopeia*. To meet these standards, the following tests must be performed:

(a) Radiochemical purity. Paper-chromatographic analysis for iodide-^{131}I and other ^{131}I ionic species. Limits: Iodate not to exceed 5% of the total activity of the iodide band. No other radioactivity bands are present.
(b) Total iodide: No detectable iodine after oxidation and extraction into chloroform.
(c) pH: 7.0–8.5.
(d) Assay: $\pm 5\%$ limit.
(e) Identification: ^{131}I radioactivity demonstrated by β-ray absorption.
(f) Sterility and pyrogen testing for parenteral formulations.

These standards are minimum requirements, and are not considered sufficient in some laboratories. Additional testing procedures employing iodine chemistry for verification of ^{131}I activity as iodide ion, and γ-ray spectrometric analysis for isotope identification, are used.

C. Iodination of Organic Compounds

Unique chemical properties and its high atomic number have placed iodine in a special position completely independent of its importance in thyroid physiology. High atomic number of iodine ($Z = 53$) means opacity to X radiation. Favorable chemical properties allow ready organic chemical synthesis. The combination of these characteristics has resulted in a wide variety of compounds used as contrast media for X-ray visualization of kidney, gall bladder, and gastrointestinal tract, as well as delineation of heart and peripheral blood vessels. It was a natural development that some of these compounds should be labeled with radioactive iodine in the hope that clinical procedures using these compounds could be carried out more quickly, more conveniently, and with less hazard to the patient. Kinetic studies, clearance rates, volumes of distribution, and so on can more readily be carried out by measuring changes in levels of radioactivity than by conventional chemical analysis. This expectation has been realized, and a variety of ^{131}I-labeled compounds are now routinely available for such clinical studies.

D. Important Iodine-Containing Compounds

1. Human Serum Albumin

The use of ^{131}I human serum albumin in measurement of plasma volume, placental localization, cardiac scanning, cardiac output, and other procedures testifies to the importance of this agent. Unlike many ^{131}I compounds which can be labeled by isotope exchange methods, the heat lability of human serum albumin-^{131}I (IHSA) requires preparation by direct iodination.

However, the problem of heat lability is only one consideration in the preparation of IHSA with suitable retention of protein integrity. Other factors are the following.

a. *Degree of Iodination.* It is essential that the extent of iodination be small, of the order of 1–2 atoms of iodine (*1*) per molecule of albumin. More heavily iodinated molecules (*4*) result in preparations whose physicochemical and pharmacological behavior are markedly different from native albumin.

b. *Specific Activity.* The ratio of labeled albumin molecules to total albumin present is an important factor in the retention of protein integrity in preparations of IHSA. Aqueous solutions of proteins are sensitive to ionizing radiation, showing marked changes in ion-binding capacity, ultraviolet absorption characteristics, and amino acid composition. Since IHSA solutions of 1 mCi/ml lead to the absorption of approximately 10,000 rad and 50,000 rad in 1 and 6 days, respectively, it is essential that steps be taken to reduce radiation damage as far as possible. These effects can be minimized by having a preponderance of unlabeled molecules present for interaction with the free radicals generated during the radiation decomposition of water.

Physicochemical systems may not readily detect alterations that may be discriminated very sensitively by a particular biological system. Thus, physicochemical testing methods of ^{131}I-labeled proteins are best used for screening purposes only; final tests of protein integrity should, where possible, be carried out with biological tests on experimental animals.

2. *o*-Iodohippuric Acid

The use of urographic agents labeled with ^{131}I for evaluation of kidney function has become a familiar clinical isotope procedure. Administration of the drug intravenously, with measurement of the rate of excretion through the kidney, often provided extremely useful information.

Of special significance in these studies is the very small weight of labeled material employed. Isotope renograms are generally carried out with material weighing only about a milligram or less. By comparison, intravenous pyelography requires 10–13 gm of material, with 8–9 gm of iodine present. Reactions to contrast material administration have been reported, some of them fatal. On the contrary, such reactions have not been reported following the administration of the small quantities involved in radioisotope studies of kidney function.

The importance of radiopharmaceutical developments is well illustrated by the history of isotope compounds used for the study of kidney function. The earliest agent widely employed, iodopyracet (Diodrast), although excreted primarily through the kidneys, was also excreted in substantial quantities through the liver. Measurement of right-kidney radioactivity was thus complicated by the amount of agent present in the liver. These difficulties were overcome when it was shown that *o*-iodohippuric acid (Hippuran) was rapidly cleared by the kidneys with little or no elimination through the liver (*19*). This has now become the agent of choice.

3. Rose Bengal

Evaluation of polygonal cell activity in the liver by measurement of the extraction kinetics of rose bengal has been described (*18*). This fluorescent red dye, which contains both iodine and chlorine atoms, is prepared by exchange of iodide-^{131}I for halogen. The presence of two kinds of halogen atoms complicates the exchange reaction, and it is not surprising that chromatographic analysis of rose bengal has indeed shown the presence of more than one component.

4. ^{131}I Fats and Fatty Acids

Since neutral fats must undergo lipolysis to fatty acids before absorption can occur, labeled fats provide a useful means of following fat metabolism. As pointed out by Van Handel and Zilversmit (*20*), however, it is essential to differentiate the requirements of a procedure designed to give clinically useful information from those needed to give definitive information concerning metabolic pathways. For the former, ^{131}I fats and fatty acids can be used; for the latter, halogen labels are unsatisfactory since deiodination occurs with resultant loss of label.

For measurement of the digestive and absorptive phases of fat metabolism, ^{131}I-labeled preparations have proven of considerable value. The addition of labeled fat to a standard fat-meal, followed by stool collection and measurement of unabsorbed fat, is a marked analytical simplification compared with standard chemical methods of fecal-fat determinations. Even this procedure has been simplified by substitution of blood levels of radioactivity as an index of absorption. However, recent work suggests the fecal-labeled fat studies to be less subject to misinterpretation.

5. CHOLOGRAFIN-^{131}I

Recent reports have described multiple areas of application of a single compound, Cholografin-^{131}I, in studies of liver function, cardiac output, and delineation of cardiac size by isotope scanning techniques. In its nonradioactive form, Cholografin serves as a contrast medium for the study of the bile ducts and gall bladder. In labeled form, the agent was shown to be useful in the selection of patients for the contrast medium studies. Of special interest was the demonstration that the labeled agent could delineate a specific hepatic metabolic defect, "Gilbert's disease" (*9*), demonstrable with depressed Cholografin-^{131}I liver uptake curves in spite of normal rose bengal data in the same patients. Thus, two agents for evaluation of liver function, totally unrelated in chemical structures, can be utilized for selective diagnostic information relative to liver disease.

The unique properties of Cholografin-^{131}I, aside from its use in liver function, depend in large part on its rate of vascular clearance. It is cleared from the blood more slowly than ^{131}I-labeled urotropic agents, but much more rapidly than labeled proteins. Thus, for clinical indications where blood retention of radioactivity is required for moderate periods of time, as in cardiac output and cardiac scanning (*15*), Cholografin-^{131}I is a logical choice. Rapid clearance of Cholografin-^{131}I through the liver and GI tract results in marked reduction in patient radiation exposure relative to similar studies using human serum albumin-^{131}I.

6. TRIIODOTHYRONINE-^{131}I (T-3)

The demonstration by Hamolsky *et al.* (*12*) of the significance of T-3 binding by erythrocytes as an index of thyroid function has stimulated considerable interest. Since the major physiological parameter in this procedure is the binding of T-3 by small amounts of plasma globulins, the red cells acting as a T-3 "sink," labeled compounds of high specific activity are required. The mass of T-3 used in this *in vitro* study is only 0.001–0.01 μg. Since only 10–20% of the radioactivity added ends up on the red cells, it is essential that sufficiently high specific activity material be used to permit statistically significant counts to be accumulated within a reasonable period of time. Material with specific activities of 20–50 mCi/mg are used. While such high specific activities are quite convenient for counting purposes, they present a serious problem for the chemical integrity of triiodothyronine.

Processes leading to labeled artifacts include deiodination of the parent compound, oxidation of iodide ion to free iodine, oxidation of amino nitrogen, and formation of labeled species other than the parent compound. Starting with T-3 labeled in the 3 position, of 25 mCi/mg radioactivity and 16 mg/ml, self-radiolysis over a 75-day period gave a number of products, with deamination of T-3 to the corresponding lactic acid as a major product. Thus, studies of T-3 binding by plasma proteins are best carried out with freshly prepared material. Corrections for contaminants can be made, if necessary, by column chromatography on starch (*16*).

In spite of the problems associated with high specific activity requirements for T-3, the test has proven so useful that it has achieved wide acceptance. However, procedural difficulties involved in handling and measuring fragile red cells led to a search for other materials that could replace erythrocytes. The most successful answer to this problem so far developed is an anion-exchange resin.

Recent experience (*8*) has shown that inorganic iodide-^{131}I present in plasma from previous diagnostic or therapeutic procedures complicates results when the resin procedure is used. Suitable corrections for inorganic iodide-^{131}I activity can be made provided the concentration of iodide does not exceed 20% of the total activity. At higher iodide-^{131}I concentrations only the Hamolsky erythrocyte uptake procedure gives consistent results.

III. CHROMIUM

The elegant procedure described by Gray and Sterling (*10*) for preparing erythrocytes labeled with radioactive chromium, ^{51}Cr, yields a tool of wide applicability. Labeled red blood cells provide significant clinical information not only in erythrocyte survival studies but in measurement of gastrointestinal blood loss (*7*), prediction of beneficial effect of splenectomy, and localization of the placenta.

During the labeling of erythrocytes, chromate ion diffuses into the cell, is reduced to chromic ion to which the erythrocyte wall is not permeable, and remains bound to hemoglobin within the cell. Although the initial reports on erythrocyte labeling with ^{51}Cr employed saline suspensions of isolated cells, the most common current practice is the use of whole blood. An anticoagulant is an obvious requirement, and a special citric acid–dextrose formulation with lower glucose and higher citrate concentrations than normally employed is the one most often used. At room temperature, with whole blood, approximately 90% of added chromate radioactivity is bound to erythrocytes within 15 min when the Strumia ACD formulation is used.

The reducing properties of glucose, and its far greater molar concentration than chromate during the tagging procedure, has led to some concern of reduced tagging efficiency due to reduction of chromate to chromic ion. At specific activities of 100 mCi/mg, 100 μCi of ^{51}Cr activity is only about 1 μg. However, over short time intervals such as addition of chromate to ACD 5 hr before addition to whole blood, no effect on erythrocyte tagging efficiency has been observed.

When desired, however, advantage can be taken of the ease with which chromate can be reduced. Once maximum tagging has occurred *in vitro,* ascorbic acid is added to convert any residual chromate ion to ineffective chromic ion. Any further inadvertent tagging *in vivo* after injection, which would vitiate the test, is thus prevented.

Some concern has been expressed at times about potential chemical toxicity of chromium. This may have been a problem with the low specific activities available at the time the method was developed, but high specific activity preparations currently available from radiopharmaceutical manufacturers have eliminated chemical toxicity of chromium. Since 30 μg of chromium per milliliter of red cells may be tolerated as an upper limit, the 1 μg of chromium in 100 μCi of a 100 mCi/mg activity preparation is far below toxic chemical levels.

IV. IRON

The unique physiology of iron has provided a fertile field for isotope tracer applications. Since iron is reutilized by the body, and there is no normal mechanism for iron excretion, a demonstrated iron deficiency is an indicator of blood loss. Demonstrated alteration of iron metabolism is, therefore, of extreme practical importance, and much use has been made of isotopes of iron in the investigation of hemopoietic disorders.

Although early work with radioactive iron involved labeling of plasma protein, this procedure has now largely been superseded by direct intravenous injection of radioactive iron salts. Measurement of the rate of initial clearance of iron, and its later appearance as hemoglobin, is useful in evaluating hematopoietic function (*14*).

The most widely used isotope of iron is ^{59}Fe, primarily because of the ease with which its β and γ radiations can be detected; on the other hand, ^{55}Fe, which decays by electron capture with emission of X rays of only 6 keV, is somewhat more difficult to detect. Nevertheless, for differential studies, methods of detection of both isotopes in the presence of each other are desirable. Several descriptions of counting techniques for simultaneous measurement of ^{55}Fe and ^{59}Fe have appeared, one using Geiger–Müller tubes of different sensitivity for the radiations of the two iron isotopes and two employing liquid scintillation techniques (*5*).

V. PHOSPHORUS

Reports on the use of ^{32}P as sodium phosphate in the treatment of certain leukemia and polycythemia gave promise of a useful role in clinical nuclear medicine. For use in human patients, uniform carefully controlled preparations are essential, and minimum standards for this product were established in *United States Pharmacopeia XVI*. The essential tests for ^{32}P, as sodium radiophosphate, are given there as follows:

(a) Identification of ^{32}P radioactivity by β-ray absorption.
(b) pH: 5–6.
(c) Assay: $\pm 5\%$ limit.
(d) Sterility and pyrogen testing of intravenous preparations.

VI. COLLOIDS: GOLD-198 AND CHROMIC PHOSPHATE-^{32}P

The early demonstration of insoluble chromic phosphate labeled with ^{32}P as a source of selective irradiation of tissues of the reticuloendothelial system suggested this material could be employed in situations where ^{198}Au was used (*11*). Furthermore, comparison of the radiation characteristics of ^{32}P, a pure β-ray emitter, and ^{198}Au, both a β- and γ-ray emitter, stimulated development of a suitable method of preparation of chromic phosphate. From the viewpoint of convenience, there can be no question concerning the advantage of inventory maintenance with long-lived ^{32}P. In addition, the complete absence of γ radiation with ^{32}P simplifies handling problems.

However, the advantage in radiation dose distribution claimed for the absence of γ radiation with ^{32}P has been challenged. The γ-ray component of ^{198}Au is claimed to contribute substantially to a better homogenization of the radiation effect. Furthermore, the higher β-ray energy of ^{32}P, 1.7 MeV, is claimed to increase the possibility of fibrosis during intraperitoneal administration, a danger less likely with the lower β-ray energy, 0.95 MeV, of ^{198}Au.

It is important to realize that a difference exists in the chemical forms of the ^{32}P and ^{198}Au preparations. Chromic phosphate, after being heated at elevated temperature, generally is further processed by continuous grinding in a ball mill. Reconstitution yields a suspension, not a true colloid. On the other hand, ^{198}Au preparations, as described in the *United States Pharmacopeia XVI*, are true colloids prepared by reduction of auric solutions with suitable reducing agents and stabilized with gelatin.

Fairly stable to heat, the colloids are precipitated at temperatures encountered during autoclaving. Although unstable toward metallic ions, particularly trivalent cations, gold colloids may generally be diluted with water, physiological saline solutions, pectin, procaine, epinephrine, and hyaluronidase. Of the two preparations, it is probable that gold colloids are more uniform and reproducible with respect to particle size. This is of importance in measurement of liver blood flow, since the liver extraction rate is dependent on particle size, with small-size colloids being extracted more slowly than those having larger mean size distributions.

VII. MERCURY

A. Mercury Compounds

From obscurity to one of the most widely used clinical isotopes in just a few years is the history of mercury-labeled chlormerodrin (Neohydrin). It is now used extensively in the detection of brain tumors and scanning of the renal areas. The greater utility of Neohydrin-^{203}Hg for brain tumor localization, its widest use, lies not so much in its chemical differentiation from human serum albumin-^{131}I, which has also been widely used, but in the particularly favorable physical characteristics of the ^{203}Hg isotope and the physiological behavior of the agent (*2*).

In the use of Neohydrin-^{203}Hg for brain tumor localization it is important to realize one is administering *intravenously* a mercurial diuretic normally given *orally*. At specific activities currently available at time of preparation, 50–100 μCi/mg, the amount of mercury administered as Neohydrin-^{203}Hg is still as small as, and often less than, the dose of mercurial diuretic used for sensitivity testing.

The success with labeled mercurials for brain tumor localization and renal scanning has led to a search for other mercurials with similar potential. One such compound, bromomercuryhydroxypropane-^{203}Hg (BMHP-^{203}Hg), (*21*) has been shown to be taken up so readily by erythrocytes that red blood cell labeling can be effected directly in whole blood in a matter of minutes. The BMHP-erythrocyte bond is a firm one and apparently alters the erythrocyte structure sufficiently to have these cells undergo splenic sequestration. As a result, it may be possible to do spleen scanning by direct erythrocyte labeling, eliminating the time-consuming heating of erythrocytes necessary when chromate-labeled red cells are employed.

B. Mercury Isotopes

One of the problems associated with the use of Neohydrin-^{203}Hg is the long time required for excretion of the compound. Kidney retention is a concomitant to the use of Neohydrin-^{203}Hg for brain scanning, one which can be accepted, considering the severity of the diagnostic problem for which the agent is being used. Nevertheless, it would still be desirable to obtain the same clinical information with reduced radiation exposure, if possible.

Since suitable chemical agents of shorter biological half-life are not currently available, the only recourse is a different isotope of mercury. Data on ^{197}Hg suggest the same studies can be carried out as with ^{203}Hg with no loss of information. Since ^{197}Hg emits no β rays and has a much shorter half-life than ^{203}Hg, the radiation energy delivered to the kidneys is markedly reduced.

As currently produced, ^{197}Hg is prepared by exposure of ^{196}Hg to neutrons. In addition to ^{197}Hg, there is also produced ^{197m}Hg and a small percentage of ^{203}Hg. It is important to appreciate the rapidity with which the *percentage* of ^{203}Hg increases with time due to the marked differences in the half-lives of ^{197}Hg and ^{203}Hg. After 2 weeks the ^{197}Hg content has been sharply reduced, and its use at this time would result essentially in the administration of ^{203}Hg as well as an undesirable amount of chemical mercury.

VIII. SELENIUM

Interest in ^{75}Se has been stimulated by the elegant studies of Blau and Bender leading to development of selenomethionine-^{75}Se for scanning of the pancreas (*3*). Biosynthesis of selenomethionine-^{75}Se, where the sulfur of methionine has been replaced by selenium, provides a preparation of high specific activity, approximately 2000 μCi/mg, suitable for clinical use. While still an investigational development, there is promise that selenomethionine-^{75}Se will be a useful agent for pancreatic scanning and possibly parathyroid scanning as well.

IX. COBALT

For uses other than teletherapy, the interest in cobalt isotopes rests on the unique physiological role of cyanocobalamin, vitamin B_{12}. This complex compound, with the molecular formula $C_{63}H_{88}CoN_{14}O_{14}P$, contains a cobalt atom as an integral part of its molecular structure. Too complex for ready chemical synthesis, vitamin B_{12} is prepared by fermentation methods through addition of radioactive cobalt to a low-cobalt medium of a vitamin B_{12}-producing strain of microorganism.

Cyanocobalamin is essential in the human dietary and is a specific therapy when administered parenterally for pernicious anemia. In its radioactive form, labeled vitamin B_{12} plays an important role in the differential diagnosis of pernicious anemia (*17*). Since part of the clinical radioisotope procedure involves parenteral administration of vitamin B_{12}, a unique situation is present where the disease, pernicious anemia, if present, is not only diagnosed but also treated at the same time.

Although vitamin B_{12} has been made available for clinical use labeled with ^{57}Co, ^{58}Co, and ^{60}Co at one time, only ^{57}Co- and ^{60}Co-labeled vitamin B_{12} enjoy widespread use currently.

REFERENCES

1. Berson, S. A., and Yalow, R. S., Radiochemical and radiobiological alterations of I^{131} labeled proteins in solution. *Ann. N.Y. Acad. Sci.* **70,** 56 (1957).
2. Blau, M., and Bender, M. A., Radiomercury (Hg^{203}) labeled Neohydrin, a new agent for brain tumor localization. Paper presented in part at 6th annual meeting, June, 1959 and 7th annual meeting, June, 1960, of the Society of Nuclear Medicine.
3. Blau, M., and Bender, M. A., Se^{75}-Selenomethionine for visualization of the pancreas by isotope scanning. *Radiology* **78,** 974 (1962).
4. Cooper, M., and Owen, C. A., Jr., Labeling human erythrocytes with radiochromium. *J. Lab. Clin. Med.* **47,** 65 (1956).
5. Dern, R. J., and Hart, W. L., Studies with doubly labeled iron. I. Simultaneous liquid scintillation counting of isotopes Fe^{55} and Fe^{59} as ferrous perchlorate. *J. Lab. Clin. Med.* **57,** 322 (1961).
6. Doctor, V. M., and Trunnell, J. B., Studies on the effect of storage on the purity of sodium iodide-I^{131}. *Endocrinology* **64,** 455 (1959).
7. Ebaugh, F. R., Jr., Clemens, T., Jr., Rodnan, G., and Peterson, R. E., Quantitative measurement of gastrointestinal blood loss. I. The use of radioactive Cr^{51} in patients with gastrointestinal hemorrhage. *Am. J. Med.* **25,** 169 (1958).
8. Foeckler, F. H., Bering, N. M., Siragusa, J., and Hunter, O. B., Jr., Comparative thyroid-function studies with the resin T-3 test. *J. Nucl. Med.* **4,** 239 (1963).
9. Galambos, J. T., and McLaren, J. R., Demonstration of a hepatic uptake defect in Gilbert's disease. *Lancet* **I,** 166 (1962).
10. Gray, S. J., and Sterling, K., The tagging of red cells and plasma proteins with radioactive chromium. *J. Clin. Invest.* **29,** 1604 (1950).
11. Hahn, P. F., Carothers, E. L., and Meneely, G. R., Production and handling of therapeutic isotopes. *In* "Theraputic Use of Artificial Radioisotopes" (P. F. Hahn, ed.), p. 77. Wiley, New York, 1956.
12. Hamolsky, M. W., Golodetz, A., and Freedberg, A. S., The plasma protein-thyroid hormone complex in man. III. Further studies on the use of the *in vitro* red blood cell uptake I^{131} 1-triiodothyronine as a diagnostic test of thyroid function. *J. Clin. Endocrinol. Metab.* **19,** 103 (1959).

13. Hughes, W. L., The chemistry of iodination. *Ann. N.Y. Acad. Sci.* **70**, 3 (1957).
14. Loeffler, R. K., Rappaport, D. A., and Collins, V. P., Radioiron citrate as tracer to determine disappearance rate of plasma iron in normal subjects. *Proc. Soc. Exptl. Biol. Med.* **88**, 441 (1955).
15. MacIntyre, W. J., Gomez-Crespo, G., and Christie, J. H., Use of radioiodinated (I^{131}) Iodipamide for cardiovascular scanning. *Am. J. Roentgenol., Radium Therapy Nucl. Med.* **89**, 315 (1963).
16. Rabinowitz, J. L., and Shapiro, B., A chromatographic method utilizing Sephadex for the separation of free iodide, protein-bound and unbound triiodothyronine in sera. *J. Nucl. Med.* **3**, 417 (1962).
17. Schilling, R. F., Intrinsic factor studies; the effect of gastric juice on the urinary excretion of radioactivity after oral administration of radioactive vitamin B_{12}. *J. Lab. Clin. Med.* **42**, 860 (1953).
18. Taplin, G. V., Meredith, O. M., Jr., and Kade, H., The radioactive (I^{131} tagged) rose bengal uptake-excretion test for liver function using external gamma ray scintillation counting techniques. *J. Lab. Clin. Med.* **45**, 665 (1955).
19. Tubis, M., Posnack, E., and Nordyke, R. A., Preparation and use of I^{131} labeled sodium iodohippurate in kidney function tests. *Proc. Soc. Exptl. Biol. Med.* **103**, 497 (1960).
20. Van Handel, E., and Zilversmit, D. B., Limitation of radioiodine as a label for fat. *J. Lab. Clin. Med.* **52**, 831 (1958).
21. Wagner, H. N., Jr., McAfee, J. G., Weiner, I. M., Iio, M., Martinez, J., and Caine, W. P., Jr., The use of Hg^{203} labeled bromomercuryhydroxypropane (BMHP) in radioisotopes scanning of the spleen. *J. Nucl. Med.* **4**, 190 (1963).

NOTE: All pertinent aspects of radiopharmaceuticals have been discussed in a recent symposium: "Radioactive Pharmaceuticals" (G. A. Andrews, R. M. Kniseley, and H. N. Wagner, Jr., eds.). Conf.-65111 U.S. Department of Commerce, Springfield, Virginia, 1966.

CHAPTER 2

THE RADIOISOTOPE LABORATORY IN THE GENERAL HOSPITAL

BEN C. CLAUNCH
RADIOISOTOPE SERVICE
VETERANS ADMINISTRATION HOSPITAL
PROVIDENCE, RHODE ISLAND

I. ESTABLISHMENT OF A RADIOISOTOPE LABORATORY

The use of radioisotopes in clinical medicine is no longer limited to large medical centers. The number of practical radioisotope procedures of proven value is growing continuously. Many community general hospitals have provided facilities for some radioisotope work. However, expansion and multiplication of radioisotope facilities in such hospitals seems inevitable.

The decision to establish a clinical radioisotope laboratory in a general hospital depends upon its size, location, use by the community and physicians, and the extent of its teaching program. The bed capacity of the hospital may be less important than other factors in determining the need of establishing a radioisotope service. The cost of establishing and running it, however, is relatively greater for smaller hospitals. General hospitals providing fairly complete diagnostic facilities will find greater need of a radioisotope laboratory than hospitals specialized to provide obstetric, pediatric, geriatric, emergency medical and surgical, or terminal care.

The teaching program of the hospital must also be considered. Training of interns and residents should include experience with radioisotope diagnostic tests and therapy, and this alone may justify the establishment of a radioisotope service. Even in the absence of a house staff, the radioisotope laboratory may become the nucleus for a dynamic postgraduate teaching program.

In areas with more than one hospital, consideration should be given to cooperative efforts. With the possible exception of blood volume determinations and scanning procedures few routine radioisotope tests are performed in an emergency situation necessitating on-premises operation of the radioisotope facility. If one hospital is used more frequently for diagnostic work-ups it may logically be chosen to incorporate radioisotope facilities. In other situations the location of one hospital or space considerations may determine the choice.

The availability of a physician who can devote the time and effort necessary to make a radioisotope laboratory a success is crucial. Present regulations controlling the use of radioisotopes require the final authority and responsibility for the administration of radioisotopes to human beings to rest with one or more physicians designated as a local radioisotope committee. A survey of community hospitals has shown that a member of the radiology department is most frequently responsible for the radioisotope service. Board certification in radiology now requires a basic introduction to nuclear physics and radiological health physics. Radiologists or pathologists are frequently the only full-time physicians on the staff of the general hospitals and therefore are available to supervise the administration of radioisotopes. Despite these advantages, a clinician familiar with the significance and limitations of radioisotope techniques should be considered for the supervision and interpretation of radioisotope tests.

The growth of radioisotope tests originates from certain advantages they offer compared with previously available methods. Radioisotope techniques frequently give increased accuracy, simplicity, and speed, besides sometimes providing unique information as in organ scanning or uptake studies. Comparison of the man hours needed to determine the mean survival of erythrocytes by the serological method of Ashby with the time required using ^{51}Cr-labeled erythrocytes demonstrates the time-saving of radioisotope techniques. The older method to diagnose pernicious anemia in a partially treated patient should be compared with the technique using radioactive vitamin B_{12} to appreciate the simplicity of radioisotope techniques.

II. STARTING AND MAINTAINING A RADIOISOTOPE LABORATORY

A. Location

The radioisotope laboratory is a clinical facility to which patients must come several times daily for some procedures. Many radioisotope procedures will be used in nonhospitalized patients. Therefore a location suitable to off-street traffic is desirable, and ease of accessibility for patients and staff is important.

The distance from the radiology area must be considered. Scattered X rays from diagnostic X-ray units seldom pose a problem if shielding is adequate for good radiological health procedures. However, operation of high-energy therapy units, including ^{60}Co or ^{137}Cs units, may vary background count-rate and cause errors in measuring specimens with low levels of radioactivity. The radioisotope laboratory should therefore be kept at least 50 ft from any therapy unit with energy above 400 kV. Similar considerations apply to locations near operating or patient rooms where radium is used.

A common cause for malfunction or failure of electronic equipment is erratic alternating line voltages, especially surges, which may occur with intermittent operation of high-starting torque electric motors found in compressors, elevators, or floor polishers. Continued operation at line voltages considerably below or above that for which electronic equipment was designed may cause failures in components. Some manufacturers may void their guarantees if this is the cause of failure. Variations in line voltage also may affect the stability of even the best high-voltage power supplies, count ratemeters, and γ-ray spectrometers. If an area of the hospital with a direct line from the main step-down transformer is not available for the radioisotope service, it is advisable to have at least one circuit used exclusively for electronic equipment, and another one for other devices such as air conditioners, adding machines, centrifuges, and so on. Anticipation of these problems will reduce servicing which may be quite expensive subsequently.

Within the limitations imposed by the *National Bureau of Standards Handbook No. 69* and the *Federal Register, Part 20* and local ordinances, the most convenient means for disposal of urine, feces, and blood containing minute quantities of radioactivity is through the sewage system. A location close to toilet facilities is therefore advisable.

Need for adequate space may influence the location of the radioisotope laboratory. The space needed for a clinical radioisotope laboratory depends upon the volume of the work, number of employees, and the variety of tests to be performed. On a minimum basis an area in which patients are received, examined, and subjected to test procedures is required. This space should have the privacy and accessibility of an examining room and may contain detection equipment used directly with patients. If a scanner is included, a separate area is strongly advised because of the time necessary to perform most organ scans. A laboratory area is needed which includes a place for a sample counter and its associated equipment, a work area for preparation of specimens, and some space for the storage of radioisotopes. An office area is also advisable. Although it is possible to combine these areas in a single large room with judicious use of screens or partitions, two or more rooms in proximity are more satisfactory. If rooms are separated by a hall or another room, even strongly radioactive sources in one room will not affect the performance of counters in the other areas.

Laboratory floors should be of a resilient substance such as vinyl asbestos tile. This simplifies the handling of spills that may unavoidably occur. Plastic floor coverings can be made quite impervious to most chemicals with plastic wax sealers. In the event of a spill wiping with paper towels may be sufficient to make the area safe. If this does not suffice for serious contamination with a long half-life radioisotope, the floor covering can be replaced easily. Sinks and bench tops should also be made of nonporous materials to minimize contamination.

An area where high-level material is received, opened, diluted, and stored should be maintained. Lead bricks arranged against a wall, distant from detection equipment and personnel areas, provide sufficient shielding for most radioactive sources received in a clinical laboratory.

B. Radiation Detection Equipment

Since subsequent chapters of this book are devoted to instrumentation, this section will deal with the subject only in general terms. Some points of advice may prove helpful in choosing equipment.

Several manufacturers produce excellent and extensive lines of clinical radioisotope detection equipment. Before a final choice is made, their products as well as their service facilities in the area should be investigated. Preference should be given to the manufacturer or dealer who maintains his own regional service department since contract service arrangements are mostly unsatisfactory.

Equipment to be used interchangeably may have to be purchased from one manufacturer. For example, if a probe and well-counter are to use the same high-voltage and scaling equipment alternately, the electronic pulse characteristics and cable connectors must be compatible.

However, purchase of separate units allows some independence in selection of manufacturers for each unit.

Minimum electronic equipment for a clinical radioisotope laboratory will include a well-counter with high-voltage and scaling circuits that are often packaged together and a probe-type detector. A survey meter and either film badges or dosimeters for personnel are required.

The equipment should be as simple in design and function as will meet the needs. Elaborate timers, automatic sample changers, built-in calculators, and other features designed primarily for sales appeal or high-volume applications should be avoided. They are seldom necessary for the volume of work in a clinical laboratory but enhance costs and frequency of service.

Transistorized equipment with a minimum number of vacuum tubes is preferable to vacuum tube equipment despite higher initial cost. It is freed of trouble, more stable, and often more easily serviced when malfunction does occur. If both transistorized and vacuum tube equipment are necessary, intermixing these units in the same mounting rack should be avoided, since heat from vacuum tube equipment may affect the operation of the transistorized equipment.

Equipment should be purchased with the understanding that it will be installed, demonstrated, and put into working condition by a factory representative before its final acceptance.

C. Maintenance Problems

In spite of excellent servicing plans offered by most manufacturers of nuclear equipment, one can anticipate some maintenance problems which must be met locally if operation is to continue without prolonged interruption. At least one of each type of vacuum tube in the instrument should be on hand. Where the same tube type is used several times, as in decade scaling circuits, it is best to have one spare for each four tubes of that type. For transistorized units one should rely upon manufacturers' service.

Electrical circuits of nuclear equipment are generally well protected by tubular fuses with close tolerances. It is important to observe the manufacturer's recommendations for replacement fuses. It is wise to keep on hand fuses of each rating listed. If a fuse burns out it should be replaced once, but if the replacement blows out this is a certain sign of some circuit failure that must be corrected.

III. RECORDS AND ECONOMICS OF THE RADIOISOTOPE LABORATORY

A. Records

For efficient and legal operation of a radioisotope service, records of business, health-personnel, radioisotope usage, and patients are necessary.

Business records are not a matter of legal responsibility and the details vary with each hospital. The last three categories are necessary to comply with the regulatory agency requirements.

1. PERSONNEL EXPOSURE

The recommendation in *NBS Handbook 69* makes it encumbent upon the supervisor or radiation safety officer of a clinical radioisotope service to keep current records of all personnel working with radioisotopes and to insure that each person's maximum permissible dose (MPD) is not exceeded (*Federal Register,* September 7, 1960, p. 8595). The maximum permissible accumulated dose in rem for occupational exposure may be calculated as $MPD = 5(N - 18)$, where N is an age greater than 18 years. It may be difficult to estimate the total accumulated exposure of a person who has spent many years working with radioisotopes. An alternative rule may be used where prior exposure is ignored and a much lower continuing dose is permitted. This amounts to 1.25 rem per calendar quarter total body radiation or about 0.1 rem per week. This is a feasible dose limitation for medical radioisotope work and can be achieved without difficulty.

Records should include a folder or page for each employee including age and date of employment. The radiation exposure as determined by film badge data and (or) dosimeters should be recorded. At the end of each calendar quarter, a total exposure for that period should be entered. When an employee leaves the service, he should be given a copy of this record stating his total accumulated exposure.

A weekly radiation survey of laboratory areas should include the general background of the laboratory, the vicinity of radioisotope storage area, work tables, and waste storage bins or cans. The dose in millirad per hour in these areas should be recorded. Any unusual change, its cause, and correction should be noted.

2. RADIOISOTOPE USAGE

The Atomic Energy Commission holds each licensee accountable for all radioisotopes which come into his possession. The licensee must be able to account for radioisotopes dispensed to patients or lost through decay.

Radioisotopes, when supplied for medical application, are assigned a lot number, an assay date, an assay of the quantity of radioactivity, and where applicable, a specific activity and expiration date. The date of each dispensation, the recipient, the quantity of radioactivity given, and the amount of the lot remaining should be entered on a record. When the entire lot has either been dispensed or the residual radioactivity has become too low to be useful, the record of that lot is balanced and closed with a notation concerning the quantity lost through decay.

3. PATIENT RECORDS

It is expedient to maintain two sets of records for work performed in the laboratory in addition to standard report forms. A bound record book is kept for each test procedure in which the patient's name, pertinent data, hospital record number, radioisotope lot number, quantity of radioisotope administered, and test data and results are entered. These records are invaluable for reviewing and evaluating one's work.

In addition, a personal file card should be prepared for each patient coming to the radioisotope laboratory. Each test performed on the patient is recorded together with the amount of radioisotope administered, the date, and the results of the test. The patient may be questioned concerning any radioisotope he had received previously and the file is checked with each request for a test procedure. Such a procedure prevents undue exposure of patients and errors in results due to previously administered radioisotopes.

4. INSTRUMENT PERFORMANCE

It is helpful to maintain a record on each detector in regular use. Daily counts of a standard source such as a cesium button or a mock iodine capsule should be recorded. Slight variations from day to day are to be expected, but significant deviation indicates the need for maintenance before a time-consuming measurement is invalidated by instrument failure. Recording component failures and required maintenance is helpful to localize subsequent failure.

B. Economics

In the spring of 1963 a questionnaire was sent to a group of randomly selected nonuniversity voluntary hospitals in many areas of the United States, inquiring about staffing of their radioisotope service and the charges made for commonly requested diagnostic and therapeutic procedures. The results based upon 23 completed questionnaires are given in Table I.

IV. FREQUENTLY PERFORMED DIAGNOSTIC PROCEDURES

The clinical tests performed with radioisotopes are well summarized in the publications listed as references at the end of this chapter. Some aspects of these tests will be discussed briefly to emphasize the complexity of even simple types of tracer studies. Each of the tests described and many new procedures not included require knowledge of clinical medicine and the limitations and artifacts that alter results for proper interpretation. The ease of performing radioisotope studies often exceeds the ability to interpret properly their significance.

TABLE I
SURVEY OF RADIOISOTOPE TESTS PERFORMED IN HOSPITALS

	Range	Average
Size of hospital (beds)	157–974	440
Admissions per year	6,500–43,300	19,583
Employees in radioisotope service, exclusive of physicians	0–6	1

	Number of tests per year		Charge per test ($)	
Tests	Range	Average	Range	Average
Iodine thyroid uptake	46–500	123	10–20	15
Uptake with TSH stimulation	0–10	3	25–40	28
Thyroid suppression	0–10	3	10–30	19
Schilling	20–169	45	15–35	23
Red cell survival	1–8	4	25–50	34
Blood volume (RISA)	25–1444	382	5–15	15
Organ scanning	41–326	174	15–50	30
Fat absorption	4–44	15	15–30	20
^{131}I thyroid therapy for hyperthyroidism	7–52	26	55–200	155

A. 24-Hour Radioiodine Uptake

Iodine is an integral part of thyroid hormone and the rate of hormone production correlates well with the rate at which iodide is trapped by the thyroid gland. In most circumstances it is possible to infer the rate of hormone production by measuring the percentage of an ^{131}I tracer dose taken up by the gland in a 24-hr period following administration. If one finds a hyperthyroid patient and therapy with ^{131}I is anticipated the 24-hr uptake should be followed by subsequent counts at 24-hr intervals for 3–5 days to establish the effective half-life of ^{131}I in the thyroid. The physician interpreting thyroid uptakes must be familiar with the situations in which uptake of ^{131}I is not representative of thyroid function. The range of normal uptake is 10–50% in 24 hr with some overlap of the hypothyroidism range at the lower end and the hyperthyroidism range at the upper end. However, a majority of hyperthyroid patients exhibit uptakes greater than 50%, and most myxedema cases fall below 10%.

Two important additions to the 24-hr uptake merit mention. A TSH* stimulation test may differentiate primary from pituitary myxedema.

* TSH, Thyroid-stimulating hormone.

If a 24-hr uptake is in the hypothyroid range and no interfering drugs are implicated, TSH is given intramuscularly on three successive days. On the fourth day, a second 24-hr uptake is performed, with appropriate corrections made for residual activity existing in the gland from the previous test. In primary myxedema it is rare for the uptake to increase by more than 5%.

A thyroid suppression test could confirm the diagnosis of hyperthyroidism in difficult cases. It is based upon the observation that the normal thyroid uptake of ^{131}I is rapidly suppressed by exogenous thyroid hormone. The hyperthyroid gland has little or no reduction in ^{131}I uptake after administration of exogenous hormone. If the results of the initial thyroid iodide uptake are above 40%, the patient is given either 75 mg of l-triiodothyronine for 1 week or 200 mg of thyroid extract daily for 4 weeks and the uptake is repeated the day following completion of administration with appropriate corrections for residual activity from the first dose. The euthyroid individual will have his uptake reduced to about one half, whereas the hyperthyroid individual shows little or no reduction in uptake.

B. Cobalt-Labeled B_{12} Tests for Pernicious Anemia and Malabsorption Syndrome

Cyanocobalamin (vitamin B_{12}) is necessary for the normal maturation of erythrocytes. Failure to absorb this vitamin, which is abundant in most diets, produces pernicious anemia. Absorption depends upon the presence of a glycoprotein (intrinsic factor) elaborated by the stomach mucosa. A person lacking this protein fails to absorb B_{12}. Administration of intrinsic factor in the form of normal human gastric juice or an extract of swine duodenal mucosa enhances the absorption of B_{12} when intrinsic factor is deficient. In disease of the intestinal mucosa the absorption may be poor or absent even when intrinsic factor is abundant.

Vitamin B_{12} contains one atom of cobalt per molecule which can be labeled to make it suitable for tracer studies. Most commonly ^{60}Co has been used to label vitamin B_{12}, but recently ^{57}Co has been recommended because of the absence of β-ray emission and its shorter half-life, which materially reduces the radiation dose. The considerably lower energy of the γ radiation of ^{57}Co also permits easier measurement in standard detectors. The failure to absorb labeled vitamin B_{12} can be demonstrated in one of several ways:

(1) By measuring the radioactivity remaining in the stool collected over a period of time after an oral dose of radioactive B_{12} (Heinle-Welch).

(2) By measuring the hepatic uptake of an oral dose of radioactive B_{12} (Glass).
(3) By measuring blood levels of radioactivity following an oral dose of radioactive B_{12}.
(4) By measuring the quantity of radioactivity excreted in the urine for a standard time (24–48 hr) after oral administration of radioactive B_{12} followed by a flushing dose of stable B_{12} administered intramuscularly (Schilling).

The Schilling procedure appears to be the most reliable test. A normal person excretes more than 7% of the administered dose in the urine in 24 hr. A total excretion of less than 7% in 48 hr is abnormal and is highly suggestive of pernicious anemia or a malabsorptive syndrome. If the total excretion is below that figure, the procedure should be repeated with the addition of intrinsic factor with the oral dose of radioactive B_{12}. This should separate abnormal tests due to intrinsic factor deficiency from those due to intestinal malabsorption. If absence of intrinsic factor is the cause of the absorptive defect, the second test should yield an increase in absorption.

C. Studies with ^{51}Cr-Labeled RBC

Chromium-51 is bound to erythrocyte hemoglobin and has no appreciable effect on red cell survival if the concentration of chromium does not exceed 5 μg per milliliter of blood. The ^{51}Cr label is removed from the circulating blood at a rate of approximately 1% per day in normal people.

A portion of the cell population is labeled *in vitro* on day zero with ^{51}Cr and reinjected into the patient. The labeled cells mix with the unlabeled cells and the disappearance rate of the labeled cells reflects the disappearance rate of the entire cell population.

The average normal half-time of ^{51}Cr-labeled red cells is 30 days. Values below 15 days indicate an active hemolytic process, provided striking changes in blood volume and hemorrhage can be excluded.

Several techniques have been reported for measuring gastrointestinal blood loss quantitatively by the use of ^{51}Cr-labeled red cells. When active splenic sequestration of red cells is suspected the ratio of the amounts of radioactivity taken up by spleen and liver, determined by external γ-ray counting, may be used to demonstrate the phenomenon.

D. Blood Volume Determination

Radioisotopes provide an ideal means for determining intravascular volumes using the simple dilution principle. Either ^{131}I-labeled human serum albumin (IHSA) or ^{51}Cr-labeled RBC can be used. For precise results, ^{51}Cr-labeled red cells from either the patient or ORh(—) cells labeled in advance and kept under refrigeration should be used. The albumin space of the body is larger than the intravascular space, and albumin slowly disappears from the circulation into this space. Therefore the sample drawn to determine the intravascular volume must be taken soon after the administration of the labeled albumin.

IHSA is supplied in disposable plastic syringes, each containing doses of about 5 μCi ^{131}I in 1–2 ml of serum albumin. After its injection, 5 to 10 min is allowed for complete mixing before withdrawal of a blood sample. Instruments have been developed recently which simplify the exact measurements of the injected dose and the resulting radioactivity in the blood sample. In addition, the instruments compute the blood volume automatically and indicate the final result in liters (Chapter 12, Section IV,C). The advantage of these instruments is their availability at the time of need to surgical, medical, or anesthesia personnel as they are simple to operate and the doses used are exempted by regulatory agencies.

E. Renal Function Studies

Iodine-131-labeled iodopyracet and *o*-iodohippurate-^{131}I (Chapter 1, Section II,D,2) are almost totally extracted from the blood by filtration and tubular secretion in one passage through the kidneys. The former is also concentrated in the liver, making it less useful to evaluate renal function. Basically the test procedure consists of recording by means of matched scintillation counters (Chapter 15, Section IV,B) the accumulation and disappearance of radioactivity over the renal areas following intravenous administration of a small dose of the tracer compound. The curves obtained from this procedure have been interpreted by intercomparison of the two kidney curves or by comparison with curves from normal people to evaluate various parameters of renal function. The technique is especially valuable as a screening procedure in hypertensive patients to detect potentially curable renovascular disease.

F. Residual Urine Measurements

The radioiodine-containing compounds used in renal function studies also make possible a rapid, simple and safe means of determining the existence of residual bladder urine while avoiding the hazards of cathertization. This procedure has proven valuable in diabetic and neurological patients in whom the dangers from diagnostic cathertization are especially great.

Either iodopyracet or iodohippurate labeled with ^{131}I is given intravenously in a dose of 5–10 μCi. From 10 to 30 min later, a count is made with a γ-ray detector positioned over the suprapubic area. Following this count the patient voids and another count is made immediately, the probe being positioned as before. A residual count greater than 10% of the original count is significant and indicative of residual urine greater than 50 ml.

G. Fat Absorption Studies

Oleic acid contains a double bond which incorporates ^{131}I relatively easily (Chapter 1, Section II,D,4). Since this label is stable under conditions found in the gastrointestinal tract, it can serve as a tracer to study absorption of lipids in the bowel.

Fatty acids may be absorbed directly by the mucosa of the small intestine whereas neutral fats must first be hydrolyzed by pancreatic enzymes before absorption can take place. In a normal subject very little ingested neutral fat or fatty acid appears in the stool. This is the basis for tests for steatorrhea that is not obvious. One group of measurements depends upon the residual activity in stool collected following oral administration of either the fat or the fatty acid. Other techniques involve measuring radioactivity found in the blood following a test meal of either the labeled fat or the fatty acid. Each technique has advantages and disadvantages which should be thoroughly evaluated before a method is set up in a new laboratory.

H. Body Scanning

Visualizing the distribution of radioactivity within an organ (thyroid, lung, kidney, liver, spleen) or a lesion (brain tumor) can yield valuable clinical information. Some time after the administration of a γ-ray emitting radioactive compound which is preferentially concentrated in the tissues of interest, counts are registered with a well-collimated detector (Chapter 17) which scans over the selected body region (Chapter 16). The various methods of presenting the registered distribution of radioactivity are also described in Chapter 16.

Unfortunately, the instrumentation required for scanning is considerably more elaborate and therefore more expensive than the smaller counters (probes and well-counters) used for the tests discussed above (Sections A–G). This has prevented many hospitals from utilizing this technique for clinical use. Until a few years ago, scanning was mainly limited to the thyroid and it is a matter of opinion whether this warrants a rather expensive setup. Lately, the instruments have been improved considerably and new compounds allow scanning of an increasing number of body sites (Chapter 16). This has made the scanner an invaluable tool in the hands of many clinicians.

SUPPLEMENTARY READINGS

Radiation physics, radioisotope production, and their medical use are covered in many publications. The books listed below are particularly useful for frequent reference and should be available to the radioisotope laboratory. A short description is given with each publication to help the selection of references.

Friedlander, G., Kennedy, J. W., and Miller, J. M., "Nuclear and Radiochemistry," 2nd ed. Wiley, New York, 1964. This is a valuable reference work for the theory and application of radioisotopes to chemical methods. It also has a succinct introductory section dealing with nuclear physics.

Handbooks of the National Bureau of Standards. Superintendent of Documents, U.S. Government Printing Office, Washington, D.C. 20402. These small but authoratative publications provide a valuable guide to safety in the operation of a radioisotope laboratory and to the determination of the radiation dose from radioisotopes.

- #42 Safe Handling of Radioisotopcs ($0.20) 1949
- #48 Control and Removal of Radioactive Contaminations in Laboratories ($0.15) 1951
- #49 Recommendations for Waste Disposal of Phosphorous-32 and Iodine-131 for Medical Users ($0.15) 1951
- #69 Maximum Permissible Body Burdens and Maximum Permissible Concentrations of Radionuclides in Air and in Water for Occupational Exposure ($0.35) 1959
- #80 A Manual of Radioactivity Procedures ($0.50) 1961
- #86 Radioactivity ($0.40) 1964
- #87 Clinical Dosimetry ($0.40) 1963

Kinsman, S. (ed.), "Radiological Health Handbook." U.S. Dept. of Health, Education & Welfare, Sanitary Engineering Center, Cincinnati, Ohio, 1960. This is a compilation of data available from no other single source. It contains many tables and monographs which are applicable in calculations concerning dosage of radioisotopes, counting techniques, and identifications of radioisotopes.

Lapp, R. E., and Andrews, H. L., "Nuclear Radiation Physics," 3rd ed. Prentice-Hall, Englewood Cliffs, New Jersey, 1963. A comprehensive yet relatively elementary nuclear physics text which can provide a foundation for the problems discussed in this book.

Overman, R. T., and Clark, H. M., "Radioisotope Techniques," 1st ed. McGraw-Hill, New York, 1960. This book contains the material presented at the Oak Ridge Institute of Nuclear Studies in the course on Basic Radioisotope Techniques. Many detailed stepwise procedures for preparation, handling, and measurement of radioisotopes are included.

This last group of books deals specifically with the application of radioisotopes to medicine. Each one of these is quite comprehensive and describes many aspects of clinical tracer techniques which are only briefly mentioned in this chapter. These books also include instrumentation sections which may be consulted before starting the detailed description presented in this book.

Behrens, C. F., and King, E. R. (eds.), "Atomic Medicine," 4th ed. Williams & Wilkins, Baltimore, Maryland, 1964.

Beierwaltes, W. H., Johnson, P. C., and Solari, A. J., "Clinical Use of Radioisotopes," 2nd ed. Saunders, Philadelphia, Pennsylvania, 1962.

Blahd, W. H. (ed.), "Nuclear Medicine," McGraw-Hill, New York, 1965.

Consalazio, C. F., Johnson, R. E., and Pecord, L. J., "Physiological Measurements of Metabolic Functions in Man." McGraw-Hill, New York, 1963. Although not dealing specifically with radioisotopes, this handboook contains many tables and techniques applicable in clinical research involving radioisotopes.

Fields, T., and Seed, L. (eds.), "Clinical Use of Radioisotopes," A Manual of Techniques, 2nd ed. Year Book Publ., Chicago, Illinois, 1961. This book is not exhaustive in content but presents stepwise procedures for most medical applications of radioisotopes.

Quimby, E. H., and Feitelberg, S., "Radioactive Isotopes in Medicine and Biology," Vol. 1, Basic Physics and Instrumentation. 2nd ed. Lea & Febiger, Philadelphia, Pennsylvania, 1963.

Silver, S., "Radioactive Isotopes in Medicine and Biology," Vol. 2, Medicine. 2nd ed. Lea & Febiger, Philadelphia, Pennsylvania, 1962.

Veall, N., and Vetter, H., "Radioisotope Techniques in Clinical Research and Diagnosis," Butterworth, London and Washington, D.C., 1958.

CHAPTER 3

BASIC CONSIDERATIONS IN NUCLEAR INSTRUMENTATION

FRANK H. LOW
PICKER NUCLEAR
WHITE PLAINS, NEW YORK

Radioisotopes have made their unique contributions to medicine because it is possible to detect the disintegration of individual nuclei and hence to locate submicroscopic quantities of a given material in body tissues or fluids. The physical amount of radioactive tracer required to follow, for example, a metabolic process is so small that it does not alter the process itself.

The extreme sensitivity of radiation detection equipment is a cardinal factor in the tracer procedures of nuclear medicine. Hence, the choice and use of nuclear instrumentation plays a vital part in the value and accuracy of the results obtained in radioisotope tests. This chapter deals with the general considerations which affect the selection and application of nuclear instruments while later chapters will discuss individual pieces of equipment in more detail. However, since all radioisotope measurements are subject to statistical variations, these are considered first.

I. STATISTICS OF RADIOISOTOPE MEASUREMENTS

A. Random Nature of Radiation

While it is possible to detect the emission of a single γ ray (or β particle), virtually nothing can be learned from a single event. A given radioactive nucleus decays in a predictable manner, but the time at which it will happen cannot be predicted. The emission of radiation from an unstable nucleus has an equal chance of occurring at any time, independent of the past history of the nucleus or its treatment. Thus, radioactive decay is a completely random phenomenon subject to the laws of probability and statistics.

Each radioisotope has a characteristic probability of decay, which determines the chance that the decay takes place during any one time interval. The most convenient way of expressing this probability is to define the length of time it takes for half of the radioactive nuclei present at time zero to decay. This time interval is called the half-life of the radioisotope. During each half-life, one half of the radioactive nuclei present at the beginning of the period undergo decay so that if there were N atoms present at the start, there would be $N/2$ present after one half-life, $N/4$ after two half-lives, $N/8$ after three half-lives, and so on.

If a radioisotope has a short half-life, a greater proportion of its nuclei decay in a minute than if it has a long half-life. The amount of radioactive material present is expressed in units called curies, which are defined as 3.7×10^{10} disintegrations per second. Thus, a curie of a long-lived material contains many more nuclei than a curie of a short-lived radioisotope.

B. Determination of Statistical Error

One must detect a number of events in order to be able to determine the rate of decay of the material or the amount of it present in a given location. The accuracy of the measurement is a function of the number of events observed. As in public opinion polls, the more data have been collected, the smaller will be the percentage of error. The error in the measurement due to the fact that only a finite number of random events have been observed is called the statistical error. There are various expressions that are used for describing the statistical accuracy, that is, the extent of the statistical uncertainty. They all are functions only of the number of events detected.

1. STATIC MEASUREMENTS

A measurement of the number of radioactive nuclei present can be obtained by counting the number of detected decays and relating this number to a time interval. For this reason almost all the scalers used for counting individual events contain a clock (electronic or mechanical) which starts and stops at the same time as the counting begins and ends. For convenience, some scalers can be made to stop automatically when a given number of counts has been accumulated. This means that the statistical error can be predetermined. In other cases time is preset because of other considerations such as the length of time a patient can sit still. Then the statistical accuracy of the measurement varies from

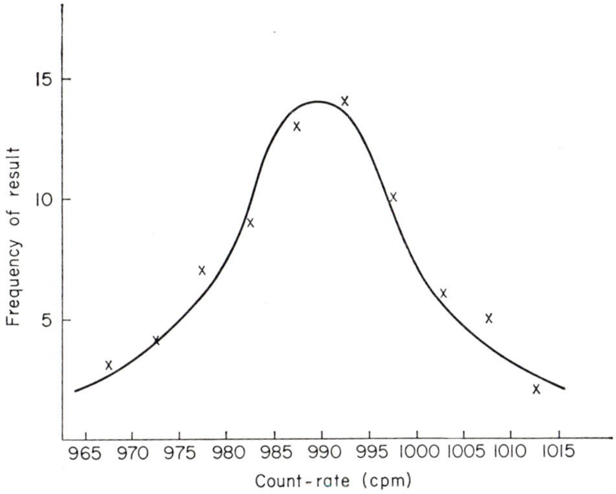

FIG. 1. Measurements with a ^{137}Cs source (half-life 33 years) from which about 1,000 cpm were detected. Each measurement was run until 10,000 counts had been accumulated; the elapsed time was read (±0.01 min) and the counts per minute were calculated. The results of 100 such measurements was plotted against the number of times that the number of counts per minute fell between successive increments of 5 (that is, between 975 and 980, or 980 and 985, and so on). The Poisson curve with best fit drawn through these points shows a mean value at the apex of 990 cpm. In a larger series, the points would fall more closely to the curve.

one set of counts to the next. The formulas for computing the statistical accuracy of scaler measurements are based on the laws of statistics.

If a count is made of a steady phenomenon, for example the cycles from a perfect frequency standard, all measurements yield identical results. A similar series made on a statistically random phenomenon, like nuclear decay, results in a variety of values. When these individual values are plotted as a function of frequency of occurrence, a bell-shaped curve is obtained (Fig. 1). The curve has its apex at the mean value of all the measurements and falls off on both sides. It is called a Poisson distribution curve.

The shape of the Poisson distribution curve depends on the number of events which were recorded in each measurement. With increasing numbers for each measurement, the bell-shaped curve becomes taller and slimmer (Fig. 2).

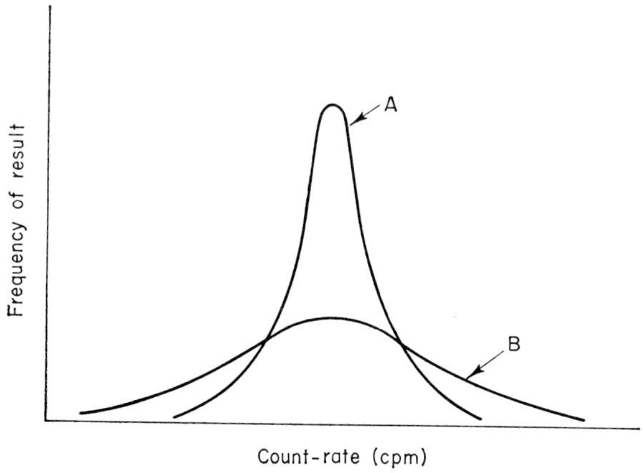

FIG. 2. Curve A is the one obtained in Fig. 1 from measurements of the time required to accumulate 10,000 counts. Curve B was obtained by measurements made on the same ^{137}Cs source, but in this case only 1,000 counts were accumulated each time. Because far fewer counts contributed to the data used to draw curve B, it is much broader and flatter than curve A.

The result of a single measurement might fall at any point on a Poisson curve drawn for the number of counts recorded in the measurement. Since the single measurement is unlikely to represent the mean value of a large series of measurements, it is not a completely accurate indication of the number of radioactive nuclei present. A study of the shape of the distribution curve can indicate the probability that the single measurement falls within a certain percentage of the mean value.

The deviation from the mean (or true) value can be expressed in several different ways to indicate the probable accuracy of the single measurement. Commonly the accuracy is expressed in terms of the deviation from the mean value to a value which is only half as likely to occur as the mean. This is the point at which the Poisson curve has fallen to half its height, and the deviation between that point and the mean is called one "standard deviation" (Fig. 3).

The *standard deviation* for a Poisson curve is the square root of the number of observed events, N.

Often it is more convenient to express the standard deviation not as a number of events but as a percentage of the result of the measurement so that the results can be recorded as N counts $\pm x\%$.

$$\text{Percent standard deviation (\% S.D.)} = \frac{\text{S.D.}}{N} \times 100 = \frac{100}{N^{1/2}}$$

In nuclear measurements a different expression for the accuracy of the data has achieved wide acceptance, even though its results do not

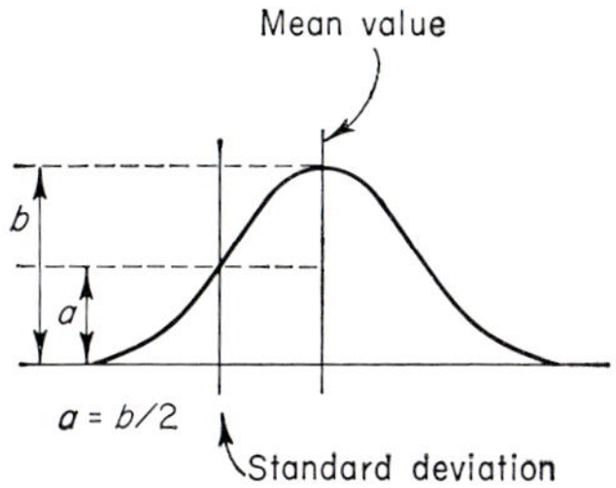

FIG. 3. The distance along the abscissa between the mean value and the point on the curve where it has fallen to half its height at the mean value is the standard deviation.

$$\text{Standard deviation (S.D.)} = N^{1/2}$$

differ greatly from those obtained by using the standard deviation. It refers to the deviation as an error in the measurement and indicates the probability that a single measurement has an error less than the defined amount. When that probability is 50%, then the deviation is called the *probable error* (Fig. 4). In that case the actual error for one measure-

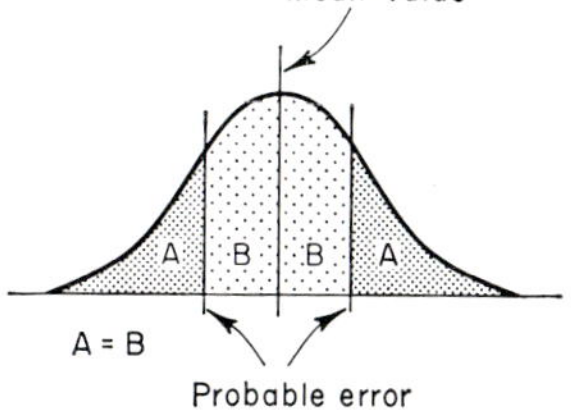

FIG. 4. The distance along the abscissa between the mean value and the point at which a vertical line cuts the area on either side of the mean value in half is the probable error.

ment has an equal chance of being greater or less than the probable error. The probable error for a Poisson curve is 0.6745 times the standard deviation.

$$\text{Probable error (P.E.)} = 0.6745(N)^{1/2}$$
$$\text{Percent probable error (\% P.E.)} = 67.45/(N)^{1/2}$$

For the data used in Fig. 1, the results in counts per minute and their percent probable error can, therefore, be expressed as follows:

$$990 \pm \frac{67.4}{10{,}000^{1/2}} \text{ \% P.E.} = 990 \pm 0.67 \text{ \% P.E.}$$

A plus or minus sign is used for the error figure since the deviation may be above or below the mean.

Some people are not satisfied to know that their error figure might be exceeded 50% of the time. They would like to know what the error would be which would have only a 1 in 10, or a 1 in 20 chance of being exceeded. Obtaining the so-called reliable (nine tenth) or the ninety five hundredth error means drawing the vertical line on the Poisson curve further from the mean value (Fig. 5).

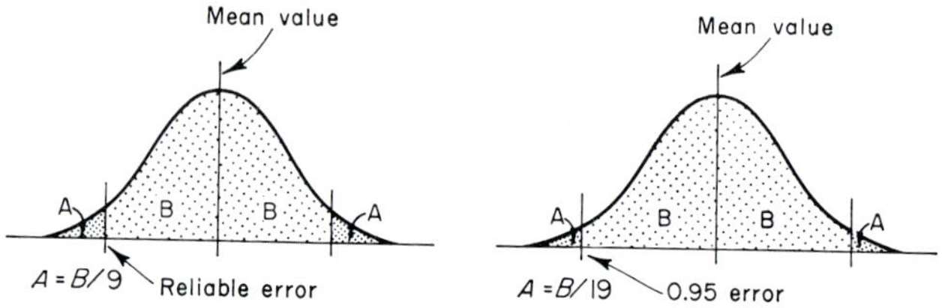

FIG. 5. The distance along the abscissa between the mean value and the point at which a vertical line cuts off only 10% of the area on either side of the mean value is the reliable error. If it cuts off only 5% of the area, it is a 0.95 error.

The formulas used for calculating these errors are:

$$\text{Reliable error (R.E.)} = 1.6949(N)^{1/2}$$
$$\text{Percent reliable error (\% R.E.)} = 169.49/(N)^{1/2}$$
$$\text{Ninety five hundredth error} = 1.9600(N)^{1/2}$$
$$\text{Percent ninety five hundredth error} = 196.00/(N)^{1/2}$$

2. BACKGROUND RADIATION

The discussion of statistics has been based so far on an ideal case where all of the detected events are the ones that one wants to measure. In practice, any detector sensitive to the radiation emitted from the material being measured also responds to similar radiation from extraneous sources such as naturally occurring radioactive material in the building, cosmic radiation, and, in the case of *in vivo* studies, radiation from other parts of the body than the one under investigation.

An estimate of the true number of counts corresponding to the radioactive material (R_{net}) being measured can be obtained by determining the background count-rate (R_{bkg}) and subtracting it from the measurements (R_{gross}).

$$\text{Count-rate}_{net} = R_{net} = R_{gross} - R_{bkg}$$

Since there is a statistical error associated with both the gross and the background measurements, the deviation in the net counts is a function of both. In accordance with the laws of statistics, this deviation is the square root of the sum of the squares of the gross and background deviations.

$$\text{Deviation in } R_{net} = [(\text{Deviation in } R_{gross})^2 + (\text{Deviation in } R_{bkg})^2]^{1/2}$$

This equation can be put into more useful form by letting K equal the ratio of R_{gross} to R_{bkg}

$$K = R_{gross}/R_{bkg}$$

and letting G equal the total number of counts measured in the gross measurement. Then if the same number of counts were taken for both the gross and the background measurements,

$$\text{Percent standard deviation of } R_{net} = [100/(G)^{1/2}][(K^2 + 1)^{1/2}/(K - 1)]$$

More often the same length of time is spent on both measurements and then the formula becomes:

$$\text{Percent standard deviation of } R_{net} = [100/(G)^{1/2}][(K^2 + K)^{1/2}/(K - 1)]$$

If, as in Fig. 1, 10,000 counts were recorded in the gross measurement in, for example, 5 min, and if in a separate measurement, 2,000 counts of background were recorded in another 5 min interval, then G would be 10,000, K would be 5, and R_{net} would be 1,600 cpm with a standard deviation of 1.4%.

$$\text{Percent standard deviation} = [100/(10{,}000)^{1/2}][(25 + 5)^{1/2}/(5 - 1)]\ \% = 1.4\%$$

Obviously, it is desirable to obtain measurements with the greatest accuracy in the shortest time. This means using the most efficient detectors available, if the cost is not prohibitive. But increasing the efficiency of the detector for the radiation emitted by the material under study may make it also more sensitive to background radiation. The above equations show that it is possible to offset the improvement in statistical accuracy which is sought by increasing the gross counts obtained, G, through a simultaneous increase in background resulting in a reduction of the gross count to background ratio K.

3. Figure of Merit

A comparison of two detectors to determine which one will give results of greater statistical accuracy in a given length of time (that is, a determination of their relative merit) must take into consideration the sensitivity of each for the radiation to be measured and for background radiation. If detector I has a net count-rate S_{I} and detector II has a net count-rate of S_{II} and if their respective background count-rates are B_{I} and B_{II} then the relative merit of detector I over detector II is given by the following equation:

$$\text{Figure of merit} = [(S_{\text{II}} + 2B_{\text{II}})/(S_{\text{I}} + 2B_{\text{I}})](S_{\text{I}}/S_{\text{II}})^2$$

If the figure of merit is greater than 1, then detector I is the better choice; otherwise detector II is preferable. If three detectors are to be compared, then the figure of merit is calculated first for one pair, and then for the superior one of that pair and the remaining detector.

The equation for obtaining the figure of merit can be simplified under two conditions. If the net count-rates are high compared with the background count-rates, it reduces to

$$\text{Figure of merit} = S_{\text{I}}/S_{\text{II}}$$

while if the net count-rates are low compared with the background count-rates, it reduces to

$$\text{Figure of merit} = (S_{\text{I}}^2/B_{\text{I}})(B_{\text{II}}/S_{\text{II}}^2)$$

Hence for low count-rates the best detector is the one with the greatest S^2/B ratio.

4. Dynamic Measurements

When measurements are made on dynamic processes, such as the uptake and clearance of material from the kidneys, then the scaler has to be operated for many short consecutive time periods to allow the detection of rapid changes in the radioactivity level of the kidneys. This can be done with special equipment which resets itself in a few microseconds and prints its readings on tape. More often it is done with a ratemeter, which is less costly. It accepts individual pulses but instead of displaying them like a scaler, averages them over a fixed period of time, and indicates the average on a meter. It does this by letting each event add a fixed amount of charge to a condenser and continuously bleeding off this charge through a resistor which is connected to the meter. The averaging time is a function of the size of the capacitor and the resistor, and is called the *RC* time constant of the circuit, because it is the product of *R* (the value of the resistor) and *C* (the value of the capacitor).

At any given moment the statistical accuracy of the meter reading is a direct function of the mean number of counts accumulated during the time represented by two successive time constants. Mathematically this is expressed as follows:

$$\text{Percent standard deviation of ratemeter reading} = 100/(2nt)^{1/2}$$
$$\text{Percent probable error of ratemeter reading} = 67.45/(2nt)^{1/2}$$

where n = mean count-rate in counts per second (cpm/60) and t = time constant in seconds.

Thus, if the meter reads 4,000 cpm and the time constant is 1 sec, the reading should be expressed as 4,000 cpm ± 5.8 %P.E. The relatively large error, of course, is due to the short averaging time of the ratemeter. If a 4 sec time constant had been used, the statistical error would have been cut in half, but the time required for the needle to go from one reading to another, the equilibrium time, would have been greater (Fig. 6).

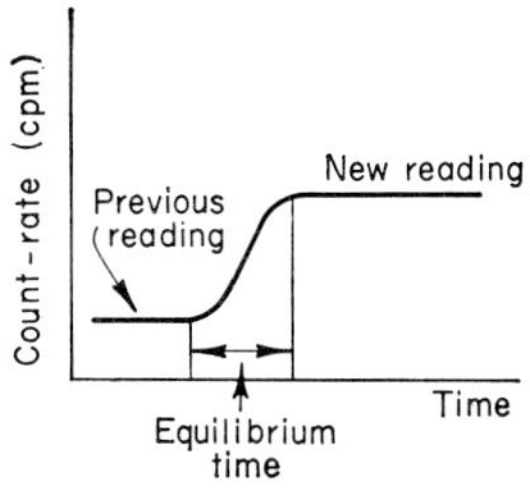

FIG. 6. Diagrammatic presentation of equilibrium time of a ratemeter.

The *equilibrium time*, T_e, is a function of both the count-rate and the time constant of the ratemeter circuitry (Fig. 7) and is given by the formula

$$T_e = t[0.5 \ln (2nt) + 0.394]$$

The compromise between long equilibrium time resulting from a long time constant or poor statistics resulting from a short time constant is best shown by comparing strip chart recordings of the ratemeter output under identical conditions, involving only a change of time constants (Fig. 8). With a short time constant the response is much more rapid, but the curve is considerably less clear.

For any time constant, curves can be drawn which show the variation of statistical accuracy and of equilibrium time with count-rate (Fig. 9). As the count-rate increases, the statistics improve, but the equilibrium time increases.

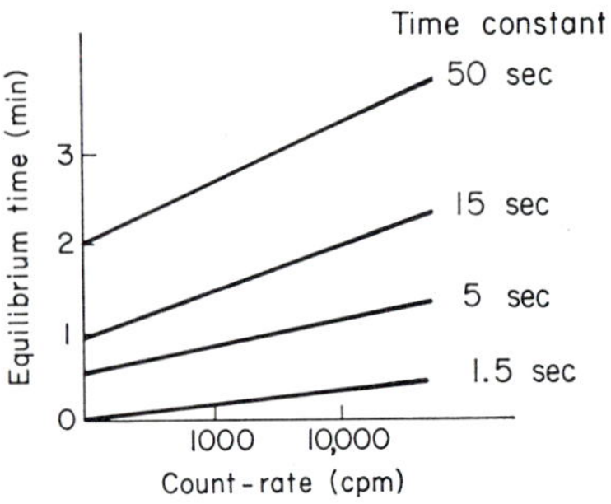

FIG. 7. Graph of equilibrium time versus count-rate for several time constant values of ratemeter.

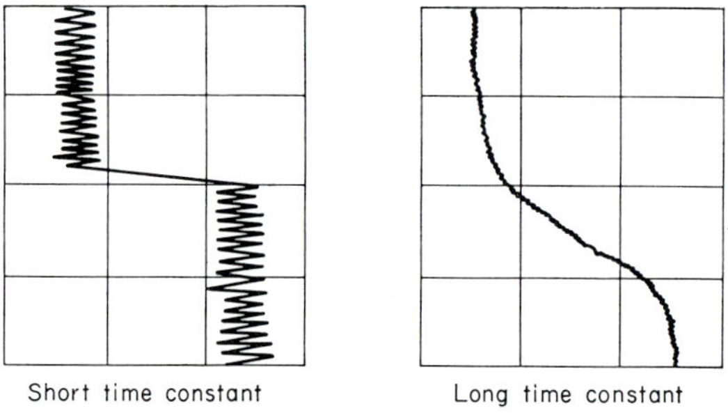

FIG. 8. Short ratemeter time constant produces a recording with many fluctuations, but with a short response to a major change in count-rate. Long ratemeter time constant produces a smooth recording, but with a slow response to a major change in count-rate.

The only way to avoid the equilibrium time problem in dynamic function studies is to use a special type of scaler called a rate computer, which counts digitally for a short period of time, resets in a few microseconds, and counts again while printing the results of the previous count. Obviously, the statistical accuracy of each printed result depends on the counts accumulated during the measurement interval.

II. RADIATION DETECTORS

A. Detection Efficiency

Determining the absolute efficiency (percentage of disintegrations detected) of a radiation detector in a given physical setup is a complex problem because of the many factors of geometry and detector performance that must be considered. For this reason, most radiation measurements are relative rather than absolute; that is, they involve obtaining count-rate data on an unknown sample (or patient) and on a standard of the same radioisotope under as nearly identical conditions as possible. For example, a dose is measured before administration to a patient, a subsequent blood sample is counted later at the same position relative to the detector, and the ratio of the two net count-rates represents the clinical data.

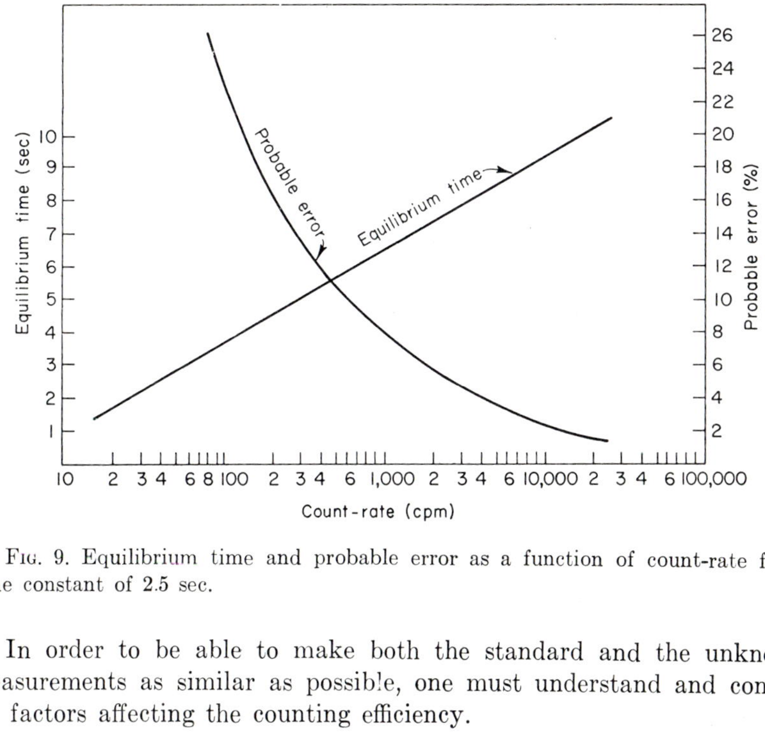

FIG. 9. Equilibrium time and probable error as a function of count-rate for a time constant of 2.5 sec.

In order to be able to make both the standard and the unknown measurements as similar as possible, one must understand and control all factors affecting the counting efficiency.

1. GEOMETRY

The first factor that must be considered is the portion of the radiation produced in the sample or organ which interacts with other atoms in the source and never gets outside. This process is called self-absorption. Obviously, the standard and the unknown should have similar self-absorption properties.

If the source is covered by inactive material, as for example the thyroid is covered by neck tissue, then absorption in the covering material must also be taken into account. It is possible that a γ ray may be only partially absorbed in the source or its covering matter and that it may emerge with reduced energy and a change in direction as a scattered ray. For this reason, the standard must be arranged to have scattering conditions similar to those of the unknown, or all scattered radiation must be eliminated from the measurement by using an energy discriminator (Section III,A,1).

Of all of the radiation emerging from the source only a fraction will be directed toward the detector. This fraction is determined by the solid angle subtended by the detector with respect to the source. It is ruled by the "inverse square law," since doubling the distance between a point source and detector reduces the solid angle by a factor of 4.

Not all of the radiation within the subtended solid angle reaches the sensitive portion of the detector because of absorption in the air and in the detector cover. This is important primarily in the case of β and low-energy γ and X radiation.

2. INTRINSIC EFFICIENCY

Radiation striking the sensitive portion of a detector may be wholly or partially absorbed or it may pass right through the detector. If a Geiger tube is used, the signal from the detector is independent of the energy of the radiation, so that partial or total absorption produce the same results. In a scintillation detector the size of the detector output pulse is a function of the energy lost by the γ ray in the crystal. Therefore, for scintillation detectors it is necessary to know both the total intrinsic efficiency (that is, the fraction of the incident rays detected) and the efficiency for total absorption, called the photofraction.

For a scintillation detector using a sodium iodide crystal, both the total and the photofraction efficiency are determined by the energy of the radiation and the size of the crystal (Chapter 6, Section III).

B. Shielding

Background radiation is present at all times in all places. It comes in part from cosmic radiation and in part from naturally occurring radioactive material incorporated in the building. For example, granite contains detectable amounts of uranium daughter products. In addition, background radiation may also come from nearby sources of radioactive material such as a cobalt-60 therapy installation, a radium safe, a supply of therapeutic or multiple diagnostic doses of radiopharmaceuticals, or patients who have received radioisotope therapy doses.

For this reason the detector should be well shielded on all sides except the one facing the patient or the sample being measured. For clinical work the shielding should be at least the equivalent of ¾ inch of lead for 1-inch diameter scintillation detectors and should go up from there to 2 inches of lead or more for 3-inch diameter scintillation detectors. It is very important that this shielding against general background extend to the back of the sensitive portion of the detector, since background radiation can come from all directions and can be scattered back even if one principal component, such as cosmic radiation, comes mainly from one direction.

The background count-rate of an unshielded scintillation detector varies with the volume of the crystal while its counting efficiency for radiation of a given energy coming from a point source varies with the frontal area of the crystal. Thus, there is no point in choosing a crystal which is thicker than required for the almost total absorption of the radiation being measured. A 1-inch thick crystal is adequate for measuring ^{131}I if all detected rays are counted, while a 2-inch thick crystal is better if only totally absorbed rays are counted. When large crystals are used (2-inch diameter or more) better ratios of efficiency to background can be obtained by using a pulse-height analyzer to limit the counted rays to those falling in the photopeak (total absorption).

C. Collimation

Detectors must be shielded not only against background radiation but also against radiation coming from parts of the patient's body other than the one under study at the moment. If a whole organ, such as a thyroid or kidney is being measured, then the front opening should be conical and subtend a solid angle just large enough to enable the detector to "see" the whole organ. For example, a 1.5-inch diameter detector requires a 36° collimator to "see" a large thyroid at a distance of 20 cm. At a distance of 35 cm the same detector needs a 20° collimator. This type of collimator is called a *flat field collimator* because it has rather uniform sensitivity across its opening (Chapter 14, Section II,C).

Images of the distribution of radioactive material in the organs of patients are formed by looking at many small areas, either one after the other (scanning), or simultaneously (camera technique). The quality, and hence the diagnostic value of the resulting image or scan depends to a large extent on the size and sharpness of outline of each of the areas or picture elements and on the statistical accuracy of the data obtained from each picture element. Obviously, the spatial definition, often called resolution, is improved if the size of each picture element is reduced, just as a printed picture looks better if a finer screen is used on the printing plate. Making the picture element smaller means that fewer counts will be recorded for that area in a given time unless the dose to the patient is increased. Thus, a compromise must be reached between spatial definition and the statistical validity of the information.

In a scanner this compromise shows up in the design of the collimator for the scintillation detector. In the early days of scanning, a straight cylindrical hole in a block of lead served as the collimator. This arrangement was very inefficient because it accepted only a very small fraction of the γ rays emitted from the area (it subtends a very small solid angle). It also had two other disadvantages. The area seen had approximately the same diameter as the collimator hole, if it was reasonably close to the front of the collimator, but it was not at all sharp because

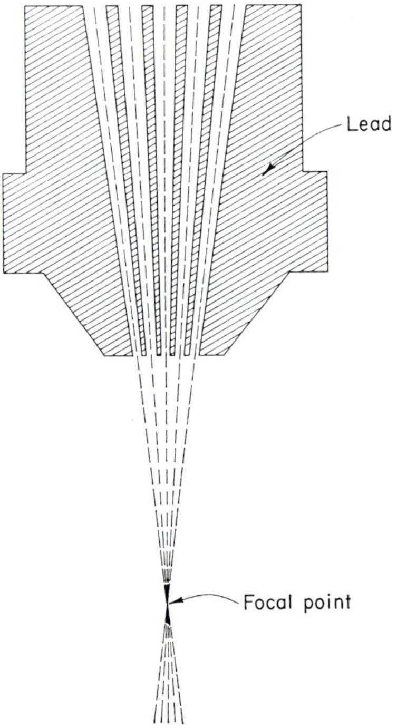

FIG. 10. Cross-sectional view of a multihole focusing collimator showing point of focus of the holes.

of the considerable penumbra inherent in the collimator shape. Furthermore, detection efficiency fell off sharply as the distance between the face of the collimator and the organ increased, owing to the inverse square law.

Subsequently, a *multihole collimator* was designed to let a large-diameter crystal subtend a large solid angle of the radiation coming from the area under study (Fig. 10). Multihole collimators have all of their holes aimed at more or less the same spot, so that they focus on the area under study; hence they are called focusing collimators. Their holes are tapered, and this feature, along with the focusing property, permits them to see the area fairly sharply, that is, their efficiency for radiation outside the area falls off quite rapidly. Also, because of the way the holes are aligned, their greatest sensitivity falls not at the surface of the collimator but in a narrow cylinder centered at the focal point and perpendicular to the collimator face (Chapter 17, Section II,F).

Focusing collimators have been designed for use with various crystal sizes. Three-inch and five-inch diameter crystals are most common for scanning. Eight inches is probably the practical maximum, because for larger crystals the path length from the focal point to the crystal for the outside holes becomes so much greater than for the inside holes that, owing to the inverse square law, the outer holes contribute little to the overall efficiency.

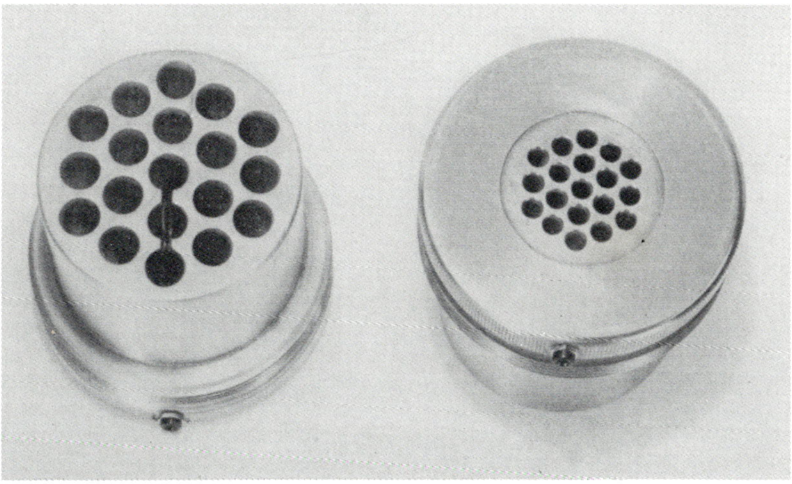

FIG. 11. Back and front view of 19-hole focusing collimator for 3-inch diameter crystal.

For a given crystal size a collimator may have more smaller holes or fewer larger holes, and they may converge at different distances from the face of the collimator. Generally, a focal distance of 2.5 to 3.5 inches is used for 3-inch diameter crystals, but many different compromises can be made between number and size of holes. These compromises must take into account the energy of the radioisotope being measured, because the thickness of the lead (or sometimes, for energetic γ-ray emitters, tungsten) between the holes, the so-called septa, must be great enough to stop virtually all rays which might cross from one hole to the other (Chapter 17, Section II,D). Most commercial collimators are designed for the principal energy of ^{131}I, since it is the most widely used radioisotope, but there are collimators available for lower and higher energies as well. Typically, a scanner has at least two interchangeable collimators, one with a larger and less sharp focal area yielding relatively high count-rates for that area (for scanning large organs) (Fig. 11), and one with a smaller and sharper focal area yielding correspondingly lower count-rates for the area (for scanning small organs).

D. Pulse-Height Resolution

Gamma radiation emitted from a radioactive isotope consists of several fixed energies which are characteristic of that radioisotope. For example, ^{131}I gives off mostly γ rays with an energy of 364 keV, and some γ rays of higher and lower energies. A graph of the spectrum of a γ-ray emitter thus has discrete lines at one or more energy levels (Fig. 12).

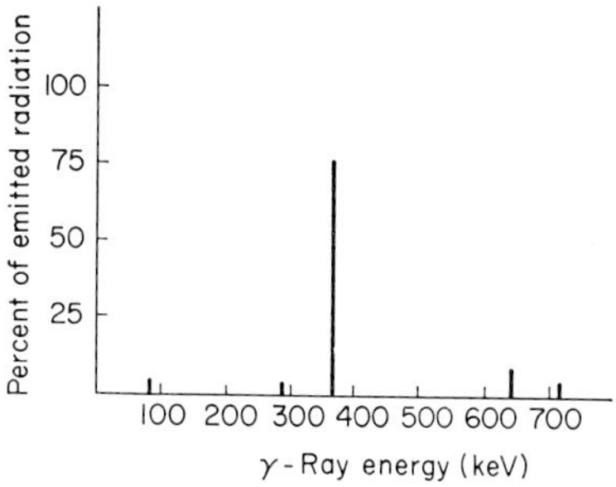

FIG. 12. The γ-ray spectrum of ^{131}I as the radiation is emitted from the nucleus.

If it were possible for a scintillation detector to put out pulses which correspond in height precisely to the energy of the detected γ ray (and if there were no scattering and every γ ray were stopped completely in the detector), then the recorded spectrum would look like Fig. 12. This does not happen because of several effects which take place in the scintillation detector, the most important of which are the collection of the light produced by the crystal scintillations and the conversion of this light to electrons by the photocathode surface of the multiplier phototube. These effects result in a spread in the size of the pulses caused by monoenergetic γ rays (Fig. 13).

The spread in the peaks introduced by the detection system is a function of the detector and of the γ-ray energy peaks. The spread itself is measured as pulse-height resolution, which is the ratio of the width of the peak at half its height to the energy at the center of the peak (Chapter 6, Section IV,A).

Normally the resolution of a detector is quoted for the single γ-ray energy of ^{137}Cs, which falls at 662 keV. It runs about 10% for a 2-inch diameter $\times$ 2-inch thick sodium iodide crystal mounted on a 2-inch diameter photomultiplier tube and about 15% for the same detector if there is a well in the crystal (due to poorer light collection). The resolution figure is worse for lower-energy γ rays and better for higher-energy rays. In general, resolution improves with increasing crystal size up to about 3 inches in diameter. After that it becomes increasingly difficult to make really uniform photocathode surfaces.

It is important to consider the pulse-height resolution of a detector system carefully in placing the selector controls on a pulse-height analyzer so that they will really bracket a peak. This becomes particularly critical if a mixture of two radioisotopes is to be measured. For example,

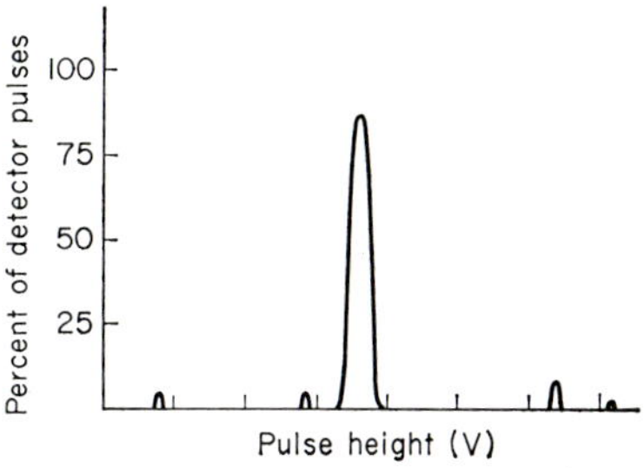

Fig. 13. The γ-ray spectrum of ^{131}I as it would appear on the recording instrument if there were no scattering of radiation and if every detected γ-ray lost all of its energy in the detector crystal.

the principal γ-ray energies of ^{51}Cr and ^{131}I are so close together that a great many detectors do not have good enough resolution to permit separate counting of one radioisotope in the presence of the other.

III. RECORDING INSTRUMENTS

A. Pulse-Height Selection

As was mentioned above, the electrical pulses produced by a sodium iodide scintillation detector as a result of the stoppage of radiation are nearly proportional in size to the energy of the detected γ rays. For example, the principal 364-keV γ rays of ^{131}I produce pulses that are about half as high as those produced by the 722-keV γ rays, which represent 2.8% of the γ rays emitted by ^{131}I.

This relationship of pulse height to radiation energy can be used to select pulses of only a given range of pulse height for recording while rejecting all others. The instrument which performs this function is called a pulse-height analyzer, or sometimes a spectrometer. If it rejects only pulses smaller than a certain size but accepts all larger ones, it is called a discriminator, and if it can look at a whole series (usually 100 or more) of adjacent pulse-height ranges at the same time, it is called a multichannel pulse-height analyzer (Chapter 7, Section III).

There are several reasons for wanting to use a pulse-height analyzer or discriminator.

1. Elimination of Scattered Radiation

The idealized spectrum of ^{131}I shown in Fig. 13 is not a true picture of the height distribution of pulses emitted by a scintillation detector. Instead, the spectrum has a continuous curve with a large contribution at the lower end due to scattered radiation and to rays which did not lose all of their energy in the crystal (Fig. 14).

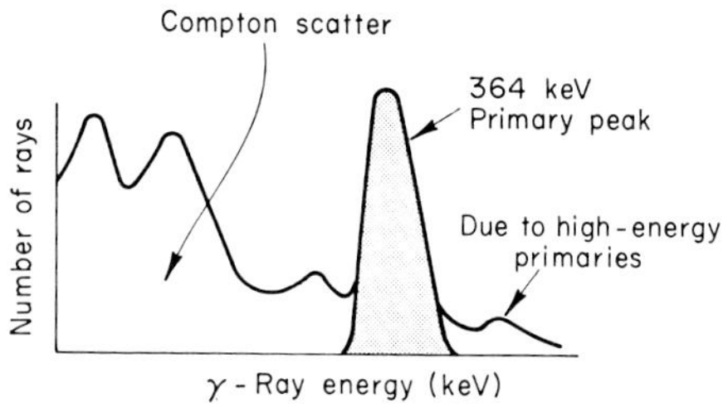

FIG. 14. The pulse-height spectrum of ^{131}I showing the direct radiation from the principal energy peak and the scattered radiation.

The scattered radiation is a source of error in the measurement either if it cannot be duplicated between standard and patient measurements, as in the case of thyroid uptake studies, or if it comes from areas of the patient outside of the one being "looked at" by a scanner at each instant. A discriminator (Fig. 15) or pulse-height analyzer eliminates the scattered radiation from the measurement.

2. Separation of Radioisotopes

Since different radioisotopes have different principal γ-ray energies, it is possible to set the "window" of a pulse-height analyzer to bracket the principal peak of one radioisotope, and thus to measure the concentration of one material in the presence of the other. The minimum difference in energy between the peaks required in order to count them separately is determined by the resolution of the detector (Section II,D). Generally, their separation must be at least twice the percent resolution times the energy of the more energetic peak, if both peaks are expected to be equally large. If one predominates, then the factor must be increased.

3. BACKGROUND REDUCTION

Background radiation is present at all energies. The use of a pulse-height analyzer in the recording system can eliminate most of this background, while a properly set window will accept much of the direct radiation from the sample (Fig. 16). In this way, a pulse-height analyzer supplements and makes more effective the lead shielding surrounding the detector.

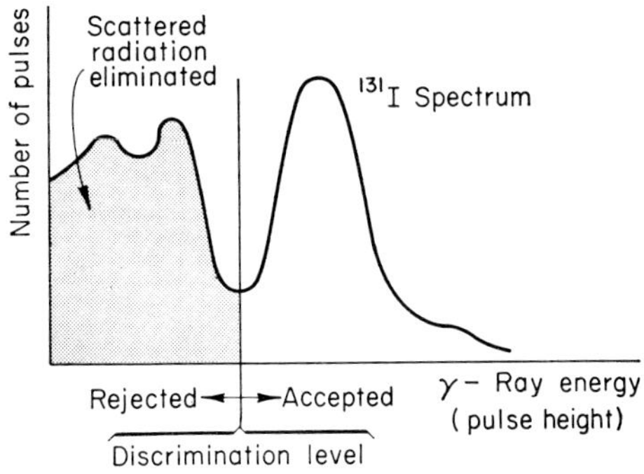

FIG. 15. The discriminator level is correctly placed when it falls in the valley between the primary peak and the scattered radiation peaks.

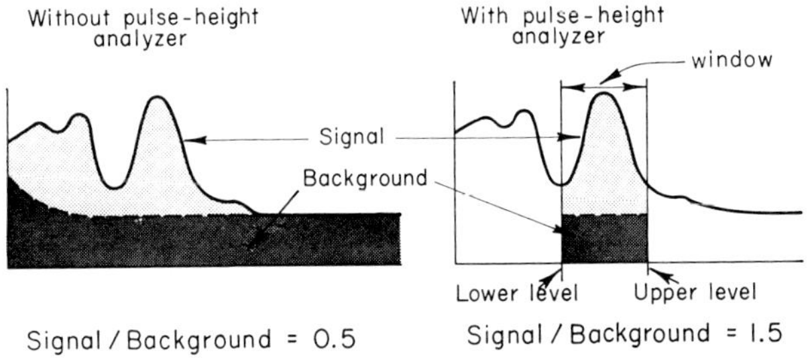

FIG. 16. Spectrum of ^{131}I and background radiation combined, showing effect on signal-to-background ratio of properly set pulse-height analyzer window.

B. Overload of Counting Circuits

Nuclear instruments can handle pulses only up to some maximum count-rate and some maximum pulse size. These limits vary from one piece of equipment to the next, and must be taken into account in radiation measurements (Chapter 7, Section II,B).

1. Resolving Time

The individual pulses produced in radiation detectors have a definite length, in terms of time, so that it is possible for a second event to occur in the detector before the pulse from the first one has disappeared. In that case, the second event will not produce a separate pulse of its own but will either be "lost" completely or will distort the pulse from the first event. This overlapping of pulses results in incorrect counting data.

The length of time it takes for a single pulse to disappear from a detector and for the detector to be ready to correctly observe the next event is called the resolving time of the detector, or the dead time. For a Geiger–Müller tube it might be anywhere from 50 to 200 μsec, depending on the design of the tube. For a scintillation detector using a sodium iodide crystal it is about 1 μsec. For a proportional counter or a scintillation detector with a plastic or liquid phosphor it is a small fraction of a microsecond.

When the detector has a short resolving time, the maximum count-rate at which the scaler can accumulate counts (the scaler resolving time) will provide the overall limit for the detection speed of the system. Most modern scalers have a resolving time of 1 μsec, which matches them to the response of the sodium iodide crystal. Such a combination can count up to 600,000 events per minute with a loss of counts due to overlap, called the coincidence loss, of less than 1%.

If a pulse-height analyzer is used between the scintillation detector and the scaler, it is likely to be the limiting factor. An analyzer must not only be able to distinguish between two successive pulses, like a scaler, but it must be able to measure the true size of each pulse. This can be done only if the second pulse does not sit on top of the last trailing edge of the preceding pulse. Usually, the resolving time of a pulse-height analyzer runs from 2 to 5 μsec.

When measurements are made on sources which give high count-rates where there is an appreciable coincidence loss, a simple equation may be used to correct for the loss:

$$N = n/(1 - n\tau)$$

where N is the true count-rate (cpm), n is the observed count-rate (cpm), and τ is resolving time (min, that is, μsec/6×10^7). Alternatively, a graph may be consulted to determine the correction factor (Fig. 17).

2. Pulse Overload

The ability of a pulse-height analyzer to correctly select pulses as a function of the radiation energy which produced them is influenced not only by the pulse-height resolution of the detector and the resolving time of the analyzer for pulses of comparable size, but also by the occasional influence of a pulse that is so large that it immobilizes the analyzer circuitry for quite a while. Such an overload pulse is most likely to result from the detection of a high-energy cosmic ray.

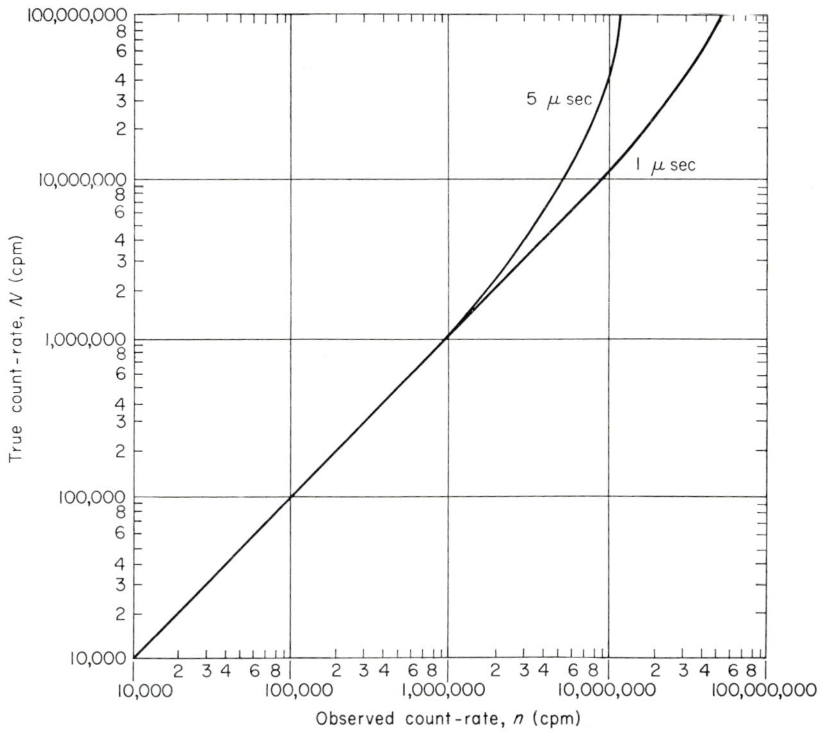

FIG. 17. Count-rate correction for resolving times of 1 and 5 μsec.

It is not practical to design a pulse-height analyzer that does not suffer some distortion due to overload, but it is desirable to keep the effects of the overload to a minimum. A good analyzer is said to overload "gracefully," that is, distortion is limited to a short time interval.

C. Instrument Stability

Once a pulse-height analyzer, or a lower-level selector, is set in relation to the radiation energy spectrum, it is important to know that its setting does not change with time. This demands good stability from the three circuits which influence pulse-height selection. Two of these (high-voltage supply and pulse amplifier) serve to amplify the electrical pulses to make them suitable for analysis, and the third one is the analyzer or discriminator itself.

The first phase of amplification takes place in the multiplier phototube and is controlled by the high voltage applied to the tube. This amplification is always linear (that is, every pulse is multiplied in height by the same factor), but the amount of amplification varies rapidly with the voltage. The second phase of amplification takes place in the preamplifier and amplifier, both of which must be carefully designed to be linear. The importance of good stability in the high voltage and amplifier circuits can be seen by observing the effect of changes in amplification on the count-rate (Fig. 18) of a fraction of a radiation spectrum.

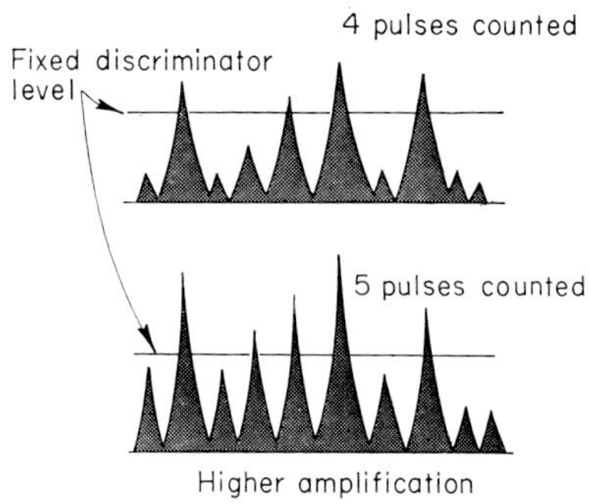

FIG. 18. Effect of increased amplification on the number of pulses out of a series which fall above the discriminator level.

In addition to maintaining the amplification as stable as possible, it is necessary to keep the lower discriminator level or the analyzer window as constant as possible. The circuits which are used in pulse-height analyzers, scalers, and ratemeters are all influenced to some degree by component aging, ambient temperature changes, and wide variations in count-rate. Transistorized equipment suffers much less from component aging and produces much less internal temperature change (which further helps component life), but at the same time transistors are more sensitive to temperature shifts produced by the external environment.

The stability of circuits in higher-quality equipment should be $\pm 1\%$ for an operating day under normal room temperatures (after warm-up) at count-rates of up to at least 100,000 cpm. The performances can be tested using a long-lived radioisotope standard of suitable energy and strength for the particular system, and making a series of measurements over several hours to determine whether the variations fall within statistical probability. It is also a good idea to check for day-to-day variations by counting the standard once daily.

IV. SELECTION OF EQUIPMENT

A. Types of Tests to Be Performed

The procedures of nuclear medicine fall into four broad categories: (1) static uptake measurements (for example, thyroid uptake), (2) dynamic function studies (such as kidney function and cardiac output), (3) radioisotope distribution imaging (scanning and autofluoroscopy, for instance) and (4) *in vitro* measurements (Schilling test, blood volume, T-3 test, and so on). In addition, some institutions engage in research work which involves laboratory equipment for counting β radiation. The latter category is not discussed here.

The *static uptake measurements* require a sealer with a discriminator and generally at least with preset time selection, a scintillation detector with a flat field collimator and at least a 1-inch diameter crystal with good side shielding, and a firm yet maneuverable support for the detector. The principal options are the size of the crystal (Section IV,B,1) and the features of the scaler. Among the optional scaler features are a pulse-height analyzer in place of the discriminator (Section IV,C) and the inclusion of a present count capability. Preset count makes the scaler useful for laboratory as well as uptake measurements (Section IV,B,2) and if the timer has infinite preset selection and a pulse-height analyzer is used to minimize background, permits the use of a simplified technique in which percent uptake can be read from the scaler decades. In this technique the standard is counted on preset count until 10,000 counts are obtained, and then the patient is measured for the same length of time as was required to obtain the 10,000 counts from the standard.

The *dynamic function studies* usually call for two or more probes (one for each kidney, one over the heart and one over the femoral artery, and so on) with good shielding and flat field collimators mounted on flexible, yet sturdy supports, and a dual-channel ratemeter connected to a two-channel strip chart recorder (Fig. 19). Again, there is a choice of crystal size and an option on the use of a dual-channel pulse-height analyzer. Also, it is possible to substitute a rate computer and printer for the ratemeter to obtain digital information and to avoid equilibrium time lag problems (Section I,B,4).

Radioisotope *distribution images* are formed by scanners or cameras (Section II,C). At this time experience with cameras is still limited but scanners have been in wide use for several years. Here again, one may choose between 3-, 5-, and even 8-inch diameter sodium iodide crystals and a variety of collimators. Most scanners use photorecording systems, but they differ in the type and extent of control over contrast enhancement that they permit. In addition, all scanners have mechanical printout systems which may use a hammer-type stylus or an electrical stylus

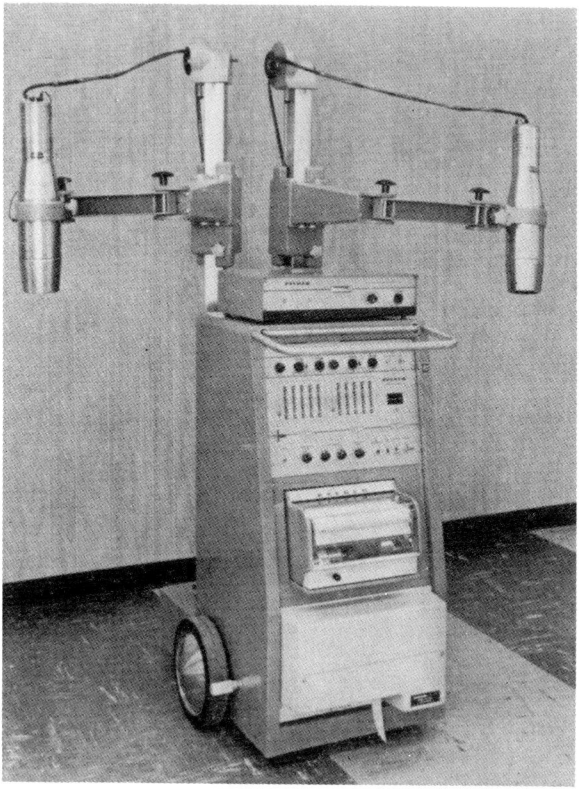

FIG. 19. Dual-channel dynamic function measuring equipment consisting of a dual-channel rate computer with dual-channel recorder, two shielded scintillation detectors, mobile probe stand, and associated components.

on Teledeltos paper, or, more recently, a color coded tapper which gives semiquantitative count-rate information depending on which of eight colors is printed at a given point.

Finally, *in vitro measurements* on liquid γ-ray emitting samples of blood or urine are carried out with a well-type scintillation detector, where the sample is actually inserted in the crystal for greater efficiency

(Fig. 20). Besides the usual option of crystal size and pulse-height analyzer, it is also possible to obtain automatic systems that will count and record many samples without attention from a technician. Recently some more specialized equipment incorporating a well-type detector and scaler circuitry, as well as a small computer, has become available; it is intended primarily for simplified, rapid blood volume measurements, but may also be used for some other tests. It has preset positions for

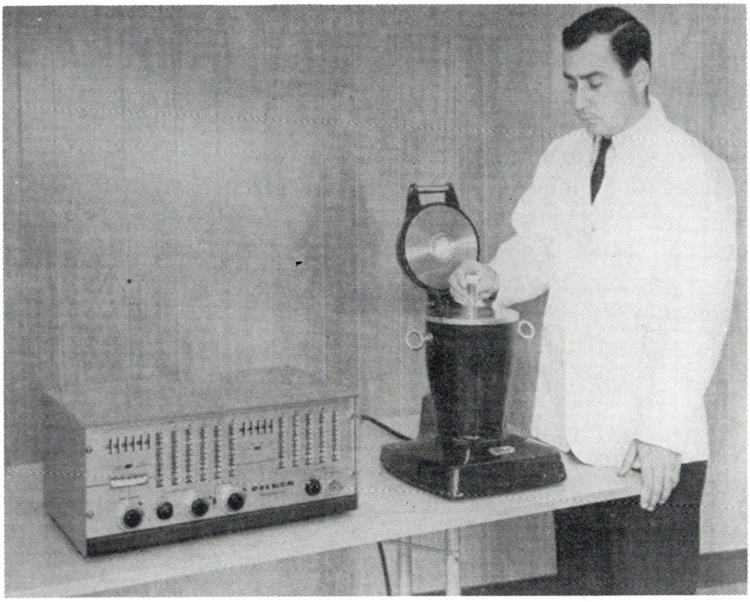

FIG. 20. Manual instrumentation for measuring liquid γ-ray emitting samples consisting of a scaler and a well-type scintillation detector.

measuring the dose, the residue after dose injection, a patient sample taken before administration of the dose, and one taken after administration. From these four measurements, the instrument automatically computes the dilution of the dose and hence the blood volume.

B. Money versus Time

Several of the important choices that can be made in selecting equipment involve a compromise between the cost of the equipment and the time required to make a measurement with a given degree of statistical accuracy.

1. Crystal Size

Detectors with large crystals are more expensive than detectors with small crystals, not only because of the substantially greater cost of the crystal and multiplier phototube, but also because the large crystal requires more shielding. As a result, the supports for the heavier detectors also must be stronger and hence cost more.

On the other hand, the count-rate of a detector goes up appreciably with increased crystal size (Section II,A,2). Specifically, for a source of ^{131}I at a fixed distance the count-rate from a 1.5-inch diameter crystal is slightly more than twice that from a 1-inch diameter crystal. A 2-inch diameter crystal in turn gives almost twice the count-rate of the 1.5-inch diameter crystal, and a 3-inch diameter crystal results in more than twice the count-rate obtained from the 2-inch diameter crystal. Similarly, the count-rate from a 3-inch diameter $\times$ 3-inch high well-type crystal for the photopeak radiation from ^{131}I is almost twice that from a 2-inch diameter $\times$ 2-inch high well-type crystal. For ^{60}Co the ratio is about 3:1 (Chapter 12, Section I).

Improvements in counting efficiency permit equal percentage reduction in counting time for the same statistical accuracy, or reduction in dose to the patient.

2. Multiple Use of Equipment

Making one instrument serve several purposes saves expense, but tends to require more operator time. One reason for this is that multiple-use equipment is apt to be less convenient for any of its applications than single-purpose instrumentation. For example, it is possible to do kidney function studies with a scanner by manually moving the probe from one kidney to the other every 30 sec and taking a reading, but this requires much more time from the operator than the use of a dual detection system, and also makes it impossible to follow accurately the rapid vascular phase at the beginning of the curve. Likewise, a well-type scintillation detector and a scaler can be used for blood volume measurements, but a blood volume computer reduces the complexity of the test to where it can be made available on a 24 hr stand-by basis without tying up a radioisotope technician.

Another reason that multiple-use equipment tends to take more operator time is that usually some work is required: moving instruments, changing connections, or recalibrating. Thus, if the same scaler is used for uptake studies and for well-type counting, it may have to be moved to the laboratory, connected to the well-type detector, and the pulse-height analyzer or discriminator will probably have to be recalibrated.

The most effective doubling-up of instruments can be achieved by including a scaler in a dual detection system so that it can be used for uptake as well as dynamic function studies. Even this arrangement needs careful thought to make certain that the more expensive dual detection system is not tied up too much of the time doing uptake measurements.

C. Future Trends

Nuclear instruments for medical work are becoming increasingly specialized, largely for the purpose of being easier to use. Accurate results can be obtained by the less specialized technicians available for routine studies only if the instruments are very nearly errorproof. This is doubly true of equipment which might have to be used in emergencies after regular laboratory hours, such as blood volume measuring devices, and of equipment operated on more than one shift.

In general, automation features cost more money and are likely to make the instrument less flexible. However, they often pay for themselves in yielding more reliable results and in requiring less of the physician's time to perform the studies. Therefore more specialized single-purpose instruments will be used in the future.

The trend to larger detectors for greater speed and accuracy and lower patient dose is likely to continue. Developments in the field of radiopharmaceuticals point toward an increasing use of low-energy γ-ray emitters such as ^{125}I, ^{197}Hg, and ^{99m}Tc, and new instruments should be selected from those capable of handling these radioisotopes. Finally, fast reset digital counting techniques will replace ratemeters for some of the dynamic function studies (Chapter 7, Section VI,B,2).

PART II

SYSTEMS FOR RADIATION ANALYSIS

CHAPTER 4

GEIGER–MÜLLER AND PROPORTIONAL COUNTERS

CHARLES V. ROBINSON*
MEDICAL PHYSICS DIVISION
MEDICAL RESEARCH CENTER, BROOKHAVEN NATIONAL LABORATORY
UPTON, NEW YORK

I. COUNTER CHARACTERISTICS

A. Pulse Formation and Registration

Geiger–Müller (G-M) and proportional counters† are similar to ionization chambers in that each consists essentially of a gas-filled volume bounded by two electrodes and an insulator. Whereas the center electrode of an ionization chamber is often a rod and may be charged with either polarity, that of a counter is a thin wire and must have positive polarity. In contrast to ionization chambers, in which only the initial ions directly associated with the ionizing events are collected, counters are characterized by collection of additional, secondary ionization produced by gas multiplication in the region of the strong electric field near the center wire. In the proportional counter the initial ionization is amplified by a constant factor, the gas multiplication. Linear amplification of the collected charge then gives an output pulse with an amplitude that is proportional to the initial ionization. In the G-M counter, on the other hand, each event that produces one or more ion

* Supported in part by U.S. Atomic Energy Commission.

† The term "counter" will be used to mean either a G-M or a proportional counter.

pairs in the sensitive volume* triggers a self-terminating discharge which produces a pulse of nearly uniform amplitude, irrespective of the number of initial ions which initiated it. The pulses from proportional counters are, in practice, several orders of magnitude smaller than those from G-M counters and hence require additional amplification before they can be registered (*3, 11, 21*).

The performance of a counting system (detector and associated circuits) is characterized by a count-rate versus anode voltage curve as shown in Fig. 1. When the counter is exposed to radiation, no counts are

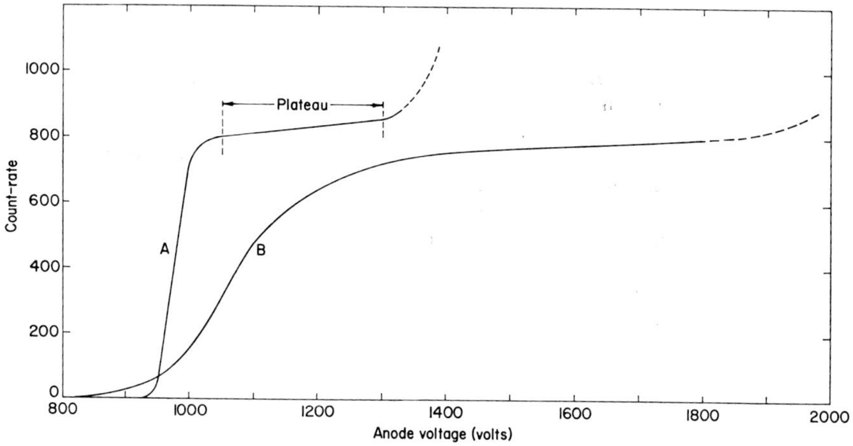

FIG. 1. Counting-characteristic curves for (A) Geiger–Müller counter and (B) proportional counter with β-ray source.

registered with anode voltages below a certain starting voltage. With increasing anode voltage the count-rate of a G-M counter increases at first rapidly until the beginning of the plateau is reached (curve A). Thereafter the count-rate rises only gradually, at a rate (the slope of the plateau) between 1 and 5% per 100 V. The counting characteristic obtained with a G-M system is an index of the performance of the counter itself since the curve is affected neither by the type of radiation detected nor by the characteristics of the associated electronics.

The counting characteristic of a G-M counter changes gradually with use, resulting in a rise in starting voltage, a steepening of the slope of the plateau, and a shortening of its length. It is therefore necessary to check the lower part of the curve occasionally and revise the oper-

* The sensitive volume is defined as that in which occurrence of an ionizing event will result in a detectable pulse. This volume is part of, but usually not the same as, the enclosed gas volume of the counter.

ating voltage for optimum operation. A G-M counter is usually operated at 50 to 100 V above the lower end of the plateau. This yields good reproducibility of counting without undue shortening of the life of the counter with use, as would occur at a higher operating voltage.

The counting characteristic of a proportional counting system exposed to a β-ray source is shown in curve B of Fig. 1. The count-rate increases with increasing voltage much more slowly than in the case of a G-M counter. With a proportional counter, events producing the greatest primary ionization are detected first, and more and more of those producing less ionization are counted as the anode voltage is increased. The counting characteristic of a proportional counting system depends not only on the type of radiation being counted, but on the characteristics of the electronics and the manner in which the gas multiplication of the counter varies with anode voltage. It is thus analogous to the counting characteristic of a scintillation counter, with the electron multiplication of the multiplier phototube corresponding to the gas multiplication in the proportional counter (*17*).

Both G-M and proportional counting systems require registering circuits such as scalers or ratemeters. Such circuits accept only pulses with amplitudes larger than their input sensitivities, which are usually 0.25 or 1 V. The pulses from G-M counters are ordinarily large enough to be fed directly into the registering circuit. Pulses from proportional counters are much smaller and usually require some amplification before they can be registered. For β-ray counting, for example, an amplifier-register combination may be used with an input sensitivity of 1 mV (for example, a gain of 1000 and a register input sensitivity of 1 V). A relatively large gas amplification of 10^5 to 10^6 would be used with such a system. The resulting pulse spectrum at the amplifier input would range up to 100 mV with less than 1% of the pulses being smaller than 1 mV and hence being rejected. In a properly designed system of this sort, only a few counts per hour are due to noise pulses from the amplifier.

B. Life of Counters

The counting life of a counter is the number of counts which can be accumulated under specified operating conditions before a certain degree of deterioration takes place. The life of a counter depends on the type and kind of gas filling and the operating conditions.

Counters may be classed either as counting tubes or as flow counters. Counting tubes have a sealed gas volume whereas the gas in flow counters is continuously replaced. In general, use of a counter causes some deterioration of the gas. In the case of a tube, this results in a cumulative adverse effect on its counting characteristics, whereas in a flow counter the effect is at most temporary. Counting also causes deterioration of the electrode surfaces, especially the anode. This effect is cumulative for either tubes or flow counters. Either type of deterioration is proportional to the accumulated number of counts and the average pulse size (more precisely the total charge collected). Since the pulse size increases with operating voltage, the latter should be kept as low as is consistent with other requirements. Deterioration with excessive voltage, or count-rate, or a combination of the two, may be disproportionately larger than that for normal operation. For example, a counting tube may be irreparably damaged by a single incident of such a nature.

One factor which indirectly affects the rate of deterioration of a counter is the total capacitative input load, which is the sum of the capacitances of the counter itself, of the connectors and cables, and of the input circuit (amplifier or register). The larger the capacitative load, the smaller is the amplitude of the pulse, since the average charge collected per pulse is independent of the input load for a fixed operating voltage. For G-M tubes the charges collected at optimum operating voltages are ample to drive the 100 to 200 $\mu\mu$F input loads usually encountered. Only an exceptionally long cable may have an unduly high capacitance. With proportional counters any increase in input load must be compensated for by a corresponding increase in gas multiplication or higher operating voltage. This causes an increase in the charge per pulse and therefore in the rate of deterioration.

Most gas fillings used in counters are one of three types: (1) mixtures of noble gases and vapors (organic gases), (2) pure organic gases, and (3) mixtures of noble gases and halogens (Cl, Br, I). Geiger–Müller tubes are filled principally with types 1 and 3, and proportional counters with types 1 and 2. The halogen fillings do not undergo significant deterioration with counting. Organic fillings vary considerably in their rates of deterioration but these are, in general, less for proportional than for G-M counters because of the smaller average charge collected.

The counting life of a counter is determined by exposing the counter to a radiation source, and accumulating counts until a specified degree of deterioration has taken place. The total time for such a measurement must be small compared with the shelf life of the counter. This is the time during which the counter will undergo the same amount of deterioration without use. Shelf deterioration may be due to slow leakage of air into the counting gas, release of gases from the counter walls, or chemical reactions within the counter. Well-made tubes have shelf lives of the order of years. The counting lives of G-M tubes filled with organic gases are ordinarily in the range 10^8 to 10^9 counts, and those of halogen-filled tubes, 10^{10} counts or indefinite. The lives of proportional tubes are 10^9 counts or more and may also be indefinite. The lives of flow counters must be considered indefinite, since the results of deterioration can be repaired completely by cleaning or replacement of parts.

II. ABSORPTION OF β RAYS AND DETECTION EFFICIENCY FOR β RAYS AND PHOTONS

If a counting system, G-M or proportional, is adjusted for optimum counting efficiency of samples containing a β-ray emitter, nearly all β rays are counted which enter the sensitive volume of the counter. The overall counting efficiency (counts per disintegration) is thus determined by the fraction of β rays which reach the sensitive volume from their points of emission, that is, the fraction of those β rays that are neither absorbed by the intervening material nor directed or scattered away from the sensitive volume.

The absorption and scattering of β rays depend on a number of factors such as the β-ray energy spectrum, the configuration of source and sensitive volume, and the chemical compositions of the sample and the window or wall of the counter. The simplified treatment of β-ray absorption given below is applicable to configurations in which the sample, the counter wall, and the sensitive volume of the counter are in close proximity (2π geometry). This is the case for several types of *in vivo* counting and for the counting of solutions (Section III). A more detailed discussion of absorption and scattering in the case of solid sample counting with less than 2π geometry is given elsewhere (*20*).

Consider a counter which has a sensitive volume bounded by a plane wall or window of thickness t_w (mg/cm^2) outside of which is a uniform layer of homogeneously active sample material of thickness t_s (mg/cm^2). The count-rate, N, is found experimentally to vary with t_s and t_w and is approximately proportional to the product of

$$\exp(-kt_w) \text{ and } [1 - \exp(-kt_s)],$$

where the constant, k, depends on the maximum energy of the β rays. If $N_{\max}$ is the count-rate extrapolated to zero wall thickness and to sample thicknesses that are greater than the maximum range of β rays, the count-rate, N, is approximately

$$N = N_{\max} \exp(-kt_w)[1 - \exp(-kt_s)] \quad \text{(cpm)} \qquad (1)$$

As will be shown below, $N_{\max}$ depends on the area common to both the sensitive volume and the sample, the specific activity of the sample material, and the energy of the β rays. The dependence of the relative count-rate, $N/N_{\max}$, on the thicknesses of the sample and the counter wall is shown in Fig. 2, which is a plot of Eq. 1. The thickness is given in units of the effective half-thickness, h, which is defined as $h = (\ln 2)/k$. For any given wall thickness, one half of the maximum count-rate (that for infinite sample thickness) is reached for a sample thickness of $t_s = h$. Increasing the wall thickness by one unit of h decreases the counts by a factor of 2.

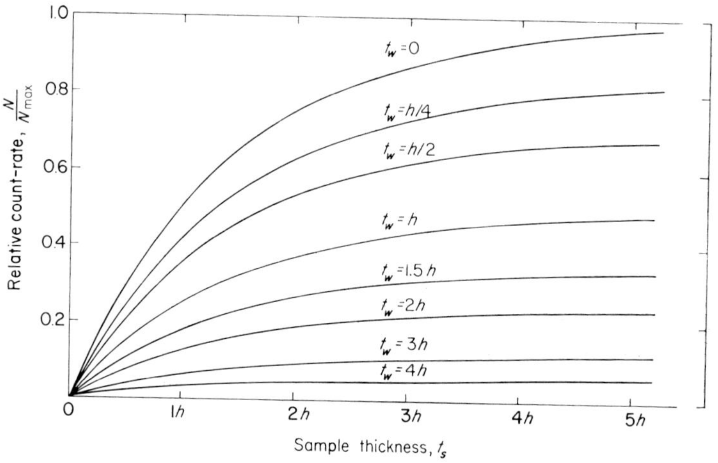

FIG. 2. Relative count-rate versus thickness of β-ray sample for various counter wall thicknesses.

If A (cm^2) represents the area of the window common to the sensitive volume and the sample, and n (dpm/mg) the specific activity of the sample, then by definition the counting efficiency, ϵ, equals

$$\epsilon = (N/At_sn) \quad \text{(counts per disintegration)} \tag{2}$$

Dividing both sides of Eq. 1 by (At_sn) yields

$$\epsilon = \epsilon_{\max} \exp(-kt_w)[1 - \exp(-kt_s)]/kt_s \tag{3}$$

where

$$\epsilon_{\max} = N_{\max}(k/An) \tag{4}$$

which is the value of ϵ when extrapolated to zero wall and sample thicknesses. A plot of Eq. 3 shows the dependence of ϵ on t_w and t_s (Fig. 3). The unit of thickness is again the effective half-thickness, h. The curves are not true exponentials and reach 50% of their maximum value ($t_s = 0$) for a sample thickness of $t_s = 2.3h$ rather than $t_s = h$.

In order to obtain numerical estimates of count-rates from these equations, it is necessary to find the value of h (or k) applicable to the

β-ray activity being counted. Let E_0 be the maximum β-ray energy of the emitter, and R_0 its range in aluminum as given by Katz and Penfold* (*9*). Values of E_0 from the literature (*15*) and the corresponding values of R_0 are listed in Table I for 9 radioisotopes of interest in medical research.

The values given for h/R_0 were obtained as follows. Experimentally determined values of the constant k applicable to the geometry considered here (2π) have been reviewed by Baker and Katz (*1*) for maximum β-ray energies E_0 from 0.155 to 3.3 MeV and for ^3H by Rydberg

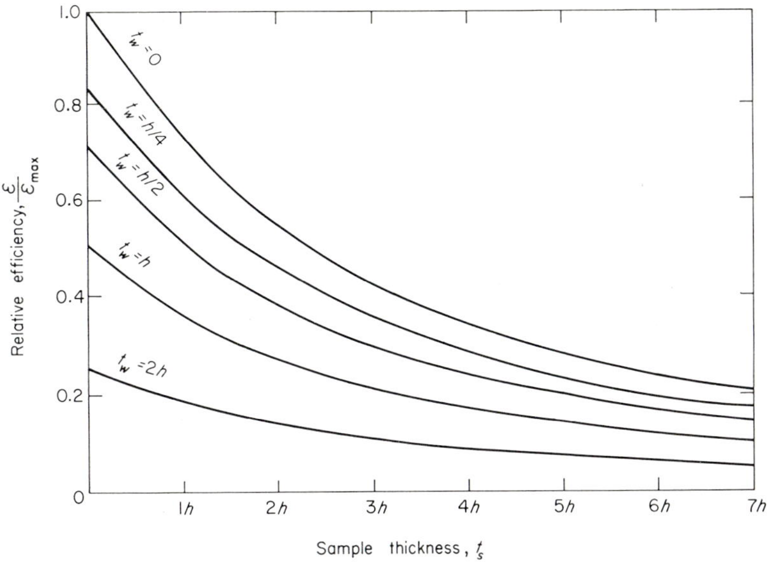

FIG. 3. β-Ray counting efficiency versus sample thickness for various counter wall thicknesses.

(*16*). For the higher energies, Baker and Katz fitted the data with the expression $k = 0.0155E_0^{-1.41}$ (cm²/mg), which gives $h = 44.7E_0^{1.41}$ (mg/cm²). The experimental values of h range from $0.09R_0$ to $0.17R_0$, and the ratio (h/R_0) tends to increase with the maximum β-ray energy. The fitted value of h, on the other hand, gives a ratio (h/R_0) which has a minimum value of $h/R_0 = 0.103$ at 0.5 MeV with higher values for energies below 0.5 MeV as well as above. By using a constant value of $h/R_0 = 0.103$ below 0.5 MeV, a better fit to the data is obtained, especially if Rydberg's ^3H data are included. This has accordingly been done for the first three values of (h/R_0) given in Table I, and the re-

* For $E_0 < 2.5$ MeV, $R_0 = 412\,E_0^{1.625-0.0954\ln E_0}$ (mg/cm²) and for $E_0 \geqslant 2.5$ MeV, $R_0 = 530\,E_0 - 106$ (mg/cm²).

TABLE I
RADIOISOTOPE DATA RELATED TO β-RAY SAMPLE COUNTING

β-Ray emitter	Maximum β-ray energy, E_0 (Mev)	Range of maximum β, R_0 (mg/cm²)	h/R_0	Effective half-absorption thickness, h (mg/cm²)	Normalized maximum count-rate, N_1 $\left(\frac{\text{cpm/cm}^2}{\mu\text{Ci/gm}}\right)$
^{3}H	0.018	0.55	0.103	0.06	90
^{14}C	0.155	28.0	0.103	2.9	4,600
^{45}Ca	0.254	60.8	0.103	6.3	10,000
^{131}I	0.608	214	0.104	22	35,000
^{198}Au	0.959	391	0.108	42	67,000
^{24}Na	1.39	618	0.115	71	110,000
^{32}P	1.70	785	0.121	95	150,000
^{90}Y	2.24	1073	0.130	140	220,000
^{42}K	3.58	1790	0.151	270	430,000

maining values are from the expression of Baker and Katz.* Although the fitted values of (h/R_0) are given to 1% accuracy in Table I, the experimental values cover a much greater range. Values applicable to this case (2π geometry) can be expected to lie within ±30% of the fitted values, or ±50% in the case of ^{3}H.

In the following columns of Table I are given the corresponding values of h and of the normalized maximum count-rate, N_1. The latter is the value of N_{max} for $A = 1$ cm² and a specific activity of 1 μCi/gm, that is, for $n = 2.22 \times 10^3$ dpm/mg. The values of N_1 are calculated on the assumption that the maximum counting efficiency ϵ_{max} in Eq. 3 is 0.5, which is the case for 2π geometry with scattering neglected. Thus $N_{max} = 0.5An/k$ (from Eq. 4). If the normalized values are used for A and n and $k = \ln 2/h$, the normalized maximum count-rate becomes

$$N_1 = 1.6 \times 10^3 h \qquad (\text{cpm/cm}^2)/(\mu\text{Ci/gm}) \tag{5}$$

As may be seen from Table I the maximum count-rate increases rapidly with increasing β-ray energy.

So far only the counts due to β rays have been considered. Bremsstrahlung produced by the absorption of the β rays (Section III,E) and γ or X rays emitted by the radioisotope may also contribute significantly to the count-rate. Such photons will be counted if they are absorbed in the gas of the sensitive counter volume or in the surrounding material

* It is suggested that for values of E_0 other than those tabulated, the same procedures be used to estimate h/R_0.

sufficiently close to the sensitive volume so that the secondary particles can ionize the gas.

The intrinsic efficiency of photon detection, ϵ_γ, is defined as the fraction of photons counted which were originally directed toward the sensitive volume. This efficiency is principally a function of the photon energy and the atomic number of the wall material of the counter (Fig. 4). It is less than 2% (for photon energies below 2.5 MeV), which is a very low photon efficiency compared with that of scintillation counters (Chapter 6, Section III,A).

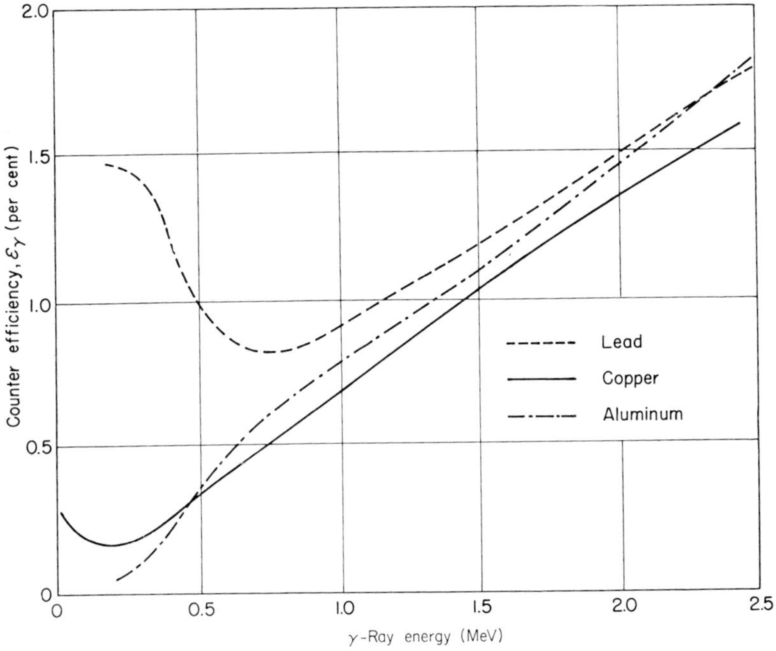

FIG. 4. Intrinsic counter efficiency as a function of γ-ray energy in counters of different wall materials (7).

Absorption of photons in the counter gas itself contributes a negligible fraction to ϵ_γ except at photon energies lower than those shown in Fig. 4 (below about 50 keV) and with gases of relatively high atomic numbers. For detection of the characteristic X rays emitted by radioisotopes decaying by electron capture, proportional counters are used which have beryllium windows and gas fillings which consist of A, Kr, or Xe plus an organic gas, usually CH_4. When used with a linear amplifier and pulse-height analyzer, such counters are well suited for detecting photons of energies below about 30 keV and for discriminating between photons of different energies in this range.

III. COUNTER SYSTEMS AND APPLICATIONS

A. Flow Counters for Solid β-Ray Samples

Several common features of commercially available counters which are operated either as G-M or as proportional counters and which detect β rays from one side of a solid sample (2π geometry) are shown in Fig. 5. The windowless type, in which the sample is placed within the gas volume, is illustrated in Fig. 5A, and the thin-window type in Fig. 5B. The windows come in two thickness ranges: (1) standard thickness (0.8 to 1.0 mg/cm^2) and (2) ultrathin (0.08 to 0.15 mg/cm^2). All windows are of plastic and have conducting metal coatings, since they must function as part of the cathode. The counters are approximately either 1 or 2 inches in diameter, corresponding to the diameters of their sample mountings which may be planchets or disks. The samples are changed either manually or by employing automatic sample changers.

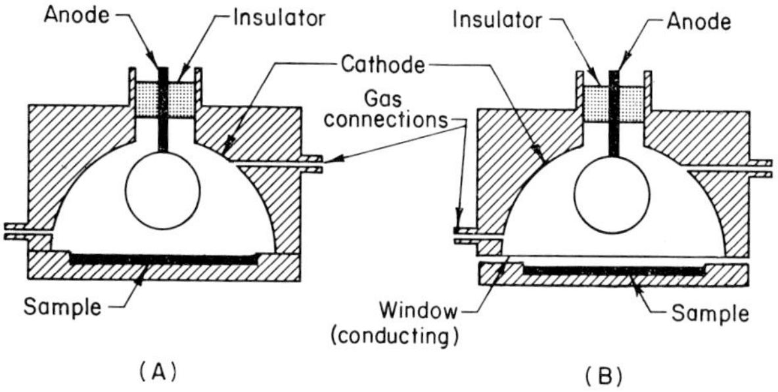

FIG. 5. Flow counters of 2π geometry: (A) Windowless counter, (B) Thin-window counter.

The anodes of flow counters are commonly loops of wire which may lie in a vertical (Fig. 5) or horizontal plane. The wire which is of stainless steel or tungsten has a 0.002-inch diameter. A thinner wire is sometimes used and gives a lower operating voltage but is more fragile.

Gases used for proportional operation are (1) 90% argon + 10% methane (P-10 gas) and (2) pure methane. Operating voltages are respectively in the ranges 1500–2000 V and 3000–4000 V. The choice of the counting gas depends on the electrical provisions made for operation at the higher voltages, and the need for high sensitivity to low-energy photons (especially in the K-capture range). Methane gives less photon sensitivity than P-10 gas. The gas mixtures used for G-M operation contain about 99% helium and 1% butane or isobutane, and, like methane, give low sensitivity to low-energy photons, but unlike methane permit operation at low voltages in the range 1000–1500 V.

For many applications there is little to choose between G-M and proportional operation. Both give good reproducibility in thin-window flow counters. In windowless counters the G-M operation is less stable. The additional circuitry required for proportional operation is a minor consideration since the necessary amplifier need not be expensive. For high count-rates, proportional systems, which have resolving times of the order of 1 μsec, are superior to G-M systems, which have resolving times of 100 to 200 μsec. Discrimination between α and β rays requires proportional operation.

In thin-window counters a steady flow of gas must be maintained throughout the counting period. This is ordinarily in the range of 50 to 100 cm^3 per minute. Windowless systems require provisions for flushing out the air which has been taken into the counter by changing the sample. A flushing period may be necessary between introduction of the sample and the beginning of the count, or the outflowing gas may be employed to preflush the sample that is to be counted next. In general, windowless counters require more gas per sample than the thin-window types.

Although windowless, flow proportional counting of ^{14}C has proven to be practical (*8*), the presently available flow counters with ultrathin windows are preferred for most routine counting of solid ^{14}C samples. Closure of the gas volume not only reduces the gas required and eliminates the flushing period, but it also decreases the likelihood of contaminating the inside of the counter and of damaging the anode. Windowless counters are used for solid samples containing ^3H or α-ray emitters.

B. Geiger–Müller Tubes for Assay and Monitoring

Geiger–Müller tubes with thin walls or windows are suitable for β-ray detection. Such tubes are mica end-window tubes, and thin-walled tubes of glass or metal. End-window tubes are available in diameters from ¼ to 2 inches, the most commonly used sizes being ¾ to 1¼ inch (Fig. 6). Available window thicknesses range from 1.4 to 5 mg/cm^2.

Thin-walled tubes are commonly available in about ¾-inch diameter and are supplied in various lengths. The thin-walled portion of the casing is approximately 30 mg/cm^2 thick in either glass or metal types. Figure 7A illustrates a thin-walled glass counter in a solution-counting arrangement (Section III,C).

Because they are inexpensive, G-M tubes are particularly well suited for portable or semiportable counting systems. The tubes are light and require no gas supply, and relatively little electronics is needed with them. They are commonly used in portable, battery-operated instruments for low-level area monitoring (Chapter 8).

The count-rate used should not exceed that recommended by the manufacturer, or the rate which gives a 10% dead-time loss (Chapter 3, Section III,B,1). In either case, this limiting count-rate is usually in the range of 10,000 to 20,000 cpm. Even with halogen tubes which are not easily damaged by high count-rates, it may be worth while to limit the count-rate to obtain satisfactory counting accuracy, since large dead-time corrections may introduce large errors in the corrected count-rates.

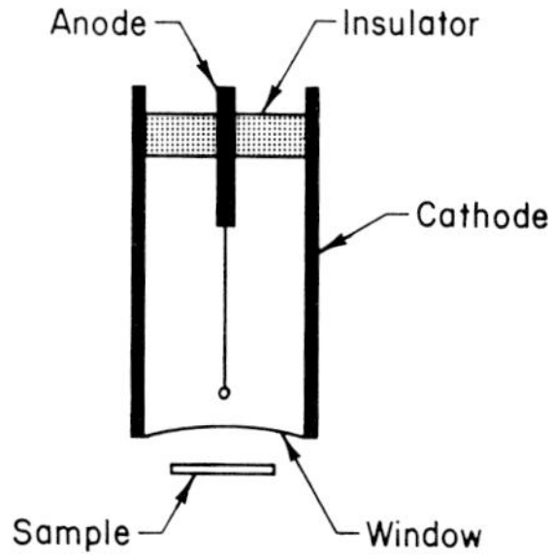

FIG. 6. End-window G-M counter.

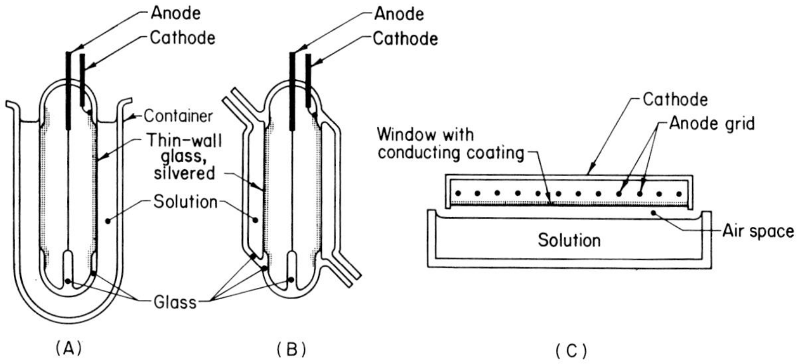

FIG. 7. Thin-walled, solution counters: (A) dip counter, (B) jacketed counter, (C) flat, gridded counter (Firma Münchener Apparatebau f. elek. Geräte, München).

Arrangements to prevent accidental overvoltage are worth while for either organic or halogen filled tubes.

C. Thin-Walled Solution Counters

One way in which solutions containing β-ray emitters may be assayed is by placing a thin-walled counter in proximity to the solution. Several forms of such counters are illustrated in Fig. 7: (A) a dip counter, (B) a jacketed counter, and (C) a flat gridded counter. Usually, types A and B are G-M tubes and type C is a proportional flow counter (*10*).

The wall thicknesses for the dip and jacketed solution counters of Fig. 7A and 7B are ordinarily about 30 mg/cm^2; that for the flat counter of Fig. 7C is 0.9 mg/cm^2, to which must be added the mass thickness of 0.5 to 2 cm of air (0.6 to 2.4 mg/cm^2) depending on the arrangement used. Types A and B cannot detect the β rays of ^{14}C. All three types of counter can detect ^{45}Ca and β-ray emitters of higher energies.

The dip counter, type A, has the advantage that the wall may be exposed for cleaning between samples. The jacketed counter, type B, may be used for continuous counting of a solution which flows through the jacket. The flat counter, type C, is available with quite a large area suitable for detecting low-activity β-ray emitters in large volumes.

One general limitation of β-ray solution counting is the small size of the volume which can be effectively counted when the β-ray energy is low. From the discussion given in Section II (Fig. 2) it follows that the fraction of the solution lying beyond 4 half-thicknesses of the counter wall can increase the count-rate due to the solution within $4h$ of the wall by at most 7%. Assuming unit density of the solution, the thickness $4h$ for ^{14}C is only $4h = 0.12$ mm, whereas for ^{32}P, $4h = 3.8$ mm. For an area of $A = 1$ cm^2, a specific activity of 1μCi/gm, and solutions of thickness $4h$, the maximum count-rate is $N_1/1.07$ which is 4,300 cpm for ^{14}C and 140,000 cpm for ^{32}P.

D. β-Ray Counting *in Vivo*

Several diagnostic procedures are based on the use of small, thin-walled counters mounted at the tips of probes or catheters to measure concentrations of β-ray emitters in tissue. Brain tumor localization at operation with ^{32}P (*18*) requires probing counters as shown in Fig. 8A,B. The counters are used in brain tissue to search for regions of increased radioactivity which are indicative of the presence of tumor. The tip-sensitive counter (Fig. 8B) is preferable to the side-sensitive one (Fig. 8A), since it gives better localization in depth and requires less penetration of tissue in the exploration. The probe diameter should preferably be about 2 mm and the probe length about 10 cm. Several companies supply side-sensitive G-M probing counters which are 2, 2.5, or 3 mm in diameter with 30 to 80 mg/cm^2 wall thicknesses and organic vapor or halogen fillings. A tip-sensitive, 2-mm diameter, proportional probing counter (*18*) has been used, and a similar 2.5-mm diameter, halogen-filled G-M tube is commercially available (Fig. 8B).

For the diagnosis of eye tumors with ^{32}P (*4, 19*), counters with end or side windows which can be placed in contact with the eyeball are used. The counters shown in Fig. 8C,D,E are suitable for anterior, equatorial, and posterior parts of the eye. These counters have mica windows of 1.4 or 2 mg/cm^2 thickness and are suitable for superficial counting of radioactive tissues. Halogen-filled G-M tubes of all three types are available commercially.

In the diagnosis of breast tumors (*2*, *6*) probing counters or small catheter counters (not illustrated) are implanted in breast tissue and left for extended periods to record variations in the level of ^{32}P. For implantation or intracavitary use, cylindrical, thin-walled tubes 5 mm

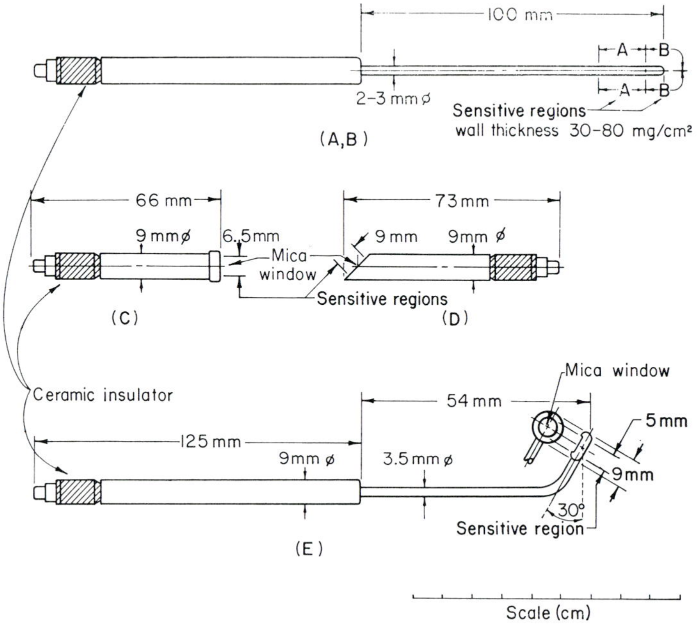

FIG. 8. Counters for *in vivo* β-ray detection: (A, B) probing counters of 2- to 3-mm diameter, *A*, side-sensitive (Eon Corp; Leighton Labs; Lionel Electronic Labs; Twentieth Century Electronics), *B*, tip-sensitive (Eon Corp. Type 5155); (C) end-window counter (6.5-mm diameter window); (D) oblique-window counter (window 6.5 $\times$ 9 mm); (E) side-window (5-mm diameter window) counter with 60° bend (Eon Corp; Lionel Electronic Labs).

or less in diameter are suitable. Several types of halogen filled G-M tubes of this description are commercially available, some with waterproof connections.

Although no routine procedure has so far been developed which utilizes intravascular β-ray counting, a feasibility study has been carried out with ^{85}Kr in dogs (*12*) which indicates that such counting is possible. A very short, tip-sensitive, proportional counter of 2-mm diameter mounted at the end of a 2-mm diameter catheter cable was used. For intracardiac catherization the cable must possess a flexibility, size, and shape similar to those of standard cardiac catheters.

The data given in Table I may be used to estimate count-rates *in vivo* for β-ray emitters homogeneously distributed in tissue as was done in Section III,C for solutions. For example, an end-window counter, as shown in Fig. 8C, may have a sensitive area of 0.25 cm^2 with a window thickness of 2 mg/cm^2. If the counter should be placed in contact with tissue containing 1 μCi/gm of ^{14}C, the expected count-rate would be about 700 cpm. For a cylindrical, side-sensitive, counter of 2-mm diameter, 1-cm sensitive length, and wall thickness 30 mg/cm^2, implanted in homogeneously active tissue containing 1 μCi/gm of ^{32}P, the expected count-rate is 75,000 cpm. Although the counting geometry in this case is not effectively planar (since h is comparable to the radius of the counter), the result agrees well with experimental values. This agreement may be due to cancellation of two opposing effects on the efficiency of counting. As the radius of a concentric layer of source material is increased, its area increases, but the solid angle subtended by the counter at points within the layer decreases.

E. Bremsstrahlung Counting *in Vivo*

Secondary photons (Bremsstrahlung) are produced by the emission or absorption of β rays. The Bremsstrahlung has much more penetration through matter than the β rays that produced it. As a source of photons, a pure β-ray emitter *in vivo* is characterized by a low photon yield per disintegration, and a broad energy spectrum (*5*). The yield of usable photons (above 20 keV) is of the order of 1 per 100 β rays for ^{32}P ($E_0 = 1.7$ MeV), and varies approximately as the square of the maximum β-ray energy, E_0. The photon energy spectrum extends as high as E_0, but there are very few photons near this upper limit. The number of photons per energy interval increases with decreasing energy until a peak is reached just above the tissue absorption cutoff, which is about 20 keV. As an example, with ^{32}P, the peak comes at about 30 keV, and the median energy of usable photons is about 100 keV.

With a suitable photon detector outside the body, concentrations of a pure β-ray emitter may be detected by means similar to those used for emitters of low-energy γ rays (*13, 14*). Low-level counting of Bremsstrahlung *in vivo* is best done either with a thin sodium iodide crystal of large area, or a large-area proportional counter employing krypton or xenon in the filling gas.

REFERENCES

1. Baker, R. G., and Katz, L., Absolute beta counting of thick planar samples. *Nucleonics* **11**, No. 2, 14 (1953).

2. Bullen, M. A., Freundlich, H. F., Hale, B. T., Marshall, D. H., and Tudway, R. C., The activity of malignant tumors and response to therapeutic agents, studied by continuous records of radioactive phosphorus uptake. *Postgrad. Med. J.* **39**, 265 (1963).
3. Curran, S. C., The proportional counter as detector and spectrometer. *In* "Handbuch der Physik" (S. Flügge, ed.), Vol. 45, p. 174. Springer, Berlin, 1958.
4. Duke-Elder, S., and Smith, R. J. H., Clinical methods of examination. *In* "System of Ophthalmology" (S. Duke-Elder, ed.), Vol. 7, Sect. III, p. 363. Mosby, St. Louis, Missouri, 1962.
5. Evans, R. D., "The Atomic Nucleus." McGraw-Hill, New York, 1955.
6. Hale, B. T., A technique for studying human tumour growth *in vivo*. *Lancet* **II**, 345 (1961).
7. Hine, G. J., and Brownell, G. L. (eds.), "Radiation Dosimetry." Academic Press, New York, 1956.
8. Karnowsky, M. L., Foster, J. M., Gidez, L. I., Hagerman, D. D., Robinson, C. V., Solomon, A. K., and Villee, C. A., Correction factors for comparing activities of different carbon-14-labelled compounds assayed in flow proportional counter. *Anal. Chem.* **27**, 852 (1955).
9. Katz, L., and Penfold, A. S., Range-energy relations for electrons and the determination of beta-ray end-point energies by absorption. *Rev. Mod. Phys.* **24**, 28 (1952).
10. Kiefer, H., and Maushart, R., Large-area flow counters speed radiation measurements. *Nucleonics* **19**, No. 12, 51 (1961).
11. Korff, S. A., Geiger Counters. *In* "Handbuch der Physik" (S. Flügge, ed.), Vol. 45, p. 52. Springer, Berlin, 1958.
12. Kreidberg, M. B., Robinson, C. V., and Chernoff, H. L., Diagnosis of shunts with intracardiac proportional-counter catheters—preliminary report. *J. Nucl. Med.* **3**, 192 (1962).
13. Lidén, K. V. H., The determination of Sr^{90} and other beta emitters in human beings from external measurements of the Bremsstrahlung. *Proc. 2nd Intern. Conf. Peaceful Uses At. Energy, Geneva, 1958* Vol. 23, p. 133. United Nations Publication, New York, 1959.
14. Lidén, K. V. H., and McCall, R. C., Low-energy-photon detectors for whole-body counting. *Proc. Symp. Whole-Body Counting, Vienna, 1961* p. 145. Intern. At. Energy Agency, Vienna, 1962.
15. Loevinger, R., Average energy of allowed beta-particle spectra. *Phys. Med. Biol.* **1**, 330 (1957).
16. Rydberg, J., Determination of the absolute activity of solid tritium samples. *Acta Chem. Scand.* **12**, 399 (1958).
17. Price, W. J., "Nuclear Radiation Detection," 2nd ed. McGraw-Hill, New York, 1964.
18. Selverstone, B., and Robinson, C. V., Localization of brain tumors with beta-emitting isotopes. *In* "Medical Physics" (O. Glasser, ed.), Vol. 3, p. 238. Year Book Publ., Chicago, Illinois, 1960.
19. Terner, I. S., Leopold, I. H., and Eisenberg, I. J., The radioactive phosphorus (^{32}P) uptake test in ophthalmology. *AMA Arch. Ophthalmol.* **55**, 52 (1956).
20. Watt, D. E., and Ramsden, D., Self-absorption and self-scattering corrections for homogeneously dispersed sources. *In* "High Sensitivity Counting Techniques," p. 232. Macmillan (Pergamon), New York, 1964.
21. Wilkinson, D. H., "Ionization Chambers and Counters." Cambridge Univ. Press, London and New York, 1950.

CHAPTER 5

SEMICONDUCTOR DETECTORS

STEPHEN S. FRIEDLAND*
DEPARTMENT OF PHYSICS
SAN FERNANDO VALLEY STATE COLLEGE
NORTHRIDGE, CALIFORNIA

AND

MICHAEL R. ZATZICK
SOLID STATE RADIATIONS, INC.
LOS ANGELES, CALIFORNIA

Though they have existed in their present form for only a few years, nuclear semiconductor detectors are rapidly finding useful applications in biology and medicine as particle detectors, nuclear spectrometers, and dosimeters. Desirable radiation detector properties such as an excellent linear response with energy that is independent of particle type, negligible entrance windows, excellent energy resolution, fast rise time pulses, variable sensitive depth, and considerable handling ease are some of the features attainable in practical devices (*9, 26*).

* Also, Solid State Radiations, Inc., Los Angeles, California.

Semiconductor radiation detectors are made of single crystals of high-purity semiconductor germanium and silicon. They include, in both silicon and germanium, the diffused p-n junction, the surface barrier structure, and the p-i-n structure. In each of these structures, there are variations in entrance and exit windows, depth of active region, physical size and mountings, and so forth, which compound the different types of detectors that may be fabricated.

Considerable information on the properties of semiconductor detectors is generally available (*6, 14, 19*). Only a brief discussion of the operational principles and characterizing properties of semiconductor detectors will be presented.

I. DETECTION MECHANISM OF SEMICONDUCTOR DETECTORS

Semiconductor detectors are essentially solid state versions of the gas-filled ionization chamber. As shown in Fig. 1A, in the gas chamber the energy of the incident charged particle is dissipated in the gas by

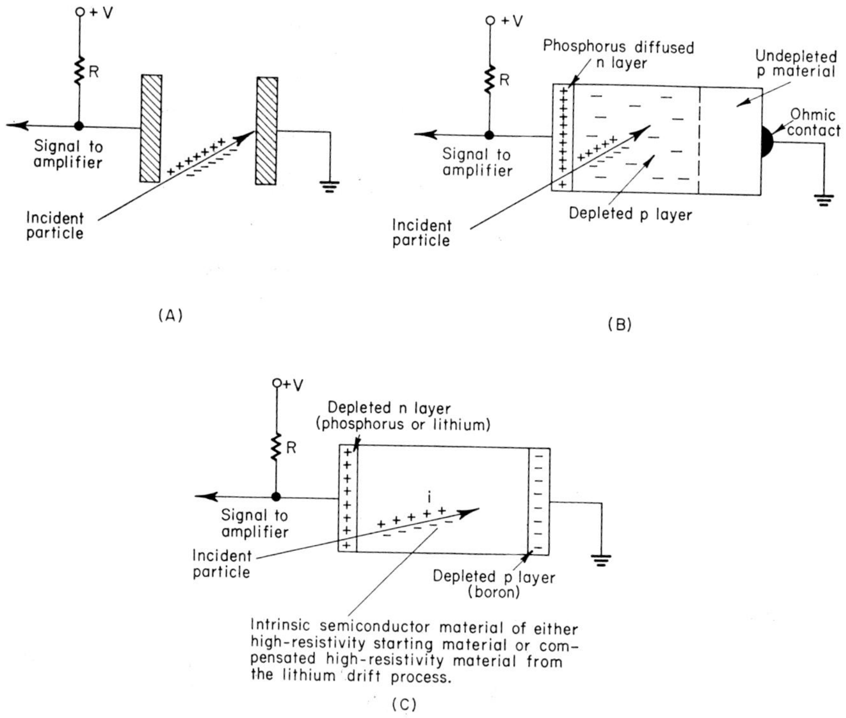

FIG. 1. Operation principle: (A) gas-filled ionization chamber; (B) the semiconductor p-n junction detector; (C) semiconductor p-i-n junction detector.

the production of electron-ion pairs, provided the dimension of the chamber and the pressure of the gas are selected to be consistent with the energy and type of the particle to be detected. In most gases, the production of each ion pair requires 35 eV of energy of the incident particle. Thus, a particle with an energy of E MeV will produce $(E/35) \times 10^6$ electron-ion pairs. The charge carriers so produced are swept out of the gas chamber by an electric field which is induced by an externally applied bias voltage. The rise time of the signal appearing in the external circuit is a function of the mobility of the electrons and ions in the gas, as well as the ratio of electric field to gas pressure. In the absence of radiation, the high resistivity of the gas to the conduction of charge results in a very small leakage current. The noise from the fluctuations in the leakage current of the gas case is small compared with the input amplifier noise.

In the semiconductor detector, the incident nuclear radiation dissipates its energy in the ionization process in which electron-hole pairs are produced. Here an electron is raised from the valence band, across the forbidden band gap, into the conduction band. If an internal electric field is present, from an external bias, the electron is free to move, thus producing a negative current flow. The electron that is now in the conduction band has left a "hole" in the valence band. A neighboring electron in the valence band will jump, under the action of the electric field, into the "hole," filling it but leaving the hole in the position from which the second electron jumped. In this way, the hole current moves through the crystal and thus represents a current flow.

If a slice of semiconductor material is placed between two electrodes, a current will flow. The current results from (a) bulk current whose magnitude depends upon the resistance of the slice and the number of electron-hole pairs that are thermally generated, and (b) surface leakage currents. The fluctuations in such currents introduce noise pulses that completely swamp any signals from nuclear particles.

In order to reduce the leakage current and the inherent noise, a barrier in the form of a p-n junction is introduced into the device to limit the bulk conductivity current. The bulk thermally generated current in silicon at room temperature can be tolerated, whereas in germanium the device must be operated at liquid nitrogen temperature. Surface leakage currents are reduced by careful cleaning, etching, and encapsulation of the crystal.

The energy required to create an electron-hole pair, which is 3.5 eV for silicon and 2.94 eV for germanium, is related to the gap between the valence and conduction bands. Here, as in the gas ionization chamber, if the dimensions of the detector's active region are consistent with the energy and mass of the particle to be detected, all of the energy of the incident particle appears in the form of electron-hole pairs. Also, the high density of a solid crystal reduces the dimensions of the path length to the order of microns.

The semiconductor counter surpasses the ionization gas chamber in energy resolution and pulse rise time (charge collection time). Since the energy loss per ion pair is 35 eV in air, approximately 10 times as much charge is collected per million electron volts of energy deposited in the semiconductor's active region. As shown below, this is responsible for the better energy resolution of semiconductor counters.

The charge collection time in a solid state ionization chamber is generally of the order of nanoseconds as compared with microseconds for gas-filled chambers. This significant improvement is due to the greater charge carrier mobilities in a semiconductor and the shorter distance for transit.

A typical semiconductor detector is shown in Fig. 1B. A p-n junction is formed by one of many processes that will be described. Selection of the process is dependent upon the ultimately desired characteristics of the detector such as sensitive depth, entrance window, and operating voltage. If the detector is made of high-resistivity p-type base material (residual impurity boron), and phosphorus or lithium diffusion is used to establish a high concentration of an n-type conducting layer on the surface, a p-n junction is formed. When the device is reverse biased a high electric field region of depth X_n on the n side and depth X_p on the p side is established. This high-field region is called either the depletion region or barrier region. The depth of the depletion region on the n side is given by *(13)*

$$X_n = \tfrac{1}{3}(\rho_n V_n)^{1/2} \qquad \text{in the n region (microns)} \tag{1}$$

and the depth of the depletion region on the p side is given by

$$X_p = \tfrac{1}{2}(\rho_p V_p)^{1/2} \qquad \text{in the p region (microns)} \tag{2}$$

where ρ_p and ρ_n are the resistivities (ohm-centimeters) of the p- and n-type layers, respectively, and where V_n and V_p are the potentials in volts across the n and p regions, respectively. The magnitude of resistivity is a measure of the impurity level in the semiconductor material: the higher the purity, the higher the resistivity.

The applied bias, V, is $V = V_n + V_p$. However, because by construction $\rho_p \gg \rho_n$, $V_n \simeq 0$ and $V \simeq V_p$. Thus Eq. 2 gives the effective depth of the depletion region which constitutes the sensitive volume. The high-field region is established because the mobile charges attached to the impurity atoms in both the n and p depletion layers are swept out by the external bias, thus leaving fixed ionized centers behind. Charge conservation requires, however, that $N_nX_n = N_pX_p$, where N_n and N_p are the electron and hole concentration densities in the n- and p-type regions, respectively. It is important to note that Eqs. 1 and 2 apply only to the diffused and surface barrier types of junctions to be described, not to compensated types such as the lithium ion drift devices to be discussed later.

When a charged particle of energy E enters through the thin front n layer and stops in the depletion region, the average number of electron-hole pairs, $\bar{n}$, created by the interaction with the atomic electrons is given by $\bar{n} = E/3.5$ for silicon and $\bar{n} = E/2.94$ in germanium. This lower energy of 3.5 or 2.94 eV to produce one electron-hole pair in a silicon or germanium semiconductor, respectively, is a result of the band structures of electron-hole energy states. Thus, almost 10 times as much charge as in the gas case is available for the same particle energy expended in the chamber. The statistical fluctuations in the actual number of n pairs formed in the depletion region about the average number $\bar{n}$ is $n^{1/2}$ in the case of a Poisson distribution. This means there is a threefold improvement in the energy resolution of the semiconductor detector over the gas chamber, subject to comparable capacitances, leakage current fluctuations, and other noise sources. The secondary electron-hole pairs produced are swept apart by the electric field. If the capacitance of the depletion region is C and no charge losses occur, the average change in potential appearing across the external resistor R is ne/C.

A. Phosphorus Diffused Junction Detectors

Phosphorus diffused junction detectors are characterized by entrance windows of 0.2 to 2.0 microns of silicon, depletion depths of 50 to 500 microns, rugged construction, and good resolution. Their drawback is that unstable surfaces, which result in excessive leakage currents, are directly related to the shallowness of the diffusion layer. Furthermore, the depletion depth is limited by the ohmic resistivity of the available p-type material and the largest potential which may be applied before excessive surface leakage occurs.

The phosphorus diffused detector is fabricated by slicing an ingot of p-type silicon (with the ⟨111⟩ plane parallel to the face of the ingot) into wafers of a thickness determined by the anticipated depletion depth and mounting. The wafers are lapped, polished, and chemically etched to remove all surface damage. The n-type dopant (phosphorus) is diffused into the wafer on all sides in the presence of a dry inert gas. The temperature and duration of the diffusion determine the depth of the n-layer diffusion. Typically, a 900°C diffusion of phosphorus for 10 min produces a diffusion depth of approximately 0.5 microns. The dopant diffused layer is lapped from all faces but one, thus forming an n-p junction. The wafer is etched, contact to the back surface is made by evaporating a p layer of aluminum or a boron alloy, and contact to the front surface is made by a method which is dictated by the mounting procedure. For applications in nuclear medicine a thin aluminum layer may also be evaporated on to the n layer to serve as a light shield and to allow for easy contact.

The long-term stability of the shallow phosphorus diffused detector leaves much room for improvement. Techniques such as oxide passivation of the surface are currently under investigation to aid in controlling the surface leakages that deteriorate the detector characteristics in time. Fortunately for nuclear medicine and biology, the existence of a 1- to 2-micron entrance window is not a limitation and long-term stability can be obtained. Thus in many of the devices to be described later, the basic detector is fabricated utilizing the above techniques.

B. Surface Barrier Detectors

The surface barrier detector is characterized by thin entrance windows (less than 10 mμ of gold), depletion depths of from 50 to 500 microns, excellent energy resolution characteristics for charged particles whose range is consistent with the detector depth, and large areas (4 cm^2 and greater have been fabricated). They suffer from the drawback that their surfaces may not be touched and the maximum depletion depth obtainable is limited by the ohmic resistivity of the available material and the largest potential that may be applied without causing excessive leakage current or noise.

The surface barrier structure (*3, 12, 15*) is a p-n junction formed by the natural formation of a strongly p-type surface on n-type silicon or germanium under normal room ambient conditions. A schematic representation is shown in Fig. 2. The wafers are formed by slicing, lapping, polishing, and chemical etching. The wafers are immediately mounted, after etching, with an epoxy resin into a lavite ring to protect the exposed edges of the junction and also give a means of physical support. The assembly is then exposed to room temperature ambient conditions for several days, thus growing an oxide on the front and back surface. The oxide, by a mechanism which is not well understood, forms a barrier junction with the n-type silicon or germanium. Gold is evaporated on to one face of the wafer forming a p contact and aluminum is evaporated on to the second side forming an n contact. The assembly is again exposed to room temperature ambient conditions for several days until its diode characteristics are stabilized. The wafer and ring are then mounted into a suitable holder with contacts made to the n and p sides for bias voltage and signal connections.

Silicon surface barrier detectors may be operated at room temperature. Germanium surface barrier detectors must be operated at liquid nitrogen temperature.

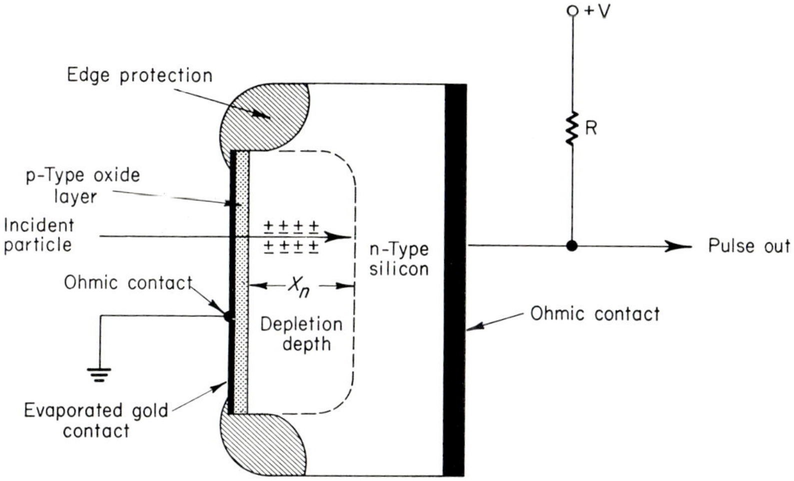

FIG. 2. Schematic representation of the surface barrier detector.

C. Lithium Ion Drift Detectors

The standard lithium ion drift detector is characterized by deep depletion regions of 1- to 10-mm depth, entrance windows of from 1 to 25 microns, and slow response times. It has excellent resolution for β-ray spectroscopy provided the range of the β rays is consistent with the depth of the detector and is large compared with the thickness of the entrance window.

The lithium ion drift process, first introduced by Pell (*21–23*), is the best known approach to obtain deep depletion regions. Here lithium is used as an interstitial n-type donor to compensate low resistivity p-type material so that the effective resistivity is comparable with that of the intrinsic material. The lithium ion drift process has been used in both silicon and germanium. Silicon devices may be used at room temperature and are recommended for charged particle detection and low-energy γ- and X-ray detection. Germanium detectors, which must be operated at liquid nitrogen temperature, have a much higher efficiency for γ- and X-ray detection and offer excellent resolution for γ rays of all energies. The improved sensitivity and resolution of the germanium lithium ion drift detector warrants the inconvenience of the low-temperature operation (*28*).

The fabrication process (*2, 13, 20*) consists of two steps: first, lithium is diffused at about 400°C into one face of a slab of low-resistivity (10 to 100 ohm-cm) p-type silicon or germanium, producing an n-p junction; second, the silicon diode is heated to about 125°C to increase the lithium mobility and is placed under reverse bias. Positively charged lithium ions drift into the depletion region under the influence of the applied electric field, and compensate the negatively charged boron acceptor ions, of the p-type material. This produces a layer of intrinsic material which is the radiation sensitive region of the detector. As the depth of the depletion region increases, the effective drift field strength at the uncompensated boundary decreases. Finally, the drift rate becomes so slow after the first 4–5 mm that as much as 6 to 8 weeks may be required to compensate to depths of 10 mm. After the wafer has been compensated to the desired depth, it is cut to the required size and shape and mounted in a suitable housing.

Such a compensated detector behaves more precisely as a gas-filled ionization chamber, that is, the applied bias serves only to provide a field for rapid collection of the electron-hole pairs produced by the incident radiation. The depth of the depletion region and its capacitance are virtually independent of the applied bias; they are fixed by the drifting depth.

An entrance window, or dead layer of less than 25-micron thickness,

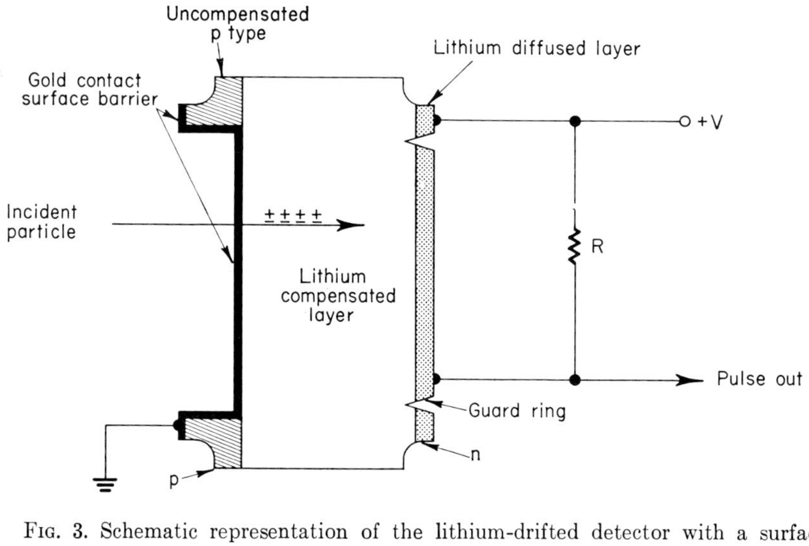

FIG. 3. Schematic representation of the lithium-drifted detector with a surface barrier entrance window and guard ring structure.

is seldom attained at the lithium surface because of the large diffusion constant and the high solubility of lithium in silicon. By extending the depletion region to a thin back contact, particles which enter from the back side may see a thinner entrance window.

In order to remove the entrance window from the lithium ion drift detector, a structure as shown in Fig. 3 is used. Such a detector is called a lithium ion drift detector with surface barrier entrance window and guard ring structure (*27*). It combines most of the excellent features of the deep depletion region detectors and the high-resolution properties of the surface barrier detectors.

The guard ring, long used with gas-filled ionization chambers and proportional counters, helps to carefully define the active region of the detector and to by-pass the leakage current through an external path so that it will not affect the noise level of the system.

In its fabrication the lithium is first drifted into a p-type silicon. Then the guard ring is cut and the uncompensated p-type silicon is removed by physical lapping or grinding. A p-type surface barrier gold contact is applied into the lapped well to supply contact to the exposed intrinsic region.

For charged particles incident on the surface barrier there is a minimum entrance window. The surface leakage effects are effectively reduced by the guard ring structure. This type of detector is capable of providing the best possible energy resolution consistent with a large area and a great depletion depth.

Because of the somewhat lower electric field intensity available in deeply depleted regions and the reduction of hole mobility, owing to increased scattering from the higher impurity concentration in the base material, the effective collection time is somewhat reduced. Therefore, thick lithium ion drift detectors are seldom used where extremely fast rising pulses are required. Low-temperature operation partially obviates this problem.

A high reliability of performance has generally been experienced with lithium ion drift detectors, as they are much less sensitive to ambient conditions than diffused junction and surface barrier types.

D. p-i-n Structure

The p-i-n structure (*31*) shown in Fig. 1C consists of an n-type layer from a lithium or phosphorus diffusion, an i or intrinsic layer from lithium compensation or from available high-resistivity material, and a p-type layer from a boron diffusion or an aluminum evaporation. It may be fabricated either by the lithium drift approach, as described above, or by a double diffusion of phosphorus (n) on one side and boron (p) on the other side of a high-resistivity (intrinsic) silicon wafer. In the first approach, the lithium may be drifted right up to the p layer. Since such p-i-n structure detectors usually have thinner p windows than n windows, they are mounted with the p side exposed to the incident radiation.

Thin wafers of p-i-n structures, 250 microns or less, provide the best possible rise times (< 2 nsec) because the transit distance is small and the high-resistivity silicon can support a very high field intensity, up to 5000 V/mm. They are recommended for recording pulsed radiation fields such as those produced by pulsed X-ray generation, betatrons, and linear accelerators (*18*).

II. DETECTOR PERFORMANCE

The specific characteristics of interest which determine the usefulness of a detector are now discussed.

A. Pulse Output

The average energy required to produce a charge pair in silicon is 3.5 eV. A particle losing 1 MeV of energy creates $10^6 \div 3.5 \simeq 3 \times 10^5$ charge pairs. They in turn give rise to a charge $Q = 3 \times 10^5 \times 1.6 \times 10^{-19} = 5 \times 10^{-14}$ coulombs.

The *output voltage* is $V_0 = Q/C$, where C is the counter capacitance, which is the simple parallel plate capacitance. For a silicon p-n junction, on p-type base material, the capacitance, C, per unit area, is about 10 pF/cm^2 for a 1-mm depletion depth. The output voltage for a 1-cm^2 diode follows as $V_0 = 5 \times 10^{-14} \times 10^{11} = 5$ mV.

With increasing depletion depth, the capacitance decreases (inversely proportional), which results in a higher output voltage. However, the signal-to-noise ratio may not increase for a given detector. It should be noted also that a charge-sensitive preamplifier (*4, 8, 10*) is frequently used in counting applications so that the output signal is nearly independent of the counter and cable capacitance.

The transit time of the slowest carriers in a given type of base material determines the maximum possible *signal rise time* from a given detector. It may be calculated from the transit time of the carriers across the depletion region of thickness X. The rise time is given as $t_r \simeq (X^2/\mu V)$, where μ is the mobility of the majority charge carrier (that is, electrons in n-type material) and V is the applied potential. The mobilities of holes and electrons as majority carriers are 500 and 1450 cm^2/V-sec, respectively, for intrinsic silicon at room temperatures. For a diffused junction a particle counter having a depletion depth of 100 microns with an applied bias of 100 V, for example, one would expect a pulse rise time of about 2 nsec. In a thick, compensated detector of perhaps 5 mm, the rise time would be much longer, approximately 5 μsec.

B. Energy Resolution

The increase in charge pairs produced in silicon compared with that in an ionization chamber for a given energy expended in the medium reduces the statistical fluctuations of change production. If we assume again an energy loss of 1 MeV, producing 3×10^5 charge pairs, their standard deviation is about $(3 \times 10^5)^{1/2}$ or ± 500, giving a percent standard deviation of 0.2. In most practical cases, the limiting factor

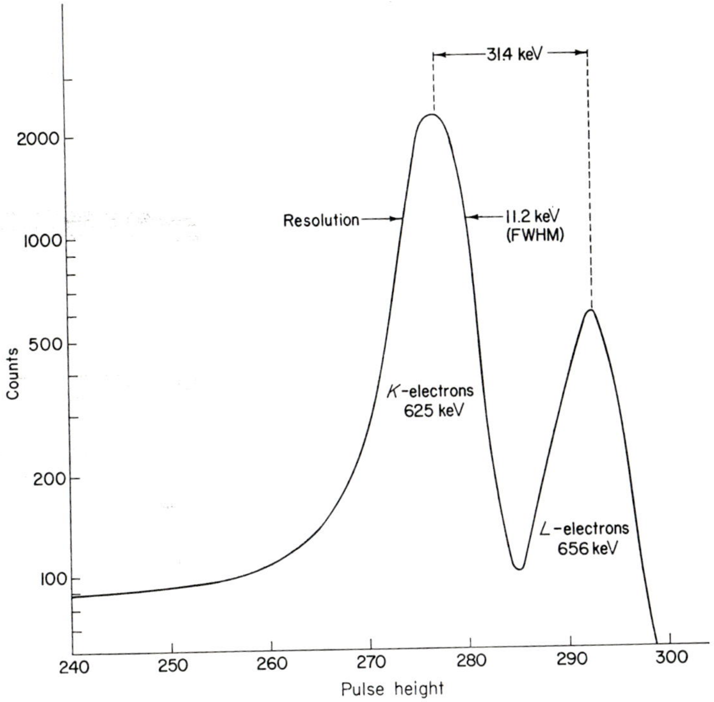

FIG. 4. Spectrum of K and L conversion electrons from ^{137m}Ba, obtained with lithium-drifted silicon detector at room temperature.

for the attainable energy resolution of a solid state detector is the electronic noise associated with the preamplifier which may be 1 keV, full width at half-maximum (FWHM) for a constant energy input.

A lithium ion drift detector, as shown in Fig. 3, and operated at room temperature, was used to obtain the spectrum of the ^{137m}Ba conversion electrons as shown in Fig. 4. The resolution (FWHM) for the 625-keV electrons is 11.2 keV. This is over a factor of 4 better than that which can be obtained routinely for γ rays of corresponding energy absorbed in sodium iodide crystals. The K and L conversion lines are well resolved in Fig. 4 though their energy difference of 31.4 keV is only 5% of their total energy.

The energy resolution for the γ rays of ^{139}Ce, in a 1-mm deep lithium-drifted germanium detector operated at liquid nitrogen temperature, as shown in Fig. 5, is 5.2 keV (FWHM) at 166 keV. The resolution

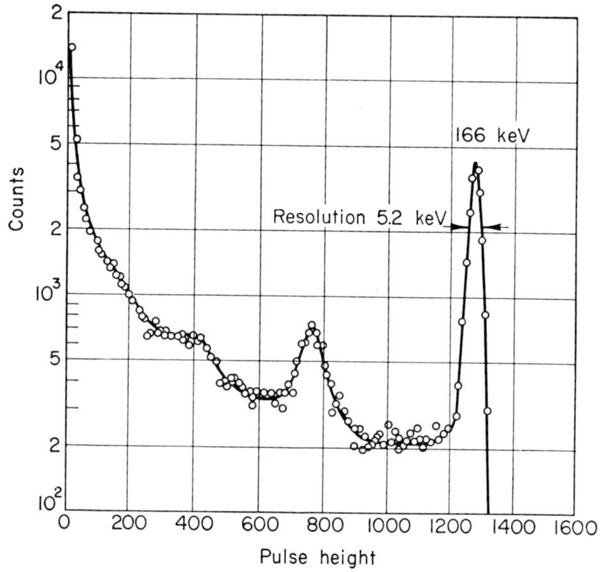

FIG. 5. Spectrum of the ^{139}Ce γ rays (166 keV) obtained with a lithium ion drift germanium detector at liquid nitrogen temperature. (Courtesy of Heath, Cline and Marsh, Phillips Petroleum Co., Idaho Falls, Idaho.)

of a surface barrier detector on silicon at room temperature is shown in Fig. 6 for 6.04-MeV and 6.08-MeV α rays as 16 keV (FWHM). No other types of radiation detectors of equivalent simplicity can achieve nearly as good an energy resolution.

C. Linearity

Unlike scintillators, the semiconductor detector is not sensitive to the specific ionization of the charged particle. Its response is linearly proportional to the energy deposited by nearly all types of particles in the depletion region. Only fission fragments and other very heavy ions have been found to exhibit a slight charge defect (*5, 11*).

The linearity of pulse height for a 1-mm thick detector for electrons, protons, and α particles of various energies is shown in Fig. 7. At energies above 700 keV, 11 MeV, and 55 MeV, the pulse heights for electrons, protons, and α particles, respectively, begin to decrease, because the 1-mm thickness of silicon is just equal to the range of the different particles with the above energies.

D. Sensitive Area and Depletion Depth

Sensitive areas of 1 mm^2 to 6 cm^2 and depletion depths of from 15 microns to 1 cm have been fabricated. The choice of a suitable detector area and depth depends on the application, that is, source-detector geometry, particle type and range, background radiation, count-rate, and

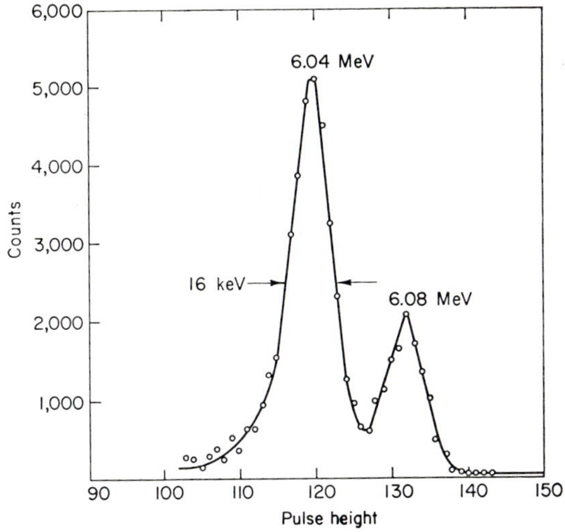

FIG. 6. Spectrum of the ^{212}Pb α rays (6.04 and 6.08 MeV) obtained with a silicon surface barrier detector at room temperature (bias voltage is 50 V).

required energy resolution. Structures of the surface barrier and diffused junction detectors are generally limited to depletion depths of less than 0.5 mm by the upper limits of applied voltage for the available high-resistivity material (Eqs. 1 and 2). For example, an applied potential of 200 V is almost excessive for low leakage current in most devices and 10,000 ohm-cm material is considered to have high resistivity. These parameters produce a 0.5-mm depletion depth in p-type base material. To obtain depletion depths up to 1 cm, one must use the lithium ion drift detectors.

E. Entrance Window

Before reaching the radiation-sensitive depletion area, the incident particles must pass through the entrance window (Figs. 1 and 2). In the case of the p-n junction detector, the surface layer which is heavily doped with a donor impurity to form the n-type region is 0.2- to 2.0-microns thick. The gold oxide layer of the surface barrier detector and the gold contact surface barrier of the lithium ion drift detector can both be made less than 100 $\mu g/cm^2$ aluminum equivalent (*29*). Entrance windows of 0.5 micron present no problem in charged particle spectroscopy except in the case of heavy ions and fission fragments.

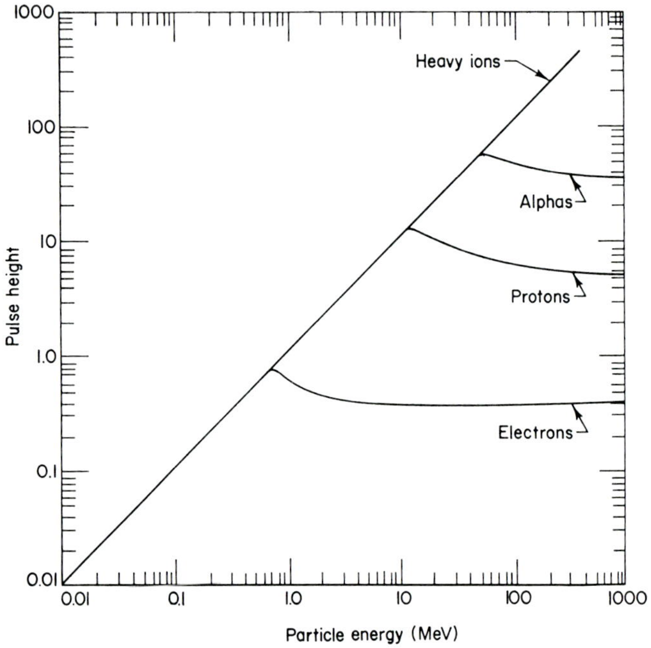

FIG. 7. Linearity of pulse height with energy for particles of different mass for a 1-mm thick detector.

F. γ-Ray Sensitivity

While the detection efficiency for all charged particles is essentially 100%, the low atomic number of silicon and the small sensitive volume of semiconductor detectors result in a very low detection efficiency for γ rays. Since photoelectric absorption is approximately proportional to Z^4, it is greatly increased by using diodes of germanium ($Z = 32$) instead of silicon ($Z = 14$).

Germanium semiconductors are operated with the detectors continually cooled to liquid nitrogen temperature. For germanium detectors the intrinsic photopeak efficiency has been measured (*7*) using γ-ray standards with known disintegration rates. The results are shown in Fig. 8

for γ rays with energies up to 3.0 MeV. The estimated accuracy of the points is $\pm 5\%$. At low energies the efficiency drops off because of absorption in the detector housing and detector entrance window.

Gallium arsenide detectors with atomic numbers comparable with that of germanium have been tried with limited success as γ-ray detectors (*16, 24*). These detectors may be operated at room temperature.

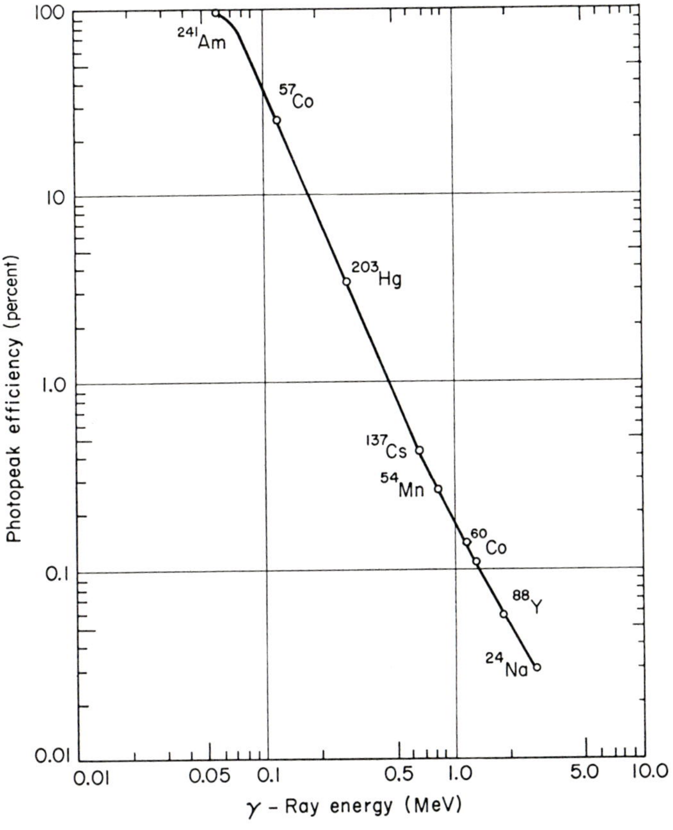

Fig. 8. Intrinsic photopeak efficiency of a germanium detector as a function of γ-ray energy (*7*). The efficiency becomes essentially 100% below 50 keV.

However, the material is not yet sufficiently pure to achieve useful energy resolution.

III. MEDICAL AND BIOLOGICAL APPLICATIONS

Several medical applications until now accomplished with miniature G-M counters, proportional counters, tissue equivalent ionization chambers, and scintillation counters are performed more conveniently and efficiently with semiconductor detectors. New applications can now be developed because of the unique characteristics of these detectors.

A. Brain Probes

Geiger–Müller probes have been used for over a decade for localization of brain tumors. A patient is given an injection of 1 mCi of ^{32}P in the form of sodium phosphate 24 hr before surgery. Because of the degeneration of the blood brain barrier around tumor tissue and the

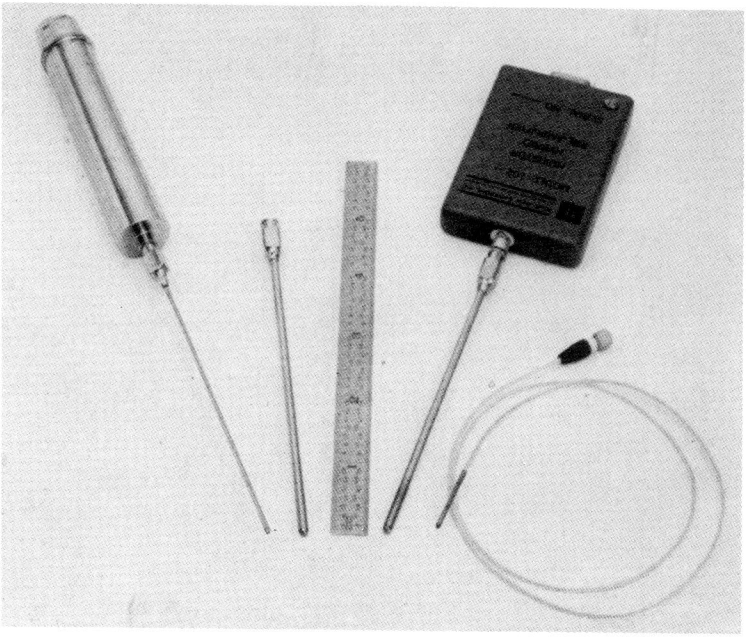

FIG. 9. Semiconductor detectors for *in vivo* tracer work. From left to right, detectors are 1-mm diameter lithium drifted detector, 3-mm diameter lithium drifted detector, 3-mm diameter phosphorus-diffused detector, and 1-mm lithium drifted detector in catheter.

rapid generating rate of tumor cells there exists a large differential uptake of ^{32}P in tumor tissue as compared with normal brain tissue. Thus the tumor may be localized for burr-hole biopsy and possible additional surgery by the insertion of a nuclear radiation detector through a burr hole into the region of interest.

An improved Selverstone–Robinson probe (*25*) has been developed that has a negligible background count rate in nontumor tissue and produces several hundreds of counts per minute in the tumor tissue. The probe shown on the left of Fig. 9 is a silicon lithium drift detector mounted in a 2-mil stainless steel wall tubing of 1-mm diameter. A low-noise charge-sensitive amplifier is mounted in the handle of the needle-like probe. A discriminator ratemeter has been designed and constructed to obtain the highest possible sensitivity from the semiconductor probe consistent with the requirement for simplicity of operation and freedom from spurious counts. The threshold of γ-ray detection is typically above 200 keV energy and the background is less than 2 cpm.

The recording system is contained in a stainless steel housing which is leakproof under normal cleaning procedures. The detector probe and amplifier assembly is capable of gas sterilization. The entire system is self-contained, deriving power for its preamplifier and probe from two 9-V batteries, which have a useful life of at least 20 hr of continuous operation.

B. Gastrointestinal Probes

Gastrointestinal probes are being developed to aid in several types of clinical problems, such as the determination of the intestinal vascular insufficiencies. The method is based upon intravenous administration of ^{32}P and monitoring the appearance of the activity in the intestinal mucosa with a probe located intraluminally. The effective tissue penetration of the ^{32}P β rays permits intraluminal detection of activity only in the volume of the mucosal capillary bed scanned, thus eliminating all background interference. The probe has an *in vivo* background of 0.2 cpm and a sensitivity of 0.5 nCi per milliliter.

In dogs, after an intracaval injection 70–120 nCi (2.5–4.7 nCi/kg) of sodium ^{32}P phosphate, a prompt increase in activity was recorded in 9–14 sec with a peak activity level of 18–250 cpm (*30*). Recession to accumulated residual activity levels of 20–30 cpm occurred within 30–45 sec. After superior mesenteric artery (SMA) flow reduction of 40–60%, appearance of the activity was delayed, peak activity was lower, and prolonged regression slopes of activity indicated reduced and slowed mucosal capillary blood flow.

A "cold" response was readily apparent when the SMA was occluded or a high grade flow reduction (60–80%) was produced. Activity levels accumulated very slowly after superior mesenteric vein ligation, which is consistent with the picture of obstructive hemorrhagic infarction that occurred. Thus, the preliminary results indicate the feasibility of this technique as a diagnostic method in intestinal vascular insufficiency. The final probe is to take the form of a semiconductor detector of 2.5-mm diameter and 12-mm length inserted with a miniaturized preamplifier into the tip of a Miller–Abbott tube.

Intestinal bleeding of unknown origin is a frequent clinical emergency, requiring precise diagnosis in order to institute treatment. Frequently the origin of such bleeding is not evident from radiography or fluoroscopy owing to the pathological changes that may obscure the site. By using labeled red cells with ^{32}P and a gastrointestinal probe capable of traversing the complete intestinal tract, a maximum count-rate is to be anticipated in close proximity to the bleeding site. The necessity for free passage of the detector in the intestinal tract requires that the detector be capable of transmitting its signals through 5 to 25 ft of cable. Satisfactory performance is obtainable with such long cables only by including a one-stage preamplifier at the detector site. In addition, because of the extreme sensitivity requirements set upon the system, extreme care must be used to shield from pickup from normal broadcast stations and other such radio frequency interference. Results to date indicate preliminary feasibility of the method.

C. α-Ray Probes

A proposed method for the treatment of malignant brain tumors consists of loading the tumor with ^{10}B through the differential uptake of the borate ion from general circulation and the bombardment of the tumor with slow neutrons from a nuclear reactor. The resulting nuclear reaction produces α particles of high ionizing power at the site of the ^{10}B concentration. Estimates of the radiation dose due to the α particles are most difficult to obtain. Their range, concentration, and energy are desirable quantities to ascertain to correlate therapeutic results. Determination of these properties has been most difficult because of the effect of the intense γ radiation upon the radiation detector.

A detector and electronic system have been developed which hopefully overcome the obstacles previously encountered. The detector is an exposed shallow diffused p-n junction of low resistivity, thus resulting in a narrow depletion region (100 microns) and nanosecond rise time at low operating potentials. The amplifier has a nanosecond response and is operated in the current mode. Thus the detector may be separated from the amplifier by a cable up to 100 meters in length. The fast rise time and subsequent clipping of the signals prevent pulse pile-up from γ-ray intensities as high as 10^{10} γ rays/cm^2-sec. The noise from the system is in the range of 0.5 MeV, requiring that the α particle deposits at least that amount of energy in the detector to be counted.

D. Circulation Probes

The diagnosis of congenital anomalies of the circulatory system is greatly facilitated by the use of intracardiac catheterization procedures.

In the detection of such anomalies the ability to observe the transport of a bolus of radioactive material through the various parts of the circulatory system would greatly simplify the procedure, which currently involves the withdrawal and analysis of a series of samples. The delays and dilutions associated with such withdrawal samples render the accuracy of measurement marginal. On the right of Fig. 9 a lithium ion drift detector which has been mounted at the tip of a standard intracardiac catheter is shown. Difficulties in noise levels due to the large capacitance of the cable have obscured positive results. Improvements in cable construction and further miniaturizing of preamplifiers will shortly lead to operational models. Since the bolus of radioactive material is relatively undiluted, small radioisotope dosages should be suitable even with very small detectors.

E. Dosimetry

1. Dose and Dose-Rate

There are three basic types of signals which may be utilized from a semiconductor detector to obtain dose and dose-rate information. The first type is the ordinary pulse signal produced by individual particles or the interaction products of single photons in the silicon. The amount of charge collected, as shown above, in each of the pulses is proportional to the energy deposited in the active region of the device for each interaction. These pulses are generally amplified by means of low-noise, charge-sensitive preamplifiers, which produce an output signal that is independent of bias voltage or detector capacitance.

The second type of signal that can be obtained from the detector is an open-circuit voltage (*1*) given by the relationship

$$V_0 = (2kT/e)\ln(K_1 D)$$

where V_0 is the open-circuit voltage, k the Boltzmann constant, e the electronic charge, T the absolute temperature, K_1 a constant of the detector, and D the dose-rate.

The third type of signal is the short-circuit current

$$I_s = K_2 D$$

where K_2 is a constant of the detector.

The open-circuit voltage is essentially logarithmic with dose-rate while the short-circuit current is linear. In any actual situation, the diode is operated in an intermediate region between these two extremes, since any current through the detector requires some voltage drop and any voltage drop across the detector requires some current flow.

Each of the detectors shown in Fig. 9 may be used for dose and dose-rate measurements. If the pulse counting method is utilized, it is necessary to keep the detector-amplifier cable short. For open-circuit voltage and short-circuit current measurements, the detector leads may be many feet in length.

2. Dynamic Range and Sensitivity

When the semiconductor detector is used in the pulse counting mode, radiation fields of 10 rad/hr may be measured. The upper limit is determined by the pulse pair resolution of the counting equipment. The count-rate corresponding to a fixed dose-rate for γ-ray energies from 70 keV to 1.4 MeV has been determined using diffused detectors (*17*). The variation was found to be less than 50% for all energies above 100 keV, while larger variations occur at lower energies.

The open-circuit voltage measured in a γ-ray field was found to be logarithmic for dose-rates from 10^{-2} to 400 rad/min, and the signal continued to increase with dose-rate up to at least 5000 rad/min (*1*). Using a 2-mm diameter by 1-mm long lithium ion drift detector enabled measurement of the dose-rate in the rectum of a patient receiving ^{60}Co therapy. A reading of 2.7 mV corresponding to a dose-rate of 41 rad/min was obtained. The results were reproducible and stable, despite the use of a 30-ft cable between the detector and the microvoltmeter in the presence of a high-level electric noise background. The readings were quite stable even at the level of a few microvolts during calibration with ^{60}Co and radium γ rays.

When the semiconductor detector is used in the mode of short-circuit current measurement, the minimum dose-rate sensitivity is set by the stability of the detector leakage current. In practice, a field of 10^{-3} rad/min is the lower limit. For all practical purposes, even in the case of intense fields from accelerator beams, no upper limit of sensitivity has been found (*31*).

Dose information may be obtained from the pulse counting method and the short-circuit current method by integrating the detector charge for the period of interest. In the pulse counting method only pulses above a given threshold are permitted to contribute charge to the integrating circuitry. In the short-circuit current method a null current is obtained in the absence of a nuclear field by utilizing suitable balanced bridge circuitry (*1*).

REFERENCES

1. Baily, N. A., and Norman, A., Miniature p-i-n junctions for *in vivo* dosimetry. *Nucleonics* **21**, No. 10, 64 (1963).
2. Blankenship, J. L., and Borkowski, C. J., Improved techniques for making p^{+}-i-n^{+} diode detectors. *IRE, Trans. Nucl. Sci.* **9**, No. 3, 181 (1962).

3. Blankenship, J. L., and Borkowski, C. J., Performance of silicon surface barrier detectors with charge sensitive amplifiers. *IRE, Trans. Nucl. Sci.* **8,** No. 1, 17 (1961).
4. Blankenship, J. L., Design of low-noise vacuum-tube pulse amplifiers for semiconductor radiation-detector spectroscopy. *IEEE Trans. Nucl. Sci.* **11,** No. 3, 373 (1964).
5. Britt, H. C., and Wegner, H. E., Multiplication phenomenon for fission fragment response in semiconductor detectors. *Rev. Sci. Instr.* **34,** 627 (1963).
6. Brown, W. L., Introduction to semiconductor particle detectors. *IRE, Trans. Nucl. Sci.* **8,** No. 1, 2 (1961).
7. Camp, D. C., and Armantrout, G. A., Lithium-drifted germanium detectors for high-resolution β- and γ-ray spectroscopy. UCRL-12245. Univ. Calif. Radiation Lab. Rept. (1965).
8. Chase, R. L., Higinbotham, W. A., and Miller, G. L., Amplifiers for use with p-n junction radiation detectors. *IRE, Trans. Nucl. Sci.* **8,** No. 1, 147 (1961).
9. Dearnaley, G., and Northrop, D. C., "Semiconductor Counters for Nuclear Radiations," 2nd ed. Wiley, New York, 1966.
10. Fairstein, E., Considerations in the design of pulse amplifiers for use with solid state radiation detectors. *IRE, Trans. Nucl. Sci.* **8,** No. 1, 129 (1961).
11. Flicker, H., Response of semiconductor detectors to fission fragments. *Rev. Sci. Instr.* **34,** 822 (1963).
12. Fox, R. J., and Borkowski, C. J., Silicon surface barrier detectors with high reverse breakdown voltages. *IRE, Trans. Nucl. Sci.* **9,** No. 3, 213 (1962).
13. Friedland, S. S., Katzenstein, H. S., and Ziemba, F. P., Advances in semiconductor detectors for charged particle space spectrometry. *IEEE, Trans. Nucl. Sci.* **10,** No. 1, 190 (1963).
14. Friedland, S. S., and Ziemba, F. P., Special detectors. *In* "Methods of Experimental Physics" (L. C. L. Yuan and C.-S. Wu, eds.), Vol. 5, Pt. A, p. 265. Academic Press, New York, 1961.
15. Hansen, N. J., Encapsulated surface barrier particle detectors, some methods and techniques. *IRE, Trans. Nucl. Sci.* **9,** No. 3, 217 (1962).
16. Harding, W. R., Hilsum, C., Moncaster, M. E., Northrup, D. C., and Simpson, O., Gallium arsenide for gamma-ray spectroscopy. *Nature* **187,** 405 (1960).
17. Jones, A. R., The measurement of gamma dose with silicon junction counters. *IRE, Trans. Nucl. Sci.* **9,** No. 5, 17 (1962).
18. Kuckuck, R. W., Bernescut, R., Zatzick, M. R., and Jupiter, C. P., Response function and sensitivity of double-diffused silicon detectors in high γ-dose rate fields. *IEEE, Trans. Nucl. Sci.* **13,** No. 1, 111 (1966).
19. Miller, G. L., Gibson, W. M., and Donovan, P. F., Semiconductor particle detectors. *Ann. Rev. Nucl. Sci.* **12,** 189 (1962).
20. Miller, G. L., Pate, B. D., and Wagner, S., Production of thick semiconductor radiation detectors by lithium drifting. *IEEE, Trans. Nucl. Sci.* **10,** No. 1, 220 (1963).
21. Pell, E. M., Ion drift in an n-p junction. *J. Appl. Phys.* **31,** 291 (1960).
22. Pell, E. M., Study of Li-O interaction in Si by ion drift. *J. Appl. Phys.* **32,** 1048 (1961).
23. Pell, E. M., The ion drift process. *In* "Semiconductor Nuclear Particle Detectors," Publ. No. 871, p. 136. Natl. Acad. Sci.—Natl. Res. Council, Washington, D.C., 1961.
24. Rediker, R. H., GaAs diodes. *In* "Semiconductor Nuclear Particle Detectors," Publ. No. 871, p. 164. Natl. Acad. Sci.—Natl. Res. Council, Washington, D.C., 1961.

25. Selverston, B., Sweet, W. H., and Robinson, C. V., Clinical use of radioactive phosphorus in surgery of brain tumors. *Ann. Surg.* **130,** 643 (1949).
26. Taylor, J. M., "Semiconductor Particle Detectors," Butterworths, London, 1963.
27. Wang, L., Zatzick, M. R., and Ziemba, F. P., A lithium-drifted silicon surface barrier detector with guard ring. *IEEE, Trans. Nucl. Sci.* **11,** No. 1, 314 (1964).
28. Webb, P. P., and Williams, R. L., Gamma ray spectroscopy using a germanium lithium-drifted diode. *Nucl. Instr. Methods* **22,** 361 (1963).
29. Williams, R. L., and Webb, P. P., The window thickness of diffused junction detectors. *IRE, Trans. Nucl. Sci.* **9,** No. 3, 160 (1962).
30. Wright, W., Radioisotopic determination of intestinal vascular insufficiency. *Clin. Res.* **12,** 289 (1964).
31. Ziemba, F. P., Pelt, G., Ryan, G., Wang, L., and Alexander, R., Properties of an n^+-i-p^+ semiconductor detector. *IRE, Trans. Nucl. Sci.* **9,** No. 3, 155 (1962).

CHAPTER 6

SODIUM IODIDE SCINTILLATORS

GERALD J. HINE
INTERNATIONAL ATOMIC ENERGY AGENCY
VIENNA, AUSTRIA

The usefulness of thallium-activated sodium iodide crystals—NaI(Tl)—as γ-ray detectors is based on a combination of several of their advantageous physical properties. Sodium iodide has a density of 3.67 gm cm^{-3}, and the high atomic number of iodine ($Z = 53$) makes it a very effective absorber for low- and medium-energy γ rays. Sodium iodide crystals are now available in sizes up to 11 or 12 inches in diameter. Finally, though the resolution of the photoelectric lines of NaI(Tl) is only moderate compared with those of semiconductor detectors (Chapter 5), sodium iodide is the most widely used detector for γ-ray spectroscopy.

The scintillation properties of sodium iodide crystals have been extensively investigated. Some of their characteristics will be described briefly; for more details the reader is referred to recent editions of five books dealing with the subject (*1, 2, 7, 9, 10*).

I. SCINTILLATION CHARACTERISTICS

A. Light Output

Pure sodium iodide crystals, without thallium activator, do not scintillate at room temperature. However, they are efficient scintillators at liquid-nitrogen temperature, because the sodium iodide crystal lattice proper becomes luminescent at very low temperatures.

The incorporation of crystal imperfections, such as impurity atoms, produces luminescent centers which can be excited by ionizing radiation even at room temperature. These impurities are known as activators. A thallium concentration of 0.1 to 0.4 mole percent serves as activator for sodium iodide crystals.

Direct excitation of the luminescent centers by γ rays is not possible. When a γ ray is absorbed in the sodium iodide crystal, its energy, or a fraction of it, is transferred to a secondary electron (Section III). These high-energy electrons lose their energy mainly by ionization. Only a fraction of their energy gives rise to luminescence, while most of it is lost as heat. For a 1×1 inch NaI(Tl) crystal, the absolute luminescence efficiency for ^{137}Cs γ rays was measured as 13% (*12*). In general, only a fraction of the luminescent light can actually be collected.

The number of luminescence quanta produced by an electron is proportional to its energy loss in the scintillator. About 20–30 photons are produced per 1 keV of energy loss. At low electron energies the efficiency of light quanta production is reduced because of the high ion density at the end of an electron track (*5, 13*). Otherwise, the luminescence intensity is a unique measure of the energy of a γ ray that is totally absorbed in the scintillator (Section IV).

The luminescent radiation shows a *spectral distribution* with a maximum at 420 mμ at room temperature (Fig. 1). This matches closely the spectral sensitivity of type S-11 photocathodes used for all common multiplier phototubes (Fig. 1). About 7–10 photons are required for the release of one photoelectron from the photocathode. Therefore, in order to produce a pulse with a magnitude distinctly above the noise level of the multiplier phototube, the secondary electron must have an energy of a few keV.

For several applications, such as coincidence counting (Chapter 18), the *decay time* of the luminescent light is of importance. To a first approximation, the number of light quanta emitted after the passage of an ionizing particle can be represented by a simple exponential function of time. The time interval required for the emission of 67% of the photons is referred to as the decay time, which in the case of NaI(Tl) is 0.25 μsec. However, a fraction of the total light from a sodium iodide crystal is emitted with a much longer decay time of 1.5 μsec (*8*). This makes sodium iodide a very slow scintillator compared with organic scintillators, which are of the order of 100 times faster.

The light emission of sodium iodide crystals diminishes linearly with increasing *temperature*. Between 0° and 270°C an average temperature coefficient of 0.12% per degree Centigrade has been observed. There-

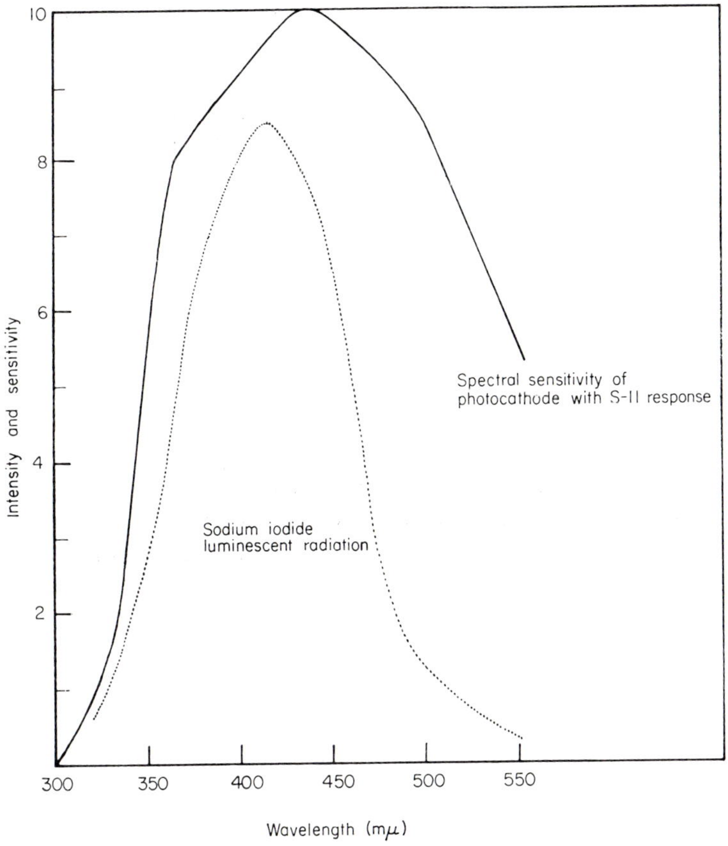

FIG. 1. Spectral distribution of luminescent radiation and photocathode response.

fore, a 10°C change in room temperature causes more than a 1% change in light output (pulse height).

B. Light Collection

The atomic structure of the thallium activated sodium iodide crystal determines the intrinsic scintillation characteristics described above. The collection of the induced luminescent light and its transmission to the multiplier photocathode is highly dependent on the crystal preparation.

Sodium iodide is highly hygroscopic and, on exposure to a humid atmosphere, it shows a yellow surface discoloration, which is probably due to free iodine. Crystals used as scintillators should be transparent and free from discolorations. It is therefore important to prepare the crystal in a moisture-free atmosphere and also to keep it permanently in such an environment during its use as a radiation detector.

For this purpose the crystal is encased in a metal container which is hermetically sealed by an optical window (Chapter 12, Fig. 1). The container, which is frequently made of $\frac{1}{32}$-inch thick aluminum, protects the crystal also from ambient light. This is of great importance since even a minute amount of light reaching the multiplier photocathode from the outside would produce an extremely high noise level.

Instead of the crystal container being sealed by a glass window, the sodium iodide crystal is frequently mounted directly on the multiplier phototube. The aluminum container is then extended from the crystal to the base of the phototube. This type of integral mounting of crystal and multiplier phototube has several advantages. The elimination of the window enhances the light collection since two reflecting surfaces (the front and back of the window) have been eliminated. Furthermore, the crystal and phototube form now a mechanically stable unit. A single seal between container and base of the multiplier phototube protects the unit against the outside atmosphere and ambient light at the same time. However, the manufacturing costs of these *integral units* are greater than those for the sealed crystal and the phototube as two separate entities.

The fraction of the light originating in the scintillator which ultimately reaches the photocathode of the multiplier phototube depends on the transparency of the optical system and its light collection efficiency. Monocrystalline sodium iodide has practically unit optical transparency for its own luminescent radiation. However, since sodium iodide has a high index of refraction (1.85), the light collection is very much affected by the nature of the crystal surface. In general, specular reflection at the surface is avoided since it can cause the trapping of some of the light in the scintillator. Diffuse reflection yields a greater and more uniform light output than specular reflection. Therefore, all surfaces of the sodium iodide crystal with the exception of the light-exit face are roughened with emery paper to obtain a diffuse surface. As a reflector, α-aluminum oxide or magnesium oxide powder is packed in a $\frac{1}{16}$-inch thick layer between the crystal surface and the encasing container. Both Al_2O_3 and MgO are excellent reflectors for light with wavelengths greater than 350 mμ. They absorb moisture easily and must therefore be kept thoroughly dry.

Finally, it is necessary to ensure good optical contact between the various polished interfaces of crystal, container window, and multiplier phototube. For sodium iodide, with a spectral distribution of the luminescent light as shown in Fig. 1, the refractive index of a highly viscous silicone compound such as Dow Corning QC-2-0057 makes it a suitable coupling agent. A thin layer of it between each interface minimizes light losses by reflection.

II. GROWTH OF SINGLE NaI(TL) CRYSTALS

In order to achieve maximum density, high optical transparency, and uniform activation, it is necessary to prepare the sodium iodide scintillator in a monocrystalline form. Frequently, the user is disturbed by the high cost of sodium iodide crystals, which if not carefully handled, are easily destroyed either by mechanical or thermal shock. Some acquaintance with the manufacturing process may yield a better understanding of the problems of procuring the scintillator.

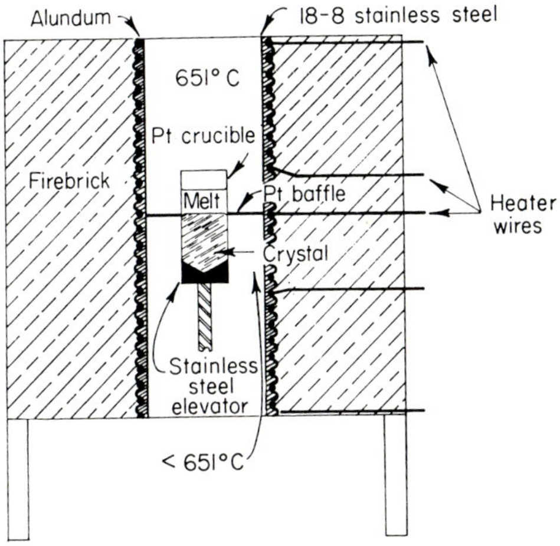

FIG. 2. Double furnace used for growing NaI(Tl) crystals by the gradient technique (*11*).

The chemical purity of the raw material is of greatest importance. It should be free of potassium which contains radioactive ^{40}K. A major effort and considerable cost are involved in obtaining sodium iodide of highest purity.

Single sodium iodide crystals are grown from the molten state. The anhydrous material is supercooled in a vacuum or inert atmosphere in a way which induces crystallization. One of two methods is generally used for crystal growing. They are known as gradient and pulling techniques.

A. The Gradient Technique

A cross section of a double furnace utilized by the gradient technique is shown in Fig. 2. The upper chamber is maintained at a temperature above the melting point of sodium iodide (651°C) while the lower half is held by its separate heater slightly below the melting point. The two halves of the furnace are separated by a platinum baffle so that a sharp temperature gradient occurs in passing through the region of the baffle. The molten salt is contained in a chemically compatible vessel (platinum crucible), which is slowly lowered through the temperature gradient within the furnace. As the tip of the conical vessel reaches the lower chamber, random nucleation of a single-crystal seed occurs. The crystal continues to grow in size with further lowering of the vessel. A typical speed is of the order of 1 inch per day.

The speed of crystal growth must be proportional to the heat conductivity of the particular material being grown. The crystal front can advance steadily only when a constant heat loss through the already formed crystal mass is maintained. With larger-diameter crystals this becomes a very difficult problem, which at present limits the crystal size to 16 inches in diameter.

Thallium iodide is added to the melt as activating impurity (Section I,A). At the melting point of sodium iodide it is toxic and volatile. This may cause an uneven distribution of the activator in the crystal owing to differences in the equilibrium concentrations in the solid and liquid phases. However, with high growth-rates or low temperature gradients in the crystallization zone, an almost homogeneous impurity distribution may be achieved.

Crystal growth defects are introduced not only by an inhomogeneous distribution of the activator, but also by the constraining effect of the growing vessel. Sticking of the crystal to the walls of the growing vessel results in a strained crystal lattice along the peripheral part of the crystal. An internal temperature gradient during the growth process may cause a further straining of the crystal mass along its growing axis.

After the crystal is grown, it has to be released from the growing vessel by careful melting of the outer layer. Afterward proper annealing and heat treatment of the crystal are important. Intense recrystallization is caused by annealing for 2–3 hr at a temperature 5°–10°C below the melting point. If this is followed by cooling through 400°–450°C over 15–20 hr, with a final cooling to room temperature over 10–15 hr, an appreciable increase in light output and in pulse-height resolution is achieved.

High-quality NaI(Tl) crystals with specified scintillation characteristics are presently produced on a large scale. It is no mean technological achievement to grow single crystals in sizes up to 16 inches in diameter weighing approximately 100 lb by the gradient technique.

B. The Pulling Technique

The molten salt is kept in a stationary crucible at several degrees above its melting point. A seed crystal, fastened to a pullrod which acts as heat sink, is lowered until the seed touches the melt. After a slight melting of the seed, growth is induced either by lowering the melt temperature, or by increasing the heat removal through the heat sink, or both.

The crystal, which grows axially as well as radially at the beginning, is slowly withdrawn from the melt by means of the pullrod after it reaches the desired diameter. It is common to rotate the crystal during its formation, to smooth out any temperature irregularities of the melt and also to insure slight stirring of the melt.

The pulling technique has some definite advantages over the gradient technique. No melt-out from the growing vessel is required since the crystal remains free of the vessel during growth and therefore its lattice should be less strained. The temperature gradient can be controlled much better and kept sharper, resulting in faster growth-rates. However, the techniques may produce sodium iodide crystals with inferior scintillation efficiency. An inhomogeneous activator distribution and crystal defects are likely to occur, caused by gravity distortion during the crystal pulling. The operator must continuously control several growth parameters and much is left to his skill and experience for the successful conclusion of a fully grown crystal. Nevertheless, several companies successfully use this technique for growing sodium iodide crystals up to 5 inches in diameter and up to approximately 15 lb in weight.

III. SODIUM IODIDE AS A γ-RAY DETECTOR

Discussing the use of NaI(Tl) crystals as γ-ray detectors only should not imply that they are insensitive to other types of radiation. Electrons or β rays with energies above 0.6–0.8 MeV can enter the crystal proper and produce pulses according to their energy just as the secondary electrons which are produced by γ rays within the crystal. However, for the needs of β-ray counting more convenient detectors have been developed (Chapters 4 and 5). These β-ray detectors may count up to 1% of the impinging γ rays and are therefore also γ-ray counters. But sodium iodide crystals are much more suitable γ-ray detectors since they commonly afford counting efficiencies in the range of 50–100%.

A. Counting Efficiency

For a γ ray to be counted, it must be absorbed in the scintillator by one of the three absorption processes: photoelectric effect, Compton scattering, or pair production. In each case a secondary electron is produced. The fraction of the γ-ray energy transferred to the secondary electron depends upon the specific absorption process. As mentioned above, the secondary electron will produce luminescent light in proportion to its energy. Finally, the scintillator light is converted into an electric pulse, which is amplified by the multiplier phototube (Fig. 3).

In the case of *photoelectric absorption,* the incident γ ray transfers all its energy to the secondary electron, except for about 29 keV, which is the binding energy of a K-electron of iodine. Because of the high atomic number of iodine ($Z = 53$), photoelectric absorption is most

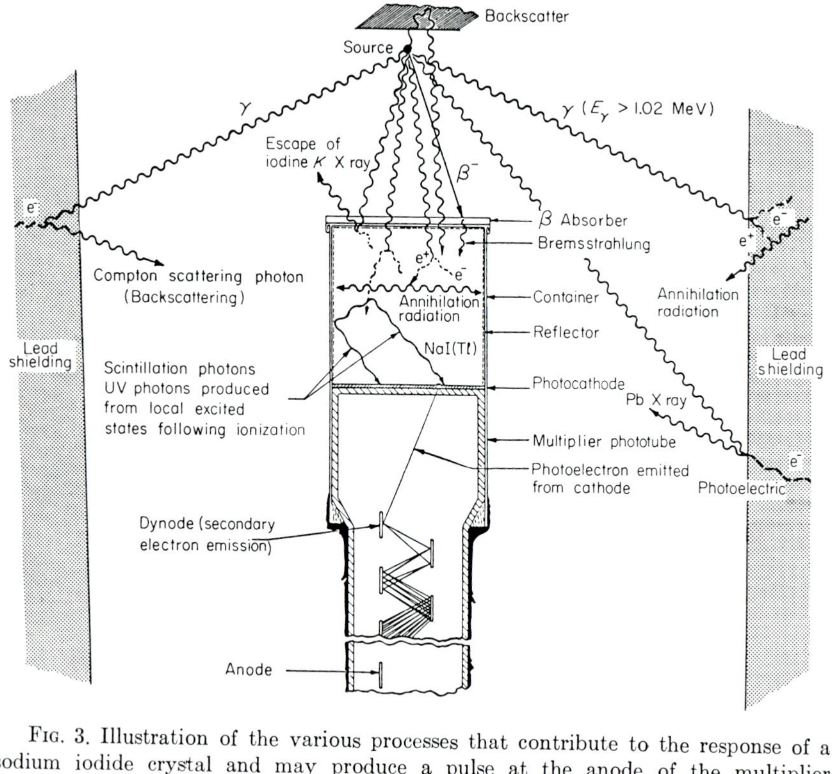

FIG. 3. Illustration of the various processes that contribute to the response of a sodium iodide crystal and may produce a pulse at the anode of the multiplier phototube (*3*).

likely to occur in one of its inner shells. Since the ejection of a photoelectron is followed by the emission of an X ray, which again is immediately absorbed in the sodium iodide crystal, the full energy of the absorbed γ ray is given to two simultaneously emitted secondary electrons. Only when the photoelectric interaction takes place close to the crystal surface is there a chance for the escape of the iodine X ray (Section IV,C,2).

In the case of *Compton scattering* the incident γ ray imparts only some of its energy to a secondary electron (Section IV,B). The scattered

γ ray will mostly escape from a small iodide crystal; it may be absorbed within the crystal if its energy is low, or if the crystal is fairly large. The result of a series of successive interactions is a single scintillation pulse whose amplitude is proportional to the sum of the energy losses from all interactions.

Pair production is possible only if the incident γ ray has an energy $E_\gamma > 1.02$ MeV, since the rest energy of the newly created electron-positron pair is 1.02 MeV. Therefore, the probability for pair production becomes significant only for very high-energy γ rays (Fig. 4) such as

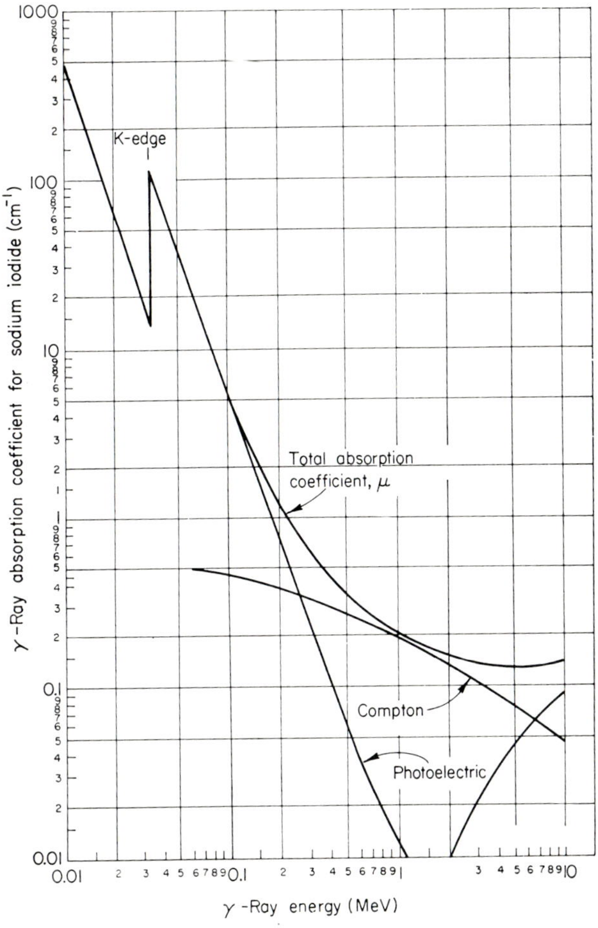

FIG. 4. Linear γ-ray absorption coefficients for sodium iodide as a function of γ-ray energy. The total absorption coefficient, μ, is the sum of photoelectric, Compton, and pair production γ-ray interaction processes.

emitted by ^{24}Na ($E_\gamma = 2.75$ MeV). A scintillation pulse is observed corresponding in amplitude to the kinetic energy of the electron pair. When the positron has lost its kinetic energy, it captures an electron and is annihilated. In this process two annihilation quanta, each with an energy of $E_\gamma = 0.511$ MeV, are emitted in opposite directions (Fig. 3). Only when the two annihilation quanta are totally absorbed within the crystal is a single pulse observed which corresponds in amplitude to the energy of the incident γ ray (Section IV,C,6).

The intrinsic counting *efficiency* of a scintillator for γ rays can be obtained by computing the fraction of the γ rays absorbed in the scintillator. The γ-ray absorption coefficients for sodium iodide versus γ-ray energy are given in Fig. 4. The total absorption coefficient μ is the sum of the three γ-ray interaction processes. If each γ-ray interaction leads to a pulse big enough to be counted, the total absorption coefficient μ can be used for calculating the intrinsic γ-ray counting efficiency.

For a parallel beam of γ rays incident normally on a sodium iodide crystal of thickness d, the intrinsic efficiency, ϵ, is the fraction of γ rays absorbed in the crystal given as

$$\epsilon = 1 - e^{-\mu d}$$

The intrinsic efficiency is practically unity if μd is greater than 2.5. At low γ-ray energies, where μ is large, this requires rather small crystal thicknesses. For γ rays with energies above 1 MeV, μ is less than 0.2 cm^{-1} and therefore only for a crystal thickness of more than 12 cm may total γ-ray absorption be observed. For example, the total absorption coefficient for the ^{60}Co γ rays with a mean energy of 1.25 MeV is $\mu = 0.188$ cm^{-1} (Fig. 4). Therefore, the intrinsic efficiency, ϵ, of a 1-inch thick NaI(Tl) crystal for counting ^{60}Co γ rays incident normally on its surface follows as

$$\epsilon = 1 - e^{-0.188 \times 2.54} = 1 - 0.62 = 0.38$$

This means that a 1-inch thick NaI(Tl) crystal absorbs only 38% of the incident ^{60}Co γ rays and therefore has a 38% counting efficiency (Table I). In practice, the efficiency of the counter will be somewhat less since some of the small pulses are rejected by the discriminator of the counting circuit (Chapter 7, Section III,B).

For a nonparallel beam of γ rays, the intrinsic efficiency depends on the source-to-crystal geometry. It has been calculated for several source-to-crystal distances as well as various crystal diameters and thicknesses, and a number of γ-ray energies *(1, 6, 10)*. The counting efficiency of well-counters is discussed in Chapter 12.

TABLE I
Calculated Intrinsic Efficiencies for NaI(Tl) Crystals for a Parallel Beam of γ Rays

γ-Ray energy (MeV)	Counting efficiency (%) — Height of sodium iodide crystal: 1 inch	2 inches	3 inches	4 inches
0.122	100	100	100	100
0.140	100	100	100	100
0.279	79	96	100	100
0.364	68	90	97	100
0.412	64	87	95	98
0.511	57	81	92	96
0.662	50	75	87	94
0.840	45	70	83	91
1.17	40	63	78	86
1.33	37	60	75	84
2.62	30	51	65	75
2.75	29	50	64	69

B. Photofraction

The three partial absorption coefficients given in Fig. 4 allow an estimate to be made of their relative importance as a function of the γ-ray energy. For γ rays with energies below 200 keV, the absorption is high and is predominantly by photoelectric interaction. Most radioisotopes now in use emit γ rays above 200 keV. They may be absorbed in sodium iodide by either photoelectric or Compton interaction (Fig. 4). In the case of photoelectric (total γ-ray energy) absorption, the scintillation pulses fall within the photopeak region, while in the case of Compton scattering they contribute to the broad Compton distribution at lower energies (Section IV). The intrinsic efficiency, as determined above, is based on counting all pulses in the photopeak as well as in the Compton region. In many instances, however, it is more useful to count the pulses in the photopeak only (Chapter 3, Section III,A).

The photofraction is the ratio of the count-rate in the photopeak region divided by the count-rate over the whole pulse-height spectrum. It approaches unity for low-energy γ rays, decreases with increasing γ-ray energy, and for a given γ-ray energy it increases with crystal size. In large crystals, the scattered γ ray produced by a Compton process has an increased chance of being absorbed by photoelectric interaction. The two processes together yield a single pulse corresponding to the total energy* of the γ ray.

For a parallel beam of γ rays incident on sodium iodide crystals of various sizes, the photofraction is given in Table II for four γ-ray energies. When a γ-ray source is placed at some distance from the crystal, the values for the photofraction are practically the same as for the parallel beam.

The photofractions given in Table II have been plotted in Fig. 5 for right cylindrical crystals of three sizes. This allows an estimate to be made of the photofraction for γ-ray energies up to 3.0 MeV. For example, for the 364-keV γ rays of ^{131}I the photofraction is 0.75 if the γ rays are absorbed in a 2-inch diameter, 2-inch thick NaI(Tl) crystal. In other

TABLE II
CALCULATED PHOTOFRACTIONS FOR NaI(TL) CRYSTALS FOR A PARALLEL BEAM OF γ RAYS (*6*)

Crystal size		γ-Ray energy (MeV)			
Radius (inches)	Height (inches)	0.279	0.662	1.33	2.62
1	1	0.816	0.399	0.233	0.147
1	2	0.855	0.481	0.286	0.199
1	4	0.869	0.530	0.334	0.232
2	2	0.894	0.576	0.385	0.282
2	4	0.913	0.663	0.477	0.361
4	2	0.919	0.631	0.452	0.346
4	4	0.943	0.752	0.592	0.474

words, 75% of the ^{131}I γ rays that are absorbed in this crystal yield pulses which contribute to the photopeak region of the pulse-height spectrum, while the remaining 25% form the continuous Compton distribution.

The photofractions for well-crystals of various sizes are given in Chapter 12, Section I,1,c. Since the wall thickness of most well-crystals is less than 2 inches, the photofractions are correspondingly smaller.

Counting the pulses in the photopeak region, instead of all pulses in the whole spectrum, results in a minor loss in count-rate if the photofraction is fairly large. The background count-rate of even a well-shielded NaI(Tl) crystal is high, especially for larger-size crystals (Chapter 20, Section II,C). Counting only the pulses in the photopeak region reduces the background count-rate considerably, maybe by a fac-

* The photopeak is frequently also called total-energy or total-absorption peak.

tor of 10 or even more. This is of great importance, especially for detecting small amounts of radioactivity (Chapter 3, Section I,B).

Counting the pulses in the photopeak region reduces not only the background count-rate but also other interferences such as back-scattered radiation (Section IV,C) or contributions from other γ-ray emitters than the one of interest. Depending on the counting problem, careful consideration should be given to choosing the pulse-height interval for counting. If the photofraction is small, 0.3 or less, the counting losses in

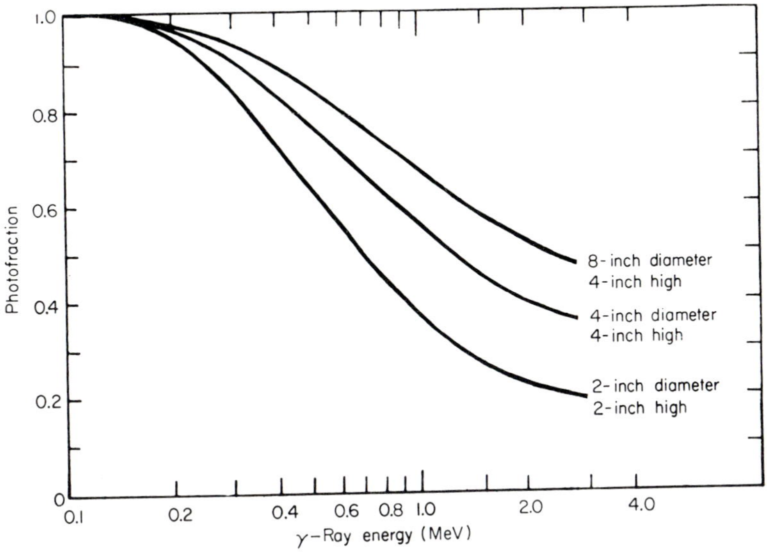

FIG. 5. Photofraction as a function of γ-ray energy for sodium iodide crystals of three sizes (*6*).

general are too severe when only the photopeak is counted. Some radioisotopes emit γ rays with more than one energy. Selecting the photopeak of one of the γ rays only might result in unnecessarily high counting losses, for instance, ^{59}Fe and ^{60}Co both emit two γ rays rather close in energy (Section IV,B).

IV. γ-RAY SPECTROSCOPY

As pointed out above, the energy of γ rays absorbed in sodium iodide crystals can be determined from the pulse height* at the photopeak (Fig. 6). This property has led in recent years to the development of

* The magnitude of a scintillation pulse is called alternatively pulse height or pulse amplitude.

many applications, usually called scintillation spectrometry. With the help of multichannel analyzers (Chapter 7, Section III,D) it is possible to measure the γ-ray spectrum of even low-activity samples or short half-life γ-ray emitters. It is not possible to discuss here all aspects of

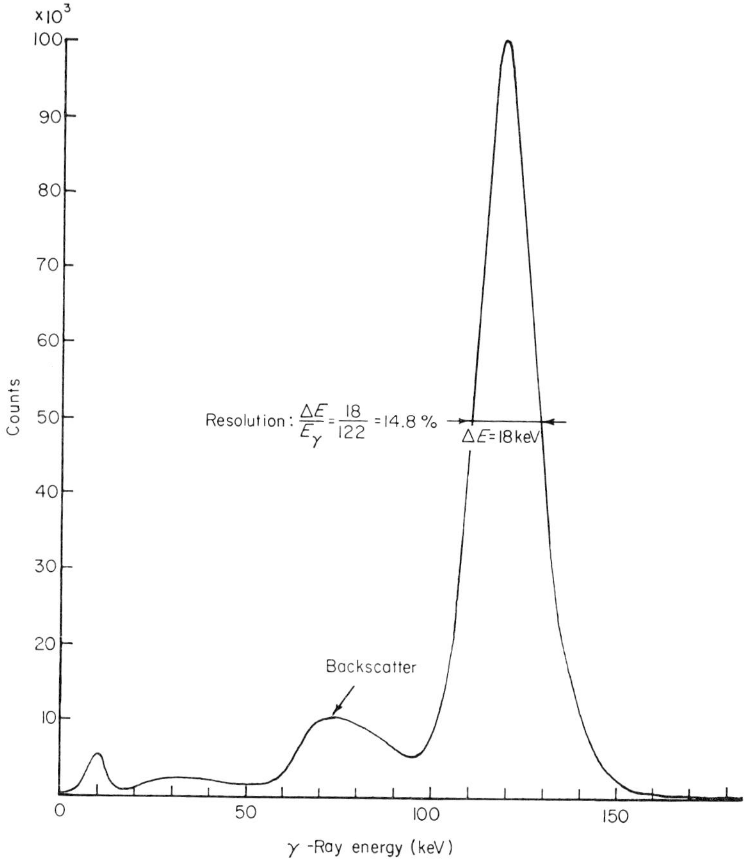

FIG. 6. Pulse-height spectrum of ^{57}Co γ rays (122 keV). The photopeak is predominant in the spectrum of such a low-energy γ-ray emitter.

γ-ray spectroscopy and the reader is referred to the extensive literature on the subject (*9*).

A. Photopeak Resolution

The wide application of γ-ray spectroscopy has been made possible by the availability of large single crystals of NaI(Tl) and the development of end-window multiplier phototubes with high resolution. The resolution of the detection systems is a measure of the extent to which the energy of a γ ray is spread in the photopeak region. The relative *full width* of the photopeak, measured at half the maximum height of the peak (FWHM) is called resolution or line width (Fig. 6). It is usually expressed as a percentage of the pulse height at the maximum of the curve. For the photopeak of ^{57}Co (122 keV) shown in Fig. 6, the resolution follows as $\Delta E/E_\gamma = 18/122 - 0.148$ or 14.8%.

The line width of the photopeak is primarily the result of the statistical fluctuations inherent in each of the multiple transitions which follow the absorption of a γ ray in the NaI(Tl) crystal. Among these are the following:

(1) The production of the luminescent light in the NaI(Tl) crystal by the secondary electron. The conversion efficiency is a function of the ionization density of the secondary electron track (*5, 13*). The light output also depends on the number of secondary electrons accompanying a given γ-ray absorption because of the nonproportional energy response of sodium iodide at low electron energies.

(2) Light collection from the NaI(Tl) crystal. Depending on the size and shape of the crystal, the fraction of the luminescent light reaching the photocathode of the multiplier phototube may vary with the location of the γ-ray absorption within the scintillator.

(3) Photoelectron production in the photocathode of the multiplier phototube. Since about 8 light quanta are required to produce one photoelectron, the statistical variation of the number of photoelectrons reaching the first dynode is the predominant factor.

(4) Electron multiplication within the multiplier phototube. The ratio of secondary electrons released from a dynode to the number of incident electrons is on the average about 4.

(5) Electronic instabilities. The amplifier stages following the multiplier phototube and the pulse-height analyzer may each exhibit minor instrumental instabilities that increase the line width of the recorded photopeak.

All these steps contribute to the statistical variance in the pulse amplitude and affect the resolution of the photopeak. For low-energy γ rays the energy spread in the photopeak is high and therefore the resolution is poor. With increasing γ-ray energy, the resolution of the photopeak improves almost linearly with $(E_\gamma)^{-1/2}$, where E_γ is the energy of the γ ray. For a 3×3 inch sodium iodide crystal, the resolution is shown in Fig. 7 as a function of the γ-ray energy. For simplicity the γ-ray energy is plotted on a logarithmic scale instead of the inverse square root of the energy.

Different γ-ray spectrometers are usually compared on the basis of their resolution for the 662-keV γ rays of ^{137}Cs. Under the best conditions with selected multiplier phototubes a resolution of 7% may be obtained. A resolution of 8–9% can be readily achieved with right cylindrical crystals, while well-crystals exhibit a somewhat poorer resolution because of greater difficulties in light collection.

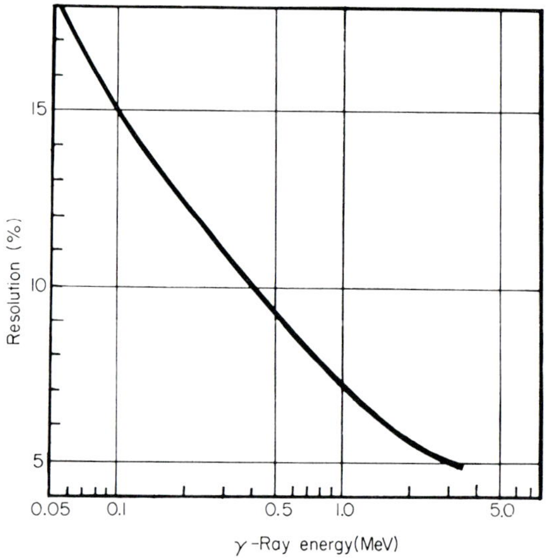

FIG. 7. Photopeak resolution of a 3 × 3 inch sodium iodide crystal as a function of the γ-ray energy (on a logarithmic scale).

B. Compton Distribution

The Compton process is an elastic collision of a γ ray with a loosely bound, essentially free, electron of the absorbing medium. Upon collision, the γ ray loses part of its energy, which is transferred as recoil energy to the electron. The maximum energy, T_{max}, is transferred to the recoil or secondary electron only when it is emitted in the forward direction.

$$T_{max} = \frac{E_\gamma}{1 + 0.511/2E_\gamma} \quad \text{(MeV)}$$

where E_γ (MeV) is the energy of the primary γ ray. Otherwise the secondary electron may have an energy from zero up to the maximum value T_{max}, known as Compton edge, given in Fig. 8 as a function of primary γ-ray energy. At low γ-ray energies, the Compton edge has an energy well below that of the γ ray while with increasing γ-ray energy the Compton edge approaches the energy of the primary γ ray.

The scintillation spectrum of the Compton distribution shows the Compton edge broadened by the resolution of the sodium iodide system (Fig. 9). For γ-ray emitters with energies below 1 MeV the Compton spectrum is well separated from the photopeak, as must be expected from the values for the energy of the Compton edge given in Fig. 8. At higher energies, the photopeak actually appears on top of the tail end of the Compton distribution. This is frequently a distinct disadvantage when

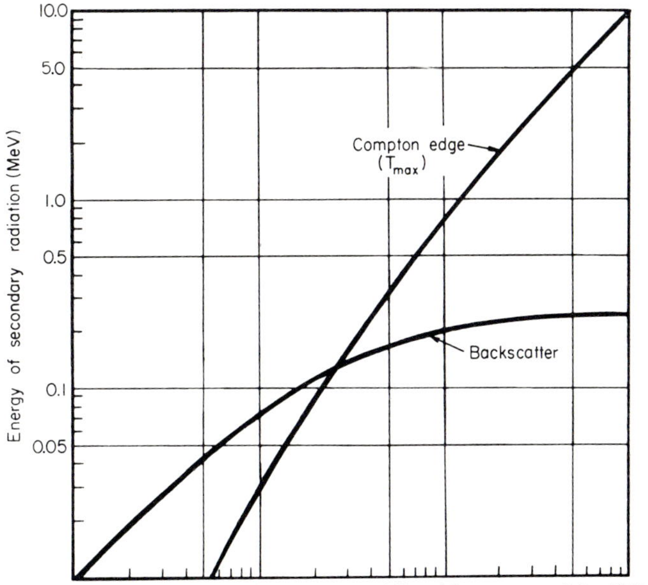

FIG. 8. Compton edge (maximum energy of Compton electrons) and backscatter (energy of 180° scattered radiation) as a function of primary γ-ray energy.

the energy or the count-rate of the photopeak has to be determined accurately.

C. Secondary Peaks

In addition to the spectrum of scintillation pulses due to the interaction of primary γ rays with the sodium iodide crystal the pulse spectrum may also include a number of additional peaks. These maxima in the pulse-height spectrum are produced by secondary effects and

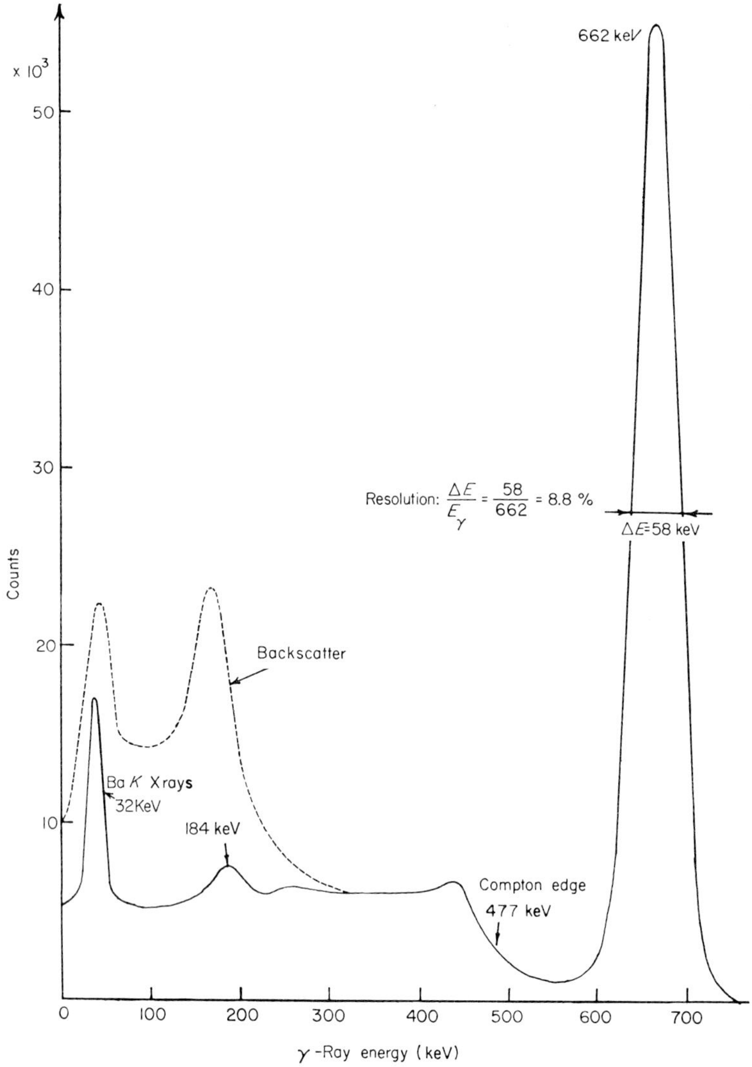

FIG. 9. Pulse-height spectrum of ^{137}Cs γ rays (662 keV). The Compton edge at 477 keV can be recognized though it is broadened by the crystal resolution. The backscatter peak at 184 keV increases when a low atomic number material is placed behind the source.

reflect only indirectly the energy of the radiation emitted by the source. The various processes that may contribute to such secondary peaks are illustrated in Fig. 3.

1. BACKSCATTER PEAK

The γ rays emitted by a source may interact with the matter of the source itself or the materials surrounding either the source or the radiation detector. With each Compton process a secondary γ ray is emitted, the energy of which depends on the angle between the direction of the primary γ ray and that of the scattered radiation. For a source at some distance from the detector, the scattering angle for radiation scattered within the source or its surroundings must be large to reach the detector (*4*). The same applies to γ rays back-scattered from the windows of the NaI(Tl) crystal and the multiplier phototube.

The energy of γ rays scattered at 180° is given as

$$E_{sc} = \frac{E_\gamma}{1 + 2E_\gamma/m_0c^2} = \frac{m_0c^2}{2 + m_0c^2/E_\gamma} = \frac{0.511}{2 + 0.511/E_\gamma} \qquad \text{(MeV)}$$

where E_γ (MeV) is the energy of the primary γ rays. The energy of this so-called backscatter is plotted in Fig. 8 as a function of the primary γ-ray energy according to the formula given above. It may be noticed that for γ rays with energies between 0.3 and 1.5 MeV, the energy of the back-scattered radiation increases only from 0.14 to 0.22 MeV. It falls into a narrow energy interval rather independent of the primary γ-ray energy. Furthermore, for scattering angles between about 140° and 180° the energy of the scattered radiation is practically the same (*4*).

Depending on the counting geometry a larger or smaller amount of backscatter will reach the sodium iodide crystal. Since the energy of the backscatter is low it is absorbed mainly by photoelectric effect (Fig. 4) and therefore a fairly sharp peak appears in the pulse-height spectrum at the energy of the backscatter (Fig. 9). The intensity of this peak can be minimized either by keeping all scattering material far away from the crystal, or by using high atomic number shielding material.

2. IODINE ESCAPE PEAK

The kinetic energy, T_e, of the photoelectron produced by a photoelectric absorption of a γ ray of energy E_γ is given as

$$T_e = E_\gamma - B_e$$

where B_e is the binding energy of the electron. The more tightly bound electrons of the K-shell have the greatest probability of photoelectric interaction and about 80% of the photoelectric processes occur in the K-shell.

The energy of the photoelectron equals that of the γ ray reduced by the binding energy of the electron. This energy subsequently appears as characteristic X rays from filling the vacancy created by the ejection of the electron. Since in sodium iodide practically all photoelectric processes occur in the iodine atom because of its high atomic number, the energy of the X rays is mainly that of the iodine K X rays, which is 29 keV. These low-energy X rays are usually absorbed within the scintillator so that in the photoelectric process the full energy of the incident γ ray is converted into secondary ionizing radiation. Therefore, the photopeak represents the full energy of the γ rays.

Low-energy γ rays such as from ^{197}Hg ($E_\gamma \sim 77$ keV) are absorbed predominantly within a thin layer close to the crystal surface. In these cases, a fraction of the iodine X rays produced with each photoelectric process may escape from the crystal. In addition to the photopeak, a second lower energy peak will then appear, which corresponds to the kinetic energy, T_e, of the photoelectron alone.

3. CHARACTERISTIC X-RAY PEAK

All nuclear γ-ray emissions must compete with the alternate mode of deexcitation of the nucleus known as *internal conversion*. This process can be visualized as a direct coupling of a bound atomic electron and the nuclear field. This results in the ejection of conversion electrons mainly from the K-shell of the atom. The kinetic energy of these electrons equals that of the nuclear transition (which is otherwise the energy of the γ ray), minus their atomic binding energy. Finally, the vacancy in the inner atomic shell will be filled by electrons from the outer shell under emission of the corresponding characteristic X rays.

An example for characteristic X rays following the emission of conversion electrons is the decay of $^{137}\mathrm{Cs} \rightarrow {}^{137\mathrm{m}}\mathrm{Ba}$. The newly formed nucleus is in an excited state in 93% of the disintegrations; of these metastable nuclei 11% decay with the emission of a conversion electron, while 89% decay with the emission of the 661.6-keV γ rays. In the pulse-height spectrum of scintillation pulses from a ^{137}Cs source, the barium K X rays with an energy of 32 keV form a distinct low-energy peak (Fig. 9).

Radioisotopes that decay by orbital electron capture always emit characteristic X rays. After the capture of an electron by the nucleus, there is a vacancy in the inner atomic shell surrounding the newly formed nucleus. Therefore, independent of its γ-ray emission, characteristic X rays are emitted following electron capture (^{51}Cr, ^{55}Fe).

4. LEAD FLUORESCENCE PEAK

Most sodium iodide crystals are surrounded by lead to reduce the background count-rate. In addition, the incident γ rays must frequently pass a lead collimator before they can reach the scintillator. Owing to the high atomic number of lead, the γ rays are absorbed mainly by photoelectric process. Some of the lead K X rays (73 keV) produced by such interactions will escape from the lead absorber. Depending on the counting geometry a fraction of these lead X rays may reach the sodium iodide crystal and produce a peak at 73 keV (Fig. 3).

5. COINCIDENCE SUM PEAK

Several radioisotopes (^{60}Co, ^{24}Na) emit more than one γ ray per disintegration. Some positron emitters, such as ^{22}Na, emit also a γ ray which accompanies the positron annihilation radiation. In all those cases, several γ rays may reach the radiation detector simultaneously. When two γ rays in coincidence are absorbed in the sodium iodide crystal, the total energy of the secondary ionizing radiation appears as a single pulse. In those cases where both γ rays are absorbed photoelectrically, a new high-energy peak appears, which is called the sum peak because it represents the full energy of the sum of the two γ-ray energies.

The intensity of the sum peak depends on the photopeak efficiencies of the crystals as well as on the counting geometry. For a source at some distance from the crystal, the probability that two coincidence γ rays reach the detector is small. For a source in contact with the surface of the NaI(Tl) crystal, the probability is 25%; for a source inside a well-counter the probability is close to 100%. Therefore, sum peaks are observed mainly in spectra recorded with a well-counter or one or two crystals close to the source (Chapter 12, Section I,4). In the case of ^{125}I, where the energies of both the γ ray (35.4 keV) and the X ray in coincidence (27.4 keV) are so low that they are absorbed always photoelectrically, only the sum peak (62.8 keV) will be observed when measured in a well-counter.

6. ANNIHILATION RADIATION PEAK

If the radiation source is a positron emitter annihilation radiation is produced whether the positrons are stopped in the source itself or the matter surrounding it. Therefore, a positron emitter is always a source of 0.511-MeV annihilation radiation which produces a pulse-height spectrum just like a γ ray of that energy. In addition a sum peak may be observed at 1.02 MeV (Section IV,C,5).

High-energy γ rays may be absorbed especially in high atomic number material by the pair production process. This may occur in the lead surrounding the detector or the sodium iodide crystal itself (Fig. 3). In each case, annihilation radiation is produced when the positron comes to rest. The annihilation radiation peak (0.511 MeV) from positron or high-energy γ-ray emitters adds to the complexity of the pulse-height spectrum.

7. β RAYS AND BREMSSTRAHLUNG

As mentioned above (Section III), high-energy β rays may penetrate the container surrounding the crystal and will then be counted. The pulse-height spectrum will not reveal the presence of β rays in the form of a peak, since the β rays have a continuous energy spectrum.

Though the β-ray pulses may not interfere with the analysis of the γ-ray pulse spectrum, they may seriously affect sample counting. When, for example, ^{42}K with a maximum β-ray energy of 3.5 MeV is being counted, the fraction of the β rays that will reach the detector depends upon the sample thickness. If the latter varies between different samples, this may cause a considerable counting error, depending on the sample mass and the fraction of the pulse spectrum used for counting.

When the high-energy β rays are stopped in an absorber, Bremsstrahlung is produced (Fig. 3). It has a continuous photon spectrum with an increasing intensity toward decreasing photon energy. The resulting pulse spectrum may have a peak at low energies because the very low-energy Bremsstrahlung photons are absorbed by the can of the crystal.

REFERENCES

1. Birks, J. B., "The Theory and Practice of Scintillation Counting." Macmillan (Pergamon), New York, 1964.
2. Crouthamel, C. E. (ed.), "Applied Gamma-Ray Spectroscopy." Macmillan (Pergamon), New York, 1960.
3. Heath, R. L., "Scintillation Spectrometry Gamma-Ray Spectrum Catalog," 2nd ed., Vols. I and II, IDO-16880. Phillips Petroleum Co., Atomic Energy Division, Idaho Falls, Idaho, 1964.
4. Hine, G. J., and McCall, R. C., Gamma-ray backscattering. *Nucleonics* **12**, No. 4, 27 (1954).
5. Iredale, P., The effect of the non-proportional response of NaI(Tl) crystals to electrons upon the resolution for γ-rays. *Nucl. Instr. Methods* **11**, 340 (1961).
6. Miller, W. F., Reynolds, J., and Snow, W. J., Efficiencies and photofractions for sodium-iodide crystals. *Rev. Sci. Instr.* **28**, 717 (1957).
7. Price, W. J., "Nuclear Radiation Detection," 2nd ed. McGraw-Hill, New York, 1964.
8. Robertson, J. C., and Lynch, J. G., The luminescent decay of various crystals for particles of different ionization density. *Proc. Phys. Soc.* (*London*) **77**, 751 (1961).

9. Siegbahn, K. (ed.), "Alpha-, Beta- and Gamma-Ray Spectroscopy," 2 vols. North-Holland Publ., Amsterdam, 1965.
10. Snell, A. H. (ed.), "Nuclear Instruments and Their Uses." Wiley, New York (1962).
11. Stockbarger, D. C., The production of large single crystals of lithium fluoride. *Rev. Sci. Instr.* **7,** 133 (1936).
12. Van Sciver, W., Spectrum and decay of NaI. *Nucelonics* **14,** No. 4, 50 (1956).
13. Zerby, C. D., Meyer, A., and Murray, R. B., Intrinsic line broadening in NaI(Tl) gamma-ray spectrometers. *Nucl. Instr. Methods* **12,** 115 (1961).

CHAPTER 7

SYSTEMS FOR DATA ACCUMULATION AND PRESENTATION

ALAN L. ORVIS
SECTION OF BIOPHYSICS
MAYO CLINIC
ROCHESTER, MINNESOTA

I. PREAMPLIFIERS

A. Preamplifiers as Part of the Counting System

The elements that are generally considered to be a part of a counting system are depicted in Fig. 1. Selection of the individual components depends on the type of detector to be used, the complexity of the counting problem, and the mode of data display. The electrical characteristics of each part of the system must be carefully considered in order to avoid mismatching and the resultant distortion of the data.

Several of the elements in Fig. 1 may be combined into one unit in simple systems. For instance, the scaler for a conventional Geiger–Müller (G-M) counter includes elements III, IV, and VII with II and VI being omitted. Scintillation and solid state detectors, however, usually demand a careful consideration of each of these elements and their relationship to each other. Although all of the detector types that will be considered in this chapter produce an output which is in the form of an electrical charge, the characteristics of this output in terms of amplitude, pulse duration, and rise time are quite different for various kinds of

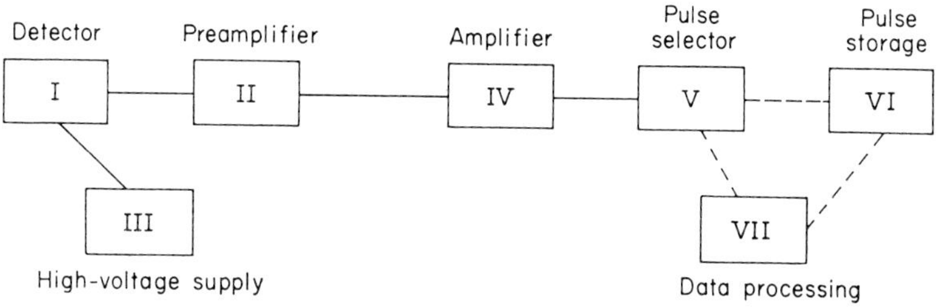

FIG. 1. Block diagram of components constituting a general counting system.

detectors and, in some cases, even for different types of incident radiations. Examples of these differences may be seen in Table I.

TABLE I
OUTPUT CHARACTERISTICS OF VARIOUS DETECTORS

Transducer	Charge (picocoulombs)	Pulse duration (microseconds)
Solid state detector	10^{-3}–10^{-1}	10^{-2}
Proportional counter	10^{-2}– 1	1
Organic scintillator	10^{-2}–10	10^{-2}
Sodium iodide scintillator	10^{-1}–10^{2}	0.25
Organic Geiger–Müller tube	10	50–300
Halogen Geiger–Müller tube	10^{3}	50–300

Radiation transducers are characteristically low-capacitance high-impedance devices. The capacitance introduced by a signal cable running from the radiation detector to the amplifier will in many cases significantly attenuate or distort the transmitted electrical impulse. Preamplifiers placed near the detector will minimize this input capacity and may be designed to provide impedance matching at their output so that cables many feet long may be used.

Preamplifiers are frequently omitted for detectors producing more than 10 pC per pulse when used with signal cables not more than 1 meter long. This situation pertains to most end-window G-M counters and also some NaI(Tl) scintillators when used to measure medium- and high-energy γ-ray emitters in conjunction with high-gain multiplier phototubes.

B. Types of Preamplifiers

The simplest type of preamplifier is called a cathode follower. This widely used device principally provides impedance matching between detector and amplifier, since its gain (ratio of output to input pulse amplitudes) is usually slightly less than one. Figure 2 shows a vacuum tube triode operated as a cathode follower.

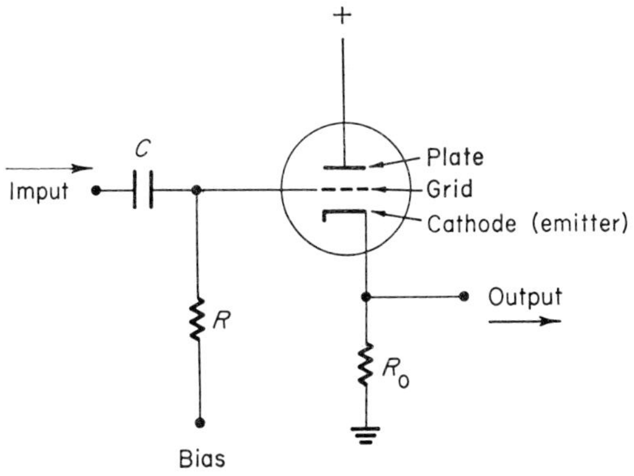

FIG. 2. Cathode follower. Impedance matching for signal transmission. See text for explanation.

The charge pulse produced by the detector as the result of a radiation interaction is impressed upon capacitor C in Fig. 2 and will have an amplitude and duration of the order of magnitude shown in Table I. Resistance R provides a leakage path for this charge and the resultant current flow through R provides an iR drop (or voltage) at the grid of the triode.

The resultant change of the current from the cathode to the plate passing through R_0 constitutes the output pulse. The cathode follower (sometimes called "emitter follower") will drive long cables at its output with little capacitance loading on the input.

The decay characteristics of the pulse are controlled by the values of C and R, which constitute the RC time constant. It should be carefully chosen to provide the proper pulse clipping, which will be considered in more detail in Section II,B. Serious mismatching in a counting system can occur if the preamplifier pulse shape is not compatible with the amplifier requirements. Likewise, components designed for optimum pulse shape for use with liquid or plastic scintillators must sometimes be modified when substituting the slower NaI(Tl) detectors.

The development of *semiconductor detectors* and the rapidly increased use of transistors in electrical circuits have been paralleled by the design and production of many charge- (or current-) sensitive preamplifiers. Semiconductor detectors (Chapter 5) require *charge-sensitive preamplifiers* because their capacitance is a variable function of the applied voltage and other external conditions. The charge collected is not similarly affected, so that pulse-height measurements with a voltage-sensitive device are subject to these capacitive variations.

Transistors are inherently current-sensitive devices, so that completely transistorized counting systems are most naturally current amplifying and current sensitive. More detailed descriptions of transistor function may be found elsewhere (*1, 5, 8, 22*), but in essence a transistor is a sandwich of three layers of semiconductor materials. If the outer layers are conductors of negative charges (n-type material), the center will be a conductor of positive charges (p-type material). The opposite configuration (p-n-p) is also widely used. The three layers are called emitter, base, and collector, respectively. The current flowing in the emitter-base circuit controls an amplified current in the emitter-collector circuit.

Current (and therefore power) gains of over 1000 are possible. The gain is a direct function of total input capacity of the preamplifier and radiation detector. Usually, however, one does not speak of the "gain" of a charge-sensitive preamplifier, but rather of the "charge sensitivity," which refers to the voltage output obtained when a given charge is produced in a high-impedance nuclear detector. Units may be millivolts per picocoulomb, or millivolts per million electron volts in a particular solid state detector (*5*).

Although some charge-sensitive preamplifiers are completely transistorized and others use only vacuum tubes, many are hybrids; that is, one or more vacuum tubes are used in the input, followed by transistors in later stages (*8*). The reason for this is that transistors have an inherently low input impedance, some temperature instability, and noise levels that are too high if good signal-to-preamplifier noise ratios are desired (*2*). Noise levels that are usually due to carrier recombination in the transistor base region are a function of input capacitance (*5*).

One recent development has been the "nuvistor," a small ceramic vacuum tube that is useful in the input stage. "Field-effect" transistors are also being increasingly used for this purpose and are making fully transistorized systems more popular. The field-effect transistor (Fig. 3) consists of a silicon crystal with contacts at each end, one called the "source" and the other the "drain." Contacts at the sides provide potential to the gates, which activate a region of space charge. The flow of current from source to drain is space charge limited and at high impedances the device functions somewhat like a vacuum tube pentode. Noise in a conventional transistor is principally caused by carrier recombination in the base region. The field-effect transistor has no p-n junction so that its noise figure is quite low (*5*).

Systems which require the use of *multiple detectors* or multiple multiplier phototubes, such as some whole-body counters, may have the

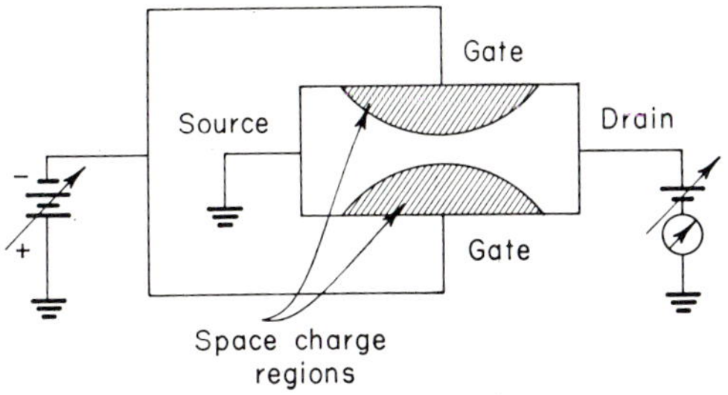

FIG. 3. Field effect transistor. Low noise and space charge limited current flow.

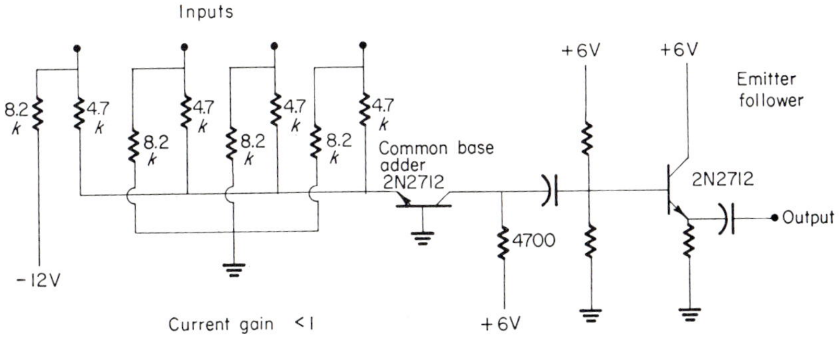

FIG. 4. Summing circuit. Pulses from multiple detectors added and fed to a single output.

several signal outputs connected in parallel to a single amplifier or preamplifier. This paralleling of the intrinsic capacitance of the cables and detector output circuits results in signal attenuation relative to the output of a single detector.

It is sometimes desirable to add detectors or multiplier phototubes without gain changes. This may be achieved by the use of a summing circuit, such as is shown in Fig. 4. The principal transistor is run in the common base mode so that the device is sometimes called a "common base adder." Four signal inputs are shown in the figure; more could be added if necessary. The adder provides a high impedance at each input so that the small impedance from each preamplifier output does not result in a gain change as the different preamplifiers are connected or disconnected. The gain of the circuit is somewhat less than one, depending mainly on the relative values of the input resistors. Scintillation detector pulses are neither significantly distorted nor inverted.

II. AMPLIFIERS

Nuclear pulse amplifiers are used to convert a low-amplitude pulse from a radiation detector (or preamplifier) to one with sufficient amplitude and the proper pulse shape to drive the pulse-selecting elements of the counting system. The amplifier must have enough gain to drive the pulse selector while still enabling the detector to operate in its most favorable operating range. Its gain must be stable against fluctuations in line voltage, ambient temperature, and other factors that might contribute to either long-term drift or transient changes. The amplifier must be relatively insensitive to both pulse amplitude and high count-rate overloads. It should have the proper rise time so that information from the detector is not lost. On the other hand, the rise time may not be so fast that unnecessary noise is introduced into the system.

General purpose amplifiers are available that excel in every aspect of performance. They have front panel controls for adjusting circuit parameters for optimal response in a variety of circumstances. These amplifiers are expensive, and more economical special purpose amplifiers designed with less rigid specifications are usually adequate for sodium iodide scintillation counters. The large volume organic detectors, however, used in whole-body counting (Chapter 21) require the most favorable noise, overload, and gain characteristics.

As with preamplifiers, amplifiers may also be classified as voltage sensitive or charge sensitive. Transistor amplifiers with low input impedance and with negative feedback in the first stage are considered to be charge sensitive. Because of the low input impedance, the associated time constant may be short compared with the decay time of the current pulse from the detector so that pulses are transmitted essentially undistorted into the amplifier. This rapid response reduces the effect of count-rate overload, allowing more intense sources to be analyzed. Preamplifiers may also be eliminated, since even long signal cables may be terminated in their characteristic impedance (*27*).

A. Pulse Shaping

The characteristics of the amplifier system determine the shape of the output pulse that it produces. The shape of a typical pulse may be seen in Fig. 5, where the amplitude, plotted as percentage of the maximum value, is shown as it changes with time. The units of amplitude are arbitrary; they may be output voltage or may represent instantaneous values of output current. The most convenient definitions of *rise time* (T_R) and *decay time* (T_D) are illustrated in the figure. Rise time is defined as the time interval during which the pulse amplitude goes from 10% to 90% of its maximum value. The decay time is taken to be the time necessary for the pulse to fall from maximum to 10% of maximum. Other characteristics that are sometimes of interest are *delay time,* the time required for the pulse to rise to 50% of maximum, and pulse duration. *Pulse duration* does not have an obvious definition for those pulses which decay exponentially, but for practical purposes may be

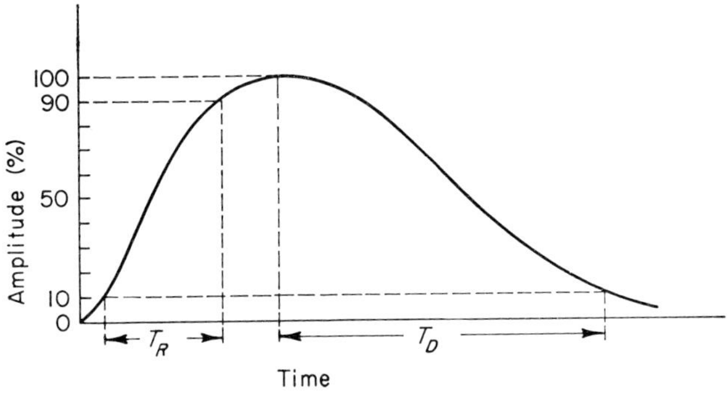

FIG. 5. Pulse shape. Variation of pulse amplitude with time.

measured from the beginning of the pulse to the time when it has decayed to 10% of the maximum.

The output pulse of a radiation detector may be characterized by the charge duration or collection time. The rise time of the amplifier should be somewhat faster than the collection time of the detector. It depends upon the differentiation and integration time constants of the amplifier. A quantitative elaboration of these factors and their interrelationships may be found in Price (*20*).

The detector output pulse consists of an ion group carrying a charge that is not instantaneous but spread out in time. The amplifier must be designed in such a way as to make the output pulse amplitude a true measure of the input pulse charge. A voltage-sensitive amplifier integrates this charge on a small capacitance. However, the pulse must be terminated after the flow of charge has ceased. This time during which charge integration is accomplished is the *pulse width* of the amplifier output, which is determined by the amplifier pulse-shaping circuits.

The pulse width must be chosen so as to integrate all the charge in one pulse but yet not to integrate two individual charge pulses which then would appear to be a larger single event. This *integration time* is a compromise between a long integration time, which would allow accurate accumulation of all ions in a single charge event, and a short integration time, which would prevent pile-up of two or more events.

A charge pulse from a sodium iodide scintillation detector has a decay time constant of approximately 0.25 μsec. This represents the time during which approximately 60% of the photons from the crystal reach the photocathode of the multiplier phototube. Since the number of photons from a single scintillation event may be rather small, it is necessary to integrate over three or four decay time constants in order to obtain a good statistical measure of the energy of the incident γ photon. Therefore, for a sodium iodide detector a good compromise would be a clipping time of 1 μsec.

In order to terminate the pulses and to provide a definite integration time (*clipping time*) a resistor must be placed in the circuit to provide

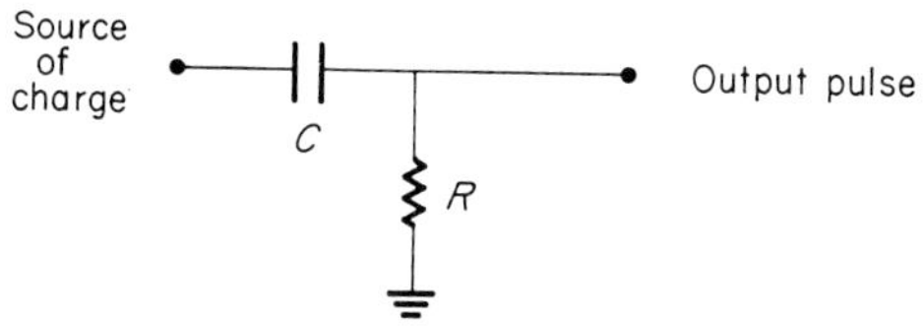

FIG. 6. *RC* clipping.

a path to ground for the accumulated charge. In a voltage-sensitive system this first *RC* clip is usually located at the detector output as shown in Fig. 6. This resistor will discharge the capacitor and the time constant will be given by the product *RC*.

The response time of the system should not be adapted to very high input count-rates by merely reducing the *RC* time constant, since resolution will be drastically reduced when the signal duration is less than the rise time of the detector. If a "slow" sodium iodide detector is to be used at high count-rates, special circuit configurations, to be considered later in this chapter, must be used. Examples where this limitation becomes important in clinical counting are when very large and efficient detectors are used for whole-body counting, or when tracer amounts of ^{132}I are being measured in the presence of therapeutic, millicurie quantities of ^{131}I.

An amplifier with a single *RC* clip (sometimes called singly differentiated) is seldom used because the base line may be depressed at high count-rates. The use of two *RC* circuits (double differentiation) in the amplifier will overcome this and other disadvantages. Double *RC* clipping produces a sharper peak in the output pulse, which makes amplitude analysis more difficult in some instances. Flat-topped pulses may be produced if a circuit element known as a delay line is used instead of an *RC* component for clipping.

An ideal *delay line* is an arrangement of circuit elements that transmits pulses unattenuated but delayed in time. A simple ladder-type delay line is shown in Fig. 7A. A delay line that employs a continuous distribution of capacitance and inductance, such as in a coaxial cable, is illustrated in Fig. 7B. Delay line shaping is achieved by short-circuiting one end of the line and terminating the other and with a resistance equal to the characteristic impedance. Open-ended delay lines may also be used in conjunction with difference amplifiers (*3*).

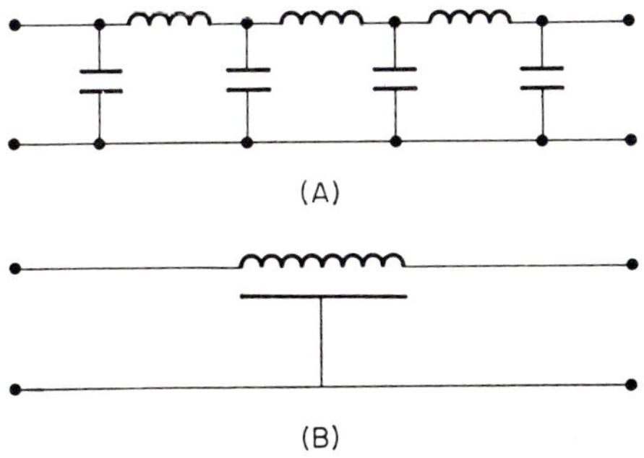

FIG. 7. Delay lines. (A) Ladder type consisting of a series of individual inductance and capacitance groups. (B) Continuous distribution of inductance and capacitance in coaxial cable.

Single delay line and single *RC* clipping are both characterized by base line shifts at high count-rates. Therefore, double delay line clipping is also frequently used (*3*). The principal advantage of delay line differentiation lies with the nearly flat-topped output pulse produced, which facilitates accurate pulse-height analysis. Also, the pulses may be produced with shorter decay times and with constant width. This leads to an advantage at high count-rates. However, delay line amplifiers are generally quite complex, and the delay lines themselves are subject to spurious responses, which can sometimes lead to poor amplitude overload characteristics.

B. Amplifier Overload

The two important functions of an amplifier are pulse shaping and pulse amplification. The actual amplification of the signal takes place in stages, which are coupled by the pulse-shaping elements.

An example of a versatile amplifier (Tennelec TC-200) is shown in Fig. 8, which has four stages of amplification. Stages 1, 3, and 4 are fixed stages of gain two. The gain of stage 2 is variable from 0.5 to 256. Thus, the overall gain of this amplifier is variable from 4 to 2048. A is the first differentiator, B is the integrator, and C is the second differentiator. In this amplifier the pulse shaping is accomplished by RC networks and an adjustment over the range of 0.05 to 12.8 μsec is possible. Thus, where maximum signal-to-noise ratio is the most important consideration, the first differentiation time constant is set equal to that of the integrator and the second differentiator is essentially inactivated.

Amplifier characteristics change with very high pulse rates and with very high input pulse amplitudes. The characteristics of count-rate overloading and amplitude overloading are not completely independent. Both are not easily specified. However, the best overloading characteristics can only be achieved by considering the entire system composed of detector, amplifier, and pulse selector. No other amplifier characteristic is as sensitive to mismatch of these three components.

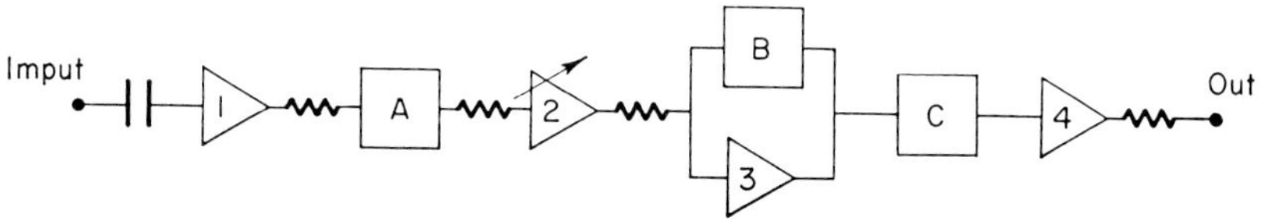

FIG. 8. Amplifier schematic diagram. Four amplifier stages coupled as in a Tennelec TC-200 amplifier. See Appendix, Section III.

The dynamical range of signal amplitude from a nuclear detector may sometimes be quite great, with some large pulses exceeding the smallest signal of interest by a factor of several thousand. This is particularly true with the background pulses from large scintillation detectors, such as might be used in a whole-body counter. All amplifiers are designed to accommodate some *pulse amplitude overloading* without serious output pulse distortion. One of the usual manifestations of this normal or design overloading in a doubly differentiated amplifier is illustrated in Fig. 9A. The smaller of the two pulses represents the nonoverloading characteristic pulse and is shown for reference. The overloading pulse has driven the amplifier to saturation output, and the return of the negative portion to the base line is somewhat delayed. This temporary depression of the base line is unimportant at low count-rates, or when the number of overloads is small relative to the normal pulses.

One of the effects of abnormal overload that is characteristic of some delay line amplifiers is shown in Fig. 9B. Small and unavoidable imperfections in the delay lines can cause an extended "ringing" or oscillation, when large overloads appear. Depending upon the characteristics of the pulse-height analyzer, one or more of the ringing peaks may be analyzed. The background count-rate will thus be increased, since these large pulses would ordinarily be rejected by the analyzer. Indeed, the ringing type of overload response may on some occasions cause spurious peaks to appear in a background spectrum. Some amplifiers, such as the A-8, a modified delay line amplifier (*6*), and the Tennelec TC-200, are specifically designed to provide "graceful" overload characteristics for high values of overload.

The situation illustrated in Fig. 9 has most frequently occurred with large crystals when the gain was adjusted so that the smaller pulse might

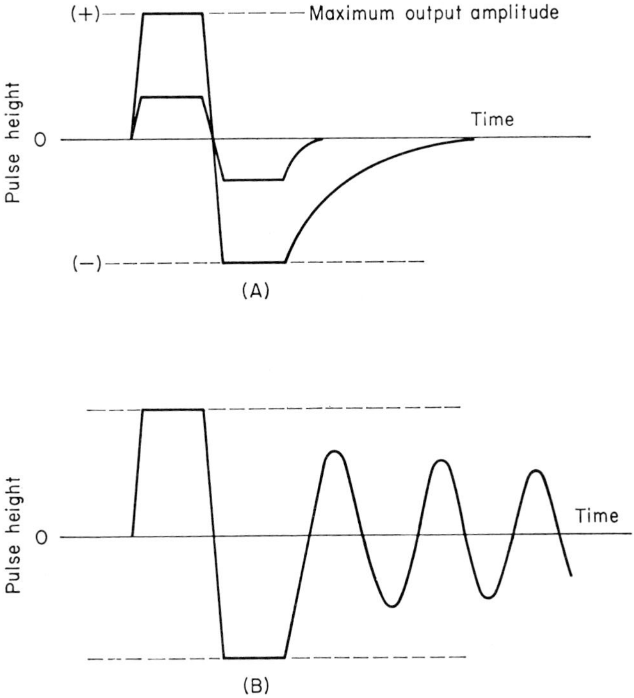

FIG. 9. Pulse height overloading. (A) Normal overload (large pulse) of a doubly differentiated amplifier. (B) Abnormal overload causing oscillations.

represent the absorption of a photon in the range of 0.5 to 1.5 MeV and the overload was caused by a very high energy meson. The recent use of low-energy γ-ray emitters such as ^{125}I makes amplitude overloading an important factor even when only modest-sized crystals of 2- or 3-inch diameter are used. The gain of the system will be such that the lower pulse might represent an energy absorption of only 0.035 MeV, which makes overloads from radiation of only a few million electron volts energy possible.

Count-rate overloading occurs when the average rate of random pulses increases to the extent that a significant number of pulses are distorted because of proximity to the previous pulse. Amplitude enhancement, usually called pile-up, is another possibility. A shorter clipping time would decrease the likelihood of the occurrence of the pile-up but, as stated earlier, would increase the noise level.

The effects of count-rate overloading depend on many factors of amplifier design and are difficult to predict. However, the inevitable result is always spectral distortion. The frequency of occurrence of these piled-up pulses is a higher order rather than a linear function of the pulse rate. For example, for the measurement of ^{59}Fe in the presence of ^{51}Cr the system is set up so that the 0.32-MeV chromium γ rays are

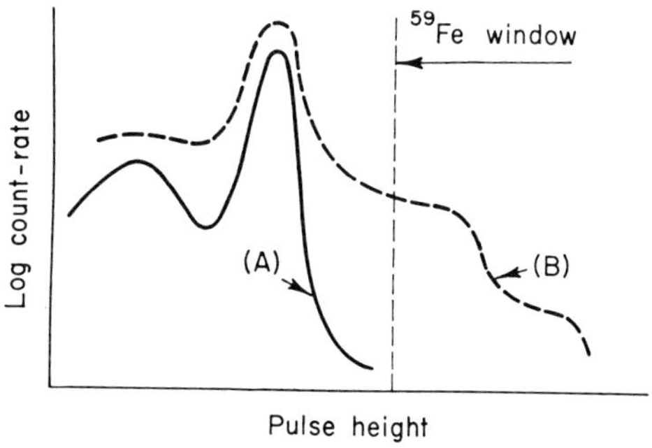

FIG. 10. Pulse pile-up. (A) Normal ^{51}Cr spectrum. (B) Distorted ^{51}Cr spectrum due to count-rate overloading.

completely excluded from the higher energy ^{59}Fe window at low count-rates. A nonlinear distortion of the iron spectrum will be caused by a high-intensity chromium background. Not only will the resolution of the iron peaks be reduced, but extraneous counts due only to the chromium will be introduced. Figure 10 shows a normal ^{51}Cr spectrum (A) and one distorted by pile-up due to count-rate overloading (B). Correction for the chromium counts registered in the iron window may only be accomplished by calibrating at the appropriate intensity levels.

Whereas pulse amplitude overloading may best be reduced by a double RC clipping amplifier, count-rate overloading is usually the least with the double-delay line types. An exception is the Fairstein amplifier (Tennelec TC-200 referred in Fig. 8), which uses active-element RC networks to provide both excellent amplitude and count-rate overloading characteristics. Pile-up may also be reduced by the use of special circuits designed to sense the distortion in pulse shape caused by the pile-up (*25*).

C. Logarithmic and Biased Postamplifiers

Simultaneous measurements of low- and high-energy emitters are sometimes required. Examples are found in liquid scintillation counting of mixtures of tritium and ^{14}C or higher-energy β-ray sources, and γ-ray counting of ^{125}I and ^{131}I. Amplifiers with *logarithmic gain* characteristics are sometimes used for this purpose (*17*). The output of such an amplifier is compared with the output of a conventional linear amplifier in Fig. 11. Analysis of peak *A* is made difficult by its compression at the low end of the spectrum of Fig. 11A. Increasing the gain of the amplifier to bring out peak *A* would result in peak *B* being lost at the upper range

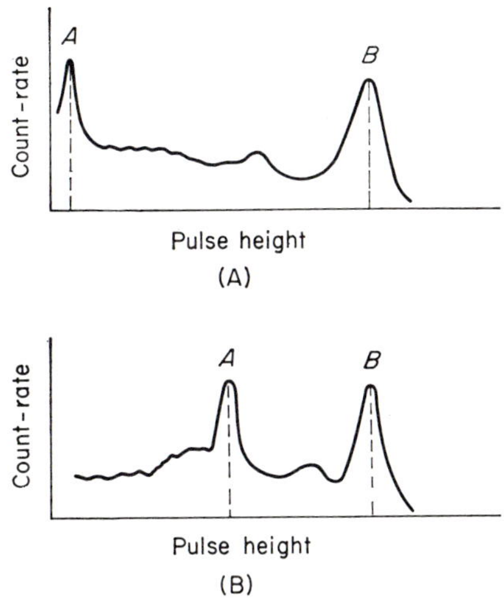

FIG. 11. Output spectra of two amplifiers. (A) Conventional linear amplifier. (B) Amplifier with logarithmic gain.

of the analyzer. One solution to the problem is shown in Fig. 11B. The logarithmic gain allows a wide range of isotope energies to be simultaneously included in the spectrum.

The problem posed by the spectrum of Fig. 11A may also be solved by connecting the inputs of a *pair of amplifiers* in parallel to the single detector output. Amplifier 1 in Fig. 12 would be run at a gain allowing optimum analysis of one peak, and amplifier 2 would be set for some other gain so that the second peak could be simultaneously counted under ideal conditions.

One other special amplifier is the so-called *biased postamplifier*. The excellent resolution of semiconductor detectors may be best realized if

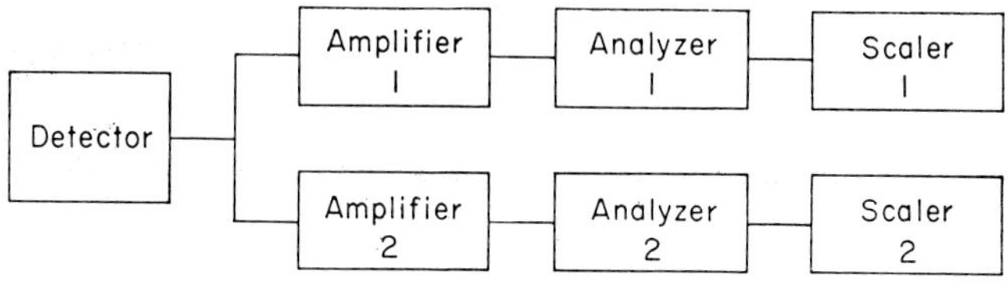

FIG. 12. Paired amplifier system. Provides optimal analysis of two widely separated pulse amplitude peaks as shown in Fig. 11.

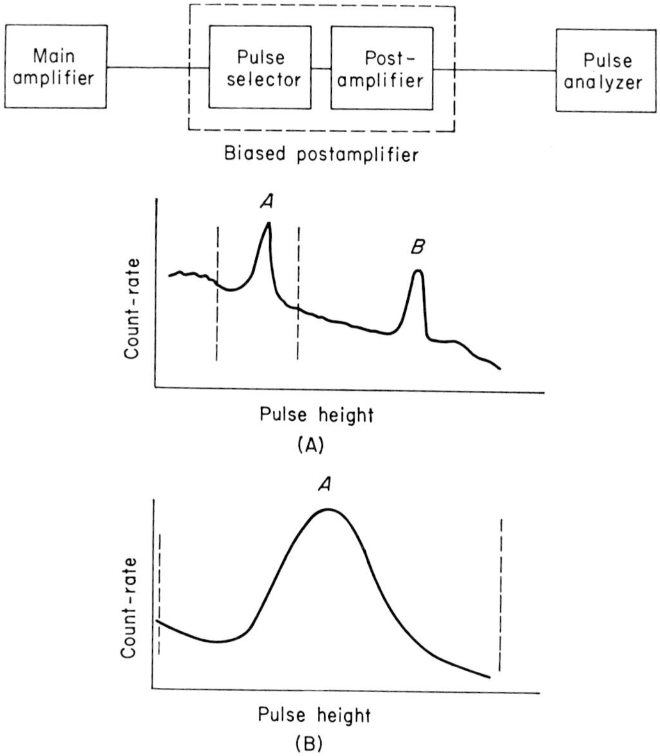

FIG. 13. Biased postamplifier system. (A) Principal spectrum showing two peaks. (B) Stretched spectrum with low-energy peak only.

the pulses in a limited region of the spectrum (around the peak of interest) are amplified separately before the final analysis. A system that includes a biased postamplifier is outlined in Fig. 13. A spectrum for the input of this selector-amplifier, with sharply defined peaks at A and B, is shown in Fig. 13A. In case the pulses in region A have been selected for postamplification, the output spectrum of the biased postamplifier is given in Fig. 13B.

This kind of system, modified by paralleling the input of the biased postamplifier with a conventional analyzing channel for counting peak B, could be used in situations similar to those in which the system in Fig. 12 would be used.

D. Checking of Amplifier Performance

The aspects of amplifier performance that need to be checked on some regular basis are *pulse shape, gain* (stability), and *noise*. Pulse shape may only be inspected with the aid of a good oscilloscope. Manifestations of poor amplifier adjustment are readily seen on an oscilloscope, as are overload-ringing, base line shift, and many kinds of transient noise. Fast, high gain oscilloscopes may be used to monitor the output signal of any of the components of the counting system so that sources of difficulty may be quickly located.

Gain stability of the detecting system as a whole may of course be checked by running a spectrum with a standard radioactive reference source at periodic intervals. Fluctuations in spectral shape, however, might be due to instabilities in some element of the system other than the amplifier. The gain of the amplifier alone may be measured with the aid of a source of electrical pulses of calibrated amplitude (a pulser) and with an output measuring device such as an oscilloscope or a pulse-height analyzer. Again, however, the pulser must be carefully matched to the input of the amplifier or preamplifier. Pulsers are also helpful when adjustments in amplifier pulse shape are necessary, and may be used to check the pulse amplitude (and sometimes count-rate) overload characteristics of the amplifier.

Certain items that are ordinarily considered to be parts of the counting system itself may also serve a dual purpose as service tools. For instance, laboratories that have a number of counters of different kinds are finding it useful to have one of the less expensive multichannel pulse-height analyzers on hand to make routine checks of the output spectra from the various counting systems.

III. PULSE-HEIGHT ANALYZERS

A. Pulse Amplitude Spectrum

The output pulses from scintillation counters, proportional counters, and solid state detectors have amplitudes that are related to the energy loss of the incident radiations. Pulse-height analyzers are used to measure the frequency distribution of these amplitudes (the pulse-height spectrum), to select portions of the spectrum for data recording, and to reject those pulses that are not desired.

Emerging from the detector output and, subsequently, from amplifier output is a train of pulses, randomly spaced with respect to time and varying in amplitude according to characteristics of the detecting system and of the incident radiations. Such a sequence of pulses is represented in Fig. 14A. An integral plot of this pulse amplitude distribution

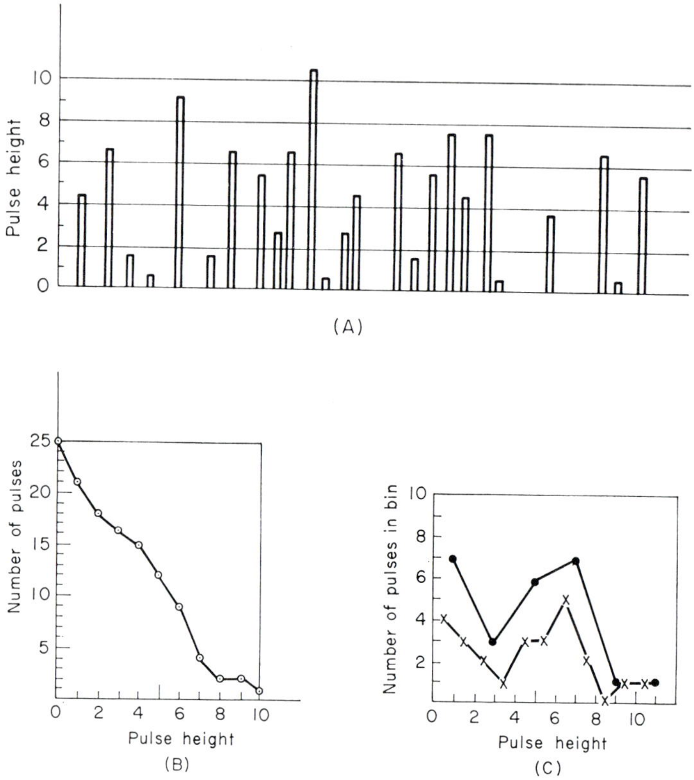

FIG. 14. Representation of a pulse spectrum. (A) Amplifier output showing time of occurrence and amplitude of individual pulses in the group to be analyzed. (B) Integral plot of pulse amplitude spectrum. (C) Differential plot of the same pulse amplitude distribution; x Bin, 1 unit of pulse height; ● Bin, 2 units of pulse height.

is shown in Fig. 14B. The number of pulses having heights greater than a particular amplitude is plotted as a function of the amplitude value. Thus, inspection of Fig. 14A reveals that there are 25 pulses having amplitudes greater than 0, 21 pulses with amplitudes greater than 1, 18 pulses with amplitudes greater than 2, and so on, and these are the coordinates of the points plotted in the integral spectrum (Fig. 14B).

Inspection of the pulse train reveals that there are four pulses with amplitudes greater than 0 but less than 1, three pulses with amplitudes between 1 and 2, two pulses with amplitudes greater than 2 and less than 3, and so on. This plot of the data (bin size equal to one unit of amplitude) gives the differential spectrum of Fig. 14C. The effect of using a larger bin when plotting the data is also shown; it yields more events per bin but reduces the resolution.

The integral and differential plots are merely two different ways of presenting the same data. Indeed, either curve may be derived from the other. Ordinate values for points above a certain value on the differential curve may be added to obtain the integral ordinate value, or successive integral ordinates may be subtracted from each other to supply the coordinates of the points on the differential curve. This is why peaks on the differential curve always correspond to regions of maximum slope on the integral curve.

B. Integral Discriminators

The pulse-height analyzer in its simplest form consists of an adjustable threshold detector, or pulse-height discriminator, which passes all pulses with amplitudes above a selected level. This level can normally be adjusted by a calibrated control, but it may also be fixed. With a calibrated control it is possible to plot the count-rate as a function of the discriminator settings and to obtain an integral spectrum. Integral pulse-height discriminators, both fixed and variable, are used in many instruments because of their simplicity.

A classical and widely used discriminator circuit is the Schmitt trigger (*21*). The circuit has an "on" or an "off" state that is determined by the potential on the input grid. Thus, potentiometric control of the triggering threshold voltage is achieved. A detailed description of this important circuit and some of its many modifications may be found in Chase (*3*). McCollom (*18*) has prepared a review of discriminators.

C. Differential Pulse-Height Analyzers

The pulse amplitude and therefore the energy information contained in a train of pulses is most readily visualized by a differential spectrum. The pulses are simultaneously fed to two discriminators connected with their inputs in parallel, and one discriminator is set to trigger at a pulse height level E_1 and the other is set to trigger at a higher level E_2. Furthermore, the output of each discriminator is connected to an anticoincidence circuit so that only those pulses that exceed the lower level, E_1, are passed. Pulses exceeding the upper level, E_2, pass through both discriminators whose output signals are in coincidence and are therefore blocked by the anticoincidence circuit.

Many single-channel analyzers use paired trigger and anticoincidence circuits that require a careful control of the timing of the trigger pulses. Therefore differential pulse-height analyzers must be considerably more complicated than the simple integral selectors. Since the input pulses have a finite rise time, a given pulse will pass the lower threshold before passing the upper. The reverse occurs during the decay phase of the pulse and the analyzer circuit must correct for these factors. The importance of trigger timing makes differential analyzers especially sensitive to the shape of the output pulse from the amplifier, and to proper matching of the components.

In many cases the *two discriminators* are biased independently of each other, one selecting the *lower level* (E_1) and the other determining the *upper level* (E_2). This arrangement is particularly useful when a relatively wide window is being used, for example, when gross counting of a particular photopeak is desired.

Fluctuations due to bias level instability become serious if very narrow windows are necessary when the settings of the two discriminators are independent of each other. Stability of *window width* is achieved by electrically tying the two discriminators to the same base line potentiometer and adding a potentiometer controlled bias to the upper trigger for controlling the width of the window (sometimes called the slit width). The position of the base line (E) is controlled by the lower discriminator and the bin, which is the distance above the base line for the upper window (ΔE), is adjusted by the window width control. In this way the bin size may be fixed when a variable base line is being used to obtain a differential pulse-height spectrum. Many commercial single-channel analyzers provide front panel controls so that either the wide window (E_1, E_2) or the fixed window (E, ΔE) modes of operation may be selected.

As with the integral discriminator, fixed window pulse-height analyzers are sometimes used. The differential spectrum is obtained by changing the high voltage on the multiplier phototube of a scintillation counter. The nonlinear characteristic of this spectrum may be observed in Fig. 15. In this system the instrumental resolution is constant for all portions of the spectrum since both base line and window width are fixed. This is advantageous when one is looking at the low-energy portions of the spectrum, especially if a group of high-energy peaks is present.

Linearity of a single-channel pulse-height analyzer relates to the precision with which the base line discriminator may be set over the energy range available. The calibrated pulse height input versus threshold setting should ideally be a straight line. The actual deviation from this line, taken at the place of maximum departure and expressed as a fraction of the base scale amplitude, is usually called the integral linearity. Analyzers are now available with integral linearity specified to be better than 0.5%. This term is somewhat misleading, however, because the absolute linearity (ratio of error of threshold to true amplitude in that region) might be quite poor at low amplitudes. Frequently the term "linearity" is used in manufacturer's specifications, and it is not clear whether "integral" or "absolute" linearity is meant.

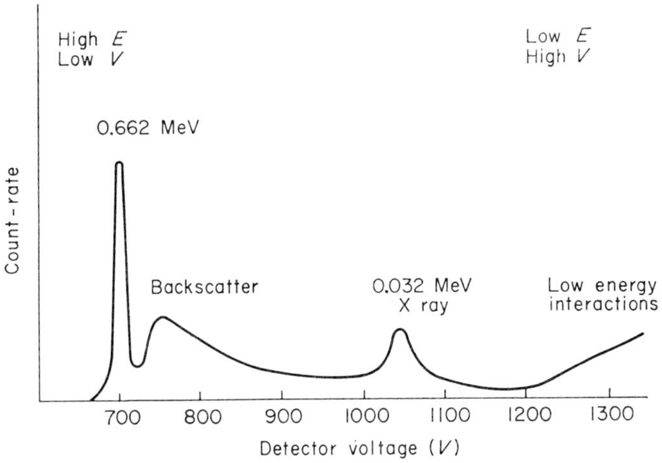

FIG. 15. Fixed window spectrum. Differential pulse-height analysis, high voltage varied with base line and window width fixed, resulting in nonlinear pulse-height spectrum.

Stability of the analyzer base line and window width is of course as important for the performance of the system as stability of the amplifier gain (*19*). Narrow window counting of photopeaks, as when mixtures of ^{131}I and ^{51}Cr are being assayed, requires the ultimate of stability. Kandiah (*15*) has described a low-level discriminator with exceptional stability characteristics which may be applied in a system with a fixed window and variable high voltage (Fig. 15).

A very stable window width is produced by a circuit designed by Gatti and Priva (*7*). This analyzer uses a single discriminator and a linear pulse reshaping circuit. In this system the window width is not independent of base line but rather is always proportional to the lower level. Thus, $\Delta E/E$ is a constant and the window width at low energies is narrower than it is at high energies. The spectrum obtained by scanning the analyzer window is thus somewhat similar in shape to the one shown in Fig. 15 for a fixed window, except that the low-energy end of the spectrum corresponds to the lower base line values. This circuit is not widely used, however, despite its advantages of slit-width stability and relatively better resolving capabilities at low energies.

Gilland (*8*) has designed a transistorized "threshold-plus-slit" type of analyzer that emphasizes the stability of the base line rather than extreme stability of window width at narrow settings. The detector is in this case the large organic scintillator of the Los Alamos whole-body counter (Chapter 21) and the analyzer windows must be designed to cover relatively broad regions of a comparatively featureless spectrum.

D. Multichannel Analyzers

Two developments made the modern multichannel analyzer possible. One was the idea (*28*) of converting pulse height (as an analog quantity) into a digital quantity (time). The other was the application of digital computer techniques for data storage (*14*). Multichannel analyzers are complex devices and contain a number of circuit elements, but the analog-to-digital converter (ADC) and the digital memory are certainly two of the most important ones.

Wilkinson's circuit (*28*), which is still basic to most *analog-to-digital converters,* employs a capacitor whose charge is made to be proportional to the amplitude of the input pulse. The capacitor is then discharged as a linear function of time. During the discharge only, an oscillator produces standard pulses at a constant rate so that the number of these pulses is proportional to the amplitude of the original pulse from the detector. Thus this number is the digital representation of the input pulse amplitude and the information may be handled by digital techniques.

A "linear-gate" is used to block the analyzer input during the time that the capacitor is charging and discharging. This is necessary in order to prevent a second signal from entering the ADC during that time and causing an error in the measurement of the first signal. The analyzer is therefore "dead" during the period that each pulse is being processed. The *dead time* is greater for pulses of higher amplitude because of the pulse height-to-time conversion feature. A typical dead time would be 0.25 μsec per channel plus a storage time of 25 μsec. In a 256-channel analyzer this means the dead time would vary from slightly over 25 μsec per pulse to 89 μsec. The variation and magnitude of the dead time dictate that a special internal timing circuit be used so that counting runs be measured only in analyzer live-time, rather than conventional clock-time.

Many types of digital data storing devices have been used, some of which will be described in Section V. The multichannel analyzers that are now being used in nuclear medicine universally make use of magnetic core storage (*3*). The basic element in a *magnetic-core memory* is a small piece of ferromagnetic material with suitable hysteresis characteristics. Current-carrying wires cause the cores to become magnetized. The polarity of this magnetism, which remains after the activating current ceases to flow, represents the digits 0 or 1. The cores are assembled in a cubic array. The x-y location of a particular core in a given plane specifies the analyzer channel that it represents, and the planes themselves are associated with the binary digits of the numbers stored in the memory. Increasing the number of cores per plane increases the number of channels in the analyzer, and increasing the number of planes increases the capacity of the memory. It is possible to read out this information stored in the core without changing the state of the core, so that the interrogation process is not a destructive one. The binary information encoded in the cores at the same x-y location in the different planes is the digital representation of the counts stored in that channel.

The linearity of a multichannel analyzer may be specified in terms of integral or absolute linearity, as with the single-channel analyzer. In addition a quantity relating to the uniformity of channel width is required, and this is called differential linearity. *Differential linearity* is defined as the percentage deviation from the average channel width in the channel for which this quantity is a maximum. The differential linearity is sometimes specified for only the upper 97% of the range, since absolute accuracy is hardest to obtain in the low-energy region.

The capacity to perform *multichannel scaling* is usually built into the analyzer. In this application the ADC is bypassed and all pulses in a given time interval are directed to the same memory position, and the channels are addressed in time sequence. The address advance controls the dwell time in each channel. In this mode of operation the analyzer functions as a fast digital ratemeter. The insensitive time during the process of switching from one channel to the next is essentially equivalent to the storage time for memory address.

Various *computer functions* can be performed with the multichannel analyzer. Punched tape may be used to read data back into the memory. For instance, background subtraction may be accomplished by reading back in the negative mode. Memory subgroups are sometimes provided. For example, a 400-channel analyzer may be subdivided into four groups of 100 channels each. Data may be interchanged between subgroups in either positive or negative modes, so that one spectrum may be subtracted from or added to another. Integration of the whole or portions

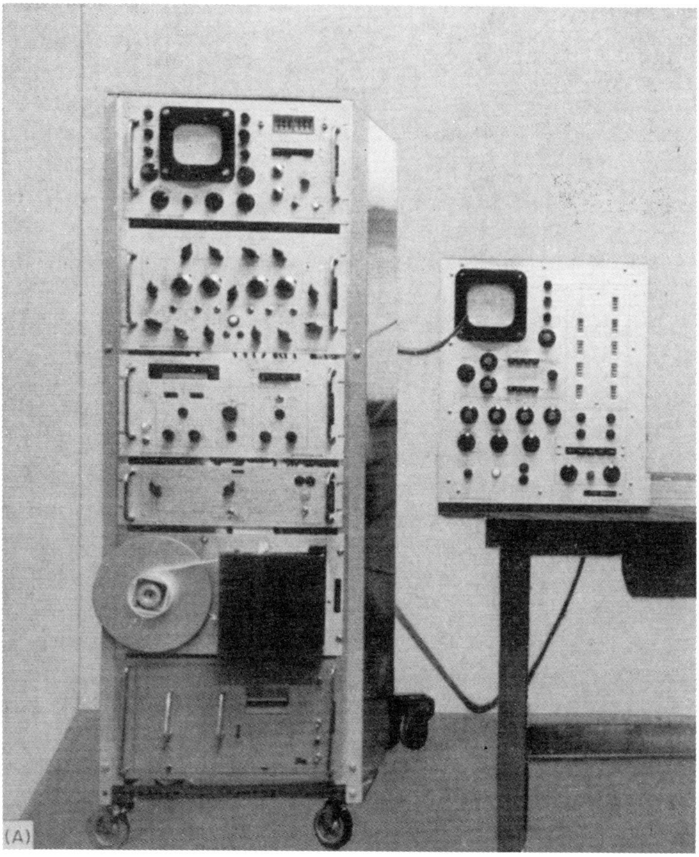
(A)

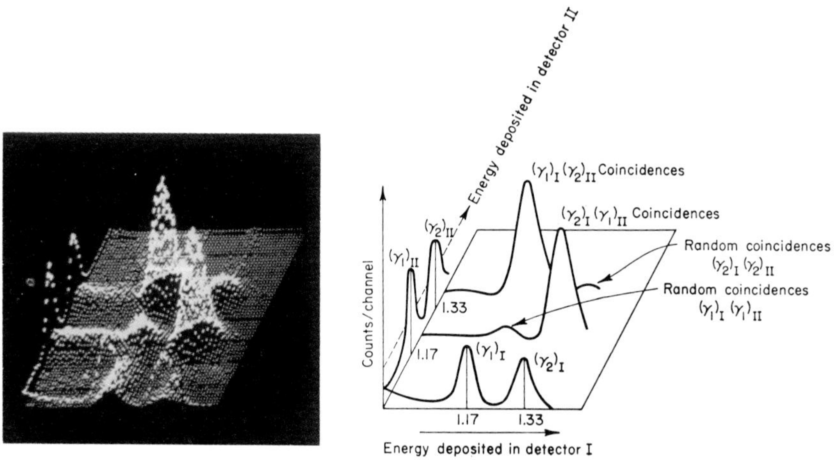
Energy deposited in detector II
$(\gamma_1)_I (\gamma_2)_{II}$ Coincidences
$(\gamma_2)_I (\gamma_1)_{II}$ Coincidences
Random coincidences $(\gamma_2)_I (\gamma_2)_{II}$
Random coincidences $(\gamma_1)_I (\gamma_1)_{II}$
$(\gamma_2)_{II}$
$(\gamma_1)_{II}$
1.33
1.17
$(\gamma_1)_I$
$(\gamma_2)_I$
Counts/channel
1.17
1.33
Energy deposited in detector I

(B)

of a spectrum is also possible. Some analyzers have auxiliary computer sections which essentially provide the specialized programming for the magnetic core memory. Others accomplish peak area integration with the printing lister, which functions as an adding machine during printout of the spectrum.

Particular portions of the spectrum may be studied in greater detail by changing the analog-to-digital conversion gain in the ADC. If 3 V represents maximum amplitude of ADC input pulses, and these pulses are stored in channel 100 with one value of conversion gain (ramp slope), then doubling the ramp slope causes this spectrum to be spread over 200 channels. Upper- and lower-level bias on the input permits still greater resolution of segments of the spectrum.

Analyzer performance specifications have been improved to the point that the overall stability of the system is most generally limited by the detector, the high-voltage supply, or the amplifier. *Stabilizing circuits* are available as auxiliary components that are able to sense fluctuations in the spectral position of a reference peak. This information is used to control the detector high voltage or the ADC ramp slope. The analog form of this instrument, which may also be used with a single-channel analyzer, monitors the count-rate on either side of the reference peak and adjusts the detector high voltage when a state of inbalance appears. Digital pulse-height stabilizers are more complicated, since the ADC zero point is stabilized in addition to overall gain regulation. If a suitable reference peak is not available in the spectra being measured, a special reference radioactive source (possibly emitting only high-energy α particles) may be incorporated in the detector (*12*). The stabilizer and analyzer will then be programmed so that counts from this peak will not be stored in the memory provided that the reference energy falls above the γ-ray energy range.

Refinements in design and in manufacturing techniques of the ADC and of the data storage have made the present transistorized multichannel analyzers fantastically reliable and relatively inexpensive. Indeed, some multichannel analyzers, the TMC "Gammascope" and the Baird-Atomic "Scintiscope," include in one package all the elements of the system shown in Fig. 1 except the detector itself. The cost is comparable with that of a high-quality amplifier, single-channel analyzer,

---

FIG. 16. (A) Two-parameter γ-ray spectrometer (Intertechnique). In its coincidence mode of operation, an event is registered only when one pulse from each of two sodium iodide crystals is received within about 0.1 μsec. This yields a very selective response from radioisotopes which decay with the emission of cascade γ rays. (B) Example showing noncoincident γ-ray spectra in each of two detectors from ^{60}Co γ rays and the two-dimensional plot of the coincident spectrum.

scaler, ratemeter, and high-voltage supply when purchased together as individual units. Multichannel analyzers are finding increasing use in nuclear medicine because of their unique capability for conserving information, their versatility of function, their computer options, and their computer-compatible output.

Large analyzers with thousands of memory channels and various operational modes for addressing the data into the memory have been developed. One such mode involves time correlations between the individual events in the spectra of two different detectors, and is called *two-parameter storage.* Each event in the differential spectrum of one detector is identified with coincident events in the spectrum of the other detector. Results may be seen in Fig. 16, which shows several presentations of the information stored in the analyzer. TMC has prepared an interesting brochure (*26*) that shows 28 ways in which this kind of two-parameter data may be viewed. Although the abundance of spectral information obtained with such a device may exceed the requirements of a nuclear medicine laboratory, programming the system to operate as a two-dimensional multichannel scaler may find applications in conjunction with such devices as the scintillation camera and the autofluoroscope. The contour plots shown in Fig. 16 might then represent the distribution of radioactivity in an organ, and these data would be in a convenient form for computer processing.

IV. HIGH-VOLTAGE POWER SUPPLIES

Because of the dependence of the output pulse amplitude of the various detectors on the value of the high-voltage bias applied to them, the high-voltage power supply is an important part of the complete electronics system for pulse amplification and analysis. Whereas the high voltage has little effect on the output in the case of G-M counters and solid state detectors, changes of only 1% in the bias of a scintillation detector will change the output pulse amplitude by 10% or more.

Stability of modern high-voltage power supplies depends on a number of factors such as time, temperature, input supply voltage, and output load. In the well-regulated high-voltage power supply, suitable for scintillation detector use, the effects of time and temperature are far more important than the effect of line voltage and load variations on the stability of the output voltage. The most meaningful specification given by the manufacturer is that of high-voltage output stability over a 24-hr period when subjected to approximately a 10°C temperature variation. The effect of line voltage and load variations on the high-voltage output should also be given so that these factors may be evaluated.

Instability will be introduced if the load inadvertently exceeds the design values. Many high-voltage supplies have been built with output ratings of 0–1 mA and are satisfactory for use with conventional sodium iodide detectors. However, this current rating is inadequate for some multiple detector systems, since their total current requirement may exceed 40 mA. In addition, maximum detector stability (particularly with organic detectors) is achieved if the multiplier phototube voltage divider network is designed to draw currents in the milliampere range. The current output rating of the high-voltage power supply must be carefully considered in these situations.

Superimposed upon the stable d.c. output of these high-voltage supplies is an a.c. component of relatively minor amplitude, called the ripple. In cases where the positive high voltage is coupled to the input circuit of the amplifier, the ripple is potentially able to contribute noise to the system because of its pulselike form. Some regulated high-voltage power supplies have a ripple that exceeds 100 mV peak to peak, and detector pulses with less than 50-mV amplitude may be lost in the background of this noise. Supplies with ripple less than 1 mV peak to peak are available and are required if the maximum detector sensitivity is to be realized.

V. PULSE STORAGE

The fundamental information in a counting experiment relates to the time interval between successive events and the energy transfer associated with each event. Conventional counting devices lump a number of events together and provide the data as events per unit time. This process is destructive in the sense that information relating to shorter averaging times is lost. Magnetic tape provides a means of preserving the time relationship between individual pulses so that the data may be run and re-run with different averaging times in order to provide the best analysis in any situation. Most experiments do not require this degree of sophistication, however, and ordinary counting, whether the measuring time be milliseconds (multichannel analyzers in multiscaler mode) or minutes and hours (conventional scaler), will suffice.

A. Fast Interim Storage

1. Delay Line Storage

A train of pulses entering the input of a delay line and emerging at the output at some later time may be said to have been stored for that period of time. Thus, components in which the output is significantly delayed relative to the input may be considered to be memory elements.

This type of memory was used in the multichannel analyzer of Hutchinson and Scarrott (*14*), although they employed an ultrasonic delay. Details relating to analog-to-digital conversion, storage, and memory addressing will not be considered at this time, since magnetic core memories have made the delay line systems obsolete for nuclear medical applications. The interested reader is referred to Chase (*3*) for a review of the subject.

Delay line memories characteristically require a long access time (if the memory capacity is large) and require active circuitry. That is to say, the memory information must be continuously recirculated through the delay line and requires continuous power. Electrical noise will of course produce data errors.

2. Charge Storage

Memory devices that involve the storage of charge on an insulated surface have been developed. *Cathode ray tubes* may be used in this manner. The electron beam, its locus of impact upon the screen controlled by the internal deflection plates, supplies the information to the storage surface under suitable conditions of secondary electron emission.

The impingement of the electron beam upon the screen causes secondary electrons to be ejected, and these return to the screen at various distances from the impact point. The net result is a positively charged "crater" surrounded by a negative rim. The absence or presence of such a crater in a given location is made to represent the binary digit 0 or 1, respectively. An external device mounted close to the screen is used to read this memory. The circumstances of reading are such that the process is destructive in the sense that the memory is caused to revert to the zero state.

Although the charge distribution on the insulator is fairly stable with time, degeneration does occur. Also, some sprinkling of secondary electrons to nonprogrammed locations occurs during data storage. For this reason it is necessary to periodically regenerate the memory by reading the information at each location and feeding it back in. The complexity of the electronic circuitry required for regeneration of the memory has limited the wider use of this type of storage system.

A cathode ray tube memory (or a similar device, a barrier-grid storage tube) may be used as part of a multichannel analyzer. Any channel of the memory of this type of charge-storing system may be read at random, whereas a delay line memory must be read in sequence.

Another kind of charge-storing memory system utilizes diodes and capacitors. *Diode-capacitor storage,* using random parallel memory access, can be made very fast, However, the cost of these units is relatively high and they are not used in nuclear medical applications.

B. Magnetic Storage

The permanence of the magnetization of ferromagnetic materials after the magnetizing field has been removed, coupled with the ease with which the degree of magnetization may be inspected and changed, has been the fundamental reason for the widespread use of magnetic materials in complex pulse storage systems.

1. MAGNETIC CORES

Magnetic cores, described in Section III,D, are of particular use in multichannel analyzers where pulses are usually stored on the basis of events per unit time rather than of time interval between pulses. Although delay line and charge-storing systems may be made faster than magnetic core devices, the latter enjoy overwhelming advantages because of simplicity, reliability, versatility, and permanence of storage.

2. MAGNETIC DRUM

Rapidly rotating cylinders with ferromagnetic surfaces may be used to store pulse information. Delays are involved for readin and readout since the computer must wait for the drum to reach the proper position each time. Magnetic drums are used in the "slow" section of some high-speed computers, in conjunction with other faster data-storing techniques.

3. MAGNETIC TAPE

Magnetic tapes are extensively used for data storage in computers, since the cost per bit is relatively small. This type of memory is quite slow because portions of the tape must be searched during readout.

Nevertheless, magnetic tapes are uniquely useful in nuclear medicine because of the fact that they are capable of storing all of the information received from the detector. Tape recorders that are used in nuclear medical counting systems commonly feature four parallel, independent recording channels. Thus, the data from four detectors may be simultaneously recorded on the same tape (multiplexed). The channels may then be individually re-run through a single data processing system. A cost savings is therefore effected when multiple probes are used since only one data processing system is required.

A selection of tape speeds is available for readin and readout. Thus, data from a fast dynamic process such as a cerebral circulation study may be readout at a slower speed, or data from a slower system may be more rapidly processed (*9, 11, 13*). Record and (or) playback speeds of 3.75, 7.5, 15, and 30 inches per second are usually available on commercial tape decks, so that a 32-min kidney clearance study could be recorded at 3.75 inches per second and played back in 4 min at 30 inches per second tape speed. On the other hand, a 20-sec recording of cephalic circulation could be extended to 160 sec in the playback.

The readout process is nondestructive so that the data may be run and re-run with different resolving times, different contrast values, and different background subtraction in order to make full use of the information content of the tape.

Tape systems can be designed to store both pulse amplitude and repetition-rate information. Most nuclear medical applications require only the latter information to be stored so the tape input is preceded by a pulse amplitude selector stage. Pulses of fixed amplitude are fed to the tape. This simplifies the design of the tape system and effects considerable savings in cost.

The paralysis time of a tape deck, analogous to the dead-time of a Geiger counter, must be considered in relation to a given counting application. Some of the earlier systems (*9*) used inexpensive tape decks with a 200-μsec paralysis time at the fastest speed ($7\frac{1}{2}$ inches per second). The magnetic impulse which activates the tape is of fixed duration and amplitude. Therefore, pulse pairs that are barely resolved at one tape speed will overlap and not be resolved at slower speeds. For this reason the paralysis time is inversely proportional to the tape speed in any system which has a selection of speeds. The maximum resolution (or maximum recording rate) is thus obtained at the fastest tape speed.

Commercially available magnetic tape recording units specifically designed for medical nuclear applications feature paralysis times of 10 μsec or less. Some provide two simultaneous outputs to analog or digital equipment, and a configuration wherein data on one track may be subtracted from any of the other channels during readout. Background subtraction is also possible.

Studies of fast dynamic systems require high count-rates so that significant data may be acquired in the short integrating time intervals. The severe limitations imposed by the paralysis time of the tape deck may be overcome if the pulses are derandomized before they are impressed upon the tape. This may be accomplished either by using buffer storage or by using a fast prescaler.

A *digital buffer memory* allows temporary storage of the second member of a pulse pair until sufficient tape has passed to assure its reliable recording. This procedure changes the statistical distribution of the time interval between successive pulses, but does not affect the measured events-per-unit-time in clinical situations, since large numbers of pulses are accumulated in each integrating time interval.

The paralysis time of a tape system may in effect be shortened if a fast decade or binary scaler precedes the recording stage. In this case each pulse on the tape will represent a number of counts equivalent to the scaling factor that has been selected. As with buffer storage, information relating to time intervals within the groups that are scaled is lost. However, this lost information is generally not useful in clinical situations since many of these groups must be lumped together in each time interval in order to minimize statistical fluctuations. Very little essential clinical information is lost if a prescaling factor of 8 or 10 is used with a tape recording system.

VI. DATA PROCESSING

A. Scalers

The term "scaler" has often been used to denote the single box containing high-voltage supply, amplifier, discriminator, binary flip-flop circuits, and mechanical register that is connected to a Geiger counter. Present usage, however, restricts the term to a mechanical or electrical device which is used to count the pulses applied to it by a radiation-detecting and analyzing system. Scalers might therefore be classified as data-storing devices. Indeed, the individual memory channels of a multichannel analyzer are very advanced scalers.

Scalers are also data processers, since they accept a series of randomly spaced pulses and produce a number. There are many kinds of scalers offering different degrees of convenience of readout, reliability, pulse-pair resolution, size, and power consumption.

1. BINARY REGISTERS

The early mechanical registers were restricted to input count-rates below 60 cps so that it became necessary to reduce or "scale down" the impulse rate at the register input by electronic means. The first electronic scalers consisted of a set of binary (scale of two) elements connected in series to provide a scaling factor of 2^n, where n represents the number of binary stages. These scale-of-two units (flip-flops) are symmetrical circuits which can be characterized by either one of two conducting states, designated 0 and 1. Such a circuit (*10*) is shown in Fig. 17. Suppose that tube B is in its conducting state. The d.c. connection insures that tube A will not be conducting at the same time. This we shall call the "0" state. When a signal is impressed upon the double diode, it will pass a pulse of one sign only, causing a flow of current in the originally nonconducting tube and a transfer of the conduction. With A conducting and B blocked the system is in the binary state "1." A neon interpolation light may be included in the system so that it will be lit in state "1." The next pulse at the diode will transfer the system back to state "0" and a pulse will appear at the output when this transition occurs. This output pulse may be used to trigger either a mechanical register or the input diode for another flip-flop circuit.

Because of the dependence upon conduction, flip-flop circuits are ideally suited for transistorization. Reliable and inexpensive transistor binary scalers are commonly available. Stoddart (*23*) has described the transistorized version of the scale-of-two circuit.

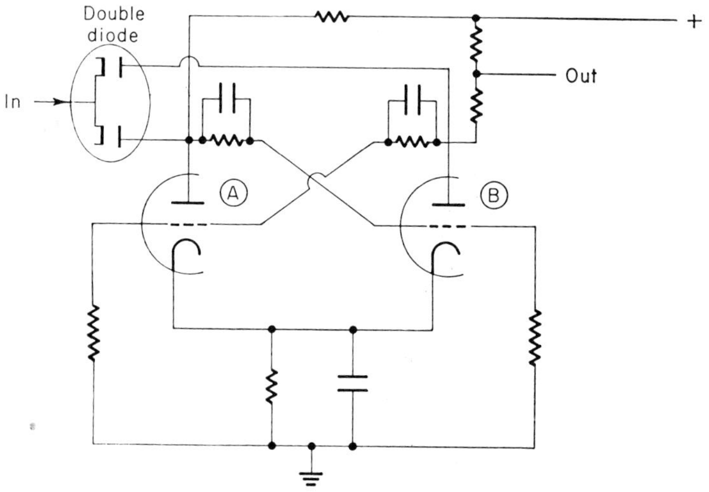

FIG. 17. Scale-of-two circuit. One output pulse for each two input pulses; called a "flip-flop" circuit.

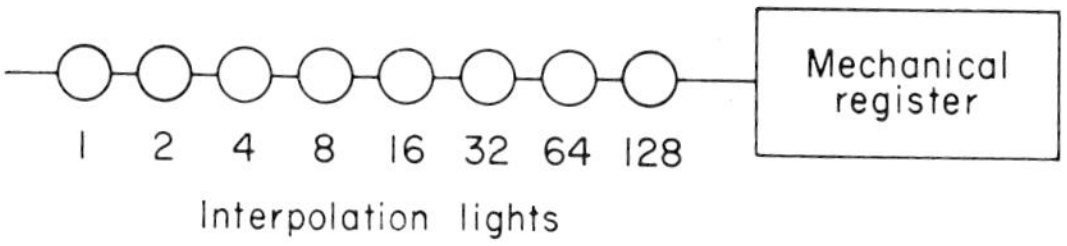

FIG. 18. Scale of 256 ($n = 8$). Eight flip-flops arranged in series to provide a scaling factor of 256.

Data from a series of n binary scaling elements must usually be converted to decimal units for computational purposes. Eight or more flip-flop circuits (scale of 256) are common because of the need to accommodate reasonably high count-rates. Each count recorded by the mechanical register of Fig. 18 represents 256 events at the scaler input, so the total count in decimal units is obtained by multiplying the register reading by the scaling factor (256) and adding to this the sum of the interpolation lights that are lit.

2. DECIMAL REGISTERS

a. *Binary-Coded-Decimal* (*BCD*). The process of converting binary information into decimal units is particularly time consuming and has been largely obviated by the so-called binary-coded-decimal systems. Binary stages may be programmed to read in decimal units in one of a number of ways. Two of the most common ones are the $16 - 6$ and $8 + 2$ systems. In the former, four flip-flop units in series (scale factor $2^4 = 16$) are made to receive false counts of 2 and 4 in the second and third stages (by the proper use of feedback), so that 10 input pulses $(16 - 6)$ are required for one output pulse. Four scale-of-two circuits are also used in the $8 + 2$ system, but an inhibit gate is included which prevents the second stage from responding to the tenth pulse but, rather, triggers the fourth stage. Thus, 8 counts are required to change the conduction state of the fourth binary element, but it reverts back to the 0 state with the addition of only 2 more counts.

BCD systems employing vacuum tube flip-flops require proportionately more complex circuitry than simple binary systems. The early decade scalers (BCD) lacked dependability and used excessive amounts of power, especially those fast scalers that claimed pulse pair resolution of better than 5 μsec. Transistor technology has dramatically changed this situation. One transistorized decade scaler (Fairchild CUL 958, BCD $8 + 2$ systems) is quite inexpensive, is very fast (2 Mc), is small (⅓ inch maximum dimension, 1.12 gm weight) and only consumes 0.19 watt of power.

b. *Beamswitching*. Beamswitching devices are vacuum tubes that employ an electron beam so constrained that input pulses cause the beam to move sequentially through a series of stable positions. These tubes may be made to be fundamentally decade in nature by building them with ten beam positions. Therefore no binary-to-decade conversion is necessary, as with the flip-flop circuits.

Figure 19 illustrates one of the early vacuum decade tubes, the Philips E1T. Focus electrodes *F* form the electron beam which is deflected by electrodes *D* and *D′*. *D′* is initially adjusted so that the beam passes into slit *O* of target *T*. The target has 10 slots and screen *S* provides a numerical identification of the slit through which the beam is passing. Stable operation is achieved when the beam grazes one side of the aperture in *T*, with the electrons that are collected on *T* being used in a feedback circuit with *D′*. The other electrons pass through to activate the numerical indication on the screen *S*. A properly controlled electrical impulse on deflector *D* will cause the beam to move over one slit and "lock-in" in a stable configuration there. Successive impulses cause the beam to move from slit to slit to the right, eventually reaching slit 9. The tenth impulse puts the full beam on T, causing the device to reset at 0 and also supplying an output pulse to the next stage of the scaler.

The E1T is capable of satisfactory service at moderately high count-rates, up to 10^5 cps. The associated electronic circuits are initially critical to adjust, but are considerably simpler than the vacuum tube BCD systems.

Another beamswitching tube is the trochotron, which uses crossed magnetic and electric fields to provide stable beam configurations. The Burroughs Beam-X switch shown in Fig. 20 is a sophisticated trochotron

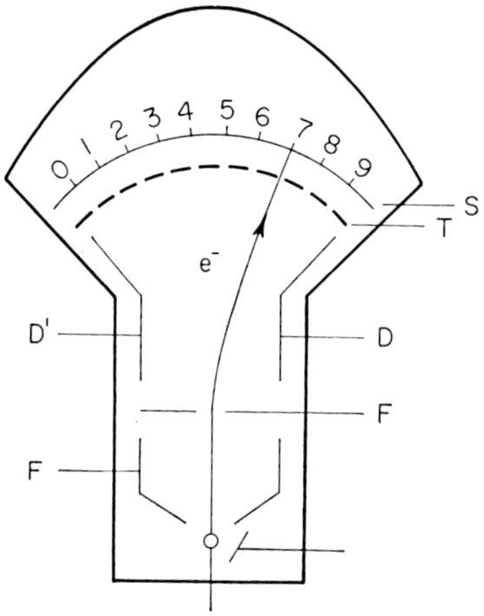

FIG. 19. Decade beamswitching tube (Philips E1T). A special cathode ray tube in which the beam is restricted to one of 10 possible trajectories.

of recent design. Small rod magnets form part of each target and provide a longitudinal magnetic field. A radial electric field is maintained between the cathode and the peripheral elements in the tube. Electrons emanating from the cathode move trochoidally around the cathode, not reaching the spades unless a sufficiently high potential is applied to the spades. The spades are operated at voltages below this cutoff voltage. If the potential of one of the spades is made sufficiently negative, a field condition is set up that allows the electron beam to graze that spade and reach the associated target element. The electron beam is then said to be "locked-in" on that spade. Current flow through the spade and its external resistance will maintain a reduced potential on the spade and can provide the condition necessary for a stable beam.

Switching is accomplished by applying a positive pulse to the proximal switching grid. The electron beam then moves to the next spade, reducing its potential when current flow begins and locking-in there. The switching grids are connected together in alternate groups (odd and even) so that no spade is skipped during the switching operation. In nuclear counting the odd and even grids are activated by a flip-flop circuit, which is part of the driving circuit for the Beam-X tube.

The spade current is adjusted to provide for stable operation of the tube. Nearly 85% of the beam current, however, passes the spade and is collected by the target. This target current constitutes the electrical

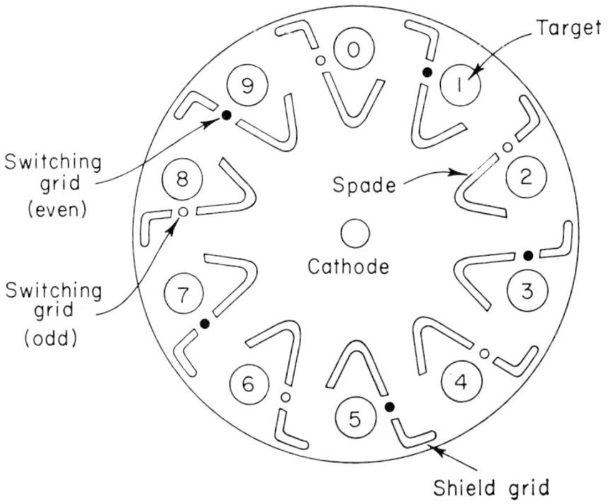

FIG. 20. Cross section of Burroughs Beam-X switching tube. The radial electron beam is controlled by crossed electric and magnetic fields.

output of the tube and may be used externally without influencing the beam characteristics.

Each target in a tube may be connected to a numerical indicating device so that direct decimal readout is possible. The output of the 0 target may also be used to drive the next stage of the scaler.

One readout device which has been designed for use with the Beam-X tube is the Burroughs "Nixie." The Nixie contains the numbers from 0 to 9 and is a gas-filled, cold cathode tube. The number corresponding to an associated Beam-X target lights up when the electron beam is locked in on that target. The Amperex decade numerical indicator is a long-life, cold cathode, gas filling indicator tube somewhat similar to the Nixie.

Beam-X tubes are available as part of decade counter modules which include the control circuitry for the beamswitching tube. These modules provide reliable decade scaling with a minimum number of component parts. The power consumption is only 2 watts and 9-μsec pulse pair resolution is achieved.

c. *Plasma Switching.* Another type of tube which is basically decade in nature is the cold cathode gas discharge tube called the glow transfer tube or Dekatron. As shown in Fig. 21, the Dekatron consists of a central anode and 30 cathodes. The cathodes labeled K_0 to K_9 are the output cathodes, those connected together to G_1 are the "first guides" and those going to G_2 are the "second guides." Nine of the cathodes (K_1–

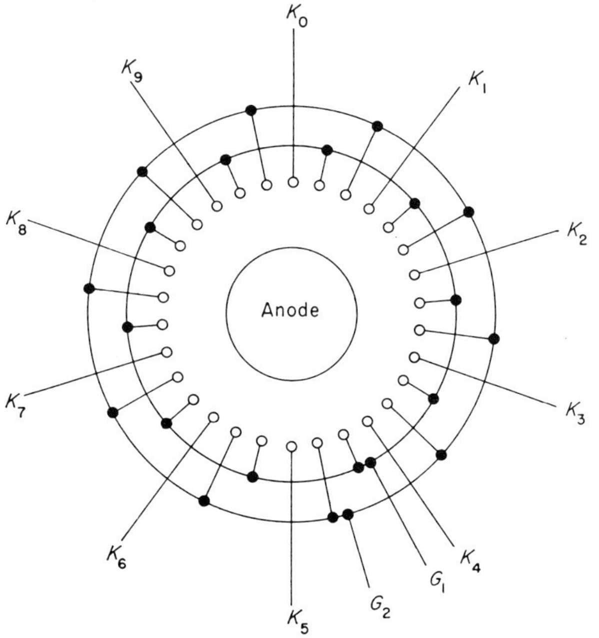

FIG. 21. Cross section of a Dekatron glow transfer decade scaling tube. The visible gas discharge between anode and a single cathode is transferred sequentially by proper application of bias potentials.

K_9) are usually connected together in a conventional decade counter, with the lead from K_0 being brought out separately. A suitable d.c. potential between anode and K_0 will cause a glow to appear in the region of K_0 because of the gas discharge. The flow of current through the external circuit during the glow drops the potential of the anode below the striking potential of the other cathodes, so that only a single discharge is maintained. The glow is transferred to the adjacent cathode by sequentially pulsing the two guide cathodes. If G_1 is first made sufficiently negative the glow will temporarily move to the nearest first guide, and will pass to the second guide when it has in turn been made negative relative to

G_1. The transfer to K_1 is completed when G_2 is returned to positive bias. In each case the transfer of the glow to an adjacent electrode is made possible because the striking potential of that electrode is influenced by the near presence of the glow.

Reversing the pulse sequence on the guides will transfer the glow in the opposite direction, which is equivalent to subtraction. The position of the glow in the tube provides a visual indication of the number of pulses that have been counted. The tenth count returns the glow to K_0 and results in an output pulse which may be used to drive subsequent decade units or a mechanical register.

The external electrical circuit for driving the Dekatrons may be vacuum tube or transistor, and is relatively simple. The counting speeds attainable with these units are limited by the time taken to sweep the heavy positive ions from the tail of the discharge as it moves along. Maximum count-rates of 5,000 cps are quoted for these tubes, with pulse pair resolution of 20–80 μsec.

The life time of these tubes is reduced if they are left on with the glow remaining in one position (usually zero), since sputtering occurs and the cathodes deteriorate. If the glow is moving continually the life time can be quite long.

BCD scalers may be designed to be self-monitoring so that component malfunction is manifested by a redundant reading. Dekatron errors, on the other hand, may be insidious in the beginning. Electrode deterioration will at first result in an occasional pulse being missed. Failure of the driving circuit can sometimes cause double or even triple pulsing. The operator must be alert to detect these errors.

d. *Mechanical.* Mechanical impulse counters are being largely replaced by electronic scalers in nuclear counting applications. The principal disadvantage of the mechanical registers, of course, is the upper limit on counting speed. Modern Sodeco impulse counters will accept up to 50 cps in a three- to six-digit model and up to 25 cps with seven digits, but this speed is poor when compared with electronic scalers.

The cost per digit and the power consumption were formerly an advantage when mechanical registers were compared with vacuum tube BCD scalers. Thus, many hybrid scalers are in use which combine electronic scales of 100 or 1000 with a mechanical register for the higher digits. However, the slow mechanical register may produce counting losses at high count-rates even though fast prescaling stages are used. The user of such a scaler should be cognizant of the limitations of the system that he is using.

As is the case with the amplifiers and analyzers discussed above, scalers have specific requirements with respect to the shape and amplitude of the input pulse. Proper functioning of the system requires careful matching of the components.

3. Timers

The assay of radioactivity requires not only the tabulation of the number of counts produced in a detector but also a measurement of the time interval during which the counts were collected. The count-rate may then be calculated and related to the radioactivity. Timing therefore plays as important a role as scaling in nuclear measurements.

The widely used electromechanical timers are driven by synchronous electric motors. Elapsed time and preset time models are available. The limitations on accuracy imposed by the clutch mechanism and by reading the smallest graduation on the dial are of a fixed nature, independent of the length of the time interval measured. Although fixed uncertainties of 0.1 to 0.2 sec are most common, errors as large as 1 sec exist with some preset timers. Therefore, 100 sec may be required for 1% precision even though the count-rate exceeds 100 counts per second.

Electronic timers feature accuracy of at least 0.01 min and in some cases as good as 10 μsec. These timers consist essentially of a fast decimal scaler, as described before, pulsed by a standard oscillator. Crystal controlled oscillators are used in some timing units. The output of the timer may be visual or may be printed automatically. The latter feature is assuming increased importance as more and more automatic counting systems are coming into use.

Most scalers measure the number of counts that appear in a fixed, preset time interval. The length of time may be chosen (1 min, 100 sec, and so forth) so that the calculation of count-rate is simplified. Replicate determinations may be made and averaged directly. Sometimes, however, the preset count mode of operation is to be preferred. The scaler measures the amount of time required to accumulate a specified number of counts. This mode is usually chosen when the same statistical accuracy is desired for each sample measured. The method used to calculate the average count-rate when replicate preset count mode data are obtained can lead to errors (*29*), however. The average of the elapsed time should be computed, rather than the average of the individually calculated count-rates.

B. Ratemeters

Ratemeters give a continuous indication of the pulse rate coming from the detector. Changes in this pulse rate (and changes in the activity of the source) may be followed by the ratemeter and may be printed out or recorded on graph paper for comparison or analysis. One application of ratemeters is, therefore, in dynamic studies, where the accumulation and transportation of radiopharmaceuticals is followed by external detectors. Another application is in the converse situation, where the radioactivity in an organ is fixed but the detector moves during a scanning procedure.

Ratemeters are also used in survey meters and laboratory monitors, since increases in activity need to be promptly indicated.

Although the term ratemeter is usually associated with analog ratemeters, a new class of rate-measuring instruments makes the distinction between analog ratemeters and digital ratemeters necessary. The fundamental difference between these two types lies in the kind of memory used to store information from the incoming pulses. A digital ratemeter is capable of storing the pulse count in digital form as binary or decimal numbers. An analog ratemeter stores a charge, which is proportional to the number of pulses received per unit time.

1. ANALOG RATEMETERS

a. *Linear Ratemeters.* The analog ratemeter that provides a response which is directly proportional to the input count-rate is by far the most commonly used type of ratemeter. Each input pulse is formed so that a fixed amount of charge is added to a "tank" capacitor (C). Charge on this capacitor is allowed to leak through a shunting resistance (R). The charge on the tank capacitor will build up until the rate at which charge leaks off is equal to the rate at which charge is supplied (equilibrium). Thus, the voltage across this integrating network will be proportional to the count-rate when equilibrium is reached.

The delay before equilibrium is reached is a function of the product RC, the time constant of the tank circuit, and of the input count-rate. If the ratemeter is initially at zero, the time necessary for the meter to come to within one standard deviation of the steady state value is given by the equilibrium time (*16*)

$$T_e = RC[0.5 \ln(2nRC) + 0.394]$$

where n is the final average count-rate. For an RC time constant of 100 sec the equation shows that T_e is 304 sec when $n = 1$ cps and T_e is 534 sec when $n = 100$ cps. Thus, significant errors in ratemeter use can occur if the RC time constant is confused with the equilibrium time (Chapter 3, Section I,B,4).

Fluctuations of the output reading of the ratemeter will occur because of the random nature of radioactive decay. The amount of fluctuations to be expected depends upon the circuit time constant and on the count-rate. Longer time constants and higher count-rates produce relatively less statistical uncertainty and therefore result in a more stable meter reading.

The fact that readings must be delayed until equilibrium has been reached implies that the ratemeter will distort the shape of curves obtained when dynamic changes are occurring. Indeed, a compromise must be reached between the curve smoothing that is obtained at higher RC values and the longer response times (Chapter 15, Section II,D). A choice of time constants is usually available on linear ratemeters so that the response times and the statistical fluctuation may have values appropriate to a given situation. As with any analog device, the zero position and the stability of the calibration of linear ratemeters must be checked at frequent intervals if artifactual results are to be avoided.

Stoddart and Berger (*24*) have shown how the lag of an analog ratemeter may be corrected by using Laplace transforms and computer programming. However, this technique does not seem likely to be useful in the average clinical radioisotope laboratory.

b. *Logarithmic Ratemeters.* If several tank circuits with diode drivers (diode pumps) are connected in parallel and the output currents summed through a current meter, the output of the ratemeter will be approximately a logarithmic function of the count-rate (*4*). As many as six decades of count-rate may be spanned on the scale of a logarithmic ratemeter, so that dynamic studies with activities which change rapidly over a wide range may be studied without the scale factor switching that would be necessary to prevent off-scale readings with a linear ratemeter. Another advantage of having a logarithmic scale is found with tracer disappearance studies, since the decrease in activity is frequently an exponential function of the time. The logarithmic ratemeter will portray such a curve as a straight line.

The accuracy of a reading depends upon the degree to which the summed tank circuits approximate a logarithmic function. Furthermore, the small nonlinearities that are present in meters become magnified when projected on a logarithmic scale of several decades. For instance, a 1% meter nonlinearity, which refers to 1% of full scale, is equivalent to about 1 degree of deflection. One degree on a four-decade logarithmic meter scale constitutes about a 10% error in the reading. Thus, the advantages of logarithmic readout are obtained at the cost of accuracy. The more elaborate and expensive logarithmic ratemeters provide scale expansion, decade suppression, and precision meters so that accuracies of 2% may be obtained. Most log-linear ratemeters, however, are restricted to 10 or 20% accuracy on the log scale.

A simplified circuit for a typical three-cycle logarithmic-linear ratemeter is shown in Fig. 22. C_1 to C_4 are the input capacitors; (C_6, $R_{\log}$),

(C_7, $R_{\log}$), and (C_8, $R_{\log}$) are the elements of the three pumps for logarithmic output, whereas (C_5, R_{lin}) constitute the linear tank. Switch S is used to select the mode of operation. The output of each pump is diode limited and the sum of the three pumps provides a logarithmic

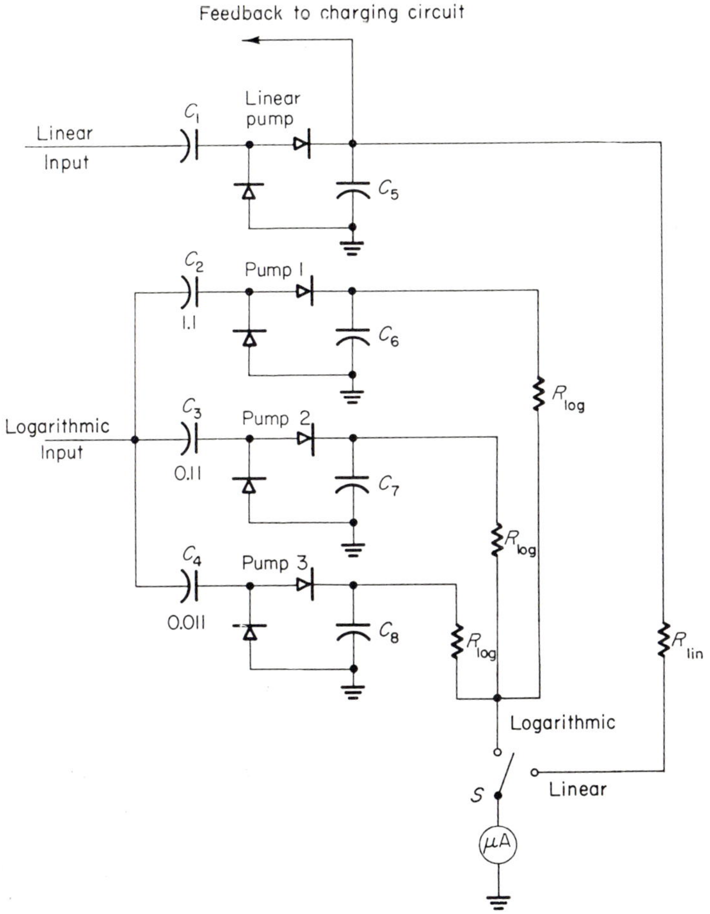

FIG. 22. Schematic of three-cycle log-linear ratemeter (*4*). The microammeter current is either directly proportional or logarithmically related to the input pulse rate. See text for explanation.

response over most of the range N_0 to 10^3N_0, with some errors at each end of the range. Because of the diode limiting feature and because of the relative values chosen for C_2, C_3, and C_4, the current output of pump 1 at an input rate of $10N_0$ is the same as the current output of pump 3 with an input of 10^3N_0. Different full scale ranges for linear operation are obtained in this case by selecting different values for C_1, a feature not shown in Fig. 22. The components of each pump are fixed so that the effective time constant is inversely proportional to the input count-rate. Under these conditions the percent probable error is a constant over the whole range of a logarithmic ratemeter. Thus, the meter fluctuations are of constant amplitude everywhere on the logarithmic scale.

2. Digital Ratemeters

A scaler preset to count for one minute could be considered to be a simple digital ratemeter, since the accumulated counts in the readout need only to be divided by unity to convert to a rate of counts per minute. A series of count-rate measurements may be obtained by repeatedly resetting and recycling the scaler. These operations are performed automatically in some scalers. However, information is lost during the inactive time, the interval when the scaler is being read out, reset, and started. Furthermore, a count to count-rate conversion is required in order to obtain the results in units of counts per minute if shorter counting times are required for rapidly changing dynamic processes.

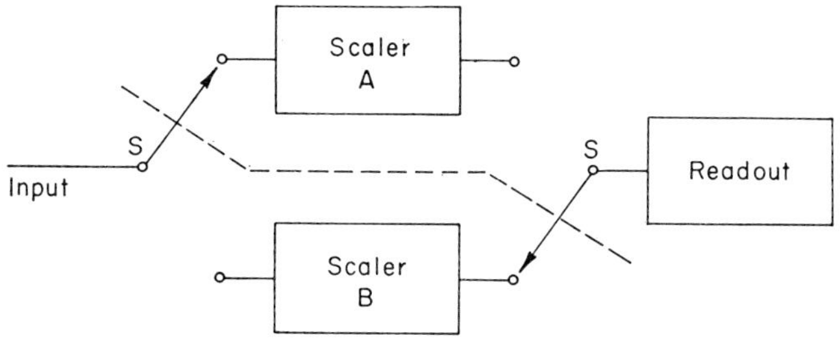

Fig. 23. Digital ratemeter using paired scalers.

The inactive time is usually made minimal by either using a pair of scalers or employing a buffer storage system. The pair of scalers in the digital ratemeter is switched so that one is accumulating counts from the input while the other is reading out its tally from the previous interval. Such a device is shown in Fig. 23. At the end of the time during which scaler A has been counting scaler B will be cleared and the switch S will reverse the roles of the two scalers.

Recycling scalers using *buffer storage* are the most common type of digital ratemeter. Figure 24 illustrates the principle of the buffer storage technique. At the conclusion of the preselected counting interval the program control causes the count to be transferred to the buffer storage, resets the scaler, and begins the next count. The buffer storage may have BCD stages like the scaler which, however, are used only for the storage of a number rather than for tabulation. The inactive time may be made fairly short in this system, typically 10 μsec. As with the paired scaler system the relatively slow readout process may make use of the complete preset counting time.

If the recycling scaler type of a digital ratemeter is to provide a readout in units of counts per unit time (and thus justify its classification as a ratemeter) the accumulated number of counts must be normalized to a rate. This procedure would require the computer capability of performing a division if an unrestricted choice of counting intervals were desired. A limited selection of intervals is usually acceptable, however, so that the design of the digital ratemeter is considerably simplified.

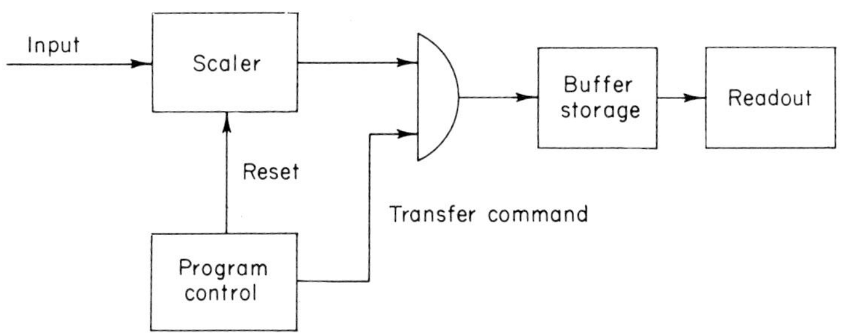

FIG. 24. Digital ratemeter using buffer storage.

In this case prescalers with scaling factors proportional to the available counting times are used. This insures that the number of pulses accumulated in the scaler at a given rate is independent of the time interval chosen, so that the readout may be in units of rate.

Readout of a digital ratemeter may be visual, as with Nixie tubes, printed, punched, or graphical. In the latter case the plot produced with a strip chart recorder appears as a histogram.

Analog ratemeters are generally less expensive than digital ratemeters, but the latter enjoy some rather important advantages. Analog devices are subject to zero drift and require calibration adjustments that are not necessary when digital techniques are used. Punched paper tape readout of digital ratemeters makes direct computer processing of the data possible. Most important, however, is the fact that there is no time lag with a digital ratemeter.

ACKNOWLEDGMENT

I would like to thank Robert Hindel and George R. Utting, who prepared a draft of part of this chapter and were kind enough to make their manuscript available to me.

REFERENCES

1. Austin, L. J., "Preamps and Amplifiers for Nuclear Instrumentation." Radiation Instrument Development Laboratory, Chicago, Illinois, 1963.
2. Blalock, T. V., A low-noise charge-sensitive preamplifier with a field-effect transistor in the input stage. *IEEE, Trans. Nucl. Sci.* **11,** No. 3, 365 (1964).
3. Chase, R. L., "Nuclear Pulse Spectrometry," McGraw-Hill, New York, 1961.
4. Cooke-Yarborough, E. H., and Pulsford, E. W., An accurate logarithmic counting-rate meter covering a wide range. *Proc. Inst. Elec. Engrs.* (*London*) *Pt. II* **98,** 196 (1951).
5. Editors of Nucleonics, Commercially available semiconductor detectors and preamplifiers. *Nucleonics* **22,** No. 5, 62 (1964).
6. Fairstein, E., Pulse Amplifier Manual. U.S. At. Energy Comm. Doc. ORNL 3348 (1962).
7. Gatti, E., and Priva, F., A new single channel elementary amplitude discriminator. *Nuovo Cimento* **10,** 984 (1953).
8. Gilland, J. R., Transistor circuitry for radiation counting. *Rev. Sci. Instr.* **30,** 479 (1959).
9. Herbert, R. J. T., and Hyde, D. B., A pulse tape-recorder for clinical radioisotope work. *Phys. Med. Biol.* **7,** 455 (1963).
10. Higinbotham, W. A., Gallagher, J., and Sands, M., The model 200 pulse counter. *Rev. Sci. Instr.* **18, 706** (1947).
11. Hine, G. J., Farmelant, M. H., Cardarelli, J. A., and Burrows, B. A., Four channel magnetic tape recording and digital analysis of radio-hippuran renal function tests in normal subjects. *J. Nucl. Med.* **4,** 371 (1963).
12. Hinrichsen, P. F., A stabilized scintillation counter. *IEEE, Trans. Nucl. Sci.* **11,** No. 3, 420 (1964).
13. Huff, R. L., Parrish, D., and Crockett, W., A study of circulatory dynamics by means of crystal radiation detectors on the anterior thoracic wall. *Circulation Res.* **5,** 395 (1957).
14. Hutchinson, G. W., and Scarrott, C. G., A high precision pulse height analyzer of moderately high speed. *Phil. Mag.* **42,** 792 (1951).
15. Kandiah, K., A sensitive pulse amplitude discriminator. *Proc. Inst. Elec. Engrs.* (*London*) *Pt. II* **101,** No. 81, 239 (1954).
16. Kniseley, R. M., and Tauxe, W. N. (eds.), "Dynamic Clinical Studies with Radioisotopes," TID-7678. U.S. At. Energy Comm., Washington, D.C., 1964.
17. Lunsford, J. S., Logarithmic pulse amplifier. *Rev. Sci. Instr.* **36,** 461 (1965).
18. McCollom, K. E., Discriminators. *Nucleonics* **17,** No. 6, 72 (1959).
19. Orvis, A. L., Koenig, M. P., and Owen, C. A., Jr., *In-vivo* measurement of thyroidal radioiodine: effect of "neck scatter." *J. Clin. Endocrinol. Metab.* **17,** 966 (1957).
20. Price, W. J., "Nuclear Radiation Detection," 2nd ed. McGraw-Hill, New York, 1964.
21. Schmitt, O., A thermionic trigger. *J. Sci. Instr.* **15,** 24 (1938).
22. Stacy, R. W., "Biological and Medical Electronic," 1st ed. McGraw-Hill, New York, 1960.
23. Stoddart, H. F., Scalers. *Nucleonics* **17,** No. 6, 78 (1959).
24. Stoddart, L. C., and Berger, R. L., Response time corrections to data from detection and recording systems. *Rev. Sci. Instr.* **36,** 85 (1965).

25. Strauss, M. G., Solid-state pulse-height encoding system with pileup reduction for counting at high input rates. *Rev. Sci. Instr.* **34,** 335 (1963).
26. Technical Measurements Corporation, "The Many Views of Na^{22}," TMC SB2 10 M 9/63. New Haven, Connecticut, 1963.
27. Trenholme, W. M., Current-input amplifiers for nuclear pulse spectrometry. *Atomics* **18,** No. 1, 37 (1965).
28. Wilkinson, D. H., A stable ninety-nine channel pulse amplitude analyzer for slow counting. *Proc. Cambridge Phil. Soc.* **46,** 508 (1950).
29. Zilversmit, D. B., and Orvis, A. L., Calculating average counting rates. *Nucleonics* **14,** No. 7, 75 (1956).

CHAPTER 8

RADIATION SAFETY INSTRUMENTS

RICHARD C. McCALL* AND JAMES A. WALL
CONTROLS FOR RADIATION, INC.
CAMBRIDGE, MASSACHUSETTS

In every laboratory or hospital using X-ray generators or radioactive materials it is necessary to have some radiation protection instrumentation. One needs to know if personnel have received a large dose of radiation in case of an accident, if they are receiving unnecessarily large chronic doses in the course of their normal work, and if contamination has occurred. In addition it is desirable to measure doses received by patients from therapeutic or diagnostic use of X rays or radioactive materials. This chapter presents the general characteristics of a broad range of radiation dosimeters (*3*). No attempt is made to treat them in detail or to provide a complete bibliography.

I. DOSE-RATE MONITORS AND SURVEY METERS

A. Types of Instruments

A *dose-rate monitor* gives a continuous indication of the radiation intensity at one or more points within an area where the radiation intensity may change owing to the manipulation of sources of ionizing radiation, such as radioactive isotopes.

An *area monitor* is a dose-rate monitor that is usually permanently installed in a radioisotope laboratory. Its purpose is to maintain a

* Present address: Linear Accelerator Center, Stanford University, Stanford, California.

constant check on the radiation intensities in such key laboratory areas as the source storage room or the hot laboratory where intense radioactive sources are handled, and also to ascertain that the radiation intensities in other areas in and around the laboratory remain below the maximum permissible safety limits.

A *laboratory bench monitor* is a semiportable dose-rate monitor that is ordinarily kept in the laboratory work area where radiochemistry, source mounting, and so on may be performed. The primary purpose of a bench monitor is to warn the laboratory worker if he should inadvertently attempt to use an excessive quantity of radioactive material. It is also useful for making rough radioassays, for checking the worker's hands for radioactive contamination, and for checking the work area for spills of radioactive solutions.

A *personnel monitor* or personal radiation alarm is a dose-rate monitor small enough to be carried in a pocket. Its purpose is to warn the wearer, usually by an audible signal, if he should enter a region of unusually high radiation intensity or if the radiation intensity in his area should suddenly increase.

A *survey meter* is a compact, portable radiation intensity measuring instrument. They are used to check the adequacy of shielding around radioactive sources, to locate areas that may have become contaminated with radioactive materials, to determine the radiation intensities in areas in the vicinity of the laboratory that cannot or need not be continuously monitored.

Some of the commercially available dose-rate monitors and survey meters are shown in Fig. 1.

In selecting an instrument for a particular application, it must first be ascertained that the instrument has adequate sensitivity, range, and accuracy. A choice can then be made on the basis of cost, size, and ease of operation. The radiation detector used in any type of instrument determines its sensitivity, range, and accuracy. It also affects to a large extent the cost, reliability, ruggedness, and other instrument characteristics such as its response to temperature or humidity changes.

1. Geiger–Müller Counter Instruments

All commercially available *laboratory bench monitors* employ G-M counters as the radiation detecting element. Except for minor differences in cabinet design and location of controls, the basic design of bench monitors does not vary much. A typical bench monitor is shown in Fig. 1. The G-M counter is attached to the end of a 3- to 4-ft long cable and can be clipped to the instrument cabinet. The thin end-window of the counter normally supplied with the instrument is protected by a removable cover or heavy wire mesh screen.

A meter on the front panel of the monitor indicates count-rate in counts per minute. Some monitors are also calibrated in terms of dose-rate (milliroentgens per hour). A loudspeaker in the cabinet produces a click each time a pulse is produced by the G-M counter, thus enabling one to qualitatively determine the count-rate without observing the meter.

Most commercially available laboratory bench monitors presently employ vacuum tubes rather than transistors. They operate from the

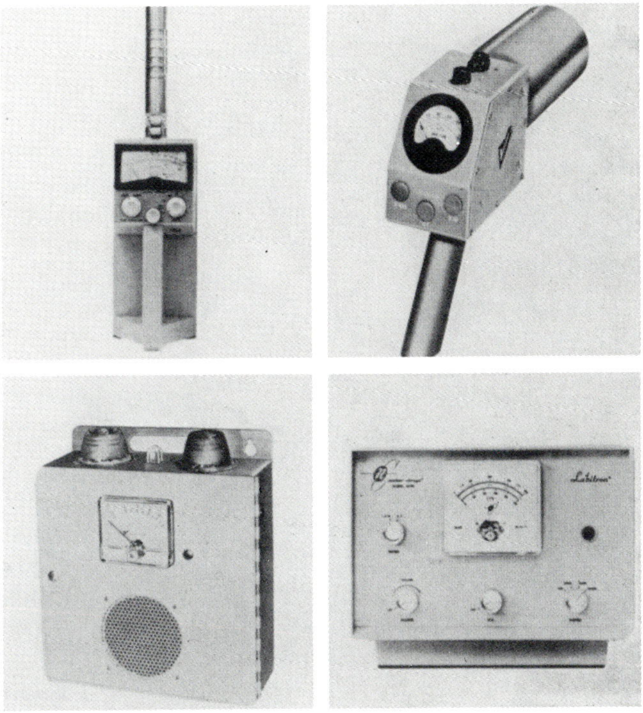

Fig. 1. *Upper left:* Nuclear-Chicago (β, γ)-ray G-M counter survey meter. *Upper right:* Victoreen Cutie Pie survey meter. *Lower left:* Victoreen Vamp area monitor. *Lower right:* Nuclear-Chicago Labitron laboratory bench monitor.

a.c. line and are light enough to be moved around the laboratory; a typical bench monitor weighs about 20 lb. Bench monitors cost between $400 and $600.

Because of their high sensitivity per unit volume and weight and the reliability attainable in their associated electronic circuitry, G-M counters are the most commonly used radiation detectors in *portable survey instruments.* Most late-model G-M survey meters are fully transistorized and can operate for 100 hr or more on a single set of flashlight or portable radio batteries. The G-M counters used in survey meters may be either thin end-window tubes or thin-walled tubes. The end-window tubes are usually provided with a screen to protect the window. The thin-walled tubes are enclosed in a metal case, a portion of which is movable to expose a section of the counter wall when α or β particles are to be counted. The G-M counter is often attached to a short length of cable to enable its use as a probe; it rests in the carrying handle of the instrument when not used. A typical G-M survey meter is shown in Fig. 1. Geiger–Müller survey meters are small in size and weigh only a few pounds; they cost from $150 to $250.

Miniature G-M counters are used in some *personal radiation alarms* such as the Numec* "Chirpie" and the Gelman† "Sparrow." These devices are small enough to be carried unobtrusively in a pocket, the Chirpie being about as long as and twice the diameter of a fountain pen. The Sparrow is about half the size of a pack of king-sized cigarettes. They employ transistorized circuits and the batteries used in them last for 50 to 100 hr of continuous operation. The Chirpie and the Sparrow emit audible chirps or pulses at a rate of about one per second under normal background conditions. The recurrence rate of the pulses increases roughly in proportion to the dose-rate. A neon lamp that flashes in synchronism with the audible pulses provides a visual indication of relative radiation intensity and is useful in noisy areas.

The Chirpie employs a special circuit to prevent the G-M counter from blocking at high dose-rates. The Sparrow, at least in its earlier versions, did not have such a provision. The commercial availability of either of these devices is questionable, owing partly to manufacturing difficulties associated with the miniature G-M counters and partly to the lack of demand for such units. When available, they cost approximately $80.

Another personal monitoring instrument employing a G-M counter is the "Nu-Tec" pocket fallout meter‡. It is actually a miniature survey meter about the size of a cigarette pack, with a meter calibrated in mR/hr over the range of 1 mR/hr to 100 R/hr. A jack is provided to which a miniature headphone can be connected. The unit is priced at less than $50.

Owing to the finite dead-time of G-M counters, an instrument can block at high dose-rates. As the radiation intensity to which a G-M counter is exposed increases, coincidence losses cause the rate at which the counter produces pulses to become less proportional to the radiation

* Numec Nuclear Instrument and Controls Corp.

† Gelman Instrument Co.

‡ Nuclear Corp. of America.

intensity. At sufficiently high radiation intensities, the count-rate decreases with increasing radiation intensity. When blocking occurs, the instrument may appear to be operating normally but could indicate a dose-rate several orders of magnitude lower than the true rate. Because of their tendency to block, G-M counter instruments should not be relied upon as the only means of measuring dose-rates above about 50 mR/hr. Nonblocking G-M counter instruments that employ special electronic circuits are available, but they are an uneconomical choice for general laboratory use. They usually cost as much as ionization chamber instruments which are much more accurate and also can be used to measure dose-rates of hundreds of R/hr.

Most G-M counters presently used in radiation safety instruments are halogen-quenched types (Chapter 4). They are preferable to the organically quenched counters primarily because of their ability to withstand exposures to excessive radiation intensities and the constancy of their characteristics over a long time.

2. Ionization Chamber Instruments

Ionization chambers are made in many different forms, each being suited to a particular application (*3*). The ionization chambers used in most health physics applications consist of a cylindrical outer electrode and a small-diameter inner electrode. The outer cylinder is closed at both ends and the connection to the inner electrode is provided through a suitable insulator. The chamber is filled with dry air at atmospheric pressure and hermetically sealed. For some special applications, such as in the Victoreen M-50 miniature γ-ray survey meter, the chamber may be filled with a monatomic gas such as argon at pressures above atmospheric to obtain greater sensitivity per unit volume. The air-filled ionization chambers are usually constructed with tissue equivalent plastic walls. This type of chamber is used to make the most accurate radiation dose-rate measuring instruments available commercially. Most argon-filled chambers are constructed with metal walls.

The ionization chamber used in the Cutie Pie *survey meter* (Fig. 1) is about 3 inches in diameter and 5 inches long, giving a volume of about 600 ml. The minimum dose-rate that can be measured with a Cutie Pie using this size chamber is approximately 1 mR/hr. By comparison, the argon-filled, metal ionization chamber used on the Victoreen Radector has about one-tenth the volume of the Cutie Pie chamber and can be used to measure dose-rates down to 0.05 mR/hr. However, this is not a strictly fair comparison because of the great differences in electronic circuitry between the two instruments. Both chambers remain useful to over 100 R/hr, although the maximum calibration on a particular instrument may be less than this by a factor of 10 or more.

The Cutie Pie type of instrument has a pistol-grip handle to which is attached a case containing the electronic circuits, indicating meter, and controls (Fig. 1). The air-filled, plastic-walled ionization chamber protrudes from the front of the case, forming a gun-type configuration to which the name Cutie Pie applies. Cutie Pie survey meters are available with a variety of full scale ranges. Victoreen, for example, supplies three Cutie Pie models, one with full scale ranges of 100, 1000, and 10,000 mR/hr; another with ranges of 50, 500 and 5000 mR/hr; and the third with ranges of 25, 250, and 2500 mR/hr. Nuclear-Chicago, on the other hand, supplies different ionization chambers that can be plugged into one basic instrument to obtain full scale ranges from 25 mR/hr to 250 R/hr.

Ionization chamber survey instruments like the Victoreen Radector and Radgun are worth noting because of their unique dose-rate range measuring capabilities. These instruments employ argon-filled, metal-walled ionization chambers with a special circuit (a vacuum tube actually mounted inside the chamber) that gives a logarithmic dose-rate scale on the indicating meter. The Radgun has three ranges, 0.01–10 mR/hr, 0.01–10 R/hr, and 10–10^4 R/hr. The Radector has two ranges, 0.05–50 mR/hr and 0.05–50 R/hr.

Ionization chambers are the most widely used radiation detectors in *area monitors* (Fig. 1). The ionization chambers are generally air filled and have aluminum walls. They are of various sizes depending on the range of dose-rates they are required to monitor and are ordinarily located remotely from the indicating and alarm control instrumentation. Vacuum tubes within the chambers amplify the minute ionization current before it is transmitted to the control station. Radioactive sources inside the chambers located behind electrically operated movable shields can be used to test and calibrate the instrument. The control instrumentation may consist of one or more channels, each channel corresponding to one ionization chamber location. A channel includes the necessary power supplies, controls, and indicating meter. Audible and visual alarms are triggered when a preset dose-rate is reached in the area being monitored.

Because of the very small electric currents available from ionization chambers at dose-rates of a few milliroentgens per hour, the "zero" setting of ionization chamber instruments tends to drift. This drift is the result of spurious currents arising from various causes such as moisture across the chamber connections, temperature changes, and so on. This is why the "zero adjust" controls are made readily accessible on most ionization chamber instruments. This drift is not severe unless an instrument is subjected to unusual conditions of shock, temperature or humidity changes, or dirty or smoky atmospheres. Generally, if an ionization chamber instrument is zeroed soon after it is turned on, then rezeroed about a half hour later, it will maintain the adjustment for several hours.

Ionization chamber instruments are slow in response, requiring some time for the indicating meter to reach its final reading after the chamber is exposed to radiation. This is because the sensitive electronic circuits necessary to measure the small electrical currents from an ionization chamber are inherently slow (*2*).

3. SCINTILLATION COUNTER INSTRUMENTS

The application of scintillation counters to radiation safety instrumentation has been limited. This is primarily because the electronic circuitry that must be used with scintillation counters is more expensive than is required with G-M counters and ionization chambers in comparable instruments. For example, scintillation counters require a high-voltage power supply similar to those used with G-M counters, but with a much more constant output voltage and capable of delivering more current.

The indicating meters and operating controls on the few commercially available, scintillation counter, health physics instruments such as the Victoreen Thyac II are similar to those used on G-M counter and ionization chamber instruments. Portable survey instruments using scintillation counters are generally somewhat larger and heavier than the other types of survey instruments.

B. Performance of Monitors and Survey Instruments

The minimum radiation intensity that can be detected with a given type of monitor or survey instrument is determined by practical considerations relating primarily to the type of detector used in the instrument. For example, the sensitivity of an instrument using an ionization chamber is limited by the leakage current across the insulators between the electrodes of the chamber and the maximum volume that the chamber can have for its intended application. In general, portable survey instruments must sacrifice some sensitivity in favor of reasonable size, weight, and ruggedness. Fixed monitors can utilize the maximum sensitivity capabilities of a detector, cost being the prime consideration. Table I lists typical sensitivities and ranges for γ- and X-radiation measuring instruments. The data in the table are representative of commercially available radiation safety instruments rather than of the maximum capabilities of the detectors.

The γ- and X-radiation energy dependence of a radiation detector is determined by several factors involved in the design of the detector

(Chapter 4, Section II). Table II lists γ-ray energy dependences for commercially available radiation safety instruments employing various detector types. The data represent the smallest typical energy dependences claimed by instrument manufacturers rather than average values.

TABLE I

PHOTON SENSITIVITIES AND RANGES FOR INSTRUMENTS EMPLOYING THE INDICATED DETECTOR TYPES

Detector	Sensitivity (mR/hr)	Range (mR/hr)	Remarks
Air-filled ionization chamber	0.1	$0.5–10^6$	Full range not obtainable with a single chamber. One chamber covers about three to four decades of dose-rate.
Argon-filled ionization chamber	0.005	$0.01–10^7$	High-pressure chamber.
G-M counters	Natural background	0–50	Upper limit in the R/hr range when antiblocking circuits are used.
Scintillation counters	Natural background	0–50	Range limited more by circuit design than by detector properties.

TABLE II

ENERGY DEPENDENCE FOR INSTRUMENTS EMPLOYING THE INDICATED DETECTOR TYPES

Detector	Percent energy dependence (γ, X rays)	Energy range (γ, X rays)	Minimum energy of detectable β rays (keV)
Air-filled ionization chamber with plastic wall	±5 ±10	80 keV to 1.2 MeV 50 keV to 2 MeV	40
Argon-filled ionization chamber with steel wall	±25	80 keV to 2 MeV	100
G-M counter in metal shield	±20	100 keV to 2 MeV	50
Scintillation counter with thick (2.5 cm) organic crystal	±10	100 keV to 5 MeV	60

Also listed in Table II is the minimum β-ray energy that can be detected by the instruments. The detectability of β rays depends upon the detector having a thin window specifically designed for β-ray detection, as does, for example, the Nuclear-Chicago Cutie Pie. Because external α radiation does not produce a significant radiation hazard, the sensitivity for α-particle detection is not listed. However, most detectors fitted with thin windows for β-ray measurement can be used to detect α particles with energies greater than 4 MeV.

Unless they have been designed for outdoor use, radiation safety instruments are not intended for use where they may be subjected to frequent mechanical shocks or vibration. Special ruggedized instruments such as the Victoreen EP 270 survey meter are available for use in such environments. Of the detectors (excluding solid state detectors), ionization chambers are most resistant to accidental damage by shock or vibration, but the electronic circuits associated with them are usually fairly delicate. Electrometer tubes can be permanently damaged by a minor shock although no apparent physical damage may occur. A slight change in the position of one of the electrodes can radically alter the characteristics of an electrometer tube, completely destroying instrument calibration.

Geiger–Müller counters vary considerably in their ability to withstand mechanical shocks. In addition to possible breakage of its window or glass wall, shock or vibration may loosen or completely disconnect the anode wire of a counter from one of its supports.

A much neglected portion of portable survey instruments is the battery clip. The battery clips in some commercial instruments hold the batteries so loosely that even in normal handling one or more batteries may become dislodged or make poor contact with the clip. A battery in poor contact with its clip can cause loss of calibration or erratic behavior of an instrument.

II. INTEGRATED DOSE INDICATORS

In many cases, particularly in personnel monitoring applications, it is not as important to know the instantaneous dose-rate as it is to know the total dose received by an individual or at a particular location over a period of time. Often the dose-rate is changing in a rapid and unpredictable manner so that it is impractical to monitor it at all times and estimate the dose from the results. In other cases, particularly at very low levels, measurement of the integrated dose for a known period of time constitutes the most accurate way of measuring the average dose-rate during that time.

A. Types of Dosimeters

1. FILM BADGES

Almost every worker who is either actually or potentially exposed to radiation now wears a film badge. Therefore, at least from the standpoint of quantity, the film badge is the most important radiation detector today. Estimates of the number of film badges processed per month in the United States fall in the range of several hundred thousands.

The film badge consists of a plastic holder containing a piece of photographic film in a light-tight paper wrapper. The paper-wrapped film is identical in construction to that used for dental X rays. The plastic holder protects the film from mechanical damage and provides a means of attaching it to the wearer.

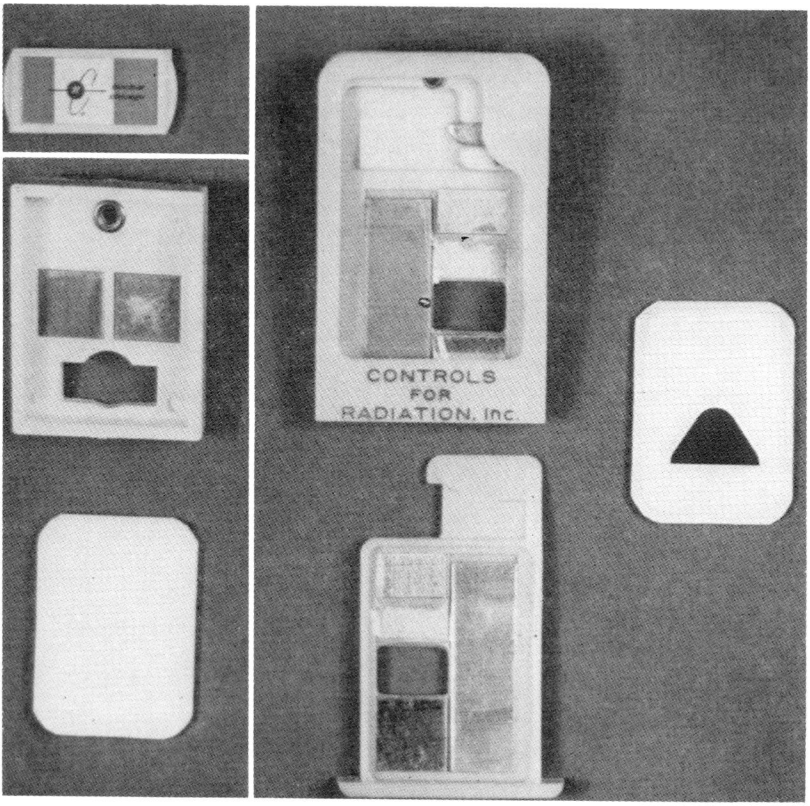

FIG. 2. Film badges. *Left:* a simple film badge with two absorbers. *Right:* the Hanford tamper-proof badge with four absorbers.

In most cases the film badge also provides some information concerning the nature of the radiation detected. In its simplest form, the film badge holder has a small window which allows β rays to impinge directly upon the film wrapping. If the radiation detected is due to β rays in addition to X or γ radiation, the film will be exposed more under the open window than on the rest of the film. A rough estimate can then be made of the fraction of the dose due to penetrating radiation and the fraction which can cause only a skin exposure. More elaborate film badge holders have one or more small metal absorbers inside the plastic to absorb the softer portion of the X and γ radiation. Measurement of the exposure under the various absorbers gives an indication of the penetration and energy of the radiation producing the exposure.

Examples of film badges are shown in Fig. 2. On the left is shown a relatively simple film badge with an open window and two metal filters. On the right is shown the Hanford film badge with an open window, and four metal absorbers. With this more complex film badge an estimate of the γ-ray energies involved would be reported. The film badge on the right is also tamper proof, that is, it requires a magnetic device to open it for film changing.

For the small laboratory, to use a commercial film badge service is simple and economical. Such services supply the customer with film badges, mail new films when it is time for changes, make regular reports of measured doses and keep records of the results. The Buyers Guide issue of *Nucleonics* (August 1965) lists 18 companies supplying film badge service in the United States.

2. Condenser Ionization Chambers

If an ionization chamber is charged to a certain voltage and the voltage source is disconnected, the ionization chamber can then be considered as a charged condenser. Exposure of the condenser ionization chamber to ionizing radiation produces ions, which are collected on the electrodes of opposite polarity, and the voltage between the electrodes decreases proportionately.

In order to use the condenser ionization chamber, it is necessary to have a device to charge it to a given voltage ready for use and a device to read the voltage after exposure. These devices are usually incorporated into a single charger-reader. Older charger-readers utilized a quartz fiber electrometer as the reading element. This is a device that measures voltage by observing the electrostatic deflection of a thin quartz filament when exposed to the voltage on the ionization chamber electrodes. By a suitable optical system, the shadow of the quartz fiber is cast upon a scale which is calibrated directly in terms of dose. Some newer charger-readers display the dose directly upon a meter. A common modification is to incorporate the quartz fiber electrometer directly into the ionization chamber. This allows the ionization chamber to be "direct reading," that is, it can be read anywhere without access to a reader.

Examples of condenser ionization chambers and readers are shown in Fig. 3. At the upper left is a transistorized charger for direct reading ionization chambers. The device at the upper right is a modern transistorized charger-reader for indirect reading chambers. It can be used for the 0–200 mR pencil-sized chambers (personnel dosimeters, lower left) and also for the larger ionization chambers for low-dose measurements (lower right). The pocket chamber shown is accurate for dose-rates up to

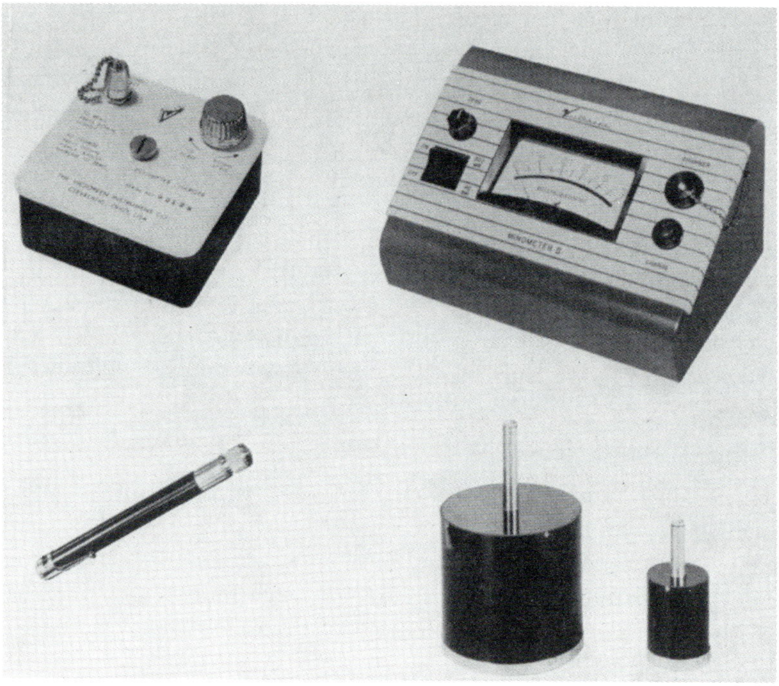

FIG. 3. Condenser ionization chambers and readers (Courtesy of the Victoreen Instrument Company). *Upper left:* A charger for direct-reading ionization chambers. *Upper right:* A charger-reader for indirect-reading ionization chambers. *Lower left:* An indirect-reading pocket ionization chamber for personal dosimetry. *Lower right:* Two large indirect-reading ionization chambers for low-dose measurements.

100 R/hr. The major advantage of condenser ionization chambers is that the dose can be ascertained in a few seconds.

3. THERMOLUMINESCENT DOSIMETERS

A new method of dosimetry is based upon the property of thermoluminescence. When exposed to ionizing radiation, certain materials have the ability to store a portion of the absorbed energy in the form of trapped electrons. If these trapped electrons later receive sufficient thermal energy, they can escape from the trap and return to the ground state, often emitting light in the process. This process is referred to as thermoluminescence.

Many natural materials such as calcite and limestone are thermoluminescent and have received very large amounts of natural radiation since their formation. The thermoluminescent light from these is bright enough to be seen if they are heated in a dark room. The light output can be measured with a photomultiplier and is a measure of the absorbed radiation dose. The thermoluminescent materials most used for dosimetry are CaF_2, LiF, and $CaSO_4$.

Since CaF_2 reacts with the atmosphere it must be used enclosed in an inert atmosphere. Several forms of this dosimeter have been developed at the U.S. Naval Research Laboratory (*6*) but are not commercially available. LiF is relatively inert and is used as a dosimeter in the form of a loose powder (*1*). Several commercial dosimetry systems employing LiF are now available.* LiF heated to readout temperature in the presence of oxygen produces a luminescence unrelated to radiation history. This causes a sort of background of several hundred milliroentgens and prevents measurement of doses lower than about 100 mR. Use of a nitrogen atmosphere in the reader, however, allows measurement down to below 10 mR (*4*).

B. Performance of Dose Indicators

A variety of dosimeters is needed to cover the range from studies of natural environmental dose-rates of about 0.25 mR/day to radiation damage experiments at dose-rates in excess of 10^7 R/sec. Workers risk exposure to an equally wide range of doses. In addition, requirements of accuracy, number of dosimeters, energy response, and detector size vary widely in different applications (*2, 3*).

The approximate range over which some types of dosimeters are useful is shown in Fig. 4. The bars representing the Victoreen roentgen meter and the Stephen pocket ionization chambers are composites since it requires several different chambers used with a single reader to cover that range. The Victoreen roentgen meter utilizes nine overlapping chambers to cover the range from a few milliroentgens to 250 R and Stephen offers pocket ionization chambers ranging from 0.2 to 1000 R full scale. A single condenser ionization chamber usually has a range of less than two decades.

Most film badges use both high- and low-sensitivity emulsions, either as two separate films or as a single film with a different emulsion on each side. Normally, the high-sensitivity emulsion is read (range 0.03 to 10 R).

* Controls for Radiation, Inc.; Madison Research & Development Laboratories, Inc.

If it is so exposed as to be too opaque for accurate measurement it is scraped off and the low-sensitivity emulsion is used. The LiF thermoluminescent dosimeter is linear up to about 10^3 R. Doses up to 10^5 R can be read by reference to a calibration curve.

If dosimeters would absorb radiation in exactly the same manner as it is absorbed in air, they would yield true dose measurements independent of the radiation energy. This occurs for all common dosimeters for photon energies from 500 keV to a few MeV. Below 500 keV, the photoelectric effect causes an energy absorption in many dosimeters

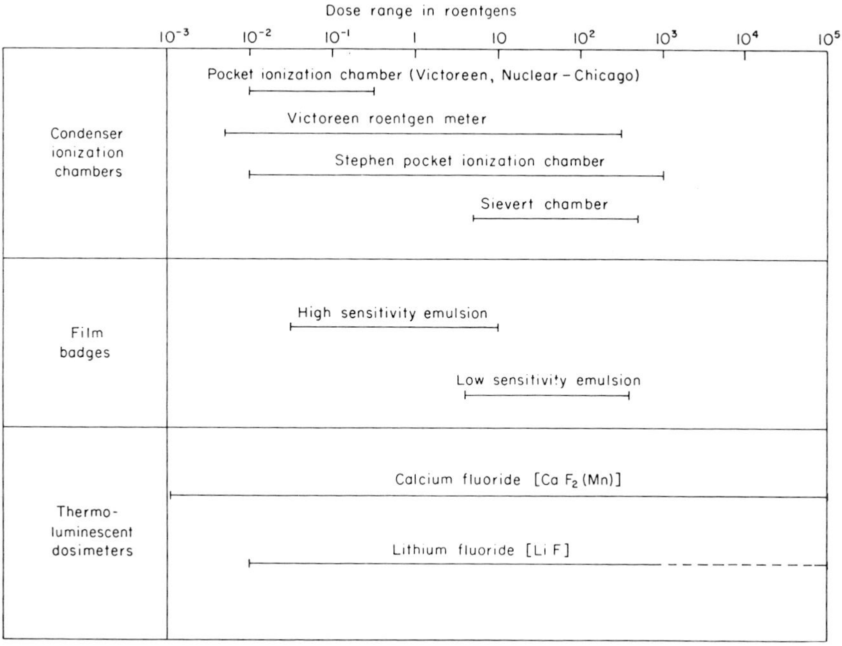

FIG. 4. Dose ranges for various types of dosimeters.

different from that of air. This may result in a large error, especially for low-energy X-ray dosage. For example, a 100-mR dose of 100 keV (effective) X rays would read about 110 mR on a Victoreen Model 362 pocket ionization chamber and about 400 mR on a film badge (read under the thin cadmium shield). Therefore, if possible, radiation dosimeters should always be calibrated against the same type of radiation as that to be measured.

For routine personnel dosimetry a delay of 1 or 2 weeks encountered in commercial film badge services is usually not important. By contrast, workers in a high radiation level area need to know their exposure immediately in order not to exceed the permissible limit. For most medical work it is usually desired to obtain the dose data in a comparatively short time. Essentially all dosimeters discussed can be read out in a few minutes, with the exception of the film badge, which requires several hours. The direct reading condenser ionization chamber is the

TABLE III
Readout Methods for Dosimeters

Dosimeter type	Treatment	Type of measurement	Auxiliary equipment required
Film badge	Developing, drying	Optical densitometry	Dark room and associated equipment, calibration source, densitometer
Condenser ionization chambers	None	Voltage measurement with an electrometer	Charger or charger-reader
Thermoluminescent dosimeter	Heating	Measurement of emitted light	Reader, phosphor dispenser

fastest since it is not necessary to move it from the exposure site to a reader. The readout methods for the dosimeters and the type of measurements required are summarized in Table III.

In considering the cost of a dosimeter system such factors as the number of exposures to be made at one time, the number of exposures over long periods of time, and the length of time the entire dosimetry system will be usable must be considered. Some of the economics of

TABLE IV
Economics of Dosimeter Systems

Dosimeter type	Initial cost ($) for 10 dosimeters and auxiliary equipment	Initial cost ($) for 100 dosimeters and auxiliary equipment
Condenser ionization chambers		
Direct reading	420	3840
Indirect reading	210	880
Thermoluminescent dosimeter		
Con-Rad LiF	4713	4785

representative dosimeter systems with reusable dosimeters are shown in Table IV. The prices given are for representative dosimeter systems of that type and are not necessarily the least expensive systems available. The center column would be representative of the costs for a small laboratory or hospital while the right-hand column would be applicable to a larger installation with 50–100 employees in positions involving possible radiation exposure. For a still larger installation requiring 1000 dosimeters, the thermoluminescent dosimeter system becomes the most economical.

The cost of a system for doing film dosimetry on a small scale, for example, 100 badges per month, is estimated at $800 initial investment, exclusive of a dark room, plus materials charges of about $0.05 per film and about $3 each for the plastic film badge itself. The small laboratory often finds it most economical to use a commercial film badge service. Typical costs of such a service are $15 per month for 10 film badges read biweekly and $85 per month for 100 film badges read at the same interval. Cost estimates for other dosimeter systems are given by Schall (*5*).

III. CALIBRATION OF INSTRUMENTS

It is not sufficient to rely on a dosimeter system without occasional recalibration. All dosimeter and dose-rate measuring devices can have failures in which the equipment will operate but give incorrect results. One solution is to return the instrument regularly to the manufacturer or to the National Bureau of Standards for recalibration. Since this requires considerable time, most installations prefer to have some method of their own for periodical recalibration.

One of the simplest methods of calibrating a radiation detector is to expose it to a radioactive source whose strength, decay scheme, and half-life are well known. For example, 1-mg (1 mCi) radium source emits γ rays that produce dose-rates of 8.26 R/hr, 83 mR/hr, and 0.8 mR/hr at 1, 10, and 100 cm, respectively. In principle, it should be possible to calibrate a radiation detector over a wide dose range by exposure to a standard source and by making use of the inverse square law. However, this holds only for conditions where scattering of the γ rays is negligible and where the dimensions of the detector are small compared with the distance to the source. This method calibrates the detector only for the γ-ray energy spectrum of that particular isotope and the instrument calibration in terms of dose-rate has little meaning when α and β radiation are measured.

When it is not possible to make an absolute γ-ray dose calibration, it is worthwhile to make relative checks. For example, a simple jig can be made to hold dosimeters and survey meters in a precise geometrical relationship to an uncalibrated source of some long-lived radioisotope. If the instruments are tested periodically and records kept for each instrument, calibration accuracy can be maintained quite well. Corrections must be made, of course, for radioactive decay of the source.

Film badge dosimetry offers special problems in calibration. Each batch of film differs in sensitivity and should be calibrated separately by exposing one or more badges to a γ-ray source or to an X-ray machine. During the exposure a good condenser ionization chamber should be exposed at the same time to measure the dose received by the film.

Some dosimeters have a built-in calibration system such as the light sources provided with thermoluminescent dose readers. Some dose-rate indicators have a built-in β-ray source for calibration purposes, such as the Victoreen remote area monitor, using ionization chambers as detectors. Each ionization chamber contains a ^{90}Sr source, which is normally shielded. By pressing a button at the control console, a relay can be made to uncover the ^{90}Sr source and provide a calibration exposure. The Victoreen Radgun is an example of a survey meter with a similar provision. Other survey meters supply a separate β-ray source to be used in checking the instrument's calibration. An example of this type is the Nuclear-Chicago Cutie Pie survey meter which provides a ^{14}C source for calibration purposes.

All such devices are subject to errors and should be used only as secondary calibration. For example, fluorescence standards and light sources can deteriorate with time or be contaminated with a fluorescent material producing excess light. β-Ray sources can be damaged and lose part of their activity or may not be positioned properly each time. The standard light source in a thermoluminescence dosimeter checks only the light detection and not the heating system.

β-Ray detectors are best calibrated by exposure to a known β-ray flux such as the surface dose of a uranium plaque. Most β-ray detectors are quite sensitive to the energy of the β rays, mostly due to absorption in the β-ray window. Allowance should be made for this in working with low-energy β-ray emitters (Chapter 4, Section II).

REFERENCES

1. Cameron, J. R., Daniels, F., Johnson, N., and Kenney, G., Radiation dosimeter utilizing the thermoluminescence of lithium fluoride. *Science* **134,** 33 (1961).
2. Handloser, J. S., "Health Physics Instrumentation." Macmillan (Pergamon), New York, 1959.
3. Hine, G. J., and Brownell, G. L. (eds.), "Radiation Dosimetry." Academic Press, New York, 1956.
4. McCall, R. C., and Fix, R. C., A sensitive LiF dosimeter for routine beta and gamma personnel monitoring. Health Physics Society Meeting, Cincinnati, Ohio, 1964, *Health Physics* **10,** 602 (1964).
5. Schall, P., Jr., A comparison of dosimetry methods. *Nucleonics* **17,** No. 10, 68 (1959).
6. Schulman, J. H., Attix, F. H., West, E. J., and Ginther, R. J., Thermoluminescence methods in personnel dosimetry. Symposium on Personnel Dosimetry Techniques for External Radiation, Madrid, Spain. OECD European Nuclear Agency, Paris, p. 319, 1963.

PART III
MEASUREMENTS OF BIOLOGICAL SAMPLES

CHAPTER 9

PREPARATION OF SAMPLES FOR LIQUID SCINTILLATION COUNTING

EDWARD RAPKIN

CONSULTANT

INTERTECHNIQUE, S.A.

PLAISIR (S. ET O.), FRANCE

A sample prepared for liquid scintillation counting includes at least three components—the material being counted, a solvent, and a scintillator. Often a fourth component—ideally an inert additive—is added to facilitate sample preparation. Usually the physical or chemical nature of the sample, rather than the particular radioisotope in question, determines solvents and additives used in sample preparation.

In the subsequent discussion there are occasional performance figures taken from the literature. The reader is advised that recent developments both in instrumentation and, particularly, in multiplier phototube quality have made for significantly improved counting performance, especially for ^3H and quenched ^{14}C samples. Therefore the user of modern instrumentation should anticipate achieving better results for these isotopes than are cited in any paper dated prior to 1965.

I. SCINTILLATORS

The characteristics of a good scintillator are easily specified:

(1) When acted upon by β or α rays it should be an efficient light producer. Light output should be of a wavelength to which the multiplier phototube is adequately responsive.

(2) It should be sufficiently soluble at the working temperature of the system to permit incorporation of an adequate quantity.

(3) It should be chemically stable for reasonable time periods.

(4) It should be economical to employ at the required concentration.

A. *p*-Terphenyl

Though many scintillators have been described since liquid scintillation counting became a practical reality in the early 1950's, few are of importance today. The first scintillator of any significance was *p*-terphenyl (*67, 99*). It performs well and is still a standard against which the performance of other scintillators is compared. It is inexpensive and it is stable. Unfortunately, it has limited solubility at the reduced temperatures employed in most liquid scintillation counters. The emission maximum of *p*-terphenyl is 3406 Å, which is a shorter wavelength than the response maximum (4200–4400 Å) of most glass-faced multiplier phototubes used in commercial liquid scintillation counters. If, however, quartz-faced multiplier phototubes are employed, *p*-terphenyl is more closely matched to their response maxima, which fall at about 3600 Å.

A good liquid scintillator, under ideal conditions, emits about 7 photons per kiloelectron volt of β-ray energy absorbed in the scintillator. Therefore, for a low-energy β-ray emitter such as tritium ($\bar{E}_\beta = 5.6$ keV) the most energetic β rays cause emission of perhaps 130 photons while about half of the events give rise to less than 45 photons. This light output is distributed over the fluorescence emission spectrum of the scintillator (Fig. 1).

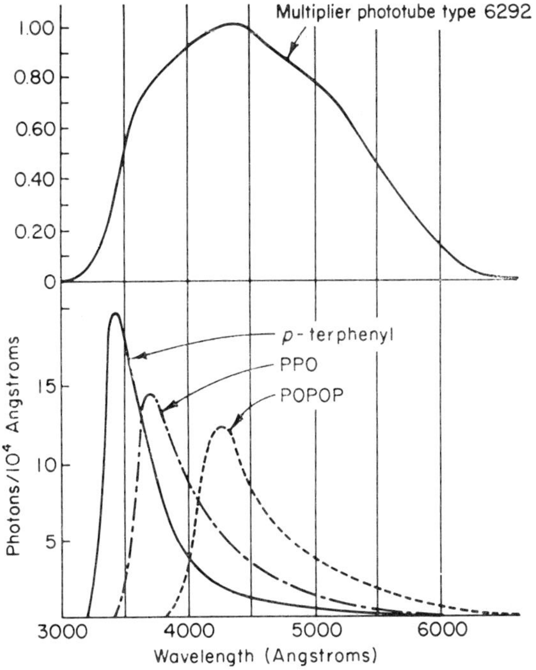

FIG. 1. Sensitivity spectrum for a type 6292 multiplier phototube and emission spectra of three liquid scintillators. Robert K. Swank *et al., Rev. Sci. Instr.* **29**, 279 (1958).

When *p*-terphenyl is used to measure fairly energetic β-ray emitters such as ^{14}C ($\bar{E}_\beta = 50$ keV), enough photons are produced at the longer wavelengths so that adequate counting results are obtained even though the scintillator is not well matched to multiplier phototube response. However, when measuring a low-energy β-ray emitter such as tritium where total light output is considerably less, *p*-terphenyl by itself is not an adequate scintillator.

In routine liquid scintillation counting of biological samples *p*-terphenyl has not been used primarily because of solubility limitations. However, with the new tendency toward construction of liquid scintillation counters capable of satisfactory operation at higher temperatures, it is expected that the use of *p*-terphenyl for measurement of more energetic β-ray emitters will increase.

B. 2,5-Diphenyloxazole (PPO)

The next important scintillator, 2,5-diphenyloxazole (PPO) (*45*), is still the most widely used scintillator today. It is an efficient photon emitter and is quite soluble in all solvents of interest even at temperatures below 0°C. It is stable and it is relatively inexpensive. The fluorescence maximum of PPO is 3800 Å. It is therefore better matched to multiplier phototube response than is *p*-terphenyl. While PPO is a somewhat poorer light emitter than *p*-terphenyl, its performance is almost identical because of its fluorescence maximum at longer wavelengths. By itself, PPO is a very adequate scintillator for ^{14}C and more energetic β-ray emitters.

For ^{3}H counting it has always been considered advantageous to add a secondary scintillator (see Section I,E) in order to produce a fluorescence spectrum having an emission maximum of longer wavelength. However, this has been true largely because of the response characteristics of the glass-faced multiplier phototubes in common use. Now that most commercial liquid scintillation counters are being furnished with quartz-faced multiplier phototubes that have peak response at shorter wavelengths, PPO, by itself, is likely to be quite adequate for routine ^{3}H determination.

C. 2,5,-Bis-2-(5-*t*-Butylbenzoxazolyl)-Thiophene (BBOT)

Recently a new scintillator, 2,5-bis-2-(5-*t*-butylbenzoxazolyl)-thiophene (BBOT), has received attention as a suggested replacement for PPO. With a fluorescence maximum of 4350 Å BBOT is better matched to typical glass-faced multiplier phototube response than is PPO or *p*-terphenyl and the need for a secondary scintillator is eliminated. BBOT is also reported to be more chemically stable than PPO; it is also claimed that it performs better than PPO in highly quenched situations where high scintillator concentrations might be advantageous. However, careful study has demonstrated that for routine use PPO continues to give superior performance. Therefore BBOT must be regarded as a scintillator of primary interest only when convenience outweighs other considerations.

D. Other Scintillators

Attempts have been made to prepare more effective scintillators than *p*-terphenyl and PPO but over the years no other material has come into widespread use. 2-Phenyl-5-biphenyloxadiazole (PBD) is among the best scintillators ever described (*89*) and has long been known to be superior to PPO. However, for optimum performance it is employed at twice the concentration required for PPO and, since its cost until April, 1966 was 4 times greater, it was eight times as expensive to use. Recent price reductions bring the cost of PBD, on a per gram basis, to the same as that of PPO; the use cost differential is therefore reduced to a factor of 2. On this basis it is believed that there will be renewed interest in PBD, particularly where the utmost in sensitivity is required.

A group of methyl- and methoxy-substituted *p*-quaterphenyls has been described by Wirth (*127*). Some of these materials are apparently superior scintillators to even PBD. However, none of them is commercially available and if they were it is likely that they would be expensive to employ in the quantities required for optimum performance.

E. Secondary Scintillators

Another group of materials must now be considered. Certain substituted oxazoles have been described which, by virtue of their lack of solubility, are not suitable for use as scintillators despite the fact that their fluorescence maxima fall in the region where the multiplier phototube is most responsive. However, advantageous use of these materials has been made. They are commonly added in trace quantities to a solution containing one of the more common scintillators. Their function is to absorb photons emitted at shorter wavelengths and reemit at longer wavelengths. This process has been unfortunately termed "wavelength shifting." The principal solute is generally known as the "primary scintillator" while the trace material is commonly called the "secondary scintillator."

Use of a secondary scintillator usually results in improved counting efficiencies for low-energy β-ray emitters or for quenched samples, since photon emission is more closely matched to multiplier phototube response. However, it should be recognized that in any process where energy is absorbed and reemitted there is some energy loss. If quartz-faced multiplier phototubes are available optimum performance will be achieved in the absence of a secondary scintillator, for in this case it is not necessary to accept the energy loss required to produce light of longer wavelength.

The two most important secondary scintillators are 1,4-bis-2-(5-phenyloxazolyl)-benzene (POPOP) and 1,4-bis-2-(4-methyl-5-phenyloxazolyl)-benzene (dimethyl POPOP). These materials are similar in cost and show little difference in performance. However, dimethyl POPOP is the more soluble and so finds increased favor, for in certain applications it may be advantageous to use relatively larger quantities than have come to be considered normal (*79*). The only other secondary scintillator that has enjoyed prominence has been α-naphthylphenyloxazole (α-NPO) but this material has largely been abandoned since its performance is somewhat inferior.

F. Scintillator Concentration

It is relatively simple to establish the optimum quantity of scintillator for any solvent system. A radioactive standard is dissolved in solvent and a measured quantity of primary scintillator is added. The sample is counted and then additional quantities of scintillator are added. A plot of count-rate versus scintillator concentration is constructed and that concentration at which maximum count-rate is achieved is ascertained. The optimum quantity of secondary scintillator can be estimated similarly. Usually in plotting such data a plateau is evident and it is best to work well past the starting point of the plateau so that weighing errors and effects of quenching, as discussed later, are minimized. Once optimum figures have been established they are generally applicable to all samples in that particular solvent and need not be redetermined.

It should be noted that fluorescence declines with excessive scintillator. It is evident that, at these concentrations, the scintillator itself interferes with the overall fluorescence process and normally this condition should be avoided. However, when working with highly quenched systems it is sometimes advantageous, as evidenced by increased count-rate, to employ what would normally be considered excessive quantities of scintillator. Whether or not this approach should be pursued can only be ascertained by experience with the particular sample and solvent system in question and is not subject to generalization.

II. SOLVENTS

The choice of solvents available for liquid scintillation counting is not much broader than is the choice of scintillators. The prime requisite of a good solvent is that it must efficiently transfer energy from the point of β-ray emission to a scintillator molecule. The solvent must also be transparent to the photons emitted; it must not freeze at the working temperature of the system; it must usually be capable of dissolving the sample either by itself or with the help of solubilizing agents. Surprisingly, this last characteristic is least important.

For some time the only solvents of any importance were the aromatic hydrocarbons and even today, despite the variety of materials being measured, toluene is still the most important single solvent available. Other aromatics are equally as good but have not been as widely used. Benzene freezes at too high a temperature; xylene, ethylbenzene, mesitylene, and so on are all satisfactory but offer no particular advantage and are not readily available in a sufficiently pure grade.

In its infancy liquid scintillation counting had limited applicability because of the restrictions imposed by use of aromatic solvents. Toluene is an ideal solvent for lipids, steroids, fatty acids, and hydrocarbons and the use of the liquid scintillation technique was, at first, confined to these few classes of material. Today these limitations have been overcome either by use of other solvents or by the use of additives which facilitate solution in toluene of such unlikely materials as tissue homogenates, amino acids, proteins, body fluids, inorganic salts, $^{14}CO_2$, and so on.

Potential solvents are usually rated by comparison to toluene. Hayes *et al.* (*46*) prepared a standard mixture of toluene and PPO and examined pulse height produced by excitation with an external ^{137}Cs γ-ray source. By substituting increased amounts of various solvents for toluene they were able to evaluate these materials as toluene replacements (Fig. 2).

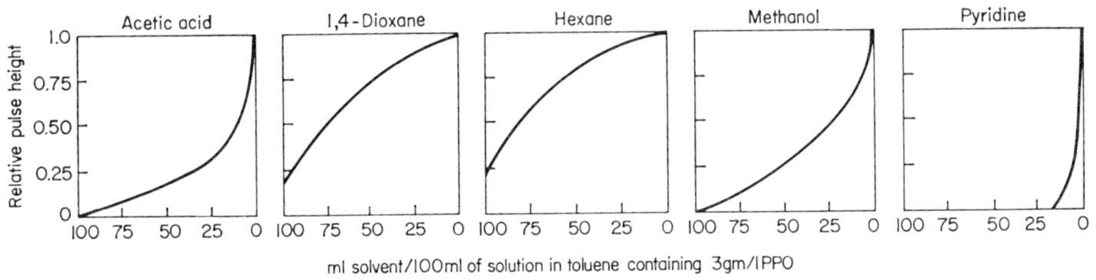

FIG. 2. Concentration versus relative pulse height for various solvents, diluters, and quenchers (*46*).

Davidson and Feigelson (*22*) directly compared performance of solvent–PPO mixtures when used to measure ^{14}C activity. The data they reported is shown in Table I. Their conclusions parallel those recorded by Hayes, though in detail the two methods give somewhat different results.

Hayes has made the useful distinction among "solvent," "diluter," and "quencher." Those materials that give rise to a pulse height equal to 80% or more of that which can be achieved in toluene are considered useful solvents and can be thought of for routine application in liquid scintillation counting. Those materials which, often in trace quantity, cause significant reduction in pulse height are quenchers and should be avoided when possible. Diluters are those materials which depress pulse height in proportion to their concentration. It is occasionally advantageous to make use of a diluter for its ability to solubilize a particular substance in a good solvent.

Apart from the aromatic hydrocarbons there are only a few other important solvents. Dioxane saturated with *p*-terphenyl can contain up

TABLE I
RELATIVE COUNTING EFFICIENCIES OF VARIOUS SOLVENTS TESTED WITH 0.3% DIPHENYLOXAZOLE AS PHOSPHOR

Compound	Freezing point (°C)	Relative efficiency
Toluene	−95	100
Methoxybenzene (anisole)	−37	100
Xylene (reagent, mixed isomers)	−20	97
1,3-Dimethoxybenzene	−52	81
n-Heptane	−90	70
1,4-Dioxane	+12	70
1,2-Dimethoxyethane (ethylene glycol dimethyl ether)	−71	60
Benzyl alcohol	−15	38
Diethyleneglycol diethyl ether (diethyl carbitol)	−44	32
Acetone	−94	12
Tetrahydropyran	−81	6
Ethyl ether	−116	4
1,1-Diethoxyethane	−100	3
Tetrahydrofuran	−65	2
1,3-Dioxolane	−10	0
Ethyl alcohol	−114	0
Diethylene glycol monoethyl ether	−10	0
Ethylene glycol monomethyl ether	−85	0
Diethylene glycol	−8	0
Ethylene glycol	−13	0
2,5-Diethoxytetrahydrofuran	−27	0
n,n-Dimethylformamide	−61	0
Diethyl amine	−49	0
n-Methyl morpholine	−66	0
2-Ethylhexanoic acid	−117	0
Tri-*n*-butyl phosphate	−80	0

to 20% water and is useful as a liquid scintillation solvent for measurement of aqueous solutions containing ^{14}C activity (*34*). Counting efficiencies are low and as dioxane has a relatively high freezing point (+11°C) it does not lend itself to use with a refrigerated detector. 1,2-Dimethoxyethane and other glycol ethers have also been investigated as potential solvents since their freezing points are lower than that of dioxane. By themselves they are inadequate even though they are capable of containing reasonable quantities of water; they fall into the category of diluters. Nevertheless these ethers have become useful as components of more widely used liquid scintillation solvent mixtures.

Furst and Kallmann (*38*) made a most valuable observation that addition of naphthalene to certain diluters, particularly dioxane, resulted in significantly increased fluorescence. This observation has been the subject of a patent (*68*), which goes into the matter in considerable detail. Dioxane systems containing naphthalene in relatively large quantities are now widely employed for the measurement of aqueous solutions. The freezing point of such mixtures may still be too high for some applications but this disadvantage can be overcome by the addition of small quantities of various other materials which lower the freezing point.

Apart from the solvents already discussed there are essentially no others being used to any extent. A discussion of various mixtures of those solvents that are of general importance follows.

III. COUNTING SOLUTIONS

Though it is possible to imagine innumerable combinations of primary and secondary scintillators and various solvents and diluters, only a few such mixtures are genuinely important. Probably, the well-equipped laboratory need be prepared to mix only two or, at most, three counting solutions in order to be able to handle almost any liquid scintillation counting problem. Therefore this discussion will be restricted to but a few of the more important solutions and a tabulation including others of lesser interest will be given.

Toluene containing 5-gm PPO/liter and 200-mg POPOP or dimethyl POPOP/liter is the single most useful general purpose counting solution. "Reagent grade" toluene should be used but there is no need for the so-called "scintillation grade." This solution should be employed whenever possible for routine counting of toluene-soluble materials. It should be used for suspension counting and for measurement of paper chromatograms; with suitable additives it is frequently the solution of choice for materials normally thought of as toluene insoluble, including $^{14}CO_2$. Toluene solutions are stable for relatively long periods when stored at room temperature in dark containers.

Measurement by liquid scintillation counting involves examination of the total sample and is not a measure of concentration. The counting efficiency of toluene-soluble nonquenching samples is expected to be independent of concentration and this has been verified by experiment (*23*). With a commercial coincidence counter utilizing glass vials having a nominal volume of 20 ml, counting efficiency was unchanged while solvent volume was varied between 5 and 15 ml, but background is least with smaller samples. Below and above these limits deviations can be attributed to changes in the optical properties of the sample rather than to any concentration effects. It therefore would seem advantageous, when working with nonquenchers, to utilize no more than 8–10 ml of solvent in the interests of economy and reduced background. However, when working with quenched systems it is generally best to work with greater solvent volumes since, as pointed out in the next section, increased dilution tends to partially overcome quenching effects.

While there has been little effort, or need, to improve the basic toluene counting system, the same cannot be said about systems primarily employed in working with aqueous solutions. In measuring radioactivity, desired statistics are achieved in the shortest possible time by obtaining the largest number of counts for any given total background. This consideration is particularly important in selecting a suitable counting solution for aqueous samples.

An outline of the techniques employed to measure *aqueous samples* must be divided in parts. If sample size is limited the system of choice should be that which permits the greatest counting efficiency. On the other hand, when sample is adequate and activities are low, the best solvent system might be that in which efficiencies are only average but which permits handling larger quantities of sample. Finally when activity levels are high, the preferred solvent system might be that which is most convenient with little importance attached to counting efficiency or to the maximum quantity of solution which can be counted.

The last situation is best handled with the aid of the standard toluene-PPO-POPOP mixture to which sufficient synthetic ethanol is added to enable achievement of the desired water concentration. Though this system was among the earliest used for counting aqueous samples (*47*) and has long been recognized to be inferior to other counting solutions, it still enjoys widespread use because of its convenience. Under the best conditions tritiated water in 1% concentration may be counted with an efficiency which in older instruments was not likely to exceed 5%.

When it is desired to maximize performance in counting aqueous solutions, mixtures of dioxane and naphthalene together with PPO and POPOP or dimethyl POPOP generally make up the counting system. Because dioxane is unstable and tends to form peroxides, "spectrochemical" grade is often employed; old solutions must be suspect. "Reagent grade" naphthalene is suitable. The best results are reported for solutions containing naphthalene almost up to its solubility limits, which, of course, vary with operating temperature. The most widely used mixture contains 100 gm naphthalene together with 7–10 gm PPO and 300 mg POPOP/liter of dioxane. Such a mixture can be used with up to 20% water concentration and at that concentration tritium counting efficiencies of over 10% may be obtained.

The simple dioxane–naphthalene system has only limited ability to solubilize salts and occasionally precipitation is noted when one is working with aqueous solutions having significant salt content. Often this precipitation is of no consequence for if no activity is carried down, the appearance of a small amount of suspended particulate matter will not interfere with counting performance. Nevertheless, there is a natural reluctance to work with suspended matter when it is not necessary to do so. Bray (*11*) has suggested a mixture of naphthalene (60 gm), PPO (4 gm), POPOP (200 mg), methanol (100 ml), ethylene glycol (20 ml), and dioxane (to make 1 liter), which has excellcnt solvent properties and permits tritium measurement with relatively high counting efficiencies. With a tritiated water concentration of 10%, tritium counting efficiency of 10% was reported. The mixture is capable of dissolving aqueous solutions of inorganic salts and also such materials as amino acids, sucrose, urine, and plasma. Bray also studied the effect of residual quantities of various protein-precipitating agents on counting efficiency and concluded that only perchloric and trichloroacetic acids in high concentrations caused significant quenching. As a general purpose counting mixture "Bray's solution" has replaced dioxane-naphthalene in many laboratories even though performance may not be quite as good.

A solvent mixture that enjoyed considerable popularity prior to the almost universal adoption of dioxane-naphthalene mixtures was the so-called "611" system (dioxane, 6 parts; anisole, 1 part; dimethoxyethane, 1 part) (*22*). It was found to be particularly advantageous for counting solutions of purines and pyrimidines. Recently its use has been suggested for the measurement of soluble ^{3}H, ^{14}C, and ^{35}S activity in blood (*60*). Addition of the "611" solvent causes both extraction of small molecules and protein precipitation. Should activity be present in solution it is, of course, readily counted; should it be present in the precipitate, it may be counted after filtration, drying, and Schöniger combustion (see Section VII). It has been demonstrated, most conclusively, that chemiluminescence, which may occur with this counting system, is a result of the presence of ether peroxides; addition of a trace quantity (1 mg/ml) of an antioxidant such as di-*t*-butyl-4-hydroxytoluene (BHT) overcomes the problem by suppressing ether peroxide formation. It is likely that this observation has considerably wider applicability than in the several examples cited in the literature.

Kinard (*72*) introduced a most useful index of the performance of counting solutions for aqueous samples which he called "figure of merit." The figure of merit for a solvent system is defined as the product of tritium counting efficiency (under conditions where the ratio of efficiency squared to background is a maximum) and tritiated water content under those conditions where the product is a maximum. Thus, Bray's solution has a figure of merit of 100 (10% efficiency × 10% concentration) while Kinard's own xylene-dioxane-naphthalene-ethanol solution has a figure of merit of 32 (4.2% efficiency × 7.7% concentration).

TABLE II
TYPICAL LIQUID SCINTILLATION COUNTING SOLUTIONS

Solvent		Scintillator			
Principal	Intermediate	Primary (gm/liter)	Secondary (mg/liter)	Figure of merit	Reference
Toluene	—	PPO (3–5)	POPOP (50–100), Dimethyl POPOP (100–200)	—	—
Toluene	—	*p*-Terphenyl (5)	Dimethyl POPOP (500)	—	—
Toluene + ethanol	—	PPO	POPOP	4.6–16.2	(*47, 87, 131*)
Xylene (5 parts) + dioxane (5 parts) + ethanol (3 parts)	Naphthalene (80 gm/liter)	PPO (5)	α-NPO (50)	32.3	(*72*)
Xylene (1 part) + dioxane (3 parts) + cellosolve (3 parts)	Naphthalene (80 gm/liter)	PPO (10)	POPOP (500)	~60	(*12*)
Dioxane	—	*p*-Terphenyl (5)	—	11.4	(*34*)
Dioxane	Naphthalene (20–120 gm/liter)	PPO (4–10)	POPOP (50–300)	100–200	(*16, 75, 123*)
Dioxane + methanol + ethylene glycol	Naphthalene (60 gm/liter)	PPO (4)	POPOP (200)	100	(*11*)
Dioxane (6 parts) + 1,2-dimethoxyethane (1 part)	Anisole (1 part)	PPO (12)	POPOP (50)	50–80	(*10, 23*)
1,2-Dimethoxyethane	Naphthalene (100 gm/liter)	PPO (7)	POPOP (300)	40–45	(*77*)
Dioxane (2 parts) + 1,2-dimethoxyethane (1 part)	Naphthalene (100 gm/liter)	PPO (7)	POPOP (300)	75–80	(*77*)

In those instances which have been discussed where sample concentration is significant, addition of further quantities of counting solution can be expected to result in increased counting efficiency. It is therefore implicit in the discussion that a total sample volume up to the limits of convenience or of the container is being considered and the possibility of increasing the volume of counting solution is precluded.

In Table II are listed various counting solutions of more than passing interest, together with leading references and, where applicable the figures of merit.

IV. QUENCHING

The term "quenching" has been applied to any process that interferes with performance of a liquid scintillation counting solution. Two distinct forms of quenching are important—color quenching arises from absorbance of colored materials in solution, while chemical quenching involves interference with the transfer of energy between the site of an event and a molecule of scintillator. Though the two processes are different, their effects are similar, and often identical procedures are used to overcome these effects.

A. Chemical Quenching

The most common quenching agent is oxygen dissolved in the counting solution (*97*). Elimination, either with the aid of ultrasonic agitation (*20*) or by purging with an inert gas (*3, 90*), results in considerable performance improvement. Nevertheless, few workers are willing to go to the trouble of deoxygenating each sample and so almost all work reported in the literature and all discussion in this chapter is based on solvent systems containing dissolved oxygen.*

As previously noted, measurement of unquenched toluene-soluble samples is essentially concentration independent. However, in situations where quenching occurs concentration becomes an important factor. By dilution of the sample the quantity of quenching agent interposed between the site of the decay event and the scintillator is reduced. Water is one of the most prominent mild quenching agents and therefore performance of systems for measurement of aqueous solutions is quite concentration dependent.

For isotopes with β rays more energetic than the tritium β rays, quenching is evidenced by a decided shift in the observed energy spec-

* Certain commercially available sealed standards for liquid scintillation counting are based upon purged solutions. Therefore they must never be used for calibration of the counting instrument but rather they are intended to provide a reference for comparison of instruments and measurement of day-to-day performance stability.

trum. As light pulses are degraded the spectrum presented is that of a seemingly lower energy β-ray emitter and, if instrument settings are not altered for the particular sample, a count loss usually results. For tritium counting, wherein only a very few photons are being measured from each event, quenching results in complete loss of many events and there is much less evidence of shift in the energy spectrum. Therefore, in performing dual-label experiments involving tritium and a more energetic β-ray emitter, severe quenching narrows the spread between the observed energy spectra.

For liquid scintillation counting to be a useful tool there must be means available either to overcome the effects of quenching or, at least, to estimate the amount of quenching for any sample. The former solution is of course best, but though possible, may not always be convenient.

A universal solution to the quenching problem is complete oxidation of the sample and collection and counting of the oxidation products. Though this may seem a drastic and time-consuming approach, in reality it is not, for simplified techniques have been devised specifically for use in liquid scintillation sample preparation. Whenever sample activities are low and quenching is suspected, oxidation should be employed for sample preparation; all other methods for dealing with quenching fall down in one way or another under these circumstances. In view of the importance of oxidative techniques, they are treated separately in Section VII.

B. Color Quenching

Color quenching can often be minimized by bleaching or decolorization and even, when color is not too intense, by dilution of the sample with additional counting solution. Blood and solutions of tissue in the solubilizing agent Hyamine 10-X have been bleached with a trace of peroxide (*53*) and sodium borohydride has also been used for the same purpose (*33*). Chlorine water has been used to bleach a prepared counting solution containing carotenoids (*110*). The bleached solution counted with the same efficiency as an unquenched standard, whereas prior to bleaching color quenching was responsible for a 50% diminution in observed count.

Other methods of eliminating color in samples being prepared for liquid scintillation counting include passage over activated charcoal (*87*), precipitation of color bodies with protein-precipitating agents including trichloroacetic acid (*75*), and azeotropic distillation of aqueous solutions if tritiated water is to be counted (*123*).

The severity of quenching caused by colored materials can also be estimated with some degree of accuracy by observing the absorption spectra over the range of the scintillator emission. Various investigators have demonstrated good correlation between color quenching and absorbance at 4000–4300 Å (*26, 42, 54, 101*). This type of measurement can be especially useful in working with count-rates which are not so high that background considerations may be disregarded.

For low-level counting it is as necessary to consider the quenching of background, just as the sample is quenched (*30*). Counting of a quenched background sample, prepared to simulate the samples of interest but without radioactivity, will almost certainly require excessive time to obtain good statistics and even then is likely to provide grossly incorrect results (*105*). Therefore it is necessary that correct values for such background samples be estimated by measurement of ultraviolet absorbance, by addition of radioactivity and actual measurement of the performance of the sample (*105*), or with the assistance of an external standard.

C. Correction Procedures

Of the methods that have been suggested for estimating the amount of quenching when chemical quenching may be present, either with or without color quenching, only a few have found widespread use. The method of *internal standardization* (*70*) is based upon the assumption that a nonquenched radioactive standard, when added to a quenched sample, will count with the same efficiency as the quenched sample. In applying this method the sample is initially counted and then a known quantity of radioactive standard is added and the sample recounted without changing instrument settings. The number of additional counts divided by the amount of activity added is taken as the counting efficiency of the original sample.

Originally benzoic acid-^{14}C was suggested as a suitable internal standard for checking ^{14}C counting efficiency but as it has been demonstrated that benzoic acid itself, in relatively large quantities, is a quenching agent (*51*) toluene-^{14}C is now the preferred internal standard for ^{14}C samples; for tritium samples, toluene-^{3}H is ideal. In a recent analysis of the statistical aspects of the internal standard technique, Herberg concluded that good counting statistics can be obtained in one minute for single- (*56*) or dual-label (*57*) samples if the standard contains 50,000 dpm of ^{14}C activity or 150,000 dpm of tritium. Dual-label samples must be counted a minimum of three times—the original count plus once for each added standard.

For radioisotopes other than ^{14}C and tritium it is frequently difficult to obtain nonquenching internal standards and other methods of estimation of absolute counting efficiency must be employed.

Baillie (*5*) has described a method for computation of quenching by determining *spectral shift* for each sample. A dual-channel instrument is employed. One channel is operated with optimum settings for the particular isotope in question while the second channel is used to examine the high-energy end of the pulse spectrum. The ratio of the counts in the two channels is constant for unquenched samples, but with quenching the ratio changes. A standard curve plotting channels ratio versus counting efficiency is constructed by successively adding increments of a quenching agent such as pyridine to a standard sample and recounting after each addition. The quenching curve can then be used to estimate counting efficiency of most samples of that same isotope counted under identical instrument settings.

Bruno and Christian (*12*) have briefly described a similar approach and Bush (*15*) has demonstrated the validity of the method for a wide variety of colored and colorless quenching agents. Bush has also shown the applicability of the "channels ratio" method to tritium counting though Baillie, in his original work, indicated that the method might not be suitable to this isotope. Probably this difference in view can be ascribed to the difference in instruments employed inasmuch as Bush worked with a modern transistorized unit with good stability whereas Baillie's instrument was of the vacuum tube type and might be expected to evidence considerable drift.

Quenching in dual-label experiments can be estimated both by using internal standards and, provided that count-rates are sufficiently high to ensure good statistics in all counting channels, by using a three-channel spectrometer (*52*). The two uppermost channels are operated with lower energy limits set to completely exclude any contribution of the less energetic β-ray emitter. The upper energy limit of one of these two channels (channel 1) is set to encompass most of the spectrum of the more energetic β-ray emitter while the upper limit of channel 2 is set to include approximately one third of the counts of channel 1. Channel 3 brackets the bulk of the spectrum of the less energetic β-ray emitter and, of course, includes a contribution from the more energetic one.

Using essentially the methods described by Baillie, the amount of quenching of the more energetic β-ray emitter may be established by observing the channel 1 to channel 2 ratio. In addition, the contribution of the more energetic emitter to channel 3 counts can be determined from a standard quench curve constructed in the absence of the less energetic β-ray emitter. The quantity of less energetic emitter is estimated after subtracting channel 3 contribution of the more energetic β-ray emitter from total channel 3 counts. The remainder is multiplied by an efficiency factor relating quenching of the more energetic emitter to counting efficiency of the less energetic one in channel 3. This factor is obtained by counting samples prepared by addition of known quantities of the less energetic β-ray emitter to previously counted standard quenched samples of the more energetic one.

Such a procedure may offer considerable convenience by eliminating the tedium and potential pipetting errors of internal standardization. Nevertheless, it must be recognized that the results obtained will have validity only if the count-rates are high in all channels.

Other methods for estimating quenching include an *extrapolation method* (*94*) wherein small increments of the sample are added to the same solution between counts and a plot of specific activity versus sample size is constructed. By extrapolation back to zero sample specific activity of an unquenched sample of the same material may be estimated. Though tedious and time consuming the extrapolation method may be more accurate and dependable than the internal standard method as the former makes use of several observations while the latter involves only a before and after determination.

Several investigators (*35, 58, 59*) have described the use of a reproducibly positioned *external standard* as an index of quenching and such was first incorporated in the Ansitron liquid scintillation counter introduced in 1964. Most often, changes in the high-energy portion of the spectrum induced by positioning a ^{137}Cs point source in close proximity to the sample have been correlated with quenching. After each initial sample count the source is reproducibly positioned and a recount is made. Regardless of the length of the initial count the recount need only be made for a short time period since a source of considerable activity may be chosen. The difference between the first and second count-rates is equal to the count-rate of the source alone and is readily related to counting efficiency through use of a calibration curve similar to that illustrated in Fig. 3. Alternatively, the change in ratio of the external standard count in two channels has been correlated with change in counting efficiency.

The external standardization technique may be successfully used for single- and multiple-labeled samples. It offers several advantages over both the internal standard and channels ratio methods for determining quenching. In contrast to internal standardization, no radioactivity need be added to the sample, thus reducing sample manipulation, eliminating pipetting errors, and leaving the sample unaltered for possible future use. Since the activity of the external standard is chosen to ensure good counting statistics in short calibration periods, counting efficiency is determined independent of sample counting statistics. One of the principal disadvantages of the channels ratio method—inaccurate results at low count-rates—is thereby overcome.

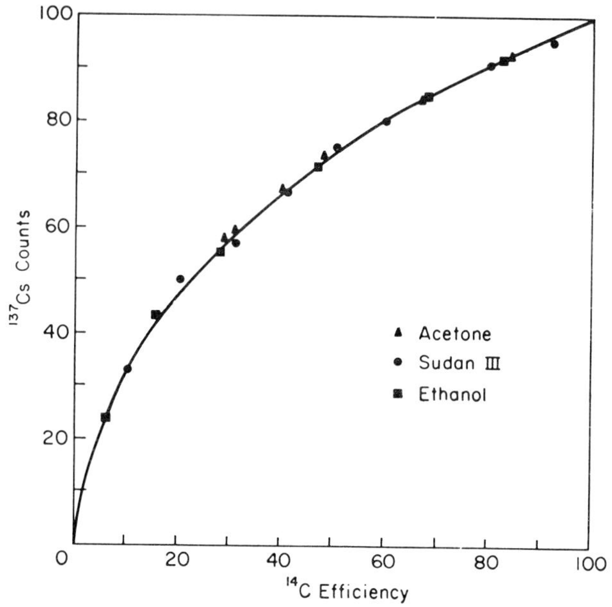

FIG. 3. Correlation curve for the ^{14}C counting efficiency versus the count-rate of a ^{137}Cs external point source by three different quenching agents (*58*).

V. SOLUBILIZING AGENTS

The liquid scintillation method would be severely limited if its use were restricted only to those substances that are conveniently solubilized in toluene or in one of the other previously discussed solvent mixtures. Fortunately, methods are available which permit solubilization of normally insoluble materials. Tissue, protein, blood, peptides, amino acids, and so on are conveniently dissolved in toluene through the use of appropriate techniques and are counted with satisfactory efficiency and acceptable reproducibility.

The first and still most widely used solubilizing agent is the hydroxide of Hyamine 10-X* (called Hyamine for convenience). Hyamine 10-X, *p*-(diisobutylcresoxyethoxyethyl)-dimethylbenzyl-ammonium chloride, a germicidal quaternary, was originally converted to the hydroxide via treatment of a methanolic solution of highly purified material with silver

* Registered trademark of Rohm & Haas, Inc.

oxide (*92*). Slight modifications of this method have been described (*31*) as has preparation by the use of sodium hydroxide (*25*).

While Hyamine originally gained prominence when it was shown to form a toluene-soluble carbonate, thereby enabling simplified $^{14}CO_2$ determination, this use is rapidly being abandoned as superior trapping agents become better known.

Proteins and amino acids are counted in toluene-PPO-POPOP using Hyamine as a solubilizing agent (*121*). Most amino acids are dissolved to the extent of 20 mg/ml of 1 *M* Hyamine in methanol, although aspartic acid and arginine are somewhat less soluble. Once complete solution has been effected the toluene-PPO-POPOP mixture (usually 15 ml) is added and the activity may then be counted. It is important that the counting solution not be added until after solution in the methanolic Hyamine has been achieved for Hyamine diluted with large volumes of toluene is not particularly effective as a solubilizing agent.

No unusual difficulties have been noted in counting amino acids in this manner so long as the prepared counting solution is dark-adapted. Counting of proteins solubilized with Hyamine has been more extensively examined (*55, 114*). Moderate quantities of protein (< 20 mg), either native or TCA precipitates, are solubilized in Hyamine without difficulty although warming may be necessary. Counting using toluene-PPO-POPOP is, for the most-part, routine. Attempts to solubilize larger amounts of protein have given unexpected results. A protein-Hyamine-toluene solution is often chemiluminescent and high count-rates may be evident even without scintillator or activity. Dark adaptation for lengthy periods may not entirely overcome this problem. However, addition of sufficient acid to neutralize the basicity of the counting solution often eliminates chemiluminescence. Generally acidification does not affect protein solubility and counting efficiency is unimpaired.

Hyamine is also used for solubilizing whole blood as well as serum and plasma (*18*) in toluene. Color may be eliminated by the addition of a trace of hydrogen peroxide. Because quenching of such solutions is a variable, even when several samples are prepared in seemingly identical fashion, one is well advised to examine each sample by the channels ratio or internal standard method.

The use of ultrasonic agitation may facilitate the solution of tissue homogenates in Hyamine (*13*). When sonication does prove effective the prepared sample frequently has less color and counts with higher efficiency than if solution had been effected by use of heat. Occasionally preliminary sonication, even if it does not result in complete solution, enables decreased heating time for total solution and consequently samples of less color and higher counting efficiency are obtained.

Enzymatic lysing of bacterial cells prior to Hyamine solubilization has been suggested as a means to facilitate determination of ^3H incorporation (*44*). Lysozyme and trypsin have been sequentially employed and after subsequent Hyamine addition complete solution in the "611" solvent system is accomplished without the need for heating or sonication.

The use of small quantities of Hyamine has also been found advantageous in preventing precipitation of biological materials from aqueous solution when such solution is added to a dioxane-naphthalene solvent mixture for counting (*119*). Solubility of such varied materials as amino acids, pyrimidines, carbohydrates, and phosphate esters is facilitated. Counting efficiencies for comparable quantities of aqueous solutions of tritiated compounds are reported to be as high in this solvent mixture as in toluene-PPO-POPOP when similar quantities of Hyamine are used to effect solution.

Other alkaline solubilizing agents appear to be as effective as is Hyamine for specific applications though none are as versatile. Ethanolic KOH has been carefully compared to Hyamine for solubilization of various lyophilized tissues (*53*) and for the most part results were quite comparable. Data for such tissues as kidney, spleen, liver, lung, muscle, and heart as well as for blood are given in terms of a merit factor—the product of counting efficiency and optimum sample weight. Though counting efficiencies, especially for tritium samples, were slightly higher

TABLE III
RECOVERY OF CHOLESTEROL-^{14}C FROM CHOLESTEROL DIGITONIDE (*108*)[a,b]

Solvent	(ml)	Dpm recovered	Recovery (%)
Original solution	—	19,514	—
Acetic anhydride–pyridine (1:1)	2	19,302	99
Phosphoric acid–*p*-dioxane (1:99)	2	19,152	98
Hyamine	0.5	18,882	97
Methanol	2	18,721	96
Ethanol	2	18,609	95
Acetic anhydride	2	18,416	94
Thixcin R	2	14,531	74
Toluene	4	13,203	68
Acetic acid	2	11,489	59
Pyridine	2	10,972	56
Cab-O-Sil	2	10,200	52
Xylene	4	6,314	32
Benzene	4	3,518	18

[a] A standard amount of digitonide (0.8 mg) was treated with the indicated solvent. After 2 minutes the solution was transferred to the scintillation counting vial and the residue was washed with ether, which was added to the solution to be assayed.

[b] Courtesy of *Analytical Chemistry*.

when Hyamine was employed, greater sample quantity could be handled with ethanolic KOH and therefore the merits are almost identical.

Aqueous KOH has also been employed in similar fashion and with comparable result (*40*). In order to solubilize digestion products it is necessary to use a toluene-methanol mixture. Plasma may be conveniently solubilized after heating with aqueous KOH; urine dissolves directly without the need for preliminary heating.

In an attempt to ascertain optimum conditions for liquid scintillation of cholesterol-^{14}C digitonide, comparison has been made of various solvent mixtures, solubilizing agents, and also suspension counting (*108*). Data given in Table III indicate that, of the conventional methods available, use of Hyamine gave the best results.

It must be emphasized that Hyamine, though convenient to employ, is a rather severe quenching agent. Therefore, it is prudent to employ the minimum quantity which will effect the degree of solubilization required and to avoid any excesses above this amount.

VI. MEASUREMENT OF $^{14}CO_2$

Measurement of $^{14}CO_2$ from respiratory gases or from Warburg-type experiments is performed routinely using the liquid scintillation method. When gas volume from which the CO_2 is to be trapped is relatively small the gas is most often absorbed by an alkaline agent which forms a toluene-soluble carbonate; when large volumes of gas must be handled and as a consequence, a large volume of trapping agent must be employed, it is usually advantageous to sequester CO_2 as $BaCO_3$, which is then isolated, dried, and counted in suspension as described in Section VIII.

Though many different trapping agents have been suggested by various authors, only a few remain of interest. Hyamine was the first reported to form a toluene-soluble carbonate and, through habit, is still the most widely used material for this purpose, though better and less costly agents are available. With Hyamine in excess, trapping of CO_2 is quantitative but as Hyamine causes significant quenching it is far from ideal to employ large quantities. The rather high viscosity of Hyamine solutions has made it difficult to effect quantitative transfer by pipetting from the center well of a Warburg flask. This problem has been overcome by use of a special flask in which the entire center well is removable (*112*). The well with its contents is dropped into the liquid scintillation vial, covered with toluene-PPO-POPOP, and the sample is counted. The presence of the glass well does not interfere with performance.

There have been numerous attempts to find trapping agents less viscous and less costly than Hyamine that also cause less quenching and have greater capacity for CO_2. 2-Phenylethylamine appears to be outstanding on all counts (*128*). It is inexpensive and has high trapping capacity. It does not quench and forms a stable carbonate which is toluene soluble. In contrast to most of the other trapping agents, which must be used by themselves and then added to a toluene-PPO-POPOP solution, phenylethylamine may first be dissolved in a toluene-methanol-scintillator solution and the entire mixture may be employed for trapping.

In a comparison between phenylethylamine and Hyamine, a Hyamine solution with a trapping capacity of 2 millimoles of CO_2 was counted with 30% efficiency while a phenylethylamine solution with the same capacity was measured with 60% efficiency; a phenylethylamine solution having a trapping capacity of 5 millimoles and a volume of 10 ml was counted with 50% efficiency while a Hyamine solution of the same volume and with the same capacity had a counting efficiency close to zero.

Monoethanolamine is another trapping agent which is replacing Hyamine in liquid scintillation work (*64*). Ethanolamine carbonate is soluble in a mixture of 2-methoxyethanol and toluene. Counting efficiencies in this system are good and slight traces of moisture which may be present along with CO_2 do not interfere with performance. Ethanolamine is inexpensive and has high trapping capacity. Count-rate is linear over a wide range of carbonate concentrations. A system containing 0.4 part of ethanolamine to 8 parts of 2-methoxyethanol and 10 parts toluene with 5.5 gm PPO per liter shows identical performance in the presence or absence of POPOP. Likewise dilution of $^{14}CO_2$ with $^{12}CO_2$ does not alter performance as long as there is sufficient ethanolamine to ensure complete trapping.

VII. COMBUSTION AND OXIDATION

Though the various techniques for solubilization and suspension of samples in preparation for liquid scintillation counting lend themselves to the handling of most materials, they are not without potential disadvantages. The possibility of quenching is ever-present; different types of samples of the same isotope must be counted with different instrument settings; sample characteristics may change on standing. In recognition of these problems several investigators have explored methods of oxidizing all samples of a particular radioisotope to a common material which can then be counted with known efficiency at one instrument setting.

In an early attempt at finding a universal method for preparing tritium-containing materials for liquid scintillation counting, samples of various biological substances, intimately admixed with copper oxide, were heated in a sealed tube (*61*). Water produced by this oxidation was carefully collected and counted in normal fashion.

Even earlier Schöniger (*106*) had described his now classic method for microanalysis of halogens and sulfur in organic compounds but it was some time until the potential of this technique for the preparation of ^{14}C and ^{3}H samples for liquid scintillation counting was recognized (*66, 69*). The Schöniger combustion method is by far the most convenient, rapid, simplest, and least expensive procedure available for converting samples to a common denominator and as such can be expected to find widespread use.

In the Schöniger method the sample to be counted is dried in a cellophane bag or wrapped in a small piece of paper and then placed in a closed flask which has been previously flushed with oxygen. The sample is ignited, usually by means of an electric spark or by focusing an infrared heat source through a wall of the flask. Combustion is rapid and complete. There is little danger involved since the amount of material combusted is comparatively small. Products of combustion are trapped by addition of a suitable scintillation counting solvent through a side arm of the flask.

If ^{14}C or ^{35}S are being measured one of the alkaline trapping agents previously discussed is suitable. Probably it is most advantageous to use phenylethylamine in a toluene-methanol solution containing PPO and POPOP (*28, 88*). For tritium measurement the bottom of the combustion flask is cooled with dry ice to freeze out water vapor (*69*). A dioxane-naphthalene scintillator solution is then added and the ice is allowed to thaw. An aliquot is taken for counting.

The Schöniger method has already had great impact on the entire field of liquid scintillation counting for it gives the investigator one method which is applicable to almost all samples. Commercially available Schöniger combustion devices available enable a single technician to prepare over 50 samples in a working day. Instrument settings for each particular radioisotope are independent of the nature of the original sample. Counting efficiency for each isotope is constant for all samples of that isotope. Quenching is eliminated and the need for routine standardization is overcome.

Occasionally it may be necessary to measure relatively large samples which cannot conveniently be made uniform (feces is a typical example). It may therefore become necessary to combust the entire sample rather than a representative portion. An oven which permits simultaneous combustion of up to 2 gm dry weight each has been described (*93*). Partial oxidation is achieved by streaming the samples at elevated temperatures with elemental oxygen. Gaseous products pass through a nickel foil–silver wool catalyst section which ensures completion of oxidation. Water vapor is collected in a dry ice trap while CO_2 may be collected by passage through a trapping agent.

Nitric acid digestion has been suggested as a means for solubilizing rat skin and insect cuticle, neither of which could be successfully solubilized with Hyamine (*86*). The acidic digests counted poorly, undoubtedly owing to the formation of nitrate salts of the scintillators employed. Neutralization with tris(hydroxymethyl)aminomethane improved the situation somewhat but the reported results (2.8% ^{3}H efficiency, 30% ^{14}C efficiency) must be considered unacceptable in light of what can be routinely achieved with combustion techniques. It is of interest to note however, that acid digestion eliminates problems of chemiluminescence that frequently accompany Hyamine solubilization. The possibility of acid digestion is cited primarily because of its potential for the assay of metal ions in various biological materials.

A modified Pirie's reagent—a mixture of nitric and perchloric acids and magnesium nitrate—capable of oxidizing sulfur-containing materials to $MgSO_4$ has been used (*62*) for measuring ^{35}S by liquid scintillation. $MgSO_4$ may then be solubilized in a scintillator solution including glycerol, ethanol, dimethylformamide, and toluene. This technique is inferior to Schöniger combustion when ^{35}S is to be measured by itself. However, it does offer the interesting possibility of enabling measurement of ^{35}S and ^{14}C in the same sample (*63*). These two radioisotopes which have essentially the same β-ray spectra cannot be differentiated by spectrometry. However, by oxidation of the sample with Pirie's reagent ^{35}S can be measured to the exclusion of ^{14}C, which is completely eliminated. By trapping the gaseous products of oxidation ^{14}C can be measured with no interference from ^{35}S.

VIII. SUSPENSION COUNTING

A. Mechanical Dispersion

Thus far emphasis has been directed to methods of sample preparation wherein solution has been achieved. It must not be thought, however, that solution is a requisite for liquid scintillation counting. Hayes *et al.* (*48*) originally noted that many completely insoluble materials could be counted after dispersion in a liquid scintillation counting medium. As settling occurred count-rate declined, thereby necessitating agitation of the sample between each count.

In an evaluation of the effects of self-absorption in individually suspended particles, a comparison was made between a sample containing

^{14}C in solution together with inert suspended matter and a sample containing the same suspended matter labeled with ^{14}C. With the liquid scintillation counter operated at low amplification there was little difference between the two samples; at higher amplification the sample containing soluble activity gave slightly higher counting efficiencies. Therefore, in such a system there must be moderate self-absorption, which acts to degrade pulses arising from the least energetic β rays but does not significantly affect those pulses arising from the more energetic ones.

Though white solids in suspension reflect most incident light with little loss, it is reasonable to expect that, as a result of multiple internal reflections, some total light loss will occur. In the case of low-energy β-ray emitters where initial light output is low, even a small loss in light incident on the multiplier phototubes results in a fairly significant loss in efficiency. It is therefore even more important in suspension counting than in solution counting to ensure optimum performance of the solvent-scintillator system. Use of a secondary scintillator therefore is a necessity in suspension counting, not only for measuring tritium but also for measuring ^{14}C, ^{35}S, ^{45}Ca, and other isotopes of similar β-ray energies. Performance of suspension counting systems is also best when the maximum volume of solvent is employed (*49*) for with increased dilution suspended particles are further separated and are less apt to interfere with photon passage through and out of the counting vial.

As has been noted, there may be self-absorption of low-energy β-rays in individual particles. It might be surmised that this effect would be overcome by reducing the sample to an extremely fine state. However, as particle size is reduced the total surface area is increased, thereby increasing internal reflection and potentially lowering counting efficiency. The two effects tend to counter one another and therefore, in a practical sense, are of little concern to the investigator.

B. Scintillating Gels

Increasing the viscosity of the counting solution should eliminate the problem of particle settling (*36*). Aluminum stearate was originally used to thicken toluene solutions and later Thixcin-R, a castor oil derivative, was introduced for the same purpose (*124*). Though Thixcin was superior to aluminum stearate in that it formed gels pourable without heating, it has largely been supplanted as a gelling agent by Cab-O-Sil (*91*), an aerated silica with an average particle size of 15 microns and a surface area of 200 meter^2/gm. Cab-O-Sil gels, fluid enough to pour, yet viscous enough to maintain stable suspensions, are prepared merely by shaking the sample together with toluene-PPO-POPOP and 4% by weight Cab-O-Sil in a counting vial. Such a gel can support up to 2 gm $BaCO_3$ in a 20-ml volume.

Measurement of $^{14}CO_2$ as $BaCO_3$ is, in fact, one of the prominent uses of suspension counting (*21, 85*). As noted in Section VI, collection of $^{14}CO_2$ as a toluene-soluble carbonate is preferred when the volume of gas to be handled is relatively small; however, when, as in the case of human breath analysis, gas volume is considerable, it is preferable to trap either directly in $Ba(OH)_2$ or in NaOH and then add $BaCl_2$ and collect and dry the $BaCO_3$ thus formed for suspension counting. It has been demonstrated that the counting efficiency of $BaCO_3$ is relatively independent of particle size provided that the sample is reduced to a reasonable fineness prior to gel preparation. Increasing the quantity of $BaCO_3$ causes decreased counting efficiency owing to greater light entrapment but, at moderate specific activities, the reduction in efficiency may show less effect on total counts than the increase brought about by added material.

$^{14}CO_2$ may also be collected and counted in NaOH solution (*43, 126*). The resulting solution may contain $NaHCO_3$ and (or) Na_2CO_3, both of which are likely to precipitate when added to any of the usual counting mixtures. However, with Cab-O-Sil present in the solvent mixture the precipitate remains uniformly suspended and is counted with ease, with good reproducibility, and with high efficiency. Possibly, all things considered, the use of NaOH in this fashion is among the best methods for $^{14}CO_2$ determination.

Cab-O-Sil gels have also been recommended for measurement of NaOH digests of tissues (*120*); dioxane-naphthalene is the suggested solvent mixture. The same gelling agent and solvent are also used for handling neutralized acid digests of fecal homogenates and neutralized urine. Dark samples may be bleached with hydrogen peroxide. The counting stability of Cab-O-Sil gels of NaOH liver digests is appreciably better than the stability of comparable preparations which do not include the gelling agent and in which phase separation will occur.

Various other toluene-insoluble materials such as inorganic salts, lyophilized tissue and bacteria, ion-exchange resin containing absorbed activity, amino acids, and polyfunctional organic compounds of all types have been counted by suspension techniques. It has been shown that certain substances that are severe quenchers in solution may be counted with superior results in suspension (*124*). Dispersion of aqueous solutions and tissue homogenates in toluene-PPO-POPOP enjoys considerable favor. Aqueous solutions containing either ^{14}C or tritium activity can be uniformly dispersed throughout a toluene-Thixcin gel using Hyamine, in the chloride form, as an emulsifying agent (*107*). Ultrasonic agitation was suggested to facilitate dispersion but others have found that sonication is not necessary. An aqueous solution of glucose-^{14}C, equivalent in volume to 5% of the total sample, was counted with an efficiency in excess of 50%; a similar volume of aqueous thymine-^{3}H solution was counted with an efficiency of 9–10%. Toluene-water emulsions of this type are reasonably stable at freezer temperature and show little change in counting performance on prolonged standing.

Cab-O-Sil has been used for the same purpose (*41*) and is probably superior in that when this gelling agent is employed it is unnecessary to add an emulsifying agent. A Cab-O-Sil–toluene–PPO-POPOP gel is prepared in the counting vial and to it the aqueous solution is added. The mixture is strongly agitated and then is ready for counting. With a water content of 6.5% it is reported that ^{14}C activity was counted with 65% efficiency while tritium was counted with 14% efficiency. In an interesting comparison of several methods of assay of ^{14}C in protein it was shown that liquid scintillation measurement of Cab-O-Sil suspensions provided higher counting efficiencies than did use of Hyamine solubilization or gas-flow measurement of the same activity adsorbed on filter paper or Millipore filters (*1*). Furthermore standard deviations of multiple determinations were least with Cab-O-Sil suspensions over a considerable weight range. However, with the minimum quantity of protein examined (0.1 mg per 10 ml toluene-PPO-POPOP) the Hyamine method showed the smallest standard deviation; in all cases the liquid scintillation method provided the greatest precision.

Special mention must be made of the possibility of measuring radioactivity in thin-layer chromatograms using suspension counting methods (*111*). The chromatogram is scored in segments; the segments are scraped into counting vials, covered with gel scintillator, and counted. Good results are obtained as long as the nature of the material being counted is such that it remains on the chromatographic support or is totally eluted into solution. If erratic counting of replicates is observed it is likely that partial elution has taken place (Chapter 11, Section II,B).

An interesting application for Cab-O-Sil is based on the observation that microgram quantities of certain labeled materials may be adsorbed from toluene on to the wall of glass counting vials (*9*). This adsorption leads to nonlinearity of observed count-rate with addition of more activity. By first adding Cab-O-Sil and then activity, the activity is preferentially adsorbed on the Cab-O-Sil rather than on the wall of the vial. This preferential adsorption leads to preservation of 4π geometry rather than the 2π geometry which occurs as a result of wall adsorption. With the materials studied it was observed that decanting the Cab-O-Sil suspension from the counting vial resulted in elimination of over 99% of the total activity. In the absence of Cab-O-Sil, decanting a toluene-PPO-POPOP solution of the activity from the vial results in substantial retention of activity on the walls of the vial. With or without the suspending agent, counting efficiencies of nonadsorbed materials were comparable, while adsorbed materials counted with one-third less efficiency in the absence of Cab-O-Sil.

C. Emulsions

True emulsions rather than gels have also been used (*82*). The detergent Triton x-100 has been employed to suspend aqueous tissue homogenates in toluene-PPO-POPOP. It is reported that ^{14}C can be measured in such a system with efficiencies comparable to those obtained in homogeneous solution and tritium counting is also done in highly efficient fashion.

Measurement of aqueous emulsions offers certain attractions. Performance is highly acceptable and sample preparation is relatively easy. It is not necessary to dry samples or to be concerned with solubility properties. With high salt content the problem of precipitation, which may occur in organic solvents, can be ignored. Dioxane is not needed, which eliminates concern regarding solvent stability and purity. Furthermore, emulsification is applicable to almost all isotopes and almost all colorless materials. Possible variations in quenching are largely eliminated by virtue of the fact that quenchers are not in the scintillation solution. The relatively large quantity of water present establishes a common performance base for all samples.

IX. COUNTING ACTIVITY ON PAPER

Liquid scintillation counting of radioactivity on paper strips or filter disks may be considered an extension of suspension counting. As first described by Roucayrol *et al.* in 1957 (*102*), strips containing ^{14}C, ^{32}P, or ^{131}I activity were moistened with toluene-PBD and then placed against the multiplier phototube of a single-tube liquid scintillation counter. Counting efficiencies for all three isotopes were satisfactory; it was also possible to measure ^{14}C simultaneously with either of the other isotopes. A patent covers modification of this system for continuous measurement of strips of great length (*103*).

Recently reports of various techniques of measuring activity on paper have appeared with increasing frequency. From the number of such reports it is obvious that this field is one of the most active areas in liquid scintillation counting, no doubt owing to the simplicity of making these measurements, the broad applicability of the method, and the good results frequently obtained.

A. Paper Strips

Measurement of radioactivity contained on paper strips must, by now, be considered routine. Strips are placed in the counting vial, either totally immersed in or merely wet by liquid scintillator, and counted. The paper acts to block some, but by no means all of the emitted light; for instrument setup the samples must therefore be regarded as being quenched and proper allowance be made. Reproducible results will be obtained when the activity is totally insoluble (the usual case with biological materials other than lipids) but if partial elution occurs the count-rate may vary with time as counting efficiency is different in solution than on paper (*122*).

Counting efficiency for colorless insoluble materials is generally constant for each isotope when counted with optimum instrument setting and with the same solvent mixture and solvent volume. This efficiency may be determined either by use of an insoluble internal standard or Schöniger combustion of representative paper strips. On occasion where considerable color is present the entire method fails and Schöniger combustion becomes a necessity (*7*); another problem may result from differences in penetration into paper fibers between large and small tritium-containing molecules (*37*) when they are filtered on paper and subsequently counted. The small molecules may penetrate further and therefore count with lower efficiency. However, in any method involving filtration an internal standard is easily incorporated in test samples; in chromatographic procedures where internal standardization is not feasible it is expected that uniform penetration does, in fact, take place.

The effects of changes in orientation of the paper strip between the two multiplier phototubes were the subject of much attention in the early literature. It was observed that counting results for ^{14}C and more energetic isotopes did not significantly vary with changes in paper positioning (*24, 39, 78, 122*) presumably because enough light is produced by higher-energy β rays to ensure that each multiplier phototube receives an adequate number of photons despite the semiopaque paper interposed between.

However, in measuring low-energy β rays from tritium, which on the average produce about 40 photons, some of which will be absorbed by the paper or lost through other processes, paper orientation seemed to significantly affect the results obtained. Therefore early investigators placed great emphasis on the attainment of reproducible orientation;

many workers suggested placing the strip flat on the bottom of the counting vial even though this resulted in considerable loss of counting efficiency. Modern instrumentation makes this unnecessary; coincidence counting systems with pulse summation provide results with tritium samples that are little more dependent on paper orientation than are results of ^{14}C counting.

Though the greatest use for paper strip counting has been for measurement of paper chromatograms, the possibility of using paper as a support for various toluene-insoluble materials has not been overlooked. An excellent example of such an application is the measurement of potassium gluconate (*8*), derived from blood glucose. An aqueous gluconate solution is applied to filter paper and dried prior to immersion in the scintillator solution. If necessary to achieve sufficient counts three or more such papers can be wedged vertically in a single counting vial. With proper instrument settings performance is independent of the specific activity of the sample. Excellent linearity between activity present and counts observed has been noted. Removal of strips from the counting vial and counting the remaining scintillator for residual activity indicated that there was no elution. Therefore, in this instance applied radioactivity may be completely recovered by washing the strips with toluene to remove scintillator, drying, and then eluting with water.

Bacterial cells labeled with thymidine-^{3}H have been supported on filter paper and counted by liquid scintillation (*2*). The bacterial culture was centrifuged and the collected cells, thoroughly washed with saline, were suspended in a suitable medium. Aliquots of the suspension were pipetted onto Whatman No. 1 paper and after drying the intact cells could be counted. Analogous methods were employed in working with thymine-^{14}C.

In paper strip counting it is often desirable to keep the activity on the paper. Therefore toluene is favored over dioxane as a solvent both because of its better energy transfer properties and its poorer solvent capability for biological material. But, for some applications there may be an even more advantageous solvent system. Nakshbandi (*84*) has demonstrated that paper strips may be counted after impregnation with the plastic scintillator Naton 136. The strips are either immersed in a viscous benzene solution of the scintillator and then dried or preferably made into a sandwich between two strips of Kleenex soaked in the scintillator solution. Using this method tritium counting efficiencies fall in the range of 10–20%, even with older instrumentation. The same compounds when counted on paper in toluene solution are likely to count with 1–2% efficiency in the same equipment.

B. Filter Disks

Measurement of activity on filter disks has also been a subject of considerable interest. For example, TCA precipitates of RNA isolated from bacterial sources have been collected on Millipore filters which are then dried and counted. Samples containing both ^{32}P and ^{14}C (*80*) and ^{32}P and ^{3}H (*29*) were counted simultaneously with only minor ^{14}C or ^{3}H in the ^{32}P channel.

Enzyme-catalyzed incorporation of amino acids into proteins has been studied by incubating the reaction mixture on a filter disk (*81*). At the conclusion of incubation the disk was immersed in a TCA solution which served both to end the reaction and fix the protein to the paper. After suitable washing to eliminate unreacted substrate the disk was counted. In this example, ^{14}C counting efficiency was comparable to that which might be obtained by solubilizing the same sample with Hyamine and counting in solution. The same methods have also been used with tritium and ^{35}S.

Millipore filters are dioxane soluble; some workers prefer to collect TCA-protein precipitates on Millipore disks which are then dissolved in dioxane-naphthalene counting solution prior to measurement (*95*).

C. Adsorbed $^{14}CO_2$

Small amounts of $^{14}CO_2$ evolved during biological oxidation are conveniently collected on filter paper moistened with an alkaline trapping agent such as aqueous KOH (*14, 19*) or Hyamine (*74*). This technique has proven to be especially effective in view of the large surface area present. Once collection is complete the strip is merely transferred to the counting vial, immersed in the scintillator, and measured. Usually the oxidation flasks include a special side arm, closed by a rubber septum, through which a hypodermic syringe needle is inserted in order to add alkali to the strip. Care must be exercised to ensure that all of the trapping agent is contained on the strip and that none is lost on the walls of the vessel.

D. Miscellaneous

Glass fiber filter paper has been suggested as a suitable support for liquid scintillation counting of precipitates. After placement in the counting vial and addition of counting solution, the filter may be broken up by vigorous agitation; the resulting suspension is conventionally counted (*65*). Alternatively the filter disk may be counted in its normal form; up to 25 such disks have been counted in a single vial with linearity between counts observed and total activity present. The linear relationship was maintained with either polar or nonpolar solvents, which caused varying degrees of elution of the activity from the paper into the solution (*96*). Counting efficiency was markedly greater on glass paper than on cellulose paper, perhaps another manifestation of the previously discussed contention that efficiency may diminish with increasing penetration of activity into the paper fibers.

Other less common forms of paper support which may be advantageous for particular applications include DEAE–cellulose paper, whose ion-exchange properties are reported to be useful in a rapid enzyme assay procedure (*109*), and Whatman No. 3 paper. The latter, being rather thick, causes diminution of counting efficiency but, especially for energetic isotopes, counting results are still significantly better than they would be if that same sample were counted by Geiger or proportional methods.

The paper strip technique is simple, time-saving, and may permit recovery of sample from the paper. There is but one serious problem. It is desirable that the nature of the radioactivity be such that it is either completely insoluble or completely soluble in the solvent system being employed. If the latter situation prevails, the strip should be removed, thereby leaving the counting vial with its solution containing the total activity. Should there be partial solubility erratic results can be anticipated. The supposition that such results can be attributed to partial solubility is easily confirmed by removing the strip and counting the remaining solvent. One method that has been suggested to overcome this problem is the use of Hyamine to completely remove various materials from paper strips (*118*). A recent mathematical treatment of the situation where partial elution occurs has been given by Willenbrink (*125*).

X. SUSPENDED SCINTILLATORS

When, for one reason or another, it has been impractical to prepare homogeneous solutions for liquid scintillation counting, emphasis has been directed to the suspension of insoluble activity in solutions containing dissolved scintillator. However, Steinberg (*115, 116*) and others (*83*) have demonstrated that for specific applications it may be advantageous to work with systems where activity is in solution while the scintillator is not.

It was originally noted that aqueous and alcoholic solutions containing ^{14}C activity could be counted using as the scintillator bundles of scintillating plastic fiber* which were merely wet with the solution.

* Pilot B, Pilot Chemical Company, Watertown, Massachusetts.

Subsequently it was found that crystalline anthracene (blue-violet fluorescence grade) was superior to plastic scintillator (*117*), giving, under comparable conditions, approximately three times the ^{14}C counting efficiency and 10 times the ^{3}H efficiency (*98*). Almost all current work in this field is being done with anthracene as no other material has been found equal in performance.

In working with suspended anthracene a trace of detergent is usually added to the solution being counted in order to ensure that the scintillator is thoroughly wet and does not float. When scintillator volume is considerably in excess of solution volume count-rate increase is linear with further addition of solution. As solution volume approaches scintillator volume the increase in count-rate falls off with further increments of solution. Finally, when the level of solution is above the level of anthracene, addition of more solution causes no increase in counts. At this point performance of the system is akin to the situation in Geiger counting known as "infinite thickness." It is generally recommended that counting with suspended anthracene be carried out under these conditions because only the quantity of scintillator employed need be measured carefully, but not the volume of the solution being counted.

Counting efficiencies of various radioisotopes using 3 ml of solution and 1 gm of anthracene, counted in a coincidence counter, for the most part with integral settings and maximum amplification are given in Table IV. Similar data but collected with a single multiplier phototube instrument are given in Table V. Sample size was 0.6 ml while 1 gm of anthracene was employed. These two tables taken together indicate the fairly broad applicability of the method together with the type of performance that can be anticipated. It should be noted that while α- and β-ray emitters can be counted satisfactorily, counting efficiency for γ-ray emitters is quite poor, as might be expected.

TABLE IV
INTEGRAL COINCIDENCE COUNTING EFFICIENCIES WITH SUSPENDED SCINTILLATOR (*116*)

Radioisotope	Max. β-ray energy (MeV)	γ-Ray energy (MeV)	Background (cpm)	Counting efficiencies (%)
^{3}H	0.018	—	99	0.5
^{14}C	0.156	—	99	16–20
^{45}Ca	0.254	—	99	49
^{32}P	1.71	—	11	78
^{131}I	0.608	0.364	99	58

TABLE V

INTEGRAL SINGLE MULTIPLIER PHOTOTUBE COUNTING EFFICIENCIES WITH SUSPENDED SCINTILLATOR[a]

Radioisotope	Max. β-ray energy (MeV)	γ-Ray energy (MeV)	α-Ray energy (MeV)	Counting efficiencies (%)
^{3}H	0.018	—	—	1
^{35}S	0.167	—	—	59
^{45}Ca	0.254	—	—	78
^{137}Cs	0.52 (92%)	—	—	80
^{137}Cs	1.19 (8%)	—	—	—
^{137}Cs	—	0.66 (92%)	—	—
^{90}Sr–^{90}Y	0.61	—	—	86
^{90}Sr–^{90}Y	2.24	—	—	—
^{32}P	1.71	—	—	91
^{210}Po	—	—	5.3	~100
^{7}Be	—	0.478	—	~6

[a] Courtesy of *Analytical Chemistry.*

Performance of the suspended scintillator method is subject to color quenching but not to the quenching of colorless materials in solution. Color quenching may be estimated either by the use of internal standards or by the channels ratio technique.

Possible advantages of the suspended scintillator technique have been summarized (*117*):

(1) It is general and applicable to virtually any compound soluble in water, salt solutions, dilute acid, or dilute alkalai.

(2) No chemical conversion or other preliminary handling is necessary, and sample preparation is simple and rapid.

(3) Samples can be recovered unaltered after radioassay and used for further characterization.

(4) Large quantities of sample can be counted, limited only by their solubility in the liquid phase, and, in the case of colored compounds, by quenching effects.

The suspended scintillator finds its greatest use where large volumes of aqueous samples with low specific activity need be handled. Literature citations include measurement of solutions of tritiated water, acetazolamide-^{3}H, $Na_2{}^{14}CO_3$, $K_2{}^{14}CO_3$, amino acids-^{14}C, proteins-^{14}C, glucose-^{14}C, benzoic acid-^{14}C, and so on, as well as inorganic salts of the various radioisotopes listed in Tables IV and V. Measurement of gross α- and β-ray activity in decolorized urine comes to mind as one potentially valuable application. However, the most important use by far is adaptation of this technique to the continuous monitoring of effluents from column chromatograms as described in Chapter 11, Section III.

XI. MEASUREMENT OF INORGANIC ELEMENTS

Wherever possible the methods used to prepare samples of inorganic materials for liquid scintillation counting are similar to those methods used for biological substances. Aqueous solutions are handled in similar fashion regardless of the isotope being measured; iodinated proteins are treated as are any proteins, and so forth. Special techniques are employed for those materials which are found in a form that does not conveniently permit simple solution or suspension.

A. Complexing Agents

Interest in many inorganic elements has been directed toward the boneseekers. Bone samples suspected of containing ^{90}Sr-^{90}Y are generally dissolved with acid and then converted to a form soluble in scintillator solution by treatment with a complexing agent such as dibutyl phosphate. This approach sets a pattern for many of the inorganic ions though the complexing agents are varied to fit specific cases. Calcium-45 is conveniently handled as the 2-ethylhexanoate; plutonium ions are soluble in a toluene solution containing dibutyl phosphate, while uranium ions may be solubilized in toluene-dioxane with methyl isobutyl ketone.

The most popular complexing agents, dibutyl phosphate, dioctyl phosphate, and 2-ethylhexanoic acid, have been used to solubilize a wide number of inorganic nuclides in toluene. They are convenient to employ for they may be admixed with toluene-PPO-POPOP and the entire mixture used as an extractant. Excess complexing agent does not cause quenching. Other isotopes aside from the aforementioned ^{90}Sr-^{90}Y, ^{241}Pu, and ^{45}Ca that lend themselves to this technique are ^{239}Pu, ^{240}Pu, ^{95}Zr, ^{95}Nb, ^{63}Ni, ^{151}Sm, ^{113}Cd, and so on.

Leffingwell *et al.* (*76*) showed that ^{59}Fe, a β- and γ-ray emitter, could be counted with approximately 50% efficiency in a liquid scintillation solution even though the iron was present as the highly colored phenanthroline complex. The intensely red complex was prepared and extracted into isoamyl alcohol; 2 ml of this solution was added to 7 ml of toluene-PPO-POPOP and the sample was counted in a coincidence-type instrument. At high concentrations of the complex some color quenching was noted but at moderate concentrations quenching problems were minimal.

Iron-55, which emits a 5.9 keV X ray in only one quarter of its total disintegrations, presents an even greater counting problem than does tritium. Nevertheless, ^{55}Fe in the ferrous state has been complexed with ascorbic acid and the complex solubilized in a toluene-ethanol-water solution for counting. Using this same technique both ^{55}Fe and ^{59}Fe have been counted simultaneously (*27*) with 14% and 50% efficiency, respectively.

B. Salt Solution

Though complex formation is the most universal method of preparing metal ions for liquid scintillation counting, it must not be thought that there is no other way. For example, though ^{45}Ca is often handled as the 2-ethylhexanoate, recent investigators prefer extraction of $^{45}CaCl_2$ by an ethanol-toluene system (*17*). Counting efficiencies in excess of 50% are reported. It has also been suggested that $^{45}Ca(NO_3)_2$ is conveniently solubilized in ethylene glycol-ethanol-toluene (*104*). Such a sample has been counted with 45% efficiency. Though this value is somewhat less than when $^{45}CaCl_2$ is measured, a greater quantity of calcium can be handled and sample preparation is simpler.

Suspension counting techniques are also applicable to solids containing various radioactive inorganic elements (*50*) and to aqueous solutions containing dissolved nuclides (*32*). Since many of these are fairly energetic β-ray emitters counting efficiencies are generally high and no special precautions or procedures need be employed.

XII. MEASUREMENT OF β, γ-RAY EMITTERS

The majority of the radioisotopes used in nuclear medicine either for therapy or for diagnosis are γ-ray emitters, though the majority of these are β-ray emitters as well and readily lend themselves to liquid scintillation counting. Certainly, for *in vivo* studies these isotopes must be counted by techniques outlined in Part IV of this book but, in specific instances when discrete samples are to be counted, the liquid scintillation method ought not be overlooked.

A. Efficiency for γ-Ray Counting

In working with individual samples of β, γ-ray emitters the investigator may be faced with deciding whether β- or γ-ray counting is preferable. Usually γ-ray counting is selected, for, in most cases, sample preparation is simpler and activity levels are such that the lower counting efficiencies of γ-ray measurement are compensated by the larger sample volume that can be handled. Furthermore, in multiple radioisotope experiments it is likely to be simpler to separate well-defined γ-ray photopeaks rather than broad β-ray spectra (Chapter 12).

Nevertheless, there are occasions when liquid scintillation counting may be preferable. When faced with many samples the investigator should keep in mind that automatic liquid scintillation counters are more common than automatic equipment for the measurement of γ-ray activity and many published methods have been designed for the equipment at hand. Also, measurement of β-ray activity is usually more efficient than measurement of γ-ray activity in a photopeak. Therefore when the sample volume is limited and the activity is low it may be more advantageous to measure β-ray decay than γ rays.

The liquid scintillator, owing to its low density and atomic number, is not an efficient system for stopping γ radiation. Measurement of an ^{35}S-^{75}Se mixture indicated that the ^{75}Se γ rays (0.405, 0.269, 0.137, 0.121 MeV) made essentially no contribution to the ^{35}S counts (*113*). This performance is typical; in measuring β, γ-ray emitters it can be anticipated that there will be little, if any, cross contribution from energetic γ-ray emission. In a single-label experiment γ-ray contribution is of little consequence even if it is measured. In a dual-label experiment cross contribution of the γ rays is corrected for in the same way that cross-contribution corrections are normally made when two β-ray emitters are counted in the same sample.

Certain low-energy γ-ray emitters such as ^{125}I (*100*) which are not β-ray emitters are conveniently counted by liquid scintillation methods. Iron-55, which has a low-energy X ray but neither γ- nor β-ray emission, may also be counted by liquid scintillation techniques (Section XI,A).

XIII. DOUBLE-LABEL COUNTING

A. Routine Measurement

The liquid scintillation method offers the possibility of counting two β-ray emitters in the same sample provided that they differ in their maximum β-ray energy by a factor of approximately 4. While those experienced in the simultaneous measurement of two or more γ-ray emitting nuclides may not think this particularly remarkable, it should be realized that β-ray spectra show a broad continuum from zero energy up to the maximum β-ray energy whereas γ-ray spectra usually involve well-defined photopeaks which are easily separated with modern instrumentation (Chapter 6, Section IV).

Techniques for preparation of samples containing two radioisotopes are usually no different than when a single isotope is involved and there is no need to cite specific examples. In most instances involving simultaneous measurement of two β-ray emitters principal concern is with proper adjustment of instrument settings so as to minimize cross contribution of either β-ray emitter to counts in the channel in which the other one is being examined. The principles of such instrument setting are discussed in Chapter 10, Section III,B.

B. Isotopic Dilution Assays

Apart from measurement of samples obtained from experimentation in which two radioisotopes are directly employed, considerable use of double-label liquid scintillation counting is made in assays where radioactivity is added as part of the assay itself. A classic example is the measurement of *aldosterone* (*73*) first described by Avivi *et al.* (*4*) based on the principles of the double isotope derivative method of Keston *et al.* (*71*). The aldosterone assay procedure has become so widely used and its principles are sufficiently general that it will be outlined in detail.

In the first step a known quantity of pure aldosterone-^{14}C is added to the mixture to be assayed and total steroids are then extracted. On occasion it may be necessary to hydrolyze the sample to release the steroids from a conjugated state. The extracted steroids are dried and then acetylated with high specific activity acetic anhydride-^{3}H. Aldosterone forms the 18,21-diacetate while various other steroids in the mixture may also be acetylated. The entire mixture is subjected to purification by paper chromatography. Carrier aldosterone-18,21-diacetate may be added to facilitate purification. After the initial paper chromatogram has been run the aldosterone-rich spot is cut out and eluted. The eluent is oxidized to a characteristic monoacetate oxidation product which is then rechromatogrammed to ensure purity. The final product is collected, dissolved in toluene-PPO-POPOP, and the ^{14}C and ^{3}H contents are measured simultaneously.

The percentage of ^{14}C recovery is taken as an index of aldosterone recovery for the entire assay procedure while from the observed tritium activity the quantity of aldosterone present is easily calculated from the knowledge of the specific activity of the acetic anhydride used for acetylation. From these two figures the initial aldosterone content is determined:

(a) $$\text{Aldosterone recovery} = \frac{\text{C}^{14}\text{ cpm recovered}}{\text{C}^{14}\text{ cpm added}}$$

(b) μmoles monoacetate

$$= \frac{\text{H}^3\text{ cpm}}{\text{H}^3\text{ eff}} \times \frac{1\ \mu\text{Ci}}{2.2 \times 10^6\text{ dpm}} \times \frac{1}{\text{spec. act. } (\mu\text{Ci/mole})}$$

(c) $$\mu\text{moles aldosterone} = \frac{\mu\text{moles monoacetate}}{\text{aldosterone recovery}}$$

The same technique has been employed for the assay of corticosterone and hydrocortisone.

A somewhat more complex procedure is required for the assay of *plasma progesterone* levels inasmuch as this steroid does not acetylate (*129*). In this instance reduction with sodium borotritide is employed to introduce the tritium label while progesterone-^{14}C is used to check overall recoveries. Because tritiation with sodium borotritide may result in variable specific activity depending upon precise reaction conditions as well as the specific activity of the reagent, it is necessary to carry along pure progesterone blanks parallel to the samples being assayed. The blanks are then used to determine the specific activity of the reduced progesterone after labile tritium has been removed by appropriate methods. It is reported that this method, though more tedious than some of the more conventional assays, is also more sensitive, permitting detection of as little as 0.1 μg of progesterone in a typical sample.

Another interesting example of double isotope counting is the recently described assay of tissue levels of *S-adenosylmethionine* (*6*), a well-known methyl group donor in several biological systems. The method is based upon isotopic dilution of *S*-adenosylmethionine-^{14}C by the unlabeled compound present in tissue extracts. The specific activity of the diluted ^{14}C compound is estimated after treatment of a crude tissue homogenate extract (to which *S*-adenosylmethionine-^{14}C has been previously added) with *N*-acetylserotonin-^{3}H and the enzyme hydroxyindole *O*-methyltransferase. Melatonin-methoxy-^{14}C-acetyl-^{3}H formed by enzymatic reaction is readily isolated and counted. A linear relation is observed between the amount of unlabeled *S*-adenosylmethionine present in the original sample and the ^{3}H to ^{14}C ratio found in the melatonin.

XIV. TRIPLE-LABEL COUNTING

Inasmuch as three-channel liquid scintillation counting units are now the most commonly sold, it would seem that there must be some interest developing in the simultaneous determination of three isotopes in the same sample. If this is in fact true, there is little evidence to be found in the literature though ^{32}P, ^{14}C, and ^{3}H have been counted in the same sample even with now obsolete equipment (*130*). With more modern instrumentation, which provides superior multiple isotope differentiation, the investigator can expect reasonably satisfactory results for good quality samples. However, for variably quenched samples considerable difficulty in achieving worthwhile results should be anticipated and it is suggested that, if at all possible, the proposed experiment should be revised to employ no more than two isotopes.

REFERENCES

1. Abell, C. W., Dirks, F. I., Delk, A. S., and Loeb, L. A., A comparison of several methods of assay of carbon-14 in protein. *Anal. Biochem.* **11**, 170 (1965).
2. Apelgot, S., and Duquesne, M., Liquid scintillation counting applied to the quantitative measurement of tritium incorporation in bacteria. *J. Chem. Phys.* **58**, 774 (1961).
3. Arnold, J. R., Scintillation counting of natural radiocarbon: I. the counting method. *Science* **119**, 155 (1954).
4. Avivi, P., Simpson, S. A., Tait, J. F., and Whitehead, J. K., The use of H^3 and C^{14} labeled acetic anhydride as analytical reagents in microbiochemistry. *Proc. 2nd Radioisotope Conf., Oxford, Engl., 1954* Vol. 1, p. 313. Butterworth, London and Washington, D.C., 1954.
5. Baillie, L. A., Determination of liquid scintillation counting efficiency by pulse height shift. *Intern. J. Appl. Radiation Isotopes* **8**, 1 (1960).
6. Baldessarini, R. J., and Kopin, I. J., Assay of tissue levels of *S*-adenosylmethionine. *Anal. Biochem.* **6**, 289 (1963).
7. Baxter, C. F., and Senoner, I., Liquid scintillation counting of C^{14}-labeled amino acids on paper, using trinitrobenzene-1-sulfonic acid, and a modified combustion apparatus. *Anal. Biochem.* **7**, 55 (1964).
8. Blair, A., and Segal, S., Use of filter paper mounting for determination of the specific activity of gluconate-C^{14} by liquid scintillation assay. *Anal. Biochem.* **3**, 221 (1962).
9. Blanchard, F. A., and Takahashi, I. T., Use of submicron silica to prevent count loss by wall absorption in liquid scintillation counting. *Anal. Chem.* **33**, 975 (1961).
10. Branson, B. M., Hagee, G. R., Goldin, A. S., Karches, G. J., and Straub, C. P., Assembly and operation of a low level counting facility. *J. Am. Water Works Assoc.* **51**, 438 (1959).
11. Bray, G. A., A simple efficient liquid scintillator for counting aqueous solutions in a liquid scintillation counter. *Anal. Biochem.* **1**, 279 (1960).
12. Bruno, G. A., and Christian, J. E., Determination of carbon-14 in aqueous bicarbonate solutions by liquid scintillation counting techniques. *Anal. Chem.* **33**, 1216 (1961).
13. Bruno, G. A., and Christian, J. E., Note on suitable solvent systems usable in the liquid scintillation counting of animal tissue. *J. Am. Pharm. Assoc., Sci. Ed.* **49**, 560 (1960).
14. Buhler, D. R., A simple scintillation counting technique for assaying $C^{14}O_2$ in a Warburg flask. *Anal. Biochem.* **4**, 413 (1962).
15. Bush, E. T., General applicability of the channels ratio method of measuring liquid scintillation counting efficiencies. *Anal. Chem.* **35**, 1924 (1963).
16. Butler, F. E., Determination of tritium in water and urine. Liquid scintillation counting and rate-of-drift determination. *Anal. Chem.* **33**, 409 (1961).
17. Carr, T. E. F., and Parsons, B. J., A method for the assay of calcium-45 by liquid scintillation counting. *Intern. J. Appl. Radiation Isotopes* **13**, 57 (1962).
18. Chen, P. S., Jr., Liquid scintillation counting of C^{14} and H^3 in plasma and serum. *Proc. Soc. Exptl. Biol. Med.* **98**, 546 (1958).
19. Chiriboga, J., and Roy, D. N., Rapid method for determination of decarboxylation of compounds labeled with carbon-14. *Nature* **193**, 684 (1962).

20. Chleck, D. J., and Ziegler, C. A., Ultrasonic degassing of liquid scintillator. *Rev. Sci. Instr.* **28,** 466 (1957).
21. Cluley, H. J., Suspension scintillation counting of carbon-14 barium carbonate. *Analyst* **87,** 170 (1962).
22. Davidson, J. D., and Feigelson, P., Practical aspects of internal-sample liquid scintillation counting. *Intern. J. Appl. Radiation Isotopes* **2,** 1 (1957).
23. Davidson, J. D., *in* "Liquid Scintillation Counting" (C. G. Bell and F. N. Hayes, eds.), p. 88. Macmillan (Pergamon), New York, 1958.
24. Davidson, J. D., "Some recent developments in liquid scintillation counting of biochemical samples." *Proc. Univ. New Mexico Conf. on Organic Scintillation Detectors* (G. H. Daub, F. N. Hayes, and E. Sullivan, eds.), TID-7612, p. 232. U.S. At. Energy Comm., Washington, D.C., 1961.
25. Davie, E. W., Hyamine hydroxide. *Biochem. Prep.* **8,** 53 (1961).
26. De Bersaques, J., Relation between the absorption and the quenching of liquid scintillation samples. *Intern. J. Appl. Radiation Isotopes* **14,** 173 (1963).
27. Dern, R. J., and Hart, W. L., Studies with doubly labeled iron. *J. Lab. Clin. Med.* **57,** 332 and 460 (1961).
28. Dobbs, H. E., Oxygen flask method for the assay of tritium-, carbon-14-, and sulfur-35-labeled compounds. *Anal. Chem.* **35,** 783 (1963).
29. Doi, R. H., and Spiegelman, S., Homology test between the nucleic acid of an RNA virus and the DNA in the host cell. *Science* **138,** 1270 (1962).
30. Domer, F. R., and Hayes, F. N., Background vs. efficiency in liquid scintillators. *Nucleonics* **18,** No. 1, 100 (1960).
31. Eisenberg, F., Jr., Round Table on preparation of the alkaline absorbent for radioactive CO_2 in liquid scintillation counting *in* "Liquid Scintillation Counting" (C. G. Bell and F. N. Hayes, eds.), p. 123. Macmillan (Pergamon), New York, 1958.
32. Erdtmann, G., and Hermann, G. Z., The counting of radioisotopes of metallic elements in liquid scintillators. *Z. Elektrochem.* **64,** 1092 (1960).
33. Fales, H. M., Discoloration of samples for liquid scintillation counting. *Atomlight* **25,** 8 (1963).
34. Farmer, E. C., and Berstein, I. A., Determination of specific activities of C^{14}-labelled organic compounds with a water-soluble liquid scintillator. *Science* **115,** 460 (1952).
35. Fleishman, D. G., and Glazunov, V. V., An external standard as a means of determining the efficiency and background of a liquid scintillator. *Pribory i Tekhn. Eksper.* **7,** No. 3, 55 (1962).
36. Funt, B. L., Scintillating gels. *Nucleonics* **14,** No. 8, 83 (1956).
37. Furlong, N. B., Williams, N. L., and Willis, D. P., Enhancement of tritium-counting efficiency on paper discs after incorporation into (^{3}H)DNA. *Biochim. Biophys. Acta* **103,** 341 (1965).
38. Furst, M., and Kallmann, H. P., Enhancement of fluorescence in solutions under high-energy irradiation. *Phys. Rev.* **97,** 583 (1955).
39. Geiger, J. W., and Wright, L. D., Liquid scintillation counting of radioautograms. *Biochem. Biophys. Res. Commun.* **2,** 282 (1960).
40. Gjone, E., Vance, H. G., and Turner, D. A., Direct liquid scintillation counting of plasma and tissues. *Intern. J. Appl. Radiation Isotopes* **8,** 95 (1960).
41. Gordon, C. F., and Wolfe, A. L., Liquid scintillation counting of aqueous samples. *Anal. Chem.* **32,** 574 (1960).

42. Halvorsen, L., Direct measurement of tritium in biological materials with the liquid scintillation counter. *Proc. Symp. Tritium Phys. Biol. Sci., Vienna, 1961* Vol. 1, p. 313. Intern. At. Energy Agency, Vienna, 1962.
43. Harlan, J. W., Liquid scintillation counting of $C^{14}O_2$ in aqueous carbonate solutions. *Atomlight* **19,** 8 (1961).
44. Hash, J. H., Determination of tritium in whole cells and cellular fractions of *Bacillus megaterium* using liquid scintillation techniques. *Anal. Biochem.* **4,** 257 (1962).
45. Hayes, F. N., Hiebert, R. F., and Schuch, R. L., Low energy counting with a new liquid scintillation solute. *Science* **116,** 140 (1952).
46. Hayes, F. N., Rogers, B. S., and Sanders, P. C., Importance of solvent in liquid scintillators. *Nucleonics* **13,** No. 1, 46 (1955).
47. Hayes, F. N., and Gould, R. G., Liquid scintillation counting of H^3-labeled water and organic compounds. *Science* **117,** 480 (1953).
48. Hayes, F. N., Rogers, B. S., and Langham, W. H., Counting suspensions in liquid scintillators. *Nucleonics* **14,** No. 3, 48 (1956).
49. Helf, S., *In* "Liquid Scintillation Counting" (C. G. Bell and F. N. Hayes, eds.), p. 96. Macmillan (Pergamon), New York, 1958.
50. Helf, S., White, C. G., and Shelly, R. N., Radioassay of finely divided solids by suspension in a gel scintillator. *Anal. Chem.* **32,** 238 (1960).
51. Helmick, M., The quenching effect of benzoic acid in a liquid scintillation system. *Atomlight* February, p. 6 (1960).
52. Hendler, R. W., Procedure for simultaneous assay of two β-emitting isotopes with the liquid scintillation counting technique. *Anal. Biochem.* **7,** 110 (1964).
53. Herberg, R. J., Determination of carbon-14 and tritium in blood and other whole tissues. *Anal. Chem.* **32,** 42 (1960).
54. Herberg, R. J., Backgrounds for liquid scintillation counting of colored solutions. *Anal. Chem.* **32,** 1468 (1960).
55. Herberg, R. J., Phosphorescence in liquid scintillation counting of proteins. *Science* **128,** 199 (1958).
56. Herberg, R. J., Statistical aspects of liquid scintillation counting by internal standard technique. *Anal. Chem.* **35,** 786 (1963).
57. Herberg, R. J., Statistical aspects of double isotope liquid scintillation counting by internal standard technique. *Anal. Chem.* **36,** 1079 (1964).
58. Higashimura, T., Yamada, O., Nohara, N., and Shidei, T., External standard method for the determination of the efficiency in liquid scintillation counting. *Intern. J. Appl. Radiation Isotopes* **13,** 308 (1962).
59. Horrocks, D. L., and Studier, M. H., Low level plutonium-241 analysis by liquid scintillation techniques. *Anal. Chem.* **30,** 1747 (1958).
60. Houtman, A. C., Liquid scintillation counting of blood. *Intern. J. Appl. Radiation Isotopes* **16,** 65 (1965).
61. Jacobson, H. I., Gupta, G. N., Ferandez, C., Hennix, S., and Jensen, E. V., Determination of tritium in biological material. *Arch. Biochem. Biophys.* **86,** 89 (1960).
62. Jeffay, H., Olubajo, F. O., and Jewell, W. R., Determination of radioactive sulfur in biological materials. *Anal. Chem.* **32,** 306 (1960).
63. Jeffay, H., and Alvarez, J., Measurement of C^{14} and S^{35} in a single sample. *Anal. Biochem.* **2,** 506 (1961).

64. Jeffay, H., and Alvarez, J., Liquid scintillation counting of carbon-14—Use of ethanolamine-ethylene glycol monomethyl ether-toluene. *Anal. Chem.* **33**, 612 (1961).
65. Johnson, D. R., and Smith, J. W., Glass filter paper suspension of precipitates for liquid scintillation counting. *Anal. Chem.* **35**, 1991 (1963).
66. Kalberer, F., and Rutschmann, J., A rapid method for determination of tritium, radiocarbon and radiosulfur in any organic sample material by means of liquid scintillation counter. *Helv. Chim. Acta* **44**, 1956 (1961).
67. Kallmann, H. P., Scintillation counting with solutions. *Phys. Rev.* **78**, 621 (1950).
68. Kallmann, H. P., Furst, M., and Brown, F. H., Scintillation solution enhancers. U.S. Patent 3,068,178 (Dec. 11, 1962).
69. Kelly, R. G., Peets, E. A., Gordon, S., and Buyske, D. A., Determination of C^{14} and H^3 in biological samples by Schöniger combustion and liquid scintillation techniques. *Anal. Biochem.* **2**, 267 (1961).
70. Kerr, V. N., Hayes, F. N., and Ott, D. G., Liquid scintillators. III. The quenching of liquid scintillator solutions by organic compounds. *Intern. J. Appl. Radiation Isotopes* **1**, 284 (1957).
71. Keston, A. S., Udenfriend, S., and Levy, M., Determination of organic compounds as isotopic derivatives. *J. Am. Chem. Soc.* **72**, 748 (1950).
72. Kinard, F. E., Liquid scintillator for the analysis of tritium in water. *Rev. Sci. Instr.* **28**, 293 (1957).
73. Kliman, B., and Peterson, R. E., Double isotope derivative assay of aldosterone in biological extracts. *J. Biol. Chem.* **235**, 1639 (1960).
74. Kobayashi, Y., Determination of histidine decarboxylase activity by liquid scintillation counting of $C^{14}O_2$. *Anal. Biochem.* **5**, 284 (1963).
75. Langham, W. H., Eversole, W. J., Hayes, F. N., and Trujillo, T. T., Assay of tritium activity in body fluids using a liquid scintillation system. *J. Lab. Clin. Med.* **47**, 819 (1956).
76. Leffingwell, T. P., Riess, R. W., and Melville, G. S., Jr., Liquid scintillation beta counting of iron-59 in clear and colored systems. *Intern. J. Appl. Radiation Isotopes* **13**, 75 (1962).
77. Loewus, F. A., The use of bis-(2-alkoxyethyl) ethers as antifreeze in naphthalene-1,4-dioxane scintillating mixtures. *Intern. J. Appl. Radiation Isotopes* **12**, 6 (1961).
78. Loftfield, R. B., Scintillation counting of C^{14} labeled paper chromatograms. *Atomlight* **13**, 1 (1960).
79. Ludwick, J. D., Liquid scintillation counting of promethium-147, bioassay procedure. *Anal. Chem.* **36**, 1104 (1964).
80. McCarthy, B. J., and Britten, R. J., The synthesis of ribosomes in *E. coli*. *Biophys. J.* **2**, 35 (1962).
81. Mans, R. J., and Novelli, G. D., Measurement of the incorporation of radioactive amino acids into protein by a filter-paper disk method. *Arch. Biochem. Biophys.* **94**, No. 1, 48 (1961).
82. Meade, R. C., and Stiglitz, R. A., Improved solvent systems for liquid scintillation counting of body fluids and tissues. *Intern. J. Appl. Radiation Isotopes* **13**, 11 (1962).
83. Myers, L. S., Jr., and Brush, A. H., Counting of alpha and beta radiation in aqueous solutions by the detergent-anthracene scintillation method. *Anal. Chem.* **34**, 342 (1962).

84. Nakshbandi, M. M., A plastic scintillator method for the radioassay of H^3- and C^{14}-labelled compounds on filter paper. *Intern. J. Appl. Radiation Isotopes* **16,** 157 (1965).
85. Nathan, D. G., Davidson, J. D., Waggoner, J. G., and Berlin, N. I., The counting of barium carbonate in a liquid scintillation spectrometer. *J. Lab. Clin. Med.* **52,** 915 (1958).
86. O'Brien, R. D., Nitric acid digestion of tissues for liquid scintillation counting. *Anal. Biochem.* **7,** 251 (1964).
87. Okita, G. T., Spratt, J., and LeRoy, G. V., Liquid scintillation counting for assay of tritium in urine. *Nucleonics* **14,** No. 3, 76 (1956).
88. Oliverio, V. T., Denham, C., and Davidson, J. D., Oxygen flask combustion in determination of C^{14} and H^3 in biological materials. *Anal. Biochem.* **4,** 188 (1962).
89. Ott, D. G., Round Table on chemistry of the counting sample scintillation solutes, *in* "Liquid Scintillation Counting" (C. G. Bell and F. N. Hayes, eds.), p. 101. Macmillan (Pergamon), New York, 1958.
90. Ott, D. G., Hayes, F. N., Hammel, J. E., and Kephart, J. F., Argon treatment of liquid scintillators to eliminate oxygen quenching. *Nucleonics* **13,** No. 5, 62 (1955).
91. Ott, D. G., Richmond, C. R., Trujillo, T. T., and Foreman, H., Cab-O-Sil suspensions for liquid scintillation counting. *Nucleonics* **17,** No. 9, 106 (1959).
92. Passman, J. M., Radin, N. S., and Cooper, J. A. D., Liquid scintillation technique for measuring carbon-14-dioxide activity. *Anal. Chem.* **28,** 484 (1956).
93. Peets, E. A., Florini, J. R., and Buyske, D. A., Tritium radioactivity determination of biological materials by a rapid dry combustion technique. *Anal. Chem.* **32,** 1465 (1960).
94. Peng, C. T., Quenching of fluorescence in liquid scintillation counting of labeled organic compounds. *Anal. Chem.* **32,** 1292 (1960).
95. Peterkofsky, A., Jesensky, C., Bank, A., and Mehler, A. H., Studies on the role of methylated bases in the biological activity of soluble ribonucleic acid. *J. Biol. Chem.* **239,** 2918 (1964).
96. Pinter, K. G., Hamilton, J. G., and Miller, O. N., Liquid scintillation counting with glass fiber paper. *Anal. Biochem.* **4,** 458 (1963).
97. Pringle, R. W., Black, L. D., Funt, B. L., and Sobering, S., New quenching effect in liquid scintillators, *Phys. Rev.* **92,** 1582 (1953).
98. Rapkin, E., and Packard, L. E., "New accessories for liquid scintillation counting." *Proc. Univ. New Mexico Conference on Organic Scintillation Detectors* (G. H. Daub, F. N. Hayes, and E. Sullivan, eds.), TID-7612, p. 216. U.S. At. Energy Comm., Washington, 1961.
99. Reynolds, G. T., Harrison, F. B., and Salvini, G., Liquid scintillation counters. *Phys. Rev.* **78,** 488 (1950).
100. Ross, H. H., Liquid scintillation counting of I^{129} and I^{125}. *Oak Ridge Radioisotope Conf., Res. Appl. Phys. Sci. Eng. Gatlinburg, Tenn., 1963.*
101. Ross, H. H., and Yerick, R. E., Quantitative interpretation of color quenching in liquid scintillator systems. *Anal. Chem.* **35,** 794 (1963).
102. Roucayrol, J-C., Oberhausen, E., and Schussler, R., Liquid scintillators in filter paper—a new detector. *Nucleonics* **15,** No. 11, 104 (1957).
103. Roucayrol, J-C., Oberhausen, E., and Schussler, R., Measurement of radioactivity emitting compounds. U.S. Patent 3,017,510 (Jan. 16, 1962).

104. Sarnat, M., and Jeffay, H., Determination of radioactive calcium by liquid scintillation counting. *Anal. Chem.* **34,** 643 (1962).
105. Scales, B., Liquid scintillation: the determination of background counts of samples containing quenching substances. *Anal. Biochem.* **5,** 489 (1963).
106. Schöniger, W., Rapid microanalytical determination of halogen in organic substances. *Mikrochim. Acta* p. 123 (1955).
107. Shapira, J., and Perkins, W. H., Liquid scintillation counting of aqueous solutions of carbon-14 and tritium. *Science* **131,** 414 (1960).
108. Shapiro, I. L., and Kritchevsky, D., Radioassay of cholesterol-C^{14} digitonide. *Anal. Biochem.* **5,** 88 (1963).
109. Sherman, J. R., Rapid enzyme assay technique utilizing radioactive substrate, ion-exchange paper, and liquid scintillation counting. *Anal. Biochem.* **5,** 548 (1963).
110. Shneour, E. A., Aronoff, S., and Kirk, M. R., Liquid scintillation counting of solutions containing carotenoids and chlorophylls. *Intern. J. Appl. Radiation Isotopes* **13,** 623 (1962).
111. Snyder, F., and Stephens, N., Quantitative carbon-14 and tritium assay of thin-layer chromatography plates. *Anal. Biochem.* **4,** 128 (1962).
112. Snyder, F., and Godfrey, P., Collecting $C^{14}O_2$ in a Warburg flask for subsequent scintillation counting. *J. Lipid Res.* **2,** 195 (1961).
113. Spencer, R. P., and Blau, M., Intestinal transport of selenium-75 selenomethionine. *Science* **136,** 155 (1962).
114. Steinberg, D., Vaughan, M., Anfinsen, C. B., Gorry, J. D., and Logan, J., The preparation of tritiated proteins by the Wilzbach method and a simple method for liquid scintillation counting of radioactive proteins, *in* "Liquid Scintillation Counting" (C. G. Bell and F. N. Hayes, eds.), p. 230. Macmillan (Pergamon), New York, 1958.
115. Steinberg, D., Radioassay of carbon-14 in aqueous solutions using a liquid scintillation spectrometer. *Nature* **182,** 740 (1958).
116. Steinberg, D., Radioassay of aqueous solutions mixed with solid crystalline fluors. *Nature* **183,** 1253 (1959).
117. Steinberg, D., A new approach to radioassay of aqueous solutions in the liquid scintillation spectrometer. *Anal. Biochem.* **1,** 23 (1960).
118. Takahashi, H., Hattori, T., and Maruo, B., Liquid scintillation counting of C^{14} paper chromatograms. *Anal. Biochem.* **2,** 447 (1961).
119. Takahashi, H., Hattori, T., and Maruo, B., Liquid scintillation counting of biological compounds in aqueous solution. *Anal. Chem.* **35,** 1982 (1963).
120. Tye, R., and Engel, J. D., Liquid scintillation counting of carbon-14 in aqueous digests of whole tissues. *Anal. Chem.* **37,** 1225 (1965).
121. Vaughan, M., Steinberg, D., and Logan, J., Liquid scintillation counting of C^{14} and H^3-labeled amino acids and proteins. *Science* **126,** 446 (1957).
122. Wang, C. H., and Jones, D. E., Liquid scintillation counting on paper chromatograms. *Biochem. Biophys. Res. Commun.* **1,** 203 (1959).
123. Werbin, H., Chaikoff, I. L., and Imada, M. R., Rapid sensitive method for determining H^3-water in body fluids by liquid scintillation spectrometry. *Proc. Soc. Exptl. Biol. Med.* **102,** 8 (1959).
124. White, C. G., and Helf, S., Suspension counting in a gel scintillator. *Nucleonics* **14,** No. 10, 46 (1956).
125. Willenbrink, J., On the quantity assay of radiochromatogram by liquid scintillation counting. *Intern. J. Appl. Radiation Isotopes* **14,** 237 (1963).

126. Williamson, J. R., Metabolic effects of epinephrine in the isolated perfused rat heart. *J. Biol. Chem.* **239,** 2721 (1964).
127. Wirth, H. O., "Syntheses and properties of substituted *p*-oligophenylenes." *Proc. Univ. New Mexico Conf. on Organic Scintillation Detectors* (G. H. Daub, F. N. Hayes, and E. Sullivan, eds.), TID-7612, p. 78. U.S. At. Energy Comm., Washington, D.C., 1961.
128. Woeller, F. H., Liquid scintillation counting of $C^{14}O_2$ with phenethylamine. *Anal. Biochem.* **2,** 508 (1961).
129. Woolever, C. A., and Goldfein, A., A double-isotope derivative method for plasma progesterone assay. *Intern. J. Appl. Radiation Isotopes* **14,** 163 (1963).
130. Wu, R., Simultaneous studies of phosphate transport and glycolysis by a simple liquid scintillation counting procedure with P^{32}, C^{14}, and H^3 compounds. *Anal. Biochem.* **7,** 207 (1964).
131. Ziegler, C. A., Chleck, D. J., and Brinkerhoff, J., Radioassay of low specific activity tritiated water by improved liquid scintillation techniques, *in* "Liquid Scintillation Counting" (C. G. Bell and F. N. Hayes, eds.), p. 185. Macmillan (Pergamon), New York, 1958.

CHAPTER 10

LIQUID SCINTILLATION COUNTING EQUIPMENT

EDWARD F. POLIC
PACKARD INSTRUMENT COMPANY, INC.
DOWNERS GROVE, ILLINOIS

The instrumentation presently employed for counting samples with liquid scintillation techniques will be described (*35*). For a review of liquid scintillation sample preparation the reader is referred to Chapter 9, to a recent book by Schram and Lombaert (*28*), to the proceedings of the 1957 (*3*) and 1960 (*12*) symposia on Liquid Scintillation Counting, and to several comprehensive reviews (*13, 14, 26*).

The liquid scintillation technique finds its primary use in counting of β-ray emitting isotopes such as ^{3}H, ^{14}C, ^{35}S, ^{32}P, and others. Many other radioisotopes commonly thought of as γ-ray emitters are also β-ray emitters and can be counted using liquid scintillation. Examples include ^{131}I, ^{137}Cs, ^{59}Fe, and ^{60}Co. The technique may also be used to count low-energy X and γ rays emitted by some radioisotopes, especially those which decay by electron capture. To simplify the present discussion however, we shall examine the use of liquid scintillation counting instruments for the measurement of ^{3}H and ^{14}C, which is by far the most important application.

I. LIGHT CONVERSION

The theoretical β-ray spectra (*19*) of ^{3}H and ^{14}C are shown in Fig. 1. Using the best present liquid scintillators one gets approximately seven photons of light per kiloelectron volt of β-ray energy in a roughly linear relationship except for added losses at low energies (below 100 keV) where the β-ray paths are relatively short. The same types of losses, due to short path lengths, are noted for α particles, which exhibit only 7–10% of the light output as compared with β rays of equal energies (*5, 6, 11*).

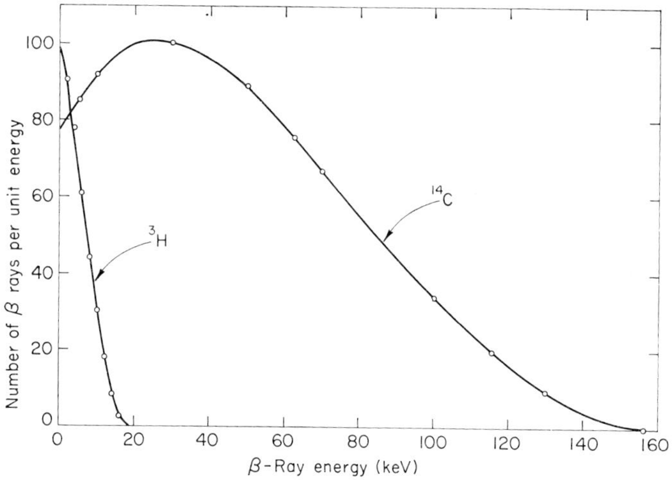

FIG. 1. Theoretical β-ray spectra of ^{3}H and ^{14}C.

Figure 2 shows the approximate light spectra of ^{3}H and ^{14}C in an idealized liquid scintillator. The average energy of ^{3}H is 5.6 keV and the number of photons emitted per decay is approximately 40. This is an extremely small light output, and it is made even smaller by the quenching agents present in most samples (Chapter 9, Section IV).

A. Light Detection

The main purpose of liquid scintillation counting instrumentation is the detection of these small quantities of light. The simplest method is to use a single multiplier phototube and associated circuitry. The block diagram of Fig. 3 is a diagram of a single multiplier phototube liquid scintillation spectrometer. It illustrates the process wherein photons of light from the sample are converted to electrons in the multiplier phototube, amplified, analyzed with respect to pulse height, and counted (*16*).

The multiplier phototube has a photosensitive surface (the photocathode) to which the photons from the sample are directed. Multiplier phototubes, usable in liquid scintillation counting systems, have quantum efficiencies (number of electrons released per photon) of about 20–30%. The electrons leaving the photocathode are multiplied by the dynode

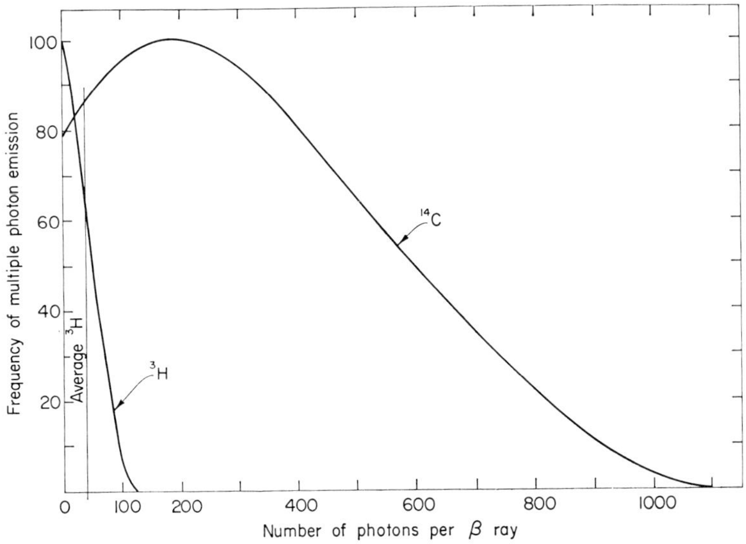

FIG. 2. Approximate light spectra of ^3H and ^{14}C in an ideal liquid scintillator.

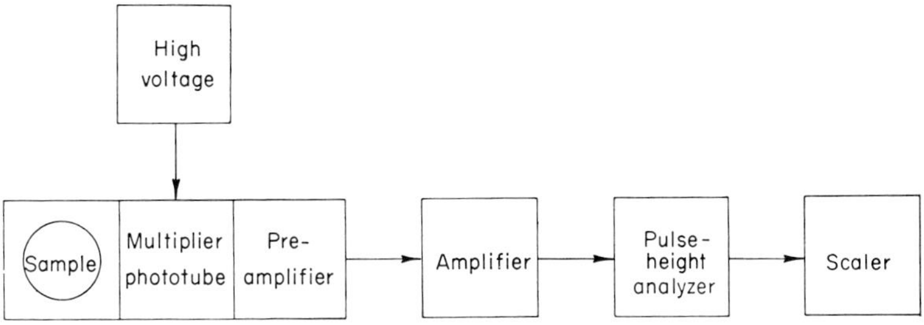

FIG. 3. Block diagram of a single multiplier phototube liquid scintillation spectrometer.

structure within the multiplier phototube so that its output is about 10^5 to 10^8 times greater than the number of electrons leaving the photocathode. Even with such large multiplication factors the output pulses of the multiplier phototube are so small that they usually require further electronic amplification before entering a pulse-height analyzer (*29*). The pulse-height analyzer, in turn, selects the pulse-height (energy) range that is desired, and the scaler counts the output of the pulse-height analyzer.

If an idealized tritium sample is introduced to such a single multiplier phototube system, and if the system is designed so that all the photons of the sample arrive at the photocathode, then the photocathode will release 0 to 25 electrons per ^{3}H decay. The average number of electrons would be only eight. The noise spectrum of the multiplier phototube, which is due mainly to thermionic emission by the photocathode, is superimposed on the tritium spectrum and results in a relatively high background even when the operating temperature of the multiplier phototube is reduced. Another disadvantage of the single multiplier phototube system is that of phosphorescence of the sample due to light

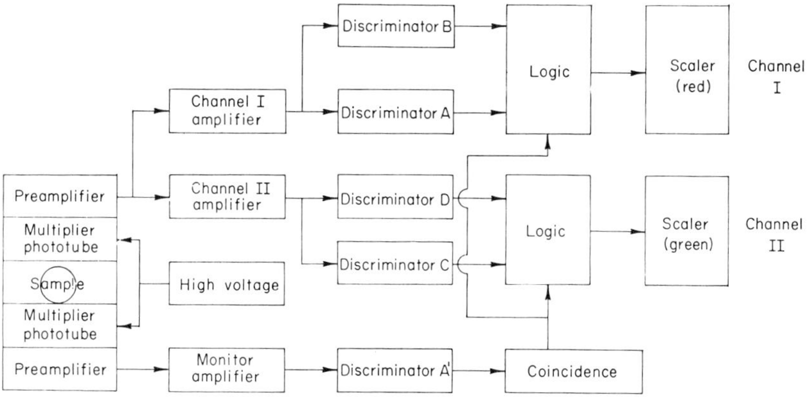

FIG. 4. Block diagram of a coincidence liquid scintillation spectrometer as used until 1963.

exposure during sample preparation. Such phosphorescence is composed of single photon events which persist for relatively long periods of time.

A coincidence system was designed to minimize the problems inherent in a single multiplier phototube system. The block diagram shown in Fig. 4 is that of commercially available liquid scintillation spectrometers as they existed from 1954 to 1963.

The coincidence system adds an additional multiplier phototube and associated circuitry, including a coincidence circuit, to the single multiplier phototube system. This allows an event to be counted only if both multiplier phototubes "observe" the event within the resolving time of the coincidence circuit. A noise event in one multiplier phototube is not correlated timewise with a noise event in the other multiplier phototube, except by chance coincidence, and is therefore not counted. Also, single photon events, as from phosphorescence, at most give rise to a pulse in only one multiplier phototube and are not counted except in such instances where the count-rate is so high that chance coincidences occur.

The coincidence system has a disadvantage in that the photons from a sample must now be distributed between two multiplier phototubes. Thus, for the idealized tritium sample each photocathode would release 0 to 12 electrons per ^{3}H decay with an average of only 4 electrons. It should be noted that in this system all the pulse-height analysis is done by one multiplier phototube, while the other one is used solely to decide whether the output of the first one is legitimate (that is, to establish coincidence).

As shown in Fig. 4, any number of channels of analysis (amplifier, pulse-height analyzer, scaler) may be added to the multiplier phototube used for analysis. Additional channels allow the user to perform simultaneous counting of two or more radioisotopes in a mixture, or to do quench monitoring on samples (Chapter 9, Section IV,C).

Recently a new concept in coincidence liquid scintillation spectrometers was introduced. The new spectrometer provides pulse-height analysis on the summed output of both multiplier phototubes instead of only one (Fig. 5). This effectively doubles the signal-to-noise ratio for pulse-height analysis and also results in a truer reproduction of the spectral shapes. With such a system, the sensitivities for counting ^{3}H and ^{14}C have doubled over the previous coincidence system. For a well-shielded, refrigerated system the figure of merit (efficiency squared: background counts per minute) for tritium is 130 or better and that for ^{14}C it is at least 300. Using glass vials tritium efficiencies of 50–60% are achieved with backgrounds of 15–25 cpm. Polyethylene vials improve tritium efficiencies a few percent (*25*). Quartz-faced multiplier phototubes are used for their low background characteristics. For instruments operated at room temperatures, the tritium efficiencies are 45–55% and the backgrounds about 35–40 cpm. The more accurate spectrum representation gives much better separation of different radioisotopes for counting double-labeled samples.

B. Light Transfer

The operation of the individual components of these liquid scintillation spectrometers must be understood in order to fully utilize the capabilities of these systems and to understand the meaning of the counts recorded by the scalers.

The detector in a liquid scintillation counting system must fulfill several requirements: The sample-counting chamber and multiplier phototube housing must be absolutely light-tight during both sample counting and sample changing. The sample-changing process should be relatively fast to maximize instrument counting time. The sample-changing mechanism must position the sample accurately. The multiplier phototubes and the sample counting chamber must be well shielded to minimize background due to cosmic rays and local radiation. Boyce and Cameron (*8*) have thoroughly discussed background contributions and background reduction.

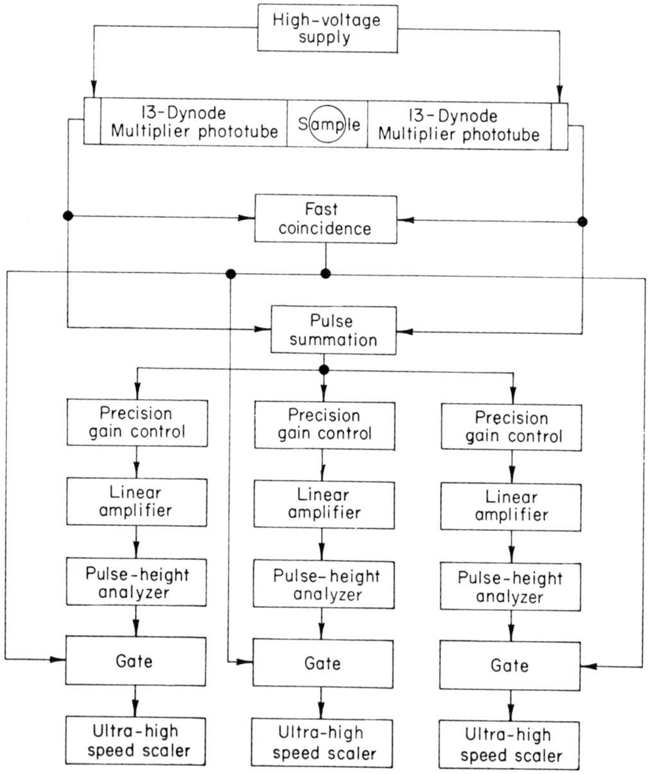

FIG. 5. Block diagram of a coincidence liquid scintillation spectrometer with pulse summation.

The sample vial plays an important part in the efficient transfer of photons from the scintillator to the photocathode (*1, 10, 25*). Glass vials, with their extremely smooth surfaces, exhibit light trapping. Polyethylene vials, with their slightly rougher surfaces, allow more light to get out of the vial because of light diffusion even though the absolute transmission of the light through polyethylene is less than that through glass. Use of polyethylene vials is particularly desirable in counting extremely low-energy radioisotopes where there are very few photons per decay and any loss results in loss of coincidence. Use of polyethylene vials with tritium samples provides some improvement in efficiency, while with higher energy β-ray emitters there is little increase in efficiency.

Polyethylene vials cause some problems that do not exist with glass vials. They are permeable to some liquid scintillation solvents (toluene but not dioxane), and cannot be heated during sample preparation as is required in some procedures. They usually cannot be reused because of adsorption of material, and exhibit much higher phosphorescence than glass vials.

The sample-counting chamber must be designed to transfer efficiently the light from the counting vials to the multiplier phototubes. The most efficient method of light transfer is a direct coupling between the counting vial and the multiplier phototubes, using an optical fluid. This is a relatively messy procedure, especially with automatic sample handling. Also, impurities introduced into the coupling fluid by the vials quickly decrease the effectiveness of light transfer. The next best system is to surround the sample vial with a light guide (*2, 4*) and to couple the light guide to the multiplier phototubes. The dimensions of a light guide are chosen so that there is sufficient clearance of any counting vials that might be used, since rubbing of the light guide gives rise to phosphorescence. The multiplier phototubes are placed as close to the counting vial as is practical to maximize counting efficiency. A minimum of material is used in the light guide to minimize Čerenkov radiation (*3*). The reflecting surfaces of the light guide are covered with a diffuse aluminum reflector for optimum dispersion of reflected light.

C. Multiplier Phototubes

The ideal liquid scintillation solution has a light output spectrum which matches the response spectrum of the multiplier phototubes being used (*27, 30*) (Fig. 1 of Chapter 9). Its photocathode is a very low work function surface composed of alkali metals such as cesium plus antimony. Approximately 2 eV of energy is required to release an electron from a Cs_3Sb surface. The amount of energy contained in a photon is dependent upon its wavelength, and may be determined approximately as follows:

$$\text{Energy (in eV)} = 1234/\text{Wavelength (in m}\mu\text{)}$$

Therefore, one photon at 400 mμ would provide about 3 eV of energy, and would result in the release of 1 electron from the photocathode in 20–30% of the events.

In practice, several problems arise. If the photocathode is too thin, it will not stop the photon. If the photocathode is too thick, electrons excited within the cathode will be unable to escape from the photocathode. Taking these considerations into account, the optimum photocathode thickness is found to be about 25 mμ (*9*). The greater the angle of incidence of photons striking the photocathode, the more likely that they will be stopped by the photocathode. In this respect, the light guide is of great benefit for it increases the critical angle at the exterior surface of the multiplier phototube, allowing a longer path length for the photon through the photocathode without increasing the path length for the excited electron.

For the multiplication of the electrons released by the photocathode, they are directed through the multiplier phototube's dynode structure. A potential is applied between the photocathode and the first dynode, between the first dynode and the second dynode, and so on. The photocathode is usually at ground potential to avoid a voltage gradient

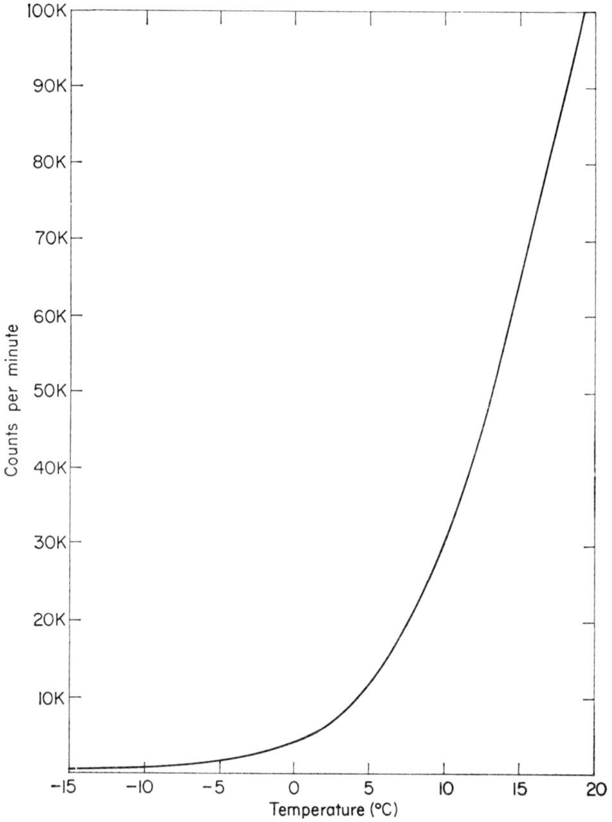

FIG. 6. Typical multiplier phototube noise versus temperature curve for an S-11 photocathode at ^{3}H counting settings.

through the multiplier phototube envelope to the surrounding environment which could cause spurious discharges at the photocathode. An electron leaving the photocathode is accelerated to the first dynode by the potential difference between the two surfaces. It strikes the first dynode and releases several secondary electrons, the number being dependent upon the applied potential difference. Each of these electrons is accelerated to the second dynode, by the potential difference between the two dynodes, and in turn releases additional secondary electrons (*18*). This process continues through all the dynode stages. From the last dynode the electrons are directed to the anode where they are collected. If the multiplication factor per dynode stage is 4, then for a 13-dynode structure the gain would be 4^{13} or approximately 67×10^6.

The multiplier phototube is also a random noise generator. Thermally excited electrons are released from the photocathode and dynodes, and those from the photocathode and first dynode cause output pulses of the same order of magnitude as the legitimate pulses to be counted. Those from the other dynodes usually cause output pulses several orders of magnitude smaller for there are fewer stages of multiplication for them. The quantity of noise events can be reduced by cooling the multiplier phototube. Figure 6 shows a typical curve of multiplier phototube noise versus temperature.

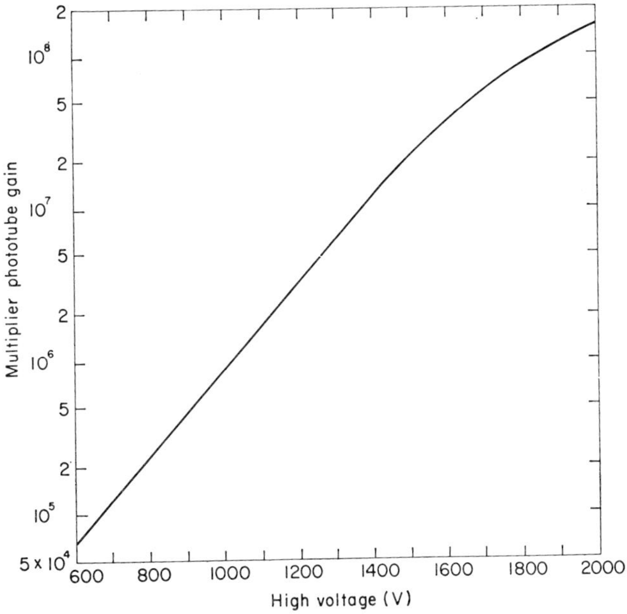

FIG. 7. Multiplier phototube gain versus applied high voltage for 6255B multiplier phototubes.

Light generated in the last stages of the dynode structure can get back to the photocathode. This is especially bad, for the photocathodes of both multiplier phototubes can "see" this light and the spectrometer can treat it as a coincident event. Radioactivity, such as ^{40}K and uranium isotopes, in the glass envelope of the multiplier phototube, particularly in the face of the tube, may cause Čerenkov scintillations which both multiplier phototubes can see. Quartz-faced multiplier phototubes practically eliminate the problem of Čerenkov radiation, and they are now available in commercial quantities with sufficiently high quantum efficiencies and low noise characteristics.

The high-voltage supply is used to supply the potential difference across the dynode resistors, and as such is the gain control for the multiplier phototube. Figure 7 shows a curve of applied high voltage versus gain of the multiplier phototube plotted on a semilogarithmic scale. It is quite obvious that the high-voltage supply must be extremely stable in order to maintain a stable gain by the multiplier phototubes.

II. ELECTRONIC CIRCUITRY

A. Pulse Coincidence

The 13-dynode multiplier phototubes provide sufficient gain so that preamplifiers are not required. This allows the use of an extremely fast coincidence circuit operating directly from the multiplier phototube outputs with no intervening electronics to degrade the pulses timewise or to add electronic jitter. The resolving time of the coincidence circuit is chosen to maximize the ratio of efficiency squared to background (E^2/B) (Chapter 3, Section 1,B,3). At present, the optimum value for resolving time seems to be approximately 30 nsec. If the resolving time is made longer, the instrument has a higher efficiency but the background due to light interaction between multiplier phototubes increases disproportionately and the E^2/B ratio decreases. If the resolving time is made shorter, the instrument has a lower background but the efficiency decreases disproportionately and the E^2/B ratio will decrease. The relationship of coincidence resolving time to the E^2/B ratio for tritium is shown in Fig. 8.

Accidentals are random coincidences between the two multiplier phototubes, because of noise or phosphorescence, which occur within the resolving time of the coincidence circuit. Accidentals can be computed as follows:

$$\text{Accidentals (cpm)} = 2N_1N_2\tau$$

where N_1 is the noise rate in counts per minute of one multiplier phototube, N_2 is the noise rate of the other, and τ is the resolving time in minutes of the coincidence circuit. Thus, for a 30-nsec resolving time this expression becomes

$$\text{Accidentals (cpm)} = N_1N_2 \times 10^{-9}$$

If the noise rates of the two multiplier phototubes are both about 30,000 cpm, the accidental count-rate would be only about 1 cpm. Therefore the

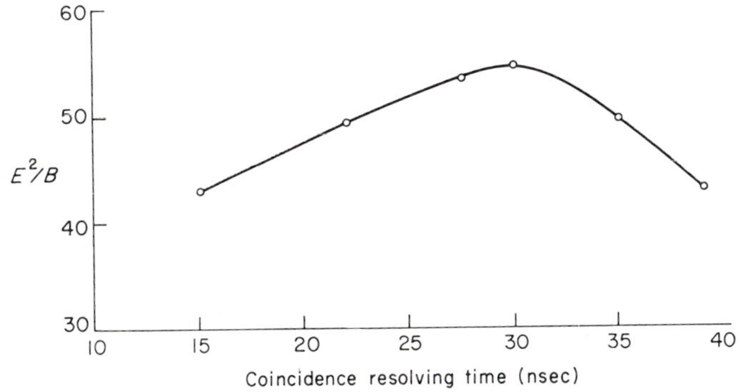

FIG. 8. Ratio of tritium efficiency squared to background as a function of coincidence resolving time for pair of 6255B 13-stage multiplier phototubes (H.V. = 1850 V).

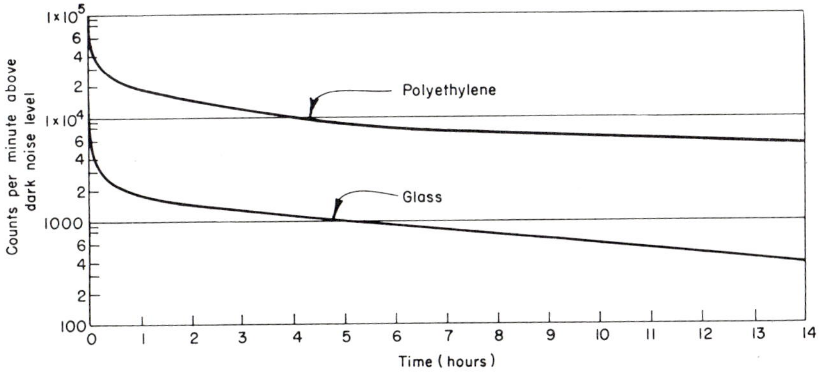

FIG. 9. Phosphorescence decay curves for glass (lower curve) and polyethylene vials (upper curve) taken under noncoincident conditions.

coincidence circuit effectively eliminates noncoincident noise sources, thermionic emission of multiplier phototubes, and phosphorescence, since these sources produce less than 1 cpm in accidentals.

The multiplier phototubes must be selected for low noise properties. Phosphorescence of the sample vial can increase the background if the level of phosphorescence is high. Therefore care should be taken to avoid undue exposure of the sample to ultraviolet light (sunlight, fluorescent light, and so on) prior to counting of the sample. Figure 9 shows phosphorescence decay curves for glass and polyethylene vials as counted in noncoincidence conditions for highly exposed vials.

B. Pulse Summation and Analysis

The output pulses of the multiplier phototubes also go to a summation circuit. If both multiplier phototubes detect the same event, their outputs arrive at the summation circuit simultaneously and are added together. The output pulse of the summation circuit is approximately twice the amplitude of either incoming pulse. If a noise event occurs in one multiplier phototube, it is not correlated with an event from the other, except by chance coincidence, and the output pulse of the summation circuit is of the same amplitude as the incoming pulse. This technique results in essentially doubling the signal-to-noise ratio.

Pulse summation also produces a much more accurate representation of the spectrum being counted, since the statistical distribution of photons between the two multiplier phototubes no longer affects the pulse spectrum to be analyzed. In the older variety of coincidence liquid scintillation spectrometers, where analysis is done on only one multiplier phototube, events of the same energy can give rise to pulses of widely differing pulse heights depending on where in the sample the events take place, and what fraction of the photons gets to the analyzer-multiplier phototube. Figure 10 illustrates the improvement in spectrum presentation by use of pulse summation.

In several types of commercially available liquid scintillation counter, the output of the summation circuit goes to separate channels of analysis in the spectrometer. Each channel of analysis consists of an amplifier with a precision gain control at its input and a pulse-height analyzer as illustrated in the simplified block diagram of Fig. 11. The precision gain control determines the energy range of the pulse-height analyzer. If the high voltage of the multiplier phototubes is set so that for a given attenuation the tritium spectrum is distributed properly within the pulse-height analysis range, then approximately one-ninth the gain would be required for ^{14}C, which is 8.7 times more energetic than ^{3}H, in order for its spectrum to be distributed properly within the pulse-height analysis range.

The pulse-height analyzer consists of two variable pulse-height discriminators and an anticoincidence circuit. If a pulse from the amplifier exceeds the lower level discriminator threshold but does not exceed the upper discriminator threshold, then a pulse appears at the output of the anticoincidence circuit. The output of the anticoincidence circuit goes to a gate and is allowed to pass through only if the output of the coincidence circuit "enables" the gate at the same time. The output of the gate goes to the scaler, which records and displays the number of analyzed coincident events. Since each separate channel of analysis has its own amplifier and precision gain control, each channel can be

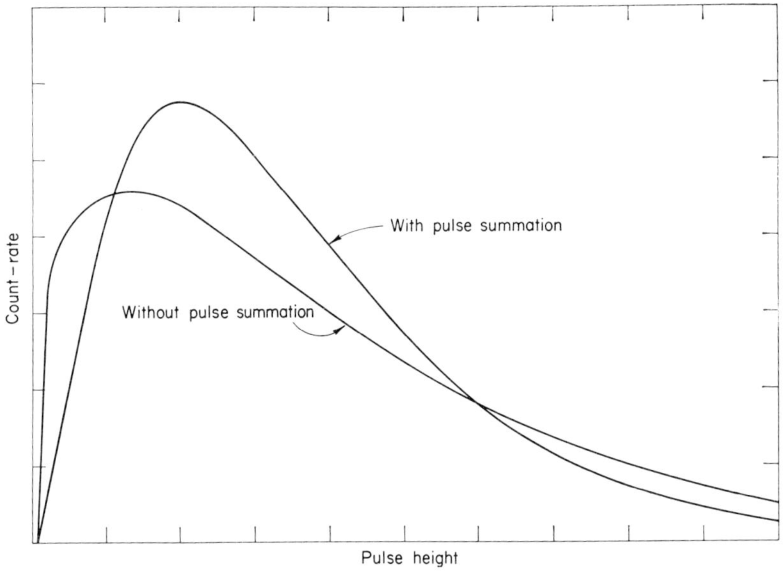

FIG. 10. Comparison of ^3H pulse-height spectra with pulse summation and without pulse summation. The spectrum without pulse summation was taken at twice the gain setting of the spectrum with pulse summation, all other conditions being the same.

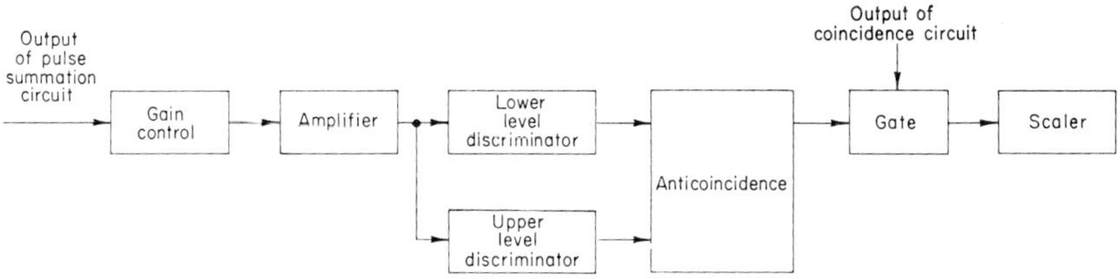

FIG. 11. Block diagram of a pulse-height analysis section.

adjusted for a different range of energies, or optimized for different radioisotopes. The dynamic range (energy range) for such a system is 10,000 to 1; the pulse-height discriminators have a range of 50 to 1 and the amplifier has a 200-to-1 gain range.

III. SAMPLE COUNTING

A. Maximum Counting Sensitivity

In order to maximize sensitivity and (or) minimize counting time the instrument should be set up to maximize the ratio of efficiency squared to background for the samples to be counted. This involves setting the two discriminator levels and the gain control for the channel of analysis to be used. The lower-level discriminator is used primarily to

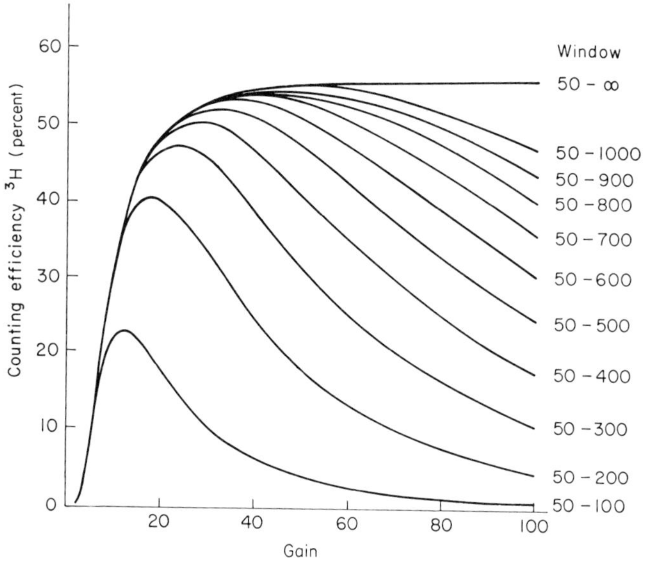

FIG. 12(A).

minimize the low-energy noise of the system and the upper-level discriminator is used primarily to minimize high-energy background counts.

The first step in starting sample counting is to introduce a calibration sample of the same consistency (quenching characteristics, and so on) as the samples to be counted. In order to minimize instrument setup time the calibration sample should be of relatively high activity. The pulse-height analyzer can be said to have a 1000 division analysis range because 10-turn, 100 division potentiometers are usually used to set the discriminator levels. The gain control determines the energy range for the 1000 divisions of the pulse-height analyzer. Initially, the lower discriminator level is set at approximately 50 divisions and the upper discriminator level is set at 1000 divisions. This is referred to as a "50–1000 window," or a 20:1 energy range. Next, the gain control is varied stepwise until a maximum count-rate is observed.

There are two reasons for selecting the gain setting that gives the maximum count-rate. First, it is desired to optimize the figure of merit. This setting gives the maximum efficiency, which is squared in deter-

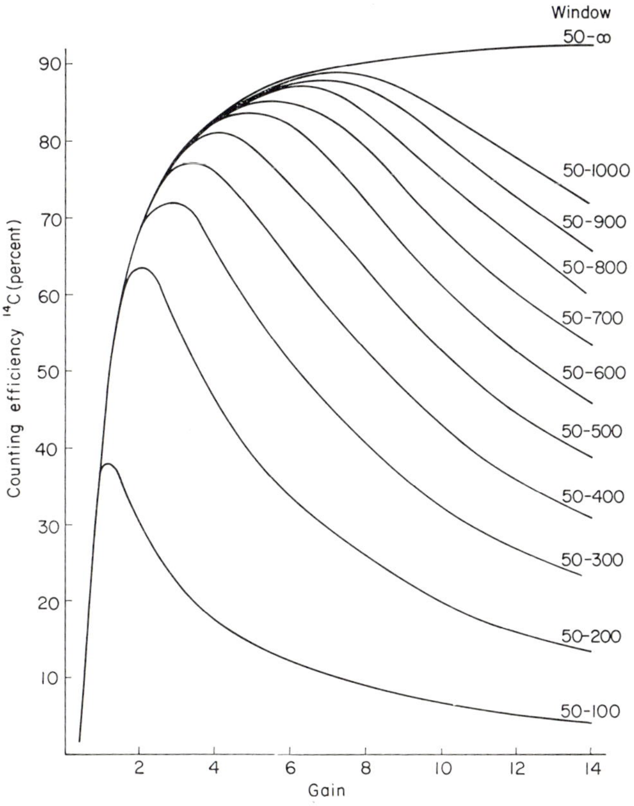

FIG. 12(B).

FIG. 12. Family of counting efficiency versus gain curves of ^{3}H (A) and ^{14}C (B) for different window widths.

mining the figure of merit for this particular window. Since the background does not vary much with change in gain, this gain setting maximizes the figure of merit for this particular window. Second, at this gain setting slight changes in the system gain, either in the sample or in the electronics, do not affect the efficiency greatly, for the gain setting is on the flattest portion of the efficiency versus gain curve (this is commonly known as balance point operation).

At the gain setting that gives the maximum efficiency, a background sample (again, having the same characteristics as the samples to be counted), is counted for a long enough period to be statistically significant. From this a figure of merit is determined for this particular window.

The calibration sample is returned to the counting chamber and the upper discriminator level is lowered to approximately 900 divisions and the gain control is varied stepwise until a maximum counting rate is achieved. Then the background sample is counted at this setting and the figure of merit for this window is determined. Obviously, the efficiency and background for this narrower window will be smaller.

The upper discriminator level is varied and the gain adjusted as described above until a maximum value is reached for the figure of merit. In general, for a low-energy radioisotope, such as tritium, a wide energy range ($\sim$20:1) is optimum; for a higher-energy radioisotope, such as ^{14}C, a narrower energy range ($\sim$5:1) is optimum. Figure 12 shows a family of efficiency versus gain curves for both ^{3}H and ^{14}C unquenched standards; the upper discriminator varies.

For practical counting of samples, where quenching occurs, the curves of Fig. 12 will be lower and displaced to the right, indicating that higher gains are required to reach a maximum efficiency in a given window and that the maximum efficiency is lower than the maximum efficiency for an unquenched sample. If a second channel of analysis is available, it can be optimized for either a different type of sample of the same radioisotope or for a different isotope, in the same way as the first channel. If only one radioisotope is used, the second channel can be used for quench monitoring (Chapter 9, Section IV,C).

B. Double Tracer Techniques

For double-labeled samples, such as those containing ^{14}C and ^{3}H, several techniques are used to establish the discriminator and gain settings (*15, 17, 21, 23*). The channel of analysis for the higher-energy radioisotope can be set so that it excludes the lower-energy isotope. However, the higher-energy radioisotope always contributes counts to the channel of analysis for the lower-energy β-ray emitter because of the overlap in spectra. It is difficult to recommend a specific procedure for setting up an instrument to do double-label counting unless the exact requirements of the experiment are known. A typical procedure is described below.

The gain of the channel of analysis for the higher energy isotope is set so that the end point energy of that isotope is positioned at the upper end of the analysis range. The upper level discriminator is set at the upper end of the analysis range. The lower level discriminator is set for an acceptable contribution of the lower energy isotope. Generally, because of spectral shapes, the best isotope separations are achieved at the lowest energies. Thus the gain of the channel of analysis for the lower energy isotope is set at its maximum. The lower level discriminator is set at the lower end of the analysis range. The upper level discriminator is set for an acceptable contribution of the higher energy isotope.

Typical results for unquenched, double-labeled ^{14}C and ^{3}H samples following the above procedure are as follows:

	^{3}H efficiency, %	^{14}C efficiency, %
^{14}C channel	<0.01	>60
	<1.0	>75
^{3}H channel	>30	<5
	>40	<8
	>50	<13

Similar techniques have been used for triple-labeled samples (*36*).

C. Liquid Flow and Gas Counting

Along with counting of individual samples the liquid scintillation technique is quit useful for the continuous monitoring of radioactivity in flowing liquid or gas streams. Applications of this kind include monitoring of amino acid analyzer streams, liquid chromatography columns, effluents from gas chromatography columns, and process streams (*22, 24*). The sample vial is replaced by a cell packed with a finely dispersed solid scintillator through which the radioactive liquids and gases flow. The most common scintillator for this purpose is anthracene. A detector designed specifically for flow measurements is shown in Fig. 13. The detector is compact enough to be installed at the fluid stream of interest while the rest of the electronics may be in a more convenient location.

In order to monitor radioactivity in the effluent from a gas chromatograph the output of the column must be combusted to CO_2 and H_2O, allowing ^{14}C compounds to be counted as $^{14}CO_2$. If tritium counting is desired, the water can be reduced by passing over hot iron filings. The $^{14}CO_2$ and (or) $^{3}H_2$ is then passed through the cell. A compact combustion furnace which provides all the combustion tubes and traps necessary is available for this purpose.

The data in the flow-monitoring systems can be presented in either analog form (ratemeter and strip-chart recorder with linear or logarithmic presentation, integration of peaks, and so on) or digital form (serial readout of 1 sec). The main advantage of flow-monitoring

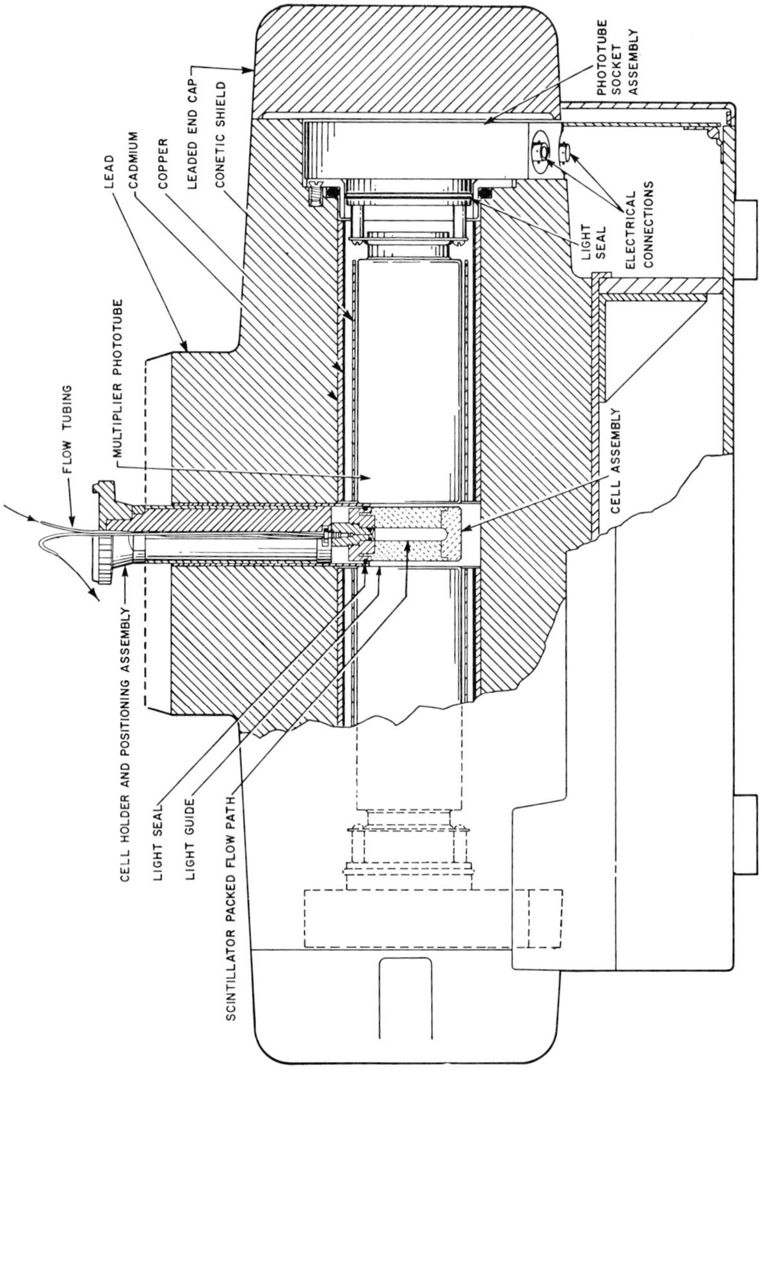

FIG. 13. Flow monitor detector for liquid or gas streams.

systems is that the data are presented immediately. It must be kept in mind that the sample counting time of the system is dependent on the flow-rate. Thus, for example, low count-rates and fast flow-rates yield poor statistical precision. If greater sensitivity and precision are required, samples should be collected and prepared in the normal fashion so that they can be counted for whatever time is required to attain the precision desired (Chapter 11, Sections III and IV).

D. Carbon Dating

Another application of liquid scintillation counting is carbon dating. In the past the biggest problem has been the preparation of the sample in a form suitable for liquid scintillation counting, that is, having both a high yield and a high concentration of carbon atoms. Recently Tamers *et al.* (*20, 31–34*) have developed a benzene synthesizer to meet these needs. This apparatus (now commercially available), converts the raw material to CO_2 by either combustion or acidification and then converts the CO_2 to benzene. The added advantages of this system are the ease and speed of sample preparation. The synthesizer may also be used to convert low-level tritium samples to benzene for subsequent counting in the liquid scintillation spectrometer.

IV. AUTOMATION AND DATA HANDLING

Liquid scintillation counting has become an extremely useful and popular tool in many laboratories using radioisotopes, with the result that automatic sample and data handling are usually required for the large volume of samples being analyzed. Two different techniques of automatic sample-changing mechanisms are illustrated in Figs. 14 and 15. The mechanism shown in Fig. 14 utilizes an endless belt for sample transport. Samples are loaded individually at the instrument location. The operating sequence starts when the belt positions a sample on the elevator and it is loaded into the counting chamber. The sample is counted for a predetermined time or count, data are printed out, and the detector unloads the sample. The belt then indexes the next sample over the elevator and the process is repeated. Empty positions in the belt are bypassed, and groups of samples may be selected for special counting through the use of appropriate programming inserts.

In the sample changer of Fig. 15 the samples may be placed in a sample changer tray right in the laboratory. Then the user simply loads the trays onto shelves in the spectrometer console. The trays, in turn, are automatically positioned over the detector by a tray elevator. The samples in each tray are counted as many times as required before the tray is changed. Empty sample and tray positions are bypassed and the sample changer may be programmed to select only trays of immediate interest.

There are many ways of presenting and handling data from a sample counting run. The high speed serial-entry readout offers the advantage of maximum actual instrument counting time (since data can be printed in only 3.5 sec), and has the added benefit that data from the readout

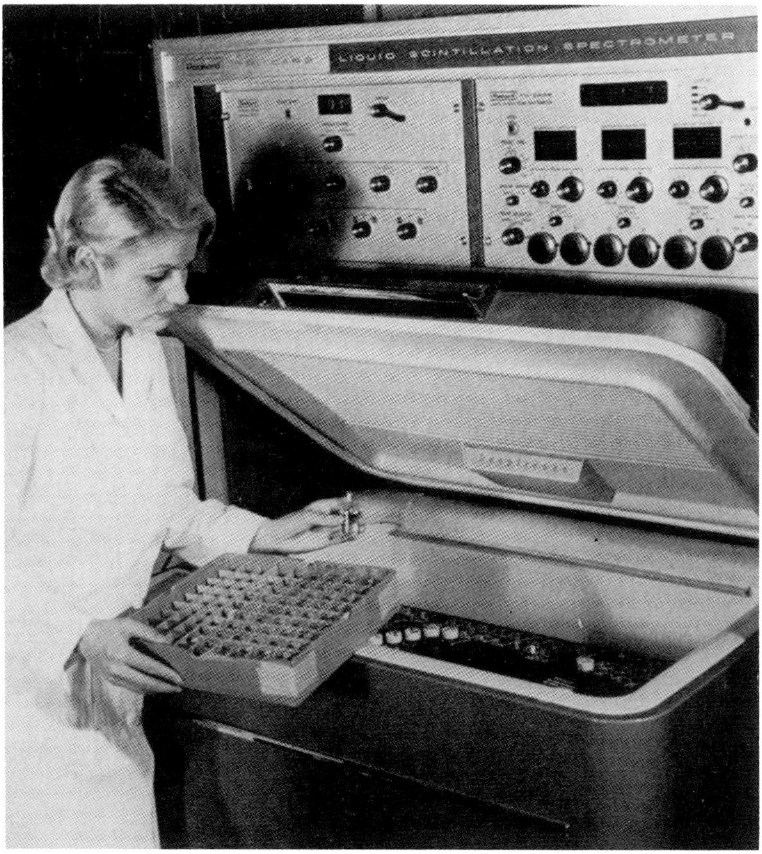

FIG. 14. Liquid scintillation spectrometer with a continuous belt sample feeder.

are available in a form suitable for computer data processing. The simplest data presentation is a straightforward listing of sample number, time of the counting period, and the accumulated counts on each channel of analysis. A more sophisticated readout also computes counts per time for each individual channel and the ratio of counts between channels for use in quench correction. In order to have valid ratios for low-level samples the background must be accurately subtracted prior to the calculation of the ratios. Tape and card punch adapters may be used with the serial entry readout, and provide a means for further handling of the data by computers (7).

Another feature of these automatic units is a low-level sample reject that allows the instrument to check the activity of the sample quickly

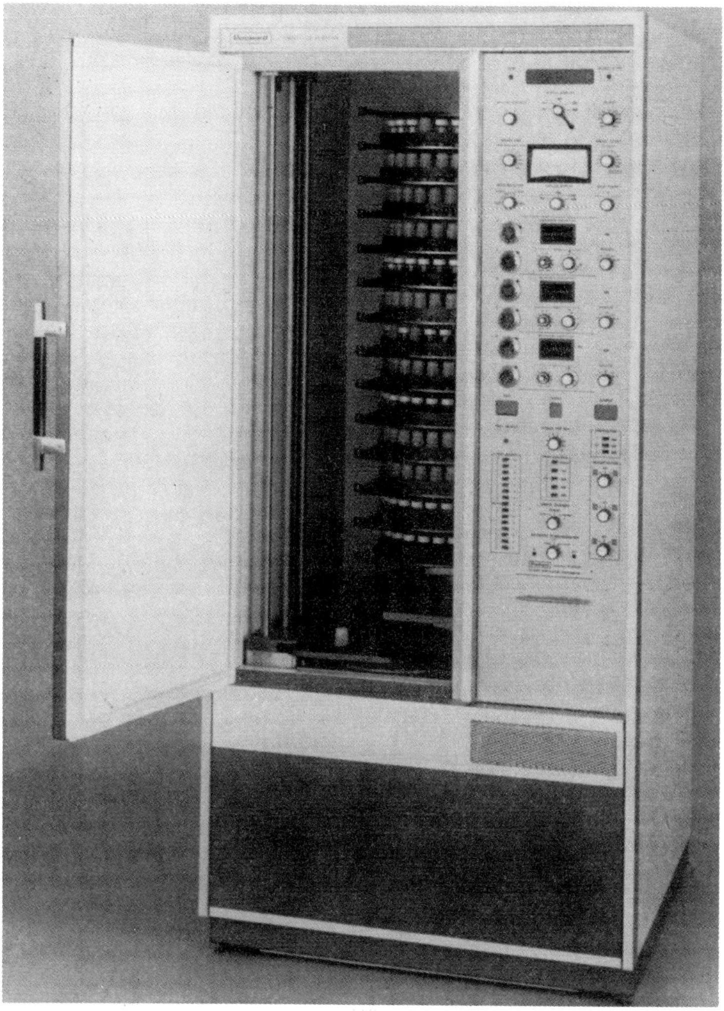

FIG. 15. Liquid scintillation spectrometer with a tray loading sample changer.

and to reject the sample if it is below a level preset by the user. This device is a great time-saver, particularly in experiments involving samples from column chromatography, where only a few samples contain material of interest.

REFERENCES

1. Agranoff, B. W., Silica vials improve low-level counting. *Nucleonics* **15,** No. 10, 106 (1957).
2. Ankenbrandt, C. M., and Lent, E. M., Increasing the light collection efficiency of scintillation counters. *Rev. Sci. Instr.* **34,** 647 (1963).
3. Bell, C. G., and Hayes, F. N. (eds.), "Liquid Scintillation Counting." Macmillan (Pergamon), New York, 1958.
4. Benson, R. H., and Maute, R. L., Liquid scintillation counting of tritium (improvements in sensitivity by efficient light collection). *Anal. Chem.* **34,** 1122 (1962).
5. Berlman, I. B., Luminescence in a scintillation solution excited by α and β particles and related studies in quenching. *J. Chem. Phys.* **34,** 598 (1961).
6. Berlman, I. B., Grismore, R., and Oltman, B. G., Study of α/β ratios of organic scintillation solutions. *Trans. Faraday Soc.* **59,** 2010 (1963).
7. Blanchard, F. A., A computer program for automated testing and reduction of liquid scintillation counting data. *Intern. J. Appl. Radiation Isotopes* **14,** 213 (1963).
8. Boyce, I. S., and Cameron, J. F., A low background liquid scintillation counter for the assay of low specific-activity tritiated water. *Proc. Symp. Tritium Phys. Biol. Sci., Vienna, 1961.* Vol. 1, p. 231. Intern. At. Energy Agency, Vienna, 1962.
9. Burton, J. A., Photoelectric and optical properties of cesium-antimony films. *Phys. Rev.* **72,** 531 (1947).
10. Cummins, D. O., Delaney, C. F. G., and McAulay, I. R., Light collection in liquid scintillation cells. *Sci. Proc. Roy. Dublin Soc.* Sect. A, **1,** 21 (1960).
11. Czirr, J. B., The α/β ratio of several organic scintillators. *Nucl. Instr. Methods* **25,** 106 (1963).
12. Daub, G. H., Hayes, F. N., and Sullivan, E. (eds.), *Proc. Univ. New Mexico Conf. Org. Scintillation Detectors, 1961* TID-7612 U.S. At. Energy Comm., Washington, D.C., 1961.
13. Davidson, J. D., and Feigelson, P., Practical aspects of internal-sample liquid-scintillation counting. *Intern. J. Appl. Radiation Isotopes* **2,** 1 (1957).
14. Hayes, F. N., Liquid scintillators: attributes and applications. *Intern. J. Appl. Radiation Isotopes* **1,** 46 (1956).
15. Hendler, R. W., Procedure for simultaneous assay of two β-emitting isotopes with the liquid scintillation counting technique. *Anal. Biochem.* **7,** 110 (1964).
16. Hodgson, T. S., Gordon, B. E., and Ackerman, M. E., Single-channel counter for carbon-14 and tritium. *Nucleonics* **16,** No. 7, 89 (1958).
17. Kliman, B., and Peterson, R. E., Double isotope derivative assay of aldosterone in biological extracts. *J. Biol. Chem.* **235,** 1639 (1960).
18. Lombard, F. J., and Martin, F., Statistics of electron multiplication. *Rev. Sci. Instr.* **32,** 200 (1961).
19. Marshall, J. H., How to figure shapes of beta-ray spectra. *Nucleonics* **13,** No. 8, 34 (1955).
20. Noakes, J. E., Isbell, A. F., Stipp, J. J., and Hood, D. W., Benzene synthesis by low temperature catalysis for radiocarbon dating. *Geochim. Cosmochim. Acta* **27,** 797 (1963).
21. Okita, G. T., Kabara, J. J., Richardson, F., and LeRoy, G. V., Assaying compounds containing H-3 and C-14. *Nucleonics* **15,** No. 6, 111 (1957).

22. Piez, K. A., Continuous scintillation counting of carbon-14 and tritium in effluent of the automatic amino acid analyzer. *Anal. Biochem.* **4**, 444 (1962).
23. Prockop, D. J., and Ebert, P. S., A simple method for differential assay of tritium and carbon-14 in water-soluble biological materials. *Anal. Biochem.* **6**, 263 (1963).
24. Rapkin, E., and Gibbs, J. A., A system for continuous measurement of radioactivity in flowing streams. *Nature* **194**, 34 (1962).
25. Rapkin, E., and Gibbs, J. A., Polyethylene containers for liquid scintillation spectrometry. *Intern. J. Appl. Radiation Isotopes* **14**, 71 (1963).
26. Rapkin, E., Liquid scintillation counting 1957–1963: A review. *Intern. J. Appl. Radiation Isotopes* **15**, 69 (1964).
27. Roser, F. X., Spectral emission of composite liquid phosphors. *Science* **121**, 806 (1955).
28. Schram, E., and Lombaert, R., "Organic Scintillation Detectors." Elsevier, Amsterdam (1963).
29. Sharpe, J., and Stanley, V. A., Photomultipliers for Tritium counting. *Proc. Symp. Tritium Phys. Biol. Sci., Vienna, 1961* Vol. 1, p. 211. Intern. At. Energy Agency, Vienna, 1962.
30. Swank, R. K., Buck, W. L., Hayes, F. N., and Ott, D. G., Spectral effects in the comparison of scintillators and photomultipliers. *Rev. Sci. Instr.* **29**, 279 (1958).
31. Tamers, M. A., Carbon-14 dating with the liquid scintillation counter: total synthesis of the benzene solvent. *Science* **132**, 668 (1960).
32. Tamers, M. A., Bibron, R., and Delibrias, G., A new method for measuring low level tritium using a benzene liquid scintillator. *Proc. Symp. Tritium Phys. Biol. Sci., Vienna, 1961* Vol. 1, p. 303. Intern. At. Energy Agency, Vienna, 1962.
33. Tamers, M. A., Stipp, J. J., and Collier, J., High sensitivity detection of naturally occurring radiocarbon—I. Chemistry of the counting sample. *Geochim. Cosmochim. Acta* **24**, 266 (1961).
34. Tamers, M. A., and Bibron, R., Benzene method measures tritium in rain without isotope enrichment. *Nucleonics* **21**, No. 6, 90 (1963).
35. Wang, C. H., and Willis, D. L., "Radiotracer Methodology in Biological Science." Prentice-Hall, Englewood Cliffs, New Jersey, 1965.
36. Wu, R., Simultaneous studies of phosphate transport and glycolysis by a simple liquid scintillation counting procedure with P^{32}, C^{14}, and H^{3} compounds. *Anal. Biochem.* **7**, 207 (1964).

CHAPTER 11

RADIOCHROMATOGRAPHIC COUNTING TECHNIQUES

FRITZ BERTHOLD
LABORATORIUM PROF. DR. BERTHOLD
WILDBAD (SCHWARZWALD)
FED. REP. OF GERMANY
AND
MARTIN WENZEL
PHYSIOLOGISCH-CHEMISCHES INSTITUT
DER FREIEN UNIVERSITÄT BERLIN
FED. REP. OF GERMANY

I. TYPES OF CHROMATOGRAPHIC TECHNIQUES

For the separation of compounds of similar chemical structure, especially in small quantities, chromatographic methods are very suitable. According to the physico-chemical properties of the compounds, the appropriate chromatographic method is chosen. The separation procedures are the same whether the compounds to be separated are radioactively labeled or not. Assay of radioactivity is in general an independent procedure, following fractionation performed by one of the standard methods. Therefore, after a short review of the fractionation methods, for which an extensive literature exists (*2, 5, 9, 11, 13, 18*), the discussion will be concentrated on the techniques for assay of radioactivity.

The well-established method of *paper chromatography* (PC) is performed by putting the solution of the compounds to be separated near the end of a strip of especially prepared paper. After a spot has been dried, the paper strip is put with the spot close to its end into a suitable mixture of solvents. This mixture moves in the paper through the action of capillary forces and the compounds to be separated are transported slowly within the network of cellulose fibers. Under suitable conditions different compounds are separated because they migrate within the paper with different velocities compared with the migration of the solvent. Their final location may be recognized, for example, by color, through chemical reactions, fluorescence, or ultraviolet absorption.

The procedure for the separation of different compounds through *thin-layer chromatography* (TLC) is basically the same as in paper chromatography, but instead of paper strips glass plates are used. They are prepared with a thin layer of an adsorbent and porous material, for example, silica gel, powdered cellulose, aluminum oxide, or similar material.

In general, paper chromatography is used more for hydrophilic compounds like amino acids, sugars, and purine derivatives, while thin-layer chromatography is better suited for lipophilic compounds, like fatty acids, steroids, and other isoprenoids. If the compounds to be separated can be brought into an ionized state, for instance, by selection of a proper pH value of the solvent, separation can be achieved in an electric field (*electrophoresis*). This method is mainly suitable for the separation of high-molecular products, like proteins.

In *gas chromatography* (GC) volatile compounds are transported by a stream of inert gas through a column of adsorbent material and the compounds to be analyzed are separated by partition and adsorption during their migration. For the determination of the separated compounds at the outlet of the column, physical methods are used, for instance, the change of heat resistance of a wire if a volatile compound is mixed with the inert gas, or flame ionization.

In *liquid chromatography* (LC) a solution of the compounds to be separated is dropped on the upper end of a column of adsorbent material, such as aluminum oxide, silica gel, ionic resins, or powdered sugar. Then the column is "developed" by adding a suitable solvent to the upper end of the column. Similarly to gas chromatography, the effluent at the lower end of the column contains in different fractions the various substances of the original mixture of compounds.

In any chromatographic method it is often difficult to locate the isolated substances and to make quantitative measurements of the separated compounds, since no method detects all substances with equal sensitivity. Therefore it is advantageous to label the compounds to be separated with radioactive isotopes. For organic substances, only the isotopes of carbon (^{14}C) and hydrogen (^{3}H) can be used rather universally. Each of these two isotopes has its special advantages. For example, ^{3}H is less expensive than ^{14}C, but the β particles of ^{14}C (maximum energy 150 keV) can often be detected with higher efficiency than those of ^{3}H (18 keV). Instruments suitable for the assay of ^{3}H and ^{14}C will in general also be capable of measuring higher-energy β-ray emitters with the best counting efficiency. When ^{3}H-labeled compounds are used it should be kept in mind that because the mass of ^{3}H is three times that of the nonradioactive ^{1}H, an isotopic effect may occur (*8*). The problem of γ-ray measurement is not often encountered in radiochromatography, but some examples will be discussed.

The detection systems used to determine radioactivity in chromatograms are not basically different from those for other kinds of sample measurements. Chromatograms, however, are characterized by their distribution in space (PC, TLC) or time (GC, LC). For their evaluation, the exact shape of this distribution is of primary interest. Therefore, instruments designed for radiochromatography show a high degree of automation, with which these data are best obtained.

II. PAPER AND THIN-LAYER RADIOCHROMATOGRAPHY

Paper chromatography and thin-layer chromatography will be discussed together because these methods are similar and many instruments are constructed to be used for both applications. The methods for the assay of radioactivity may be divided into destructive and nondestructive methods (*20*).

The most important nondestructive method is *external scanning*. The developed paper or thin-layer chromatogram is passed automatically in front of a radiation detector and the count-rate is recorded as a function of source position. If external scanning does not yield satisfactory results, a *destructive method* may be employed. For instance, a paper chromatogram strip may be cut into individual pieces and these may be measured in a liquid scintillation counter. Destructive methods are mostly tedious and time consuming and the material, which could otherwise be used for further investigations, is lost.

A. External Scanning

1. PAPER CHROMATOGRAM STRIP SCANNER

The instrument chosen as an example (Fig. 1) allows scanning of chromatogram paper of any thickness used in practice in the form of strips from 0.5 to 2 inches wide. Therefore, either chromatograms have to be developed on individual paper strips not wider than 2 inches or, if a large chromatogram paper sheet is used, this has to be cut into individual strips for scanning.

Two windowless Geiger–Müller counters with interchangeable collimators are used as radiation detectors. The paper strip passes between them so that both sides of the paper are measured simultaneously in

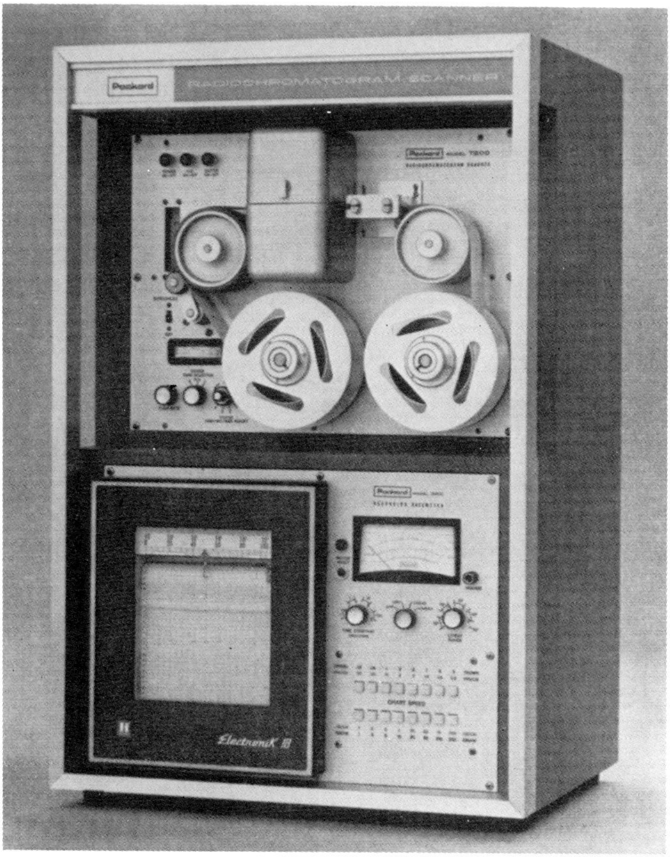

FIG. 1. Paper chromatogram strip scanner. Self-contained instrument with 4π GM counting tube for paper chromatogram strips, paper storage and transport system, ratemeter, and recorder. (Courtesy of Packard Instruments Corporation)

almost 4π geometry. The signals from the two G-M counters are amplified and fed into a ratemeter; the count-rate is displayed on a recorder. The recorder paper advances with a speed identical to that of the chromatogram strip. Therefore, the recorded count-rate can be directly related to the chromatogram.

a. *Detectors and Collimators.* A cross section of the 4π detector geometry is shown in Fig. 2. The paper strip passes between the two counters with a selected speed. The resolution of the instrument is determined by the two diaphragm slits, which in this instrument can be adjusted to widths of 2.5, 5, 7.5, and 10 mm.

The counting gas enters through an inlet tube as indicated in Fig. 2 and leaves through the diaphragm slits. Because of the long dead time of a G-M counter (about 50 μsec), counting losses of about 10% will occur at count-rates of 200,000 cpm. This already takes into account that two counters in parallel have only half the dead time of a single one.

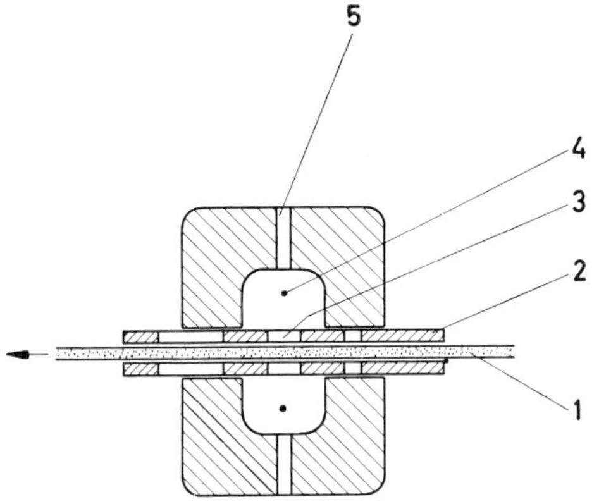

FIG. 2. Cross section of 4π counting tube for paper chromatogram strips. The paper chromatogram strip, 1, is pulled through diaphragm plates, 2. Resolution is defined by width of diaphragm slits, 3. Negative charge carriers are collected by anode wire, 4. Counting gas is provided through inlet tube, 5, and leaves through diaphragm slit, 3. Construction is symmetric with respect to PC strip.

b. *Paper Transport Mechanism.* Since a single paper chromatogram is not longer than 40–50 cm, a much simpler paper transport than shown in Fig. 1 could be employed. However, by joining several strips up to a length of 50 meters and coiling them on a storage reel, automatic data recording for longer periods (over night) becomes possible. Leaving the detector slit, the paper is pressed against the main capstan, which advances the strip at one of 16 preselected speeds between 0.02 and 5 cm per minute and 1 and 200 cm per hour.

c. *Thin-Layer Chromatogram Adapter.* The PC scanner shown in Fig. 1 can also be used for scanning TLC plates 2×8 inches if an adapter is used. It consists of a tray which holds the plates and a plastic strip feeder. The latter automatically passes the TLC plate in front of the upper radiation detector. Its main limitation is that only plates not more than 2 inches wide can be scanned while the standard dimension of TLC plates is 8 × 8 inches.

d. *A Simple Method for Paper Strip Scanning.* Short PC strips can be counted with a simple arrangement as shown in Fig. 3. If the PC

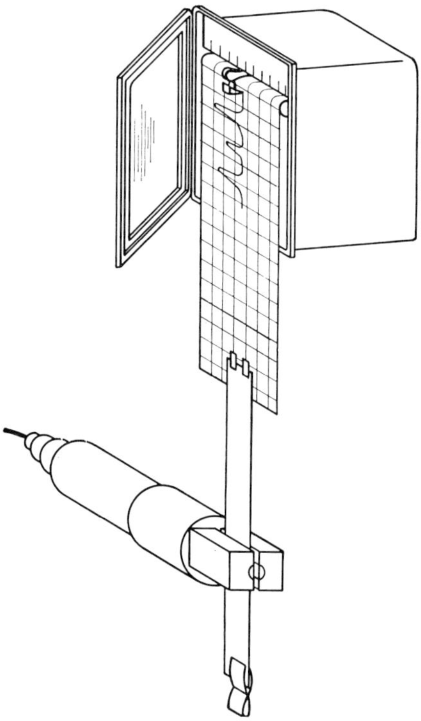

FIG. 3. Simple method for paper chromatogram strip scanning. The PC strip is fixed to the recorder paper. Both advance synchronously as the PC-strip passes through the 4π counting tube. The ratemeter curve displays the radioactivity directly as a function of position on the PC strip.

strip is brought vertically into the same plane as the recorder paper, the paper drive may move the strip past the detector slits. A small weight at the other end of the paper strip ensures its smooth movement.

Apart from being simple, this method secures perfect synchronization between chromatogram and recorder paper advance. In addition, a disturbing effect is avoided which is sometimes observed when long paper bands are stored on spools. Strongly diffusing or sublimating compounds sometimes induce pseudo-activity in the adjacent paper layer. Finally, the vertical paper travel minimizes the possibility of detector contamination by paper deposits or dust.

2. THIN-LAYER CHROMATOGRAM SCANNER

The essential elements of a TLC scanner will also be discussed by describing a typical instrument (Fig. 4). This instrument is in several respects similar to the PC scanner described above.

Since the β rays cannot penetrate the glass plate, only one counter above the adsorbent layer can be employed. Though positioned as close as possible, the counter should not touch the chromatogram because the thin adsorbent layer is easily destroyed. This requires a precise mechanical guidance of the TLC plate as well as the possibility of a

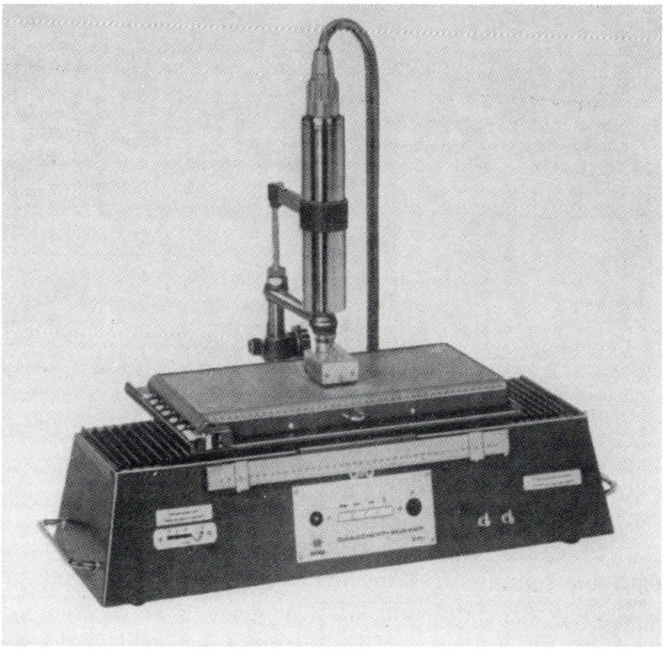

FIG. 4. Two-dimensional thin-layer chromatogram scanner (*1*). Automatic two-dimensional scanning of thin-layer and paper chromatograms with 2π gas-flow counting tube. (Courtesy Laboratorium Prof. Dr. Berthold)

vertical adjustment of the detector position. Typically, the distance between the lower detector surface and the thin layer is chosen as 0.5 mm.

Usually, up to 10 chromatograms are developed on a single 8×8 inch TLC plate. Since, in general, it is not possible to join the single tracks as in the case of PC sheets, one track has to be scanned after the other. This requires a two-dimensional scanning system (Fig. 4). Not only one or two TLC plates but also PC sheets may be scanned two-dimensionally with this instrument, but only with 2π geometry. The detector is a special type of flow proportional counter for operation with or without window. Its function is described in Section II,A,3.

A pair of adjustable end limit switches permits selection of the longitudinal movement between 10 and 400 mm. When one of the end limit switches is reached, the scanning motion is automatically reversed and the plate is advanced in the transverse direction. This scan spacing (pitch) can be selected between 2 and 160 mm. The 2 mm distance is used only in connection with a dot printer for small animal γ-ray scanning with a NaI(Tl) scintillation counter and collimator, or for histological preparations. A pitch of 10 mm is typical for two-dimensional thin-layer and paper chromatograms.

It is also possible to operate with a pitch varying from one step to the next for an efficient method of evaluating two-dimensional chromatograms (Fig. 5). The specimen with the substance to be analyzed is applied to one corner of the rectangular chromatogram carrier (paper or thin-layer plate), and then developed parallel to one edge in the

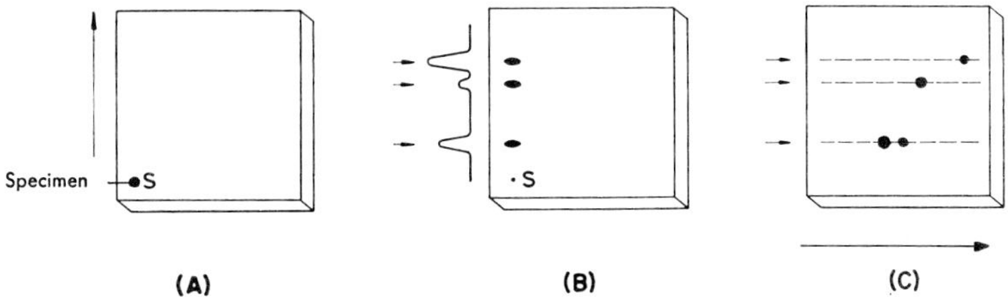

FIG. 5. Evaluation of two-dimensional chromatograms. (A) Development in mixture A. (B) First scan and setting of pitch for second scan. (C) Development in mixture B and two-dimensional scanning (*1*).

chromatographic mixture A (Fig. 5A). The activity distribution is then determined along this path (Fig. 5B). A series of adjustable contacts is set according to the positions of the maxima obtained, and thereby the instrument is adjusted for the final measurement after the second development in mixture B, transposed by 90° as compared to the first development (Fig. 5C). Now, the final evaluation is made along the paths defined by the adjustable contacts.

This method saves a lot of time because only those lines of the two-dimensional chromatogram are scanned on which there is some radioactivity. At the same time, each activity spot is covered completely in one line scanning and is not distributed between several lines.

The basic instrument performs the scanning motion automatically in one dimension only. The scanning speed is variable from 0.2 to 5 cm per minute. For scanning the next line, the chromatogram is advanced manually in the transverse direction and the next automatic scan is started. This method is actually sufficient for many applications. However, an additional carriage can be placed on the basic instrument to perform steps of the selected size in the transverse direction automatically, thus resulting in the automatic two-dimensional scanning program described above.

3. CHOICE OF RADIATION DETECTORS

In general, G-M and proportional counters are used for radiochromatogram scanners. There are no significant differences in the performance of counting tubes for β-ray emitters with a maximum energy of above 0.3 MeV. For ^{14}C and ^{35}S, however, the counting efficiencies vary considerably with different designs.

Obviously ^{3}H with a maximum energy of 18 keV is the β-ray emitter that is the most difficult to measure. The maximum β-ray range is only 0.7 mg/cm^2 and the half-value layer is about 0.04 mg/cm^2. Therefore, even the thinnest window feasible absorbs most of the β rays, and

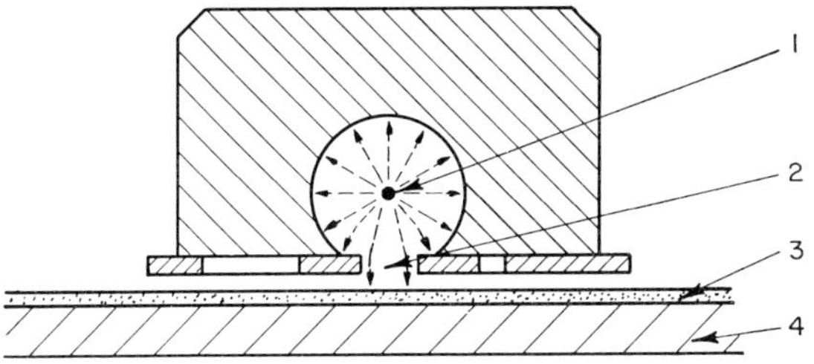

FIG. 6. Schematic of windowless 2π counting tube for scanning of thin-layer chromatograms. The electrical field from the anode, 1, extends outside the diaphragm slit, 2, down to the adsorbent layer, 3, supported by a glass plate, 4. Negative charge carriers from β particles, even those just leaving the chromatogram surface, are counted.

windowless measurements are required in the case of ^{3}H; they yield somewhat higher counting efficiencies also for ^{14}C and ^{35}S where the half-value layer is about 0.9 mg/cm^2.

Flow counters are the most convenient detectors. A standard type of flow counter with a circular cross section as it is used for planchet counting might be applied in chromatogram scanning but it does not recommend itself for these applications. The geometry of the counting problem requires diaphragms of a length between 10 and 40 mm (perpendicular to the scanning direction) and a width between 1 and 10 mm, the latter defining the (one-dimensional) resolution. To obtain minimum background, the active cross section of the counting tube should be equal to the maximum slit dimensions. This requirement is best fulfilled by a counter designed with its axis parallel to the diaphragm and the anode wire over the middle of the slit (Fig. 6).

The counting gas cannot be prevented from escaping through the diaphragm slit. However, a sufficient concentration of counting gas in the sensitive volume of the counter and the space between slit opening and chromatogram surface is maintained by extending the diaphragms horizontally beyond the slit opening by more than 1 cm in each direction, thereby reducing diffusion of air into the counter volume. The counting gas consumption is limited to about 3 liters per hour and a good counting plateau is obtained.

As shown below in Fig. 8, the counting efficiency for an infinitely thin sample is 50%. This means that all β rays emitted upward are counted. This is possible because the electric field reaches through the diaphragm to the surface of the adsorbent layer (Fig. 6), and attracts negative charge carriers from the space between diaphragm and adsorbent layer into the sensitive volume of the counter (*15*). Only with this effect does it become possible to measure ^{3}H-labeled substances in chromatograms by external scanning. Not only does the counting yield reach its theoretical optimum, but it is also independent of unavoidable fluctuations of the distance between chromatogram surface and detector.

A thin window may be used for higher energy β-ray emitters than ^{3}H. Again 2π geometry is assured by using a diaphragm of only a few tenths of a millimeter thickness which is covered by a window of 0.1 mg/cm^2 or less. This design can be used for β-ray emitters of 150 to 500 keV maximum energy. For even higher-energy β-ray emitters a thicker diaphragm is required to prevent β rays from passing through it.

An interesting possibility is the separate measurement of ^{3}H and ^{14}C in one chromatogram through successive scanning with and without a window, using the old method of range discrimination (*19, 20*). An example of this type is shown in Fig. 7. The same principle can also be used to separate other double-labeled substances, such as ^{14}C-^{32}P, using windows of different thickness.

A 4π counter for PC may simply be considered to consist of two 2π counters used for TLC, and, indeed, a number of systems are constructed in that way. The requirements for PC counters are not so stringent because for 4π counters the paper serves as a gas seal in the case of windowless measurements.

In a few cases, as for ^{125}I and ^{99m}Tc, γ-ray scanning is required. For the best geometrical resolution and the lowest background count-rates, rectangular NaI(Tl) crystals are used, 20 mm long, 5 mm wide, and 5 mm high.

4. Determination of Counting Efficiency

One of the most important specifications of a PC or TLC scanning system is the counting efficiency. In order to obtain good resolution of adjacent peaks, the diaphragm slit width is always made smaller than the radioactive spots corresponding to certain fractions separated by chromatography. The total amount of radioactivity must, therefore, be obtained by scanning and pulse integration.

The counting efficiency, ϵ, is defined as the ratio of the count-rate, N (counts per minute), and the rate of disintegrations, A (disintegrations

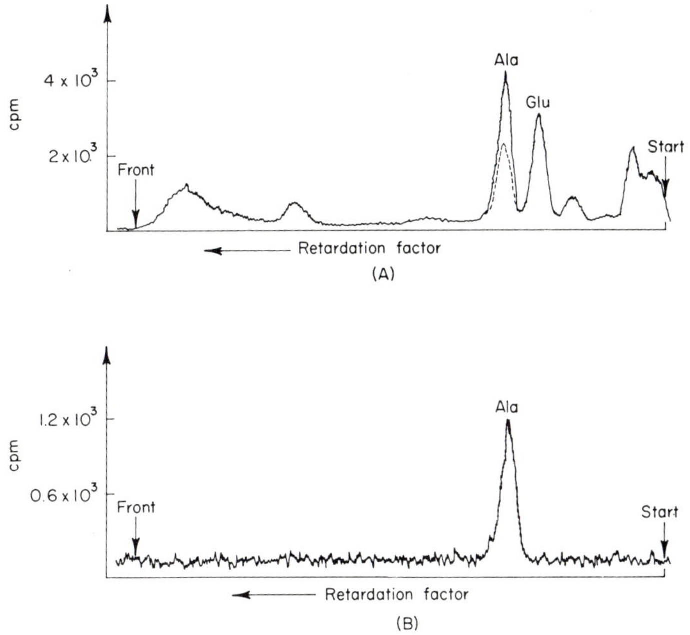

FIG. 7. Paper chromatogram of a cell extract of ascites tumor cells after incubation with glucose-1-^{3}H. (A) 4π Counter measurements without window. Separation of alanine-^{14}C (Ala) and glutamic acid-^{3}H (Glu). (B) With window detection of alanine-^{14}C only.

per minute), which occur under the diaphragm slit. If d (millimeters) is the diaphragm width, and v (millimeters per minute) the scanning speed, the total number of counts, Z, obtained in scanning a radioactive spot is

$$Z = \int N(t)\, dt = \epsilon \times \frac{d}{v} \times A \qquad \text{(counts)}$$

This equation allows the determination of ϵ from scanning an area for which the total radioactivity is known. After ϵ has been determined, the equation is used to determine the radioactivity in an unknown fraction that has been scanned.

A counting tube can never register more particles than reach the sensitive counter volume. Assuming a low-energy β-ray emitter is spread in a practically infinitely thin layer ("infinitely thin" layer for tritium about 1 $\mu g/cm^2$, for ^{14}C about 10 $\mu g/cm^2$), 50% of the particles in the sample are emitted in the upward direction. A thin-layer counting tube mounted close to such a radioactive layer can, therefore, register a maximum of 50% of the particles emitted into all directions. If the same amount of radioactivity is distributed in increasingly thicker layers, an increasingly large portion of the particles is absorbed within the layer. This means the counting efficiency for a TLC or PC counting tube de-

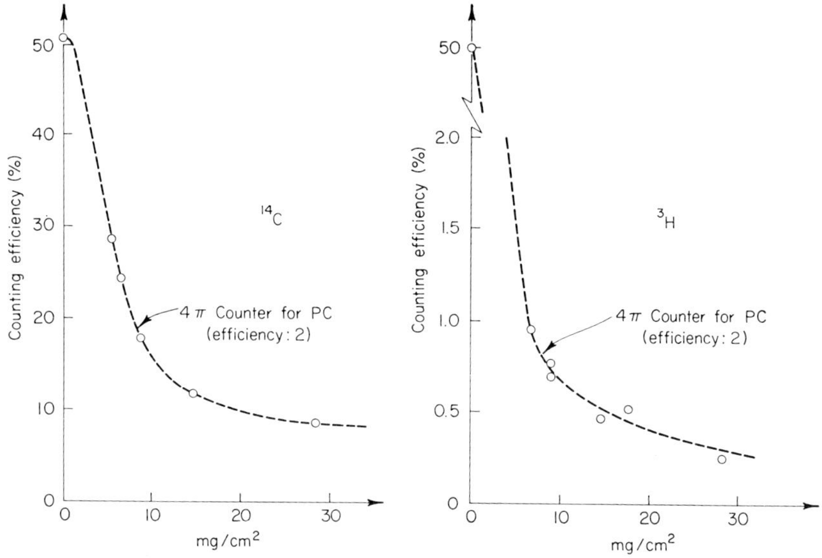

FIG. 8. Counting efficiency of 2π counting tube for thin-layer chromatograms. Dependence upon thickness of adsorbent layer is shown for ^{14}C- and ^{3}H-labeled compounds. The arrow indicates points obtained for 4π counting of paper chromatograms, where counting is twice as high as for 2π counting of thin-layer chromatograms of equal weight per unit area.

pends on the thickness of the layer containing the radioactive material (Chapter 4, Section II).

Experimental values for this dependence for the system described in Section II,A,2 are shown in Fig. 8. It can be seen that an efficiency of 50 to 10% can be obtained for ^{14}C in TLC, depending on the thickness of the adsorbent layer used. Correspondingly, the efficiency for tritium varies between 50 and 0.4%. In PC the efficiency is twice as high since the 4π counting tube measures on both sides of the radioactive paper strip.

All measurements were made without a window. Since a counting efficiency of 50% is reached for infinitely thin samples, the performance of this counting tube has reached its optimum theoretical value.

Figure 8 illustrates why the counting efficiency of commercial instruments, indicated as, for instance, "efficiency for tritium 4%," is entirely arbitrary as long as the conditions under which the measurements were made are not stated. The weight per unit area of the chromatogram carrier must be given, but it is also necessary to develop the spot before performing the efficiency determination (*4*). In view of these possible ambiguities, it would seem better if the specifications of commercial instruments would give the efficiency values for an infinitely thin sample, and with a diagram such as shown in Fig. 8 the efficiency values for the type of chromatogram carrier used could then be determined.

B. Destructive Methods

If the results obtained by external scanning are not satisfactory, the paper chromatogram strip may be cut perpendicularly to the direction of the run into small pieces. The radioactivity of each piece is then determined individually. The width of the single segments defines the geometrical resolution. A 40-cm-long PC strip may be cut into 80 pieces, each 5 mm wide, which are then counted in an automatic liquid scintillation counter (Chapter 10). Especially for ^{3}H-labeled chromatograms, the additional work required for the destructive method may be rewarding. The counting efficiency of only 1%, obtained in external scanning procedures, due to self-absorption of the low-energy β rays (Fig. 8) may be increased by a factor of 20 or more, by using liquid scintillation counting.

For the evaluation of thin-layer chromatograms, segment after segment (1–5 mm) of the adsorbent layer containing the labeled substance must be scraped off the glass plate. In this procedure the material crumbles into a powder which is then processed. The labeled substances may be eluted from the adsorbent powder and may subsequently be measured by liquid scintillation counting. Otherwise, the powder may be suspended in a scintillator solution containing a thixotropic material which secures a uniform suspension of the radioactive powder. Very good results are reported by Snyder (*17*), who has constructed an instrument that automatically scrapes off 1-, 2-, or 5-mm zones of the adsorbent layer and transfers them into liquid scintillation vials.

C. Autoradiography

Autoradiography uses the blackening of an X-ray film positioned on top of a paper or thin-layer radiochromatogram, thus producing a very detailed picture of the radioactivity distribution. The exposure time depends strongly on the energy of the β-ray emitter. For practicable quantities of radioactivity, the exposure time may be several hours in the case of ^{32}P, but it may go up to many weeks for ^{14}C and ^{3}H (*17*). Therefore, autoradiography is less applicable in nuclear medicine, if ^{3}H and ^{14}C are used as tracers.

A considerable reduction of exposure time for chromatograms of ^{3}H-labeled substances is possible if the chromatograms are impregnated with a scintillator solution sprayed onto the chromatogram. After evaporation of the solvent, the X-ray film is applied and additional film blackening is obtained by the fluorescent light from the scintillator. For thin-layer chromatography a method has been described (*10*) where a thin layer consisting of an intimate mixture of small mesh silica gel and anthracene is used.

III. GAS AND LIQUID CHROMATOGRAPHY

In paper and thin-layer chromatography, the fractionation process and the radioactivity assay are two completely separated steps. After development of the chromatogram on a paper strip or a thin-layer plate these can be scanned at any convenient time thereafter.

For continuous radioactivity assay in gas and liquid chromatography the situation is different. The separated fractions leaving the gas or liquid chromatography columns in their carrier stream must pass through, or close by, the sensitive volume of a stationary radiation detector. The standard representation of the data is again a ratemeter curve, displaying the count-rate as a function of time.

It is also possible to collect individual fractions and measure their radioactivity in a discontinuous way thereafter. This is tedious and time consuming; however, especially in the field of liquid chromatography, fraction collection is still widely used because the existing instruments for continuous measurements have several drawbacks, which will be discussed below (Section III,B).

The methods of fractionation in the gas- or liquid-chromatographic column are not different for radioactive and nonradioactive substances, and the standard chromatographic systems are generally used for separation of radioactively labeled substances as well. Therefore mainly radioactivity measuring instruments allowing on-line monitoring of the gaseous or liquid effluent from chromatographic columns will be discussed.

The definition of the *counting efficiency* of such systems may cause some problems. If, from a radioactivity, A (disintegration per minute), within the sensitive volume, v (cubic centimeters), of the detector a count-rate, N (counts per minute), is observed, the counting efficiency, ϵ, of the detector is given as $\epsilon = N/A$.

For a radioactivity that passes the detector with a flow-rate, f (cubic centimeters per minute), the resident time within the volume V as a function of the flow velocity must be taken into account. The total number of counts, Z, from the passage of a radioactive fraction follows as

$$Z = \epsilon \times \frac{V}{f} \times A \quad \text{(counts)}$$

The total number of registered counts is inversely proportional to the flow-rate, a parameter which has to be chosen according to the fractionation problem. The flow-rate must be constant, since it affects the quantitative evaluation of the radiochromatogram.

It should be pointed out that the above definition of counting efficiency is only useful for pulse counting devices like proportional and

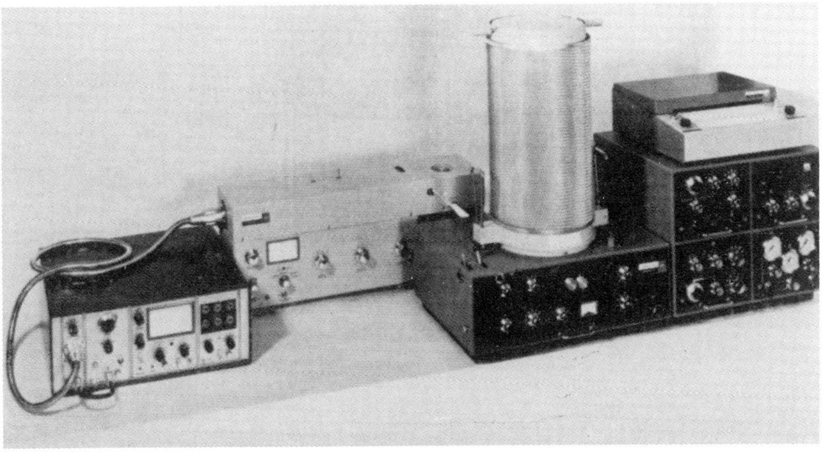

FIG. 9. Complete instrument for gas radiochromatography. *From right to left:* Gas chromatograph with outlet connected to detector block with a flow-through chemical conversion unit and proportional counting tube and radiation measuring instrument. (Courtesy Bodenseewerk Perkin-Elmer & Co. GmbH)

scintillation counters. A different definition of counting efficiency is used for ionization chamber measurements (Section III,A,2).

A. Gas Radiochromatography

1. PROPORTIONAL COUNTER SYSTEMS

The method in general will be described by discussing an advanced system which has been developed recently (Fig. 9). The fractions emerging from the gas chromatograph pass to the radiation detector unit containing a flow-through proportional counter. The output signals from the proportional counter go to a preamplifier within the detector unit. The pulses are registered by a ratemeter and recorder; the counts within a peak can be integrated automatically.

The components contained in the detector unit are indicated in Fig. 10. The effluent from the gas chromatograph enters the detector unit through a connecting tube, 1, which can be heated up to 350°C so that the fractions cannot condense if the fractionation is performed at high temperatures. From there, the substances pass a flow-through reaction tube, 2, heatable by a surrounding oven, 3, from 100 to 750°C by means

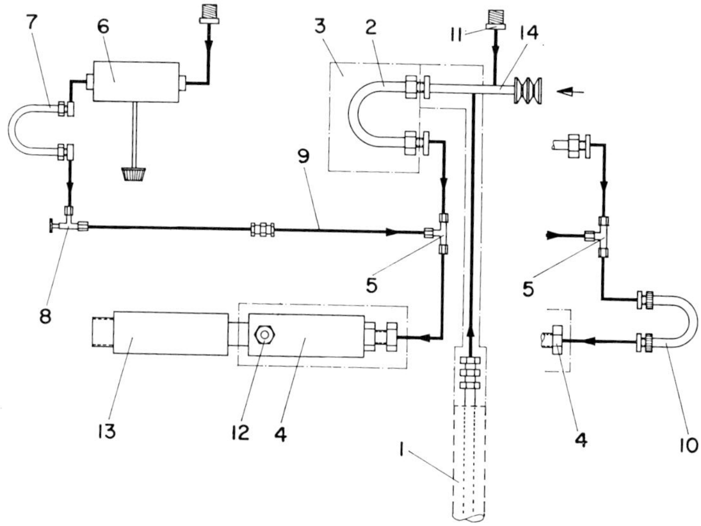

FIG. 10. Schematic of detector unit for gas radiochromatography. See text for explanation.

of a regulating transformer. The oven consists of two parts for rapid cooling and easy accessibility to the reaction tube.

The flow-through reaction tube converts the fractions chemically into a form suitable for counting in the proportional counter, 4. Before the effluent enters the proportional counter, methane is added to it, through the methane feed, 5, in proportion 1:2. This is necessary to obtain a good counting plateau. The methane feeding line has a flow regulator for a constant methane stream, 6, a filter column with a molecular sieve for prepurification of the methane, 7, a needle valve for working pressure regulation, 8, and a capillary resistance as diffusion break, 9.

It would be simpler if the gas together with methane could be brought into the counter without previous chemical transformation. This would also have the advantage of a nondestructive procedure and the samples could be collected for further use after leaving the proportional counting tube. Whenever this is possible, an empty tube is used in place of the reaction tube.

In most cases the chemical conversion is required because most substances either produce a pseudo activity or have a quenching effect in the proportional counter (*16*). Pseudoactivity produces an incorrectly high and quenching a too low count-rate.

For the conversion there is a choice between an oxidative method and hydrogenating cracking. For the *oxidative method,* used on ^{14}C-labeled substances containing only C, H, and O, the reaction tube is filled with copper or cobalt oxide. A small tube, 10, filled with a drying agent to absorb water vapor formed in the reaction tube, is placed between reactor and counting tube, since water vapor may disturb the proper functioning of the proportional counter.

For the analysis of ^{3}H-labeled compounds by the oxidative method the last down-stream part of the reaction tube is filled with an iron packing as a reducing agent so that the water vapor formed is reduced to HT and H_2. As carrier gas hydrogen, helium, or argon can be used if the system is similar to that described by James *et al.* (*6, 7*).

The oxidative method has several limitations. For the analysis of ^{14}C-labeled compounds it is reliable for substances containing C, H, and O, but not if other elements like nitrogen, halogens, or sulfur are present. In the analysis of ^{3}H-labeled substances long lasting memory effects are sometimes observed. These are probably due to the adsorption of water vapor between the combustion and the reduction part of the filling in the reaction tube.

For *hydrogenating cracking,* the reaction tube filling is composed of iron, zinc, cobalt oxide, nickel oxide, and vanadium pentoxide mixed with an inert carrier. This method does not have the shortcomings of the oxidative method. A great number of ^{3}H- and ^{14}C-labeled substances of quite different chemical structure have been tested without any disturbances being observed (*16*). Since hydrogen is required for the cracking process, either it has to be used as a carrier gas or, if another carrier gas is preferred, it has to be added through the input nipple, 11.

Counting tubes of 2-, 10-, or 80-ml active volume can be employed. The counting gas enters axially and leaves the counting tube through outlet 12. A transistor preamplifier, 13, with an amplification of 200 is connected directly to the counting tube.

The limits of detectability depend upon counting efficiency, active counter volume, and background of the counting tube as well as on the flow-rate. Counting efficiencies are 70% for ^{3}H and 85% for ^{14}C. Using a 10-ml counting tube with a background of 10 cpm and a flow-rate of 60 ml/min (40 ml/min column effluent plus 20 ml/min methane), a fraction containing 10^{-4} μCi of ^{3}H or ^{14}C can clearly be detected. For the 80-ml counting tube the detection limits are lower by about a factor of three.

An unusual feature of this system is the possibility of measuring not only gases but also *solutions* or *liquids* labeled with ^{3}H or ^{14}C. Liquids or solutions are injected with a Hamilton syringe through an injection port, 14, directly into the reaction zone of the reaction tube. This is only possible with the filling used for hydrogenating cracking. In the stream of hydrogen provided through the nipple, 11, liquid substances or substances in solution are converted within seconds into simple gases, mainly methane. From here on the procedure is the same as in radioactive gas chromatography.

2. Ionization Chamber Systems

Low-energy β-ray emitters may be measured by passing the effluent gases of the GC column through a flow-through ionization chamber. The latter does not require the addition of a counting gas such as methane and in many cases chemical conversion of the sample before measurement is not required. Nevertheless chemical conversion is frequently necessary because certain substances produce pseudo activity or quenching effects even in an ionization chamber (*3*, *12*).

The fraction of the radiation energy used to create ions times the fraction of the electrons collected determines the efficiency of the ionization chamber. Efficiencies of 33% for ^{14}C and 75% for ^{3}H have been reported. Compared with proportional counter systems, the sensitivity of ionization chamber systems is lower by about a factor of 10 for ^{3}H and a factor of 3 for ^{14}C.

3. Flow-Through Scintillation Detectors

The flow-through scintillation detectors best suited for the measurement of low-energy β-ray emitters consist of a plastic cylinder with a flow-through channel (mostly U-shaped) filled with a powder of anthracene crystals. As the effluent passes through the volume filled with anthracene, scintillations are produced by the absorption of β-particle energy.

Since the scintillation detector cannot operate at elevated temperatures, chemical conversion before counting is practically always necessary. At the same time this reduces the danger of contaminating the detector. One instrument* uses a combustion system similar to that described in connection with the oxidative method for proportional

* Packard Instrument Corporation (Chapter 10, Fig. 13).

counter systems. The effluent gas passes first over hot copper oxide in the combustion chamber to produce CO_2 and H_2O. If only ^{14}C is to be measured, the H_2O is trapped in a moisture trap, and only the CO_2 passes through the detector flow-cell. If tritium is to be measured too, hydrogen is added to the effluent after the combustion chamber, and the resulting mixture passes over hot iron to reduce the water vapor to HT and H_2 before entering the scintillation cell.

The sensitive volume of the scintillation cells is typically 10 ml and the counting efficiencies are about 10% for ^3H and 65% for ^{14}C. About 1.5×10^{-3} μCi of ^3H and 2×10^{-4} μCi of ^{14}C are detectable. These values are similar to those for ionization chamber systems. Since the multiplier phototube assembly and the electronic system—except for the ratemeters—are practically identical with that of a liquid scintillation counter, the scintillation flow-cell can also be used as an accessory to a liquid scintillation counter. The flow cell then takes the place between the two multiplier phototubes which is normally occupied by a sample vial.

4. METHODS FOR γ- AND HIGH-ENERGY β-RAY COUNTING

So far, systems primarily intended for the measurement of ^3H and ^{14}C have been discussed. For β-ray emitters of higher energies and γ-ray emitters, the problems of radiation detection are greatly reduced. No special instruments are required any longer. Effluent gases with β-ray emitters of more than 0.4 MeV maximum energy may pass the window of a radiation detector (Chapter 4). For γ-ray emitters, 4π geometry may be achieved if the gas is passed into and out of the hole in a well-counter or through a cylindrical crystal with a lead-through hole perpendicular to the crystal axis (Chapter 12, Fig. 1).

B. Liquid Radiochromatography

Liquid radiochromatographic systems have the task of monitoring and recording continuously the radioactivity in the effluents from liquid-partition columns. In contrast to gas chromatography, the liquids containing the radioactivity obviously cannot be introduced into the sensitive volume of a gas-filled radiation detector. Therefore, flow-through scintillation cells filled with anthracene powder, as described in Section III,A,3, are practically the only useful type of radiation detector. Because in liquid chromatography the single fractions follow each other with little separation, small flow-through cells with 1–4 ml active volume must be used (*20*).

For practical applications, the continuous LC systems have several drawbacks. While the method works satisfactory for aqueous solutions, it is not suitable for many chemical mixtures, like organic solvents, which may dissolve the organic scintillator. The efficiency for tritium is very low, about 1%, while it is satisfactory for ^{14}C (about 30%). If the substances are colored, the counting efficiency may be further reduced. Finally, adsorption of the radioactive material on the scintillator surface is possible; it would result in an increased background count-rate.

By using small mesh inorganic scintillators as a filling material for the flow-cell, chemical reactions between scintillator and liquid effluent are greatly avoided (*14*). Furthermore, the scintillator may easily be decontaminated by aggressive cleaning materials. However, the efficiencies are even lower than those for anthracene (1.6% for ^{14}C, 0.12% for ^{3}H), when Ce-activiated lithium glass is used.

The possibility of using plastic scintillator tubes as flow-through detectors should be mentioned. In general, these tubes are wound in the form of a flat spiral. β-Particles penetrating into the wall produce scintillations that are detected by one or two multiplier phototubes. Their main advantage is that color quenching effects are not important. The counting efficiencies for low-energy β-ray emitters are low, while in the assay of higher-energy β-ray emitters, such as ^{32}P, counting efficiencies up to about 75% can be obtained.

The methods for continuous evaluation in liquid radiochromatography do not seem very satisfying at present. Therefore, in most cases discontinuous methods are still used. The individual fractions can be collected with an automatic fraction collector and counted thereafter in a liquid scintillation counter in the usual way.

IV. ELECTRONIC AND RECORDING SYSTEMS

The simplest and in most cases the most adequate display of the radioactivity distribution in a chromatogram is the linear ratemeter diagram on a recorder (Fig. 11, upper curve). In performing gas radiochromatography, for instance, this representation corresponds directly to the familiar mass diagram and both diagrams may be correlated directly with each other.

A problem often encountered in chromatography is the *integration of the peak area* as a measure of the radioactivity contained in an individual fraction. Because the usual graphic integration methods are time consuming, automatic peak area integration systems are offered by some manufacturers.

One system* uses an integrating circuit producing a defined voltage increment for each counting pulse. The output of the integrating circuit can be recorded on a dual-chart recorder (Fig. 11, lower curve) beside the ratemeter diagram.

* Laboratorium Prof. Dr. Berthold.

The diagrams in Fig. 11 have been produced with the paper advancing from right to left. The approximately constant value of the background count-rate in the ratemeter curve results in a straight line with a constant slope in the integral representation. At the beginning of the

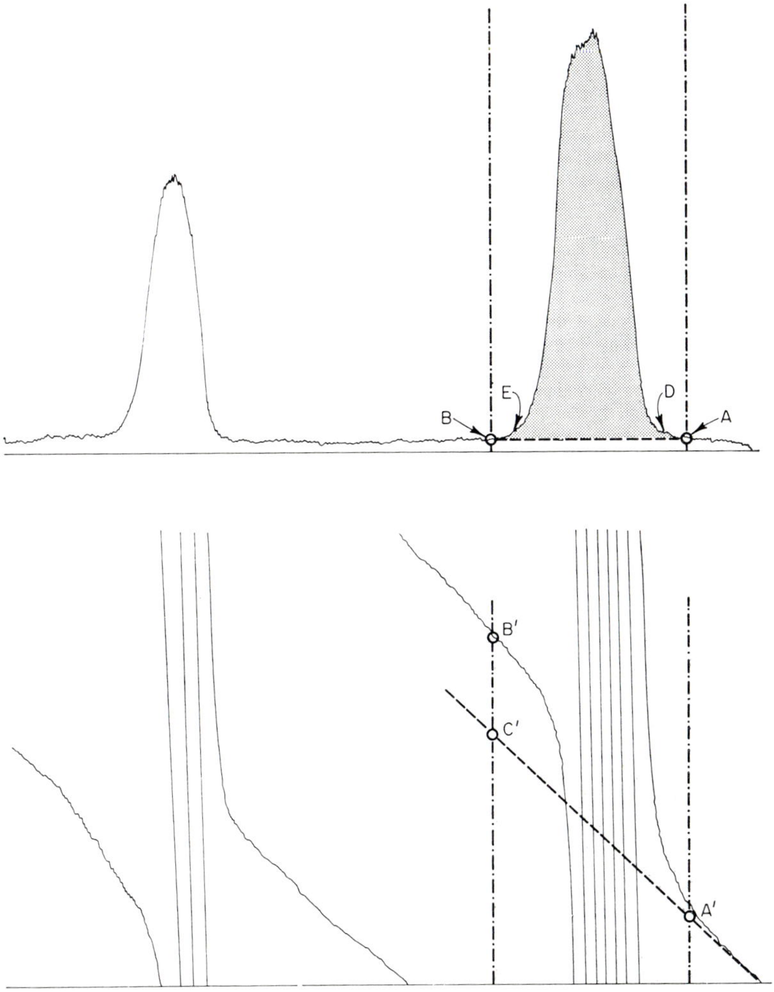

FIG. 11. Simultaneous recording and integration of chromatogram peaks (*1*). *Upper curve:* linear ratemeter display. *Lower curve:* integral count-rate diagram.

peak (point A in ratemeter diagram, A' in integral curve) the slope of the integral curve increases until full scale deflection is reached. At this point the integrating circuit is automatically reset to zero and the next cycle begins. At points B and B', respectively, only background counts are recorded again.

For integration over the shaded area in the ratemeter diagram, the straight line representing the background counts is elongated beyond point A' to point C'. Then, the total number of pulses can be read in the following way: number of intersections of the line $A'–C'$ with the integral curve plus distance $C'–B'$. For the example represented by Fig. 11, the peak area is equivalent to 7210 pulses taking into account that the sensitivity was set to 1000 pulses full scale. The background counts are already subtracted, since, without occurrence of a peak, the integral curve would have lead directly from A' to C'.

In another method,* a threshold is set to the ratemeter indication, just above the normal background count-rate including its maximum statistical fluctuations. As soon as the count-rate exceeds this threshold at point D (Fig. 11, upper curve), a scaler operated in parallel with the ratemeter starts counting and is stopped only after the intensity falls again below the set threshold at point E. The number of pulses representing the integrated area is printed out and the system is ready for the next integrating cycle.

Some special *display problems* exist for two-dimensional paper and thin-layer chromatograms. A display and a semiquantitative record of the radioactivity distribution in the chromatogram are desirable. This problem, and therefore also its solution, is the same for γ-ray radioisotope scanning of human subjects (Chapter 16, Section IV).

A dot printer is used which produces a dot on a sheet of recording paper for any preselected number of pulses counted by the detector. A carriage table may support both chromatogram and the recording paper, and one scanning mechanism provides the two-dimensional motion under the stationary detector and dot-printer, respectively.* The density of dots on the recording paper corresponds to the amount of radioactivity in the chromatogram. The picture resembles that of an autoradiograph obtained with poorer resolution but in much shorter time, especially for low-energy β-ray emitters.

REFERENCES

1. Berthold, F., Recent methods for the automatic evaluation of thin-layer and paper chromatograms of labelled substances. *Proc. Symp. Radioisotope Sample Measurement Tech. Med. Biol., Vienna, 1965* p. 303. Intern. At. Energy Agency, Vienna, 1965.
2. Burchfield, H. P., and Storrs, E. E., "Biochemical Applications of Gas Chromatography." Academic Press, New York, 1962.
3. Cacare, F., Labelled organics in gas chromatography. *Nucleonics* **19**, No. 5, 45 (1961).
4. Carlton, F. J., and Roberts, A. R., Determination of the specific activity of

* Nuclear-Chicago Corporation.

tritiated compounds on paper chromatograms using an automatic scanning device. *Intern. J. Appl. Radiation Isotopes* **10,** 79 (1961).

5. Dal Nogare, S., and Juvet, R. S., Jr., "Gas-Liquid Chromatography, Theory and Practice." Wiley, New York, 1962.
6. James, A. T., and Hitchcock, C., An improved gas-liquid radiochemical chromatogram for C-14 and tritium. *Kerntechnik* **7,** 5 (1965).
7. James, A. T., and Piper, E. A., Automatic recording of the radioactivity of zones eluted from the gas-liquid chromatogram. *J. Chromatog.* **5,** 265 (1961).
8. Klein, P. D., and Kunze-Falkner, B. A., Analysis of chromatographic peak displacement and band broadening by impurities. *Anal. Chem.* **37,** 1245 (1965).
9. Lederer, M. (ed.), *Chromatog. Rev.* **1–8** (1959–1966).
10. Lüthi, U., and Waser, P. G., Low temperature fluorography induced at tritium-labelled compounds on thin-layer chromatograms. *Nature* **205,** 1190 (1965).
11. Marini-Bettòlo, G. B. (ed.), *Proc. Symp., Thin-Layer Chromatog., Rome, 1963* Elsevier, Amsterdam, 1964.
12. Nelson, D. C., Ressler, P. C., Jr., and Hawes, R. C., Performance of an instrument for simultaneous gas chromatographic and radioactivity analysis. *Anal. Chem.* **35,** 1575 (1963).
13. Randerath, K., "Thin-Layer Chromatography." Verlag Chemie, Weinheim and Academic Press, New York, 1963.
14. Scharpenseel, H. W., and Pietig, F., Anorganische Szintillatoren zur ^{14}C- and ^{3}H-Messung in radiosäulenchromatographischen Durchflusszellen. *Atompraxis* **11,** 98 (1965).
15. Schürfeld, H., and Wegner, L. A., Zur fensterlosen Messung weicher β-Strahler *Nukleonik* **7,** 74 (1965).
16. Simon, H., Muellhofer, G., and Medina, R., A general method for the rapid determination of carbon-14- and hydrogen-3-labelled substances by gas chromatography. *Proc. Symp. Radioisotope Sample Measurement Tech. Med. Biol., Vienna, 1965* p. 317. Intern. At. Energy Agency, Vienna, 1965.
17. Snyder, F., Quantitative radioassay methods for thin-layer chromatography: zonal and autoradiographic scans. *Proc. Symp. Radioisotope Sample Measurement Tech. Med. Biol., Vienna, 1965* p. 521. Intern. At. Energy Agency, 1965.
18. Stahl, E. (ed.), "Thin-Layer Chromatography: A Laboratory Handbook." Academic Press, New York and Springer, Berlin, 1964.
19. Wenzel, M., Einfache Aktivitätsmessung doppelt-markierter Substanzen auf Chromatogrammen. *Naturwissenschaften* **52,** 129 (1965).
20. Wenzel, M., and Schulze, P. E., "Tritium-Markierung." Walter de Gruyter, Berlin, 1962.

CHAPTER 12

γ-RAY SAMPLE COUNTING

GERALD J. HINE*

RADIOISOTOPE SERVICE
VETERANS ADMINISTRATION HOSPITAL
BOSTON, MASSACHUSETTS

The idea of a scintillation well-counter for liquid or solid samples of γ-ray emitting radioisotopes was first presented by Anger (*3*). He summarized his results as follows: "The γ-ray counting efficiencies of this counter for 2-milliliter samples of ^{59}Fe, ^{60}Co, and ^{131}I are about equal to the β-particle counting efficiency for a mica-window G-M counter when counting thin samples." As recently as 1951 the end-window Geiger–Müller counter was the only efficient radiation detector. The presently available methods for γ-ray sample counting are discussed in this chapter.

I. SODIUM IODIDE WELL-COUNTERS

The best geometry is a 4π-counter, and the highest efficiency is obtained when all γ rays are absorbed within the counter. At present this is nearly obtainable for small samples of low-energy γ-ray emitters. A

* Present address: International Atomic Energy Agency, Vienna, Austria.

small hole in a 2 × 2-inch, or 3 × 3-inch sodium iodide crystal allows positioning of samples at the center of the crystal with minor losses of γ rays escaping through the hole. Essentially all γ rays with energies below 200 keV are absorbed by 1 inch of sodium iodide surrounding the source (Chapter 6, Section III,A). Most radioisotopes, however, emit

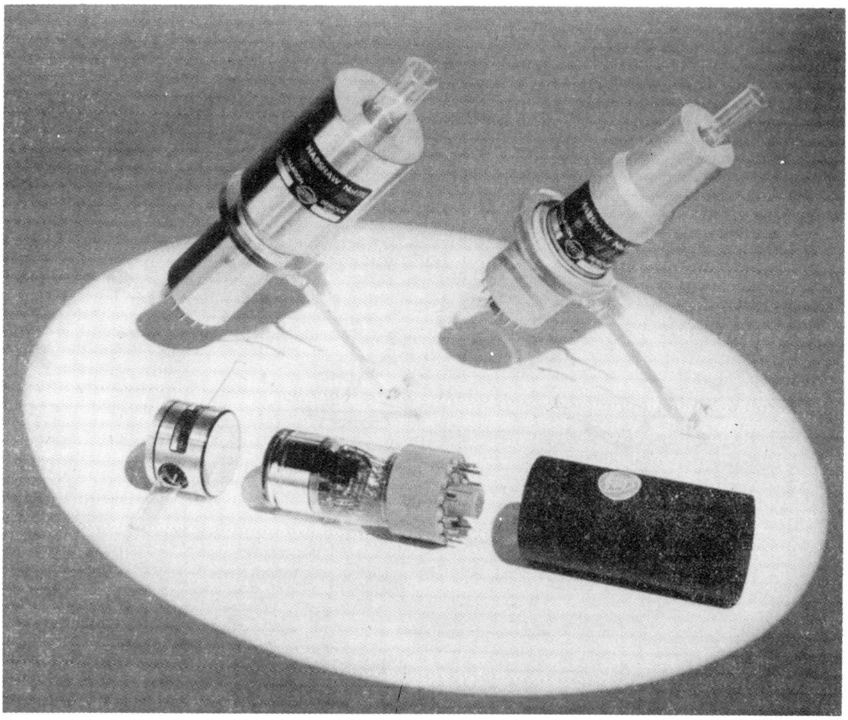

FIG. 1. Sodium iodide well-counters and multiplier phototube (Courtesy of Harshaw Chemical Company). *Upper left:* Integral line assembly of 3-inch diameter, 3-inch high crystal with 1-inch diameter, 2-inch deep well and 3-inch multiplier phototube. *Upper right:* Integral assembly of standard well-counter with 16-mm diameter test tube. *Lower left:* Components for through-hole assembly. Crystal 2-inch diameter, 1.5-inch high with the aluminum through-hole having an inside diameter of 0.68 inch or 17.2 mm, for 16-mm diameter test tube. *Center:* Multiplier phototube (2-inch diameter) for through-hole or standard well-counters. *Lower right:* Mu-metal magnetic shield for 2-inch multiplier phototube.

γ rays of higher energies. Though 9 × 9-inch and bigger sodium iodide crystals are now available, they are rarely used as well-counters for obvious economic reasons (*25*). Therefore, for different sample sizes and γ-ray energies, a variety of well-counters has been developed, representing a compromise in geometry, counting efficiency, background count-rate, and expense for each particular counting problem.

1. CRYSTAL SIZE: 1¾ INCH IN DIAMETER, 2 INCHES HIGH

Most well-counters presently in use employ sodium iodide crystals 1¾ inch in diameter and 2 inches in height, with a well ¾ inch in diameter* and 1½ inch deep (Fig. 1). Therefore, the well is surrounded by ½ inch of sodium iodide on all sides. This well-counter is often referred to as the "standard" sodium iodide well-counter. Its properties have been investigated by several authors and will be discussed here in detail.

Many variables affect the data taken with a well-counter. Therefore, the conditions of measurements must be defined clearly. The statement, "the efficiency of the standard well-counter for ^{131}I is 50%," though correct, is not sufficient. The sample volume, the fraction of the pulse-height spectrum included in the measurement, and whether the efficiency refers to the number of disintegrations or to the number of γ rays emitted must be stated.

a. *Sample Volume.* The fraction of γ rays escaping through the opening of the well without passing through any section of the sodium iodide crystal depends upon the source position. It varies between less than 2% for γ rays originating at the bottom of the well and 50% for γ rays emitted on top of the well. For sources outside the well an even smaller fraction of the γ rays reaches the crystal.

The geometrical relation of source to crystal is the same for all γ-ray emitters. In the standard well, if a glass test tube that fits in easily but not too loosely is used (the outside diameter of such test tubes is about 16 mm), a 5-ml solution just reaches the top of the well. The effect of sample volume on the count-rate is shown in Fig. 2 and Table I. For a given amount of radioisotope the count-rate decreases with increasing dilution at first slowly and then about linearly beyond 4 ml.

For the measurement of a solution of given concentration of radioactivity, the count-rate increases with increasing sample volume (Table I). While the count-rate is nearly proportional to the sample volume for the first few milliliters, it falls off rapidly as more of the sample approaches the top of the well or even exceeds it. There is only a 1% difference in count-rate between a 7- and 8-ml sample. Therefore, when enough sample is available (urine samples), filling the test tube to its top, instead of pipetting a few milliliters, is the simplest method which yields the highest count-rate. It requires, however, that the diameter and the wall thickness of all test tubes be the same. Otherwise, the amount of the sample inside the well where the count-rate varies strongly with sample volume would not be constant.

* Inside diameter of aluminum well liner is 0.656 inch or 16.5 mm.

TABLE I
EFFECT OF SAMPLE VOLUME ON COUNT-RATE OF STANDARD SODIUM IODIDE WELL-COUNTER[a]

Sample volume (ml)	Relative count-rate for constant radioactivity (%)	Relative count-rate for constant concentration (%)
0	100	—
1	99	100
2	98	195
3	94	280
4	88	350
5	82	405
6	74	440
7	66	455
8	58	460

[a] The count-rate varies with the sample volume independently of the γ-ray energy. Only for such radioisotopes as ^{125}I with γ-ray energies below 50 keV does the γ-ray absorption in the samples become significant.

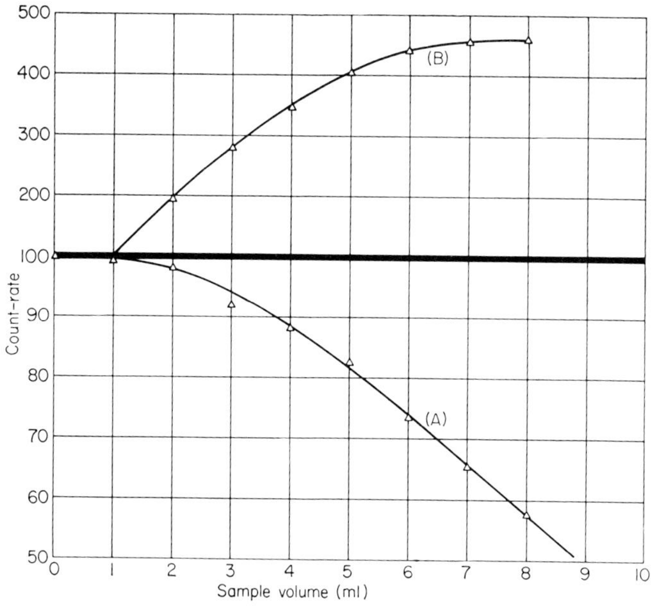

FIG. 2. Effect of sample volume on counting sensitivity of standard well-counter. (A) Dilution of a constant amount of radioactivity. (B) Increasing sample volume of constant concentration.

Variations in count-rate due to differences in test tube size can be minimized by using a 3-ml sample, though more solution may be available. This results in about a 50% reduction in count-rate from the maximum sample volume (Table I). Depending on the test tube diameter, the height of the sample varies slightly. However, since a 3- or 4-ml sample of constant radioactivity (Table I) shows only a 6% difference in count-rate, a small variation in sample height will not affect the counting accuracy.

b. *Counting Efficiency.* The most important question is that of counting efficiency. Since the count-rate varies with sample size, the efficiency should be given for a 1-ml sample; using Fig. 2 and Table I one can then calculate the efficiency for any other sample volume. From a physics viewpoint the counting efficiency (quantum-detection efficiency) can be defined as the number of counts obtainable per 100 γ rays of a given energy emitted by a 1-ml source. The counting efficiency per disintegration can then be calculated if the number and energies of the γ rays emitted by a given radioisotope are known.

Calculation or measurement of counting efficiencies requires some information about the distribution of pulse heights in the γ-ray spectrum. Depending on the type of interaction of the γ rays with the sodium iodide crystal, pulses of various sizes result (Chapter 6, Section IV). A counting efficiency can be defined if all pulses are taken into account; that means no low-energy pulses are cut off by a discriminator. In order to achieve this, the amplifier gain and the high voltage of the multiplier phototube have to be chosen so that the counter is operated near the *plateau* of the integral count-rate curve for each radioisotope (Fig. 3). If the gain of the system is increased further, the count-rate does not increase significantly, because all pulses, including the small ones, are already counted. Under these conditions the efficiency of well-counters can be determined with good accuracy.

Operating the counter at high gain results in a high background count-rate. The multiplier phototube is still operated below the point where the tube noise becomes appreciable. Nevertheless, the background count-rate might be several times that observed in ordinary laboratory use of the counter. No figures can be given because the background count-rate depends on the amount of lead shielding and the noise pulses which vary with the multiplier phototube and associated electronics. A reduction in the amplification of the system or the elimination of some low-energy pulses by a discriminator may result in a slight decrease in efficiency but a big reduction in the background count-rate.

The *quantum-detection efficiency* for a 1-ml sample in the standard sodium iodide well-counter is given in Fig. 4. Since the low-energy γ rays cannot pass through 0.5 inch of sodium iodide without interaction, the counting efficiency is close to 100% for γ rays with energies below 140 keV. Of the 350-keV γ rays, 50% are absorbed while for high-energy γ rays (2 MeV), the probability of interaction decreases to 20%. The points are experimental values obtained with calibrated radioisotope sources. Solid line (A) has been calculated using the total mass absorption co-

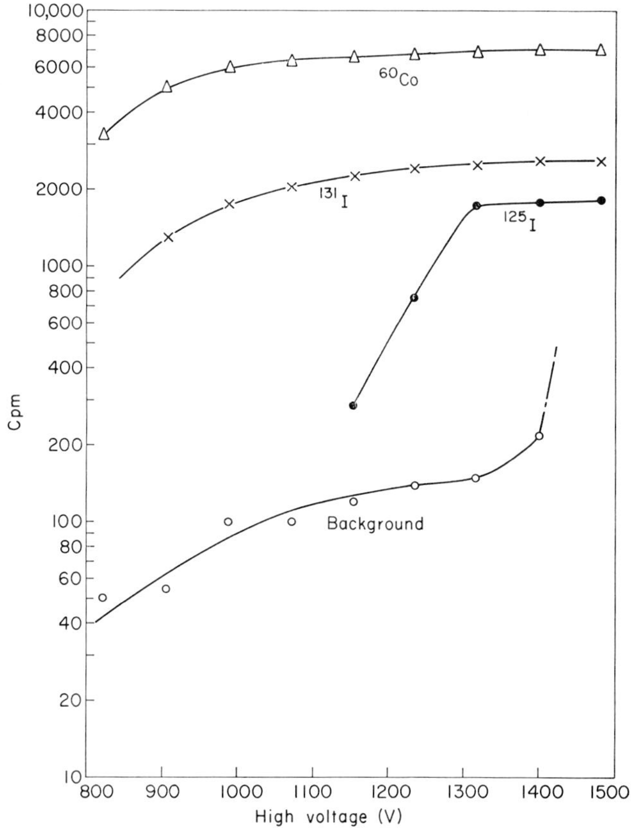

FIG. 3. Count-rate as a function of high voltage applied to multiplier phototube for different radioisotopes and counter background. The plateau is reached when the count-rate is practically independent of high voltage.

efficient for sodium iodide (*15*) and a thickness of 1.5 cm (Table II). An average path length of 1.5 cm (or 0.59 inch) for the γ rays passing through the walls of the sodium iodide well yielded the best fit with the experimental data (Fig. 4). The actual wall thickness is 0.50 inch, but since most γ rays strike the wall at some angle, the effective wall thickness is slightly larger.

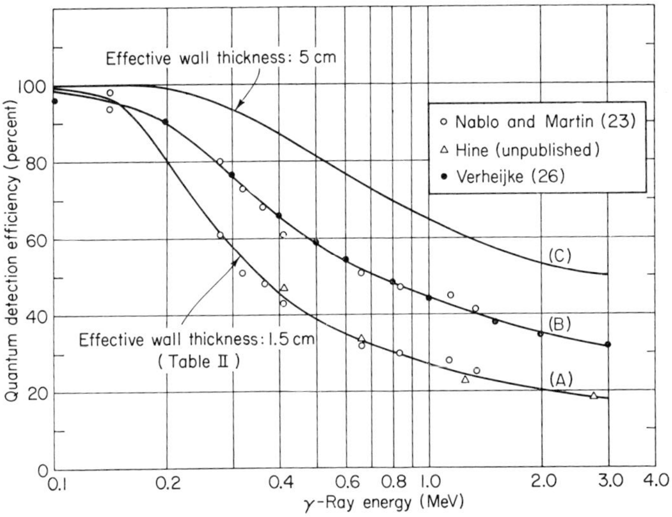

FIG. 4. Quantum-detection efficiency as a function of γ-ray energy for 1-ml samples in sodium iodide well-counters of different wall thickness. (A) Standard well-counter. The solid line calculated for an effective wall thickness of 1.5 cm is in good agreement with the experimental points. (B) 3×3 inch crystal; wall thickness of well is 1 inch. (C) 5×5 inch crystal; effective wall thickness of well is 5 cm.

TABLE II
γ-RAY ABSORPTION IN SODIUM IODIDE

γ-Ray energy (MeV)	Total mass absorption coefficient (cm^2/gm)	Absorption in 1.5 cm sodium iodide (%)
0.1	1.57	100
0.15	0.568	96
0.2	0.305	81
0.3	0.155	57
0.4	0.111	46
0.5	0.0901	39
0.6	0.0789	35
0.8	0.0657	30
1.0	0.0577	27
1.5	0.0465	23
2.0	0.0412	20
3.0	0.0367	18

The *counting efficiency per disintegration* of any radioisotope, for which the energies of the γ rays and the number of γ rays emitted per disintegration are known, can now be determined. For example, ^{131}I emits the 364-keV γ rays in 80% of its disintegrations. Since a γ ray of this energy is counted with 49% efficiency (Fig. 4), this yields a $49 \times 0.8 = 39\%$ efficiency per disintegration. The four additional γ rays of ^{131}I with much less intensity increase this value to 48% efficiency per disintegration. The counting efficiencies per disintegration for frequently used radioisotopes are given in Table III.

TABLE III
COUNTING EFFICIENCY FOR 1-ML SAMPLES IN A STANDARD SODIUM IODIDE WELL-COUNTER[a]

Radio-isotope	γ-Ray energies (MeV) (number per disintegration)	Counting efficiency per disintegration (%)	Counts per minute per microcurie
^{51}Cr	0.323 (8%)	4.3	95,500
^{60}Co	1.17 (100%), 1.33 (100%)	43	955,000
^{198}Au	0.411 (96.1%), 0.68 (1.1%), 1.09 (0.26%)	43.5	965,000
^{199}Au	0.051 (0.3%), 0.158 (41%), 0.209 (9%)	46	1,020,000
^{131}I	0.08 (2%), 0.28 (5%), 0.36 (80%), 0.64 (9%), 0.72 (3%)	48.3	1,070,000
^{59}Fe	0.19 (2.8%), 1.10 (57%), 1.29 (43%)	27.3	606,000
^{203}Hg	0.073 (17%), 0.279 (83%)	67	1,490,000
^{42}K	1.53 (18%)	4.0	89,000
^{22}Na	0.511 (200%), 1.28 (100%)	81	1,800,000
^{24}Na	1.37 (100%), 2.75 (100%)	38	844,000

[a] Calculated from Fig. 4 assuming all pulses are counted.

The *count-rate per microcurie* obtainable for a 1-ml source in the standard sodium iodide well-counter is determined by multiplying the counting efficiency by 2.22×10^6 (Table III). The counts per minute per microcurie for ^{131}I follow as: $0.483 \times 2.22 \times 10^6 = 1{,}070{,}000$ cpm/μCi. The efficiency of the standard well-counter is so high that one thousandth of a microcurie of ^{131}I or less can still be counted accurately in a short time.

Some radioisotopes emit two or more γ rays per disintegration. When two γ rays are absorbed simultaneously in a well-counter, only one pulse is registered. This reduces the counter efficiency due to coincidence losses (see Section I,4). The counting efficiencies per disintegration listed in Table III have been corrected for coincidence losses in the cases of ^{60}Co, ^{22}Na and ^{24}Na, which are radioisotopes emitting more than one γ ray per disintegration. The calculated values are in good agreement with those measured by Baskin *et al.* (4) when their efficiencies for 4-ml samples are converted to the increased efficiencies of 1-ml samples.

Since the efficiencies of the standard sodium iodide well-counter are known with good accuracy, it is possible to calibrate an unknown amount of any γ-ray emitting radioisotope by using the values given in Fig. 4 or Table III. It has to be kept in mind, however, that a correct answer is obtained only if all pulses produced by the γ rays are included in the measurements, that means no elimination of small pulses.

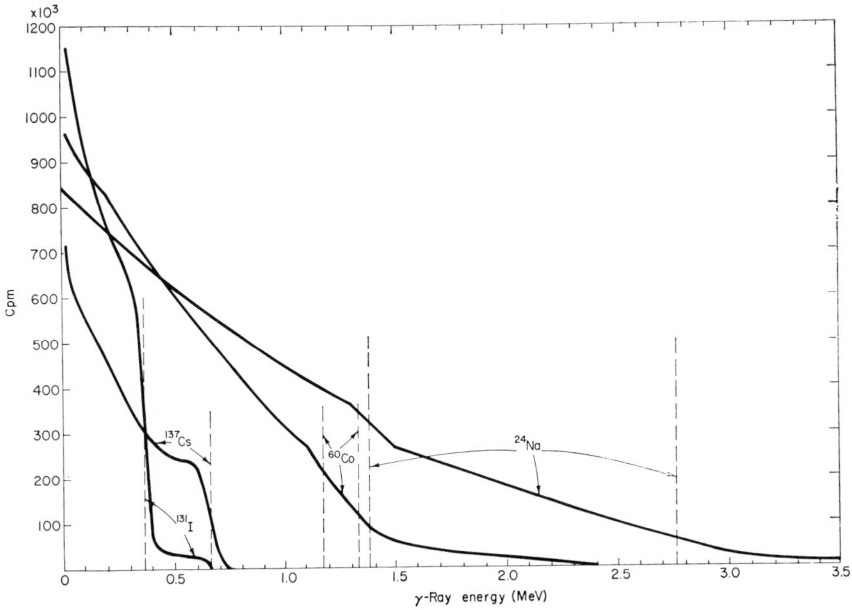

FIG. 5. Counts per minute per microcurie for 1-ml samples in standard well-counter as a function of discriminator setting. The vertical lines represent the main γ-ray energies of the four radioisotopes.

The effect of a *discriminator* on the count-rate is shown in Fig. 5 for four radioisotopes. The count-rates at zero γ-ray energy, when all pulses are counted, are equal to the cpm/μCi given in Table III. The dashed vertical lines indicate the main γ-ray energies for each radioisotope. In the case of ^{131}I, the discriminator curve shows a more rapid decrease in count-rate above 300 keV, the low-energy edge of the 364-keV peak. At 300 keV, the count-rate has decreased to about 50% of its value at zero γ-ray energy. At about 420 keV, the high-energy edge of the 364-keV peak, only 4% of the total count-rate remains. In the case of ^{60}Co, the count-rate drops to 30% of the maximum value at the low-energy edge of the two γ-ray lines and to about 8% at the high-energy edge. The high-energy tail of the discriminator curves for ^{60}Co and ^{24}Na are due to coincidence absorption of the two γ rays.

As discussed in Chapter 7, Section III, either a discriminator or a γ-ray spectrometer is employed for the selection of the pulse-height range to be counted. Discriminator curves as shown in Fig. 5 allow a good estimate to be made of the counting loss at any discriminator setting. When a γ-ray spectrometer (upper and lower pulse-height discriminator) is used, only the pulses between the two discriminators or within the spectrometer window are counted. For example, if an ^{131}I

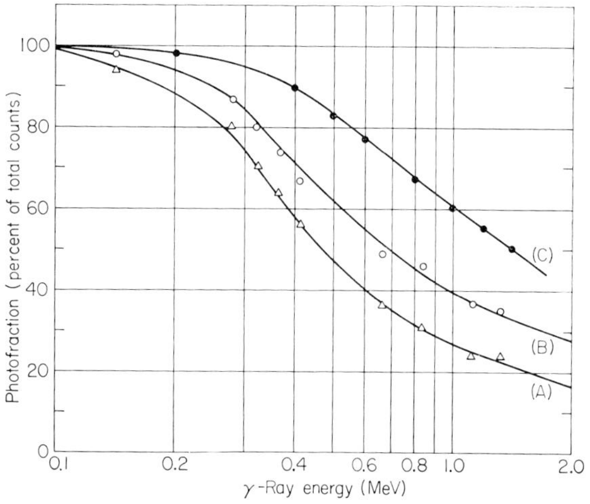

FIG. 6. Photofraction of 1-ml samples as function of γ-ray energy. (A) Standard well-counter (*23*). (B) 3×3 inch crystal with 1-inch diameter well (*16*). (C) 5×5 inch well-counter (*27*).

source is to be counted in the energy interval between 280 and 420 keV, the expected cpm/μCi can be obtained from Fig. 5 as $(660 - 40) \times 10^3 = 620{,}000$ cpm. This is about half the maximum count-rate when all pulses down to zero energy are counted. For high-energy γ-ray emitters the counting loss is more severe when only a narrow pulse-height interval is used for the measurements.

c. *Photofraction.* The counting efficiencies given above are based on the number of γ rays that interact at least once with the sodium iodide surrounding the 1-ml sample. For many reasons (Chapter 3, Section III,A), it is often desirable to know the fraction of all pulses that fall within the full-energy peak of the pulse-height spectrum (Chapter 6,

Section III,B). This so-called photofraction is given in Fig. 6 as a function of the γ-ray energy; it is expressed as percentage of the quantum-detection efficiency shown in Fig. 4. At low energies practically all pulses fall within the photopeak. In the standard well-counter, 64% of the pulses produced by the 364-keV ^{131}I γ rays fall into the photopeak, while the photofraction for the high-energy ^{60}Co γ rays is only 23% (Table IV).

TABLE IV
STANDARD SODIUM IODIDE WELL-COUNTER[a]

γ-Ray energy (MeV)	Quantum-detection efficiency (% per γ ray)	Photofraction (% of total counts)	Photopeak efficiency (% per γ ray)
0.080	97	100	97
0.142	94	94	88
0.279	61	80	49
0.321	51	70	36
0.364	48	64	31
0.411	43	56	24
0.511	38	46	17.5
0.662	32	36	11.5
0.835	30	31	9.4
0.885	29	29	8.4
1.11	28	24	6.7
1.17	25	24	6.0
1.27	24	23	5.5
1.33	23	23	5.3
2.75	18	14	2.5

[a] Crystal $1\frac{3}{4}$ inch in diameter, 2 inches high; well $\frac{3}{4}$ inch in diameter, $1\frac{1}{2}$ inch deep; 1-ml samples.

The photofraction is also a function of the sample volume (*23*). With increasing sample volume it decreases from the values given for the 1-ml samples in Fig. 6 and Table IV.

d. *Photopeak Efficiency*. The photopeak efficiency is the number of pulses in the peak of the pulse-height spectrum per γ ray emitted by the source. The quantum-detection efficiency, that is, the total number of pulses per γ ray, times the photofraction yields the photopeak efficiency (Table IV). The latter is plotted in Fig. 7 as a function of the γ-ray energy. In the case of ^{131}I, where 48% of the 364-keV γ rays from a 1-ml sample in the standard well produce a pulse, 64% of these pulses fall within the photopeak and therefore 31% of the emitted γ rays yield a pulse within the photopeak region. With increasing γ-ray energy, the photopeak efficiency decreases rapidly. At the energy of the ^{60}Co γ rays, only 5 to 6% of the emitted γ rays contribute to a photopeak (Fig. 7, Table IV).

The counting properties of the standard 1¾-inch diameter well-counter are discussed here in detail, because this is the most commonly used well-counter. Recently, well-counters of larger dimensions have found more frequent applications. Their properties are discussed briefly below.

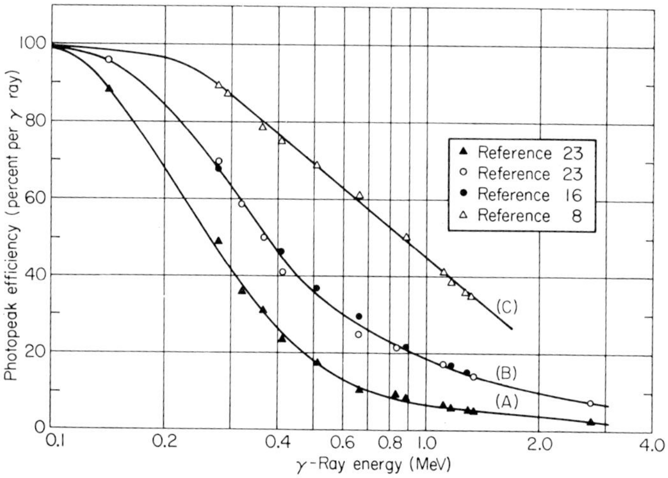

FIG. 7. Photopeak efficiency of 1-ml samples as function of γ-ray energy. (A) Standard well-counter. (B) 3×3 inch crystal with 1-inch diameter well. (C) 5×5 inch well-counter.

2. CRYSTAL SIZE: 2 INCHES IN DIAMETER, 2 INCHES HIGH

Since the count-rate of the standard sodium iodide well-counter does not increase appreciably for sample volumes larger than 5–6 ml (Table I), Baskin *et al.* (*4*) suggested the use of a 2-inch diameter, 2-inch high crystal with a hole 1⅜ inch in diameter and 1⅝ inch deep. A well with these dimensions holds a 20-ml vial and a plastic protective liner.

The wall thickness of this larger well is only $\frac{5}{16}$ inch instead of ½ inch, and therefore its efficiency is less than that of the standard well-counter. For example, a 1-ml sample of ^{131}I in the larger well counts only 85% of what it counts in a standard well. For high-energy γ-ray emitters the reduction in counting efficiency is somewhat greater. Since the top of the well is approached much slower in the larger well as the sample volume increases, its sensitivity exceeds that of the standard well for volumes larger than 6 ml. For ^{131}I, a 20-ml sample yields about 3 times the count-rate of a 4-ml sample of equal concentration in the standard well.

Though the larger well seems to be superior, in practice it is rarely used. Test tubes for the standard well are easily available and can be heated for chemical reactions. For many biological samples, such as blood or serum, only a few milliliters are available for which the standard well has a higher sensitivity. Its greater wall thickness results not only in a higher efficiency, but also in a greater photofraction and slightly improved photopeak resolution. Finally, for urine and other samples, where a large volume is available, the 20-ml vial still holds only a small fraction of the total volume. Therefore, even larger sodium iodide crystals are now used as well-counters.

3. Crystal Size: 3 Inches in Diameter, 3 Inches High

A crystal of these dimensions appears to be ideal for many applications. As a well-counter, it allows a wide choice of well sizes. The 3-inch multiplier phototubes secure maximum efficiency for light collection. Finally, the weight of shielding material required for background count-rate reduction is not excessive.

Well sizes of various dimensions have been used for 3 × 3-inch crystals. The smallest practical well has about the same dimensions as that of a standard well-counter. This leaves a little more than 1 inch of sodium iodide on all sides surrounding the well, resulting in a good quantum-detection efficiency and a high photofraction. The other extreme would be a large well (2 inches in diameter, 2.5 inches deep) which leaves 0.5 inch of sodium iodide as wall thickness, the same as that of the standard well. Such a well gives a high counting sensitivity for large samples (50 ml or more) but shows a small photopeak with poor resolution, owing to poor light collection from the U-shaped crystal.

A well about 1 inch in diameter and 1.5 to 2.5 inches deep would be a good compromise. The radiation properties of such well-counters have been determined by several investigators (*16, 23, 26*). Though the actual dimensions were somewhat different in each case, the counting efficiencies do not vary much with small changes of the well dimensions. Representative values (*23*) are given in Table V for the quantum-detection efficiency, the photofraction, and the photopeak efficiency for 1-ml samples. They are plotted in Figs. 4, 6, and 7 together with the values for the standard sodium iodide well-counter. For high-energy γ rays all values have increased by nearly a factor of 2 because the wall thickness has been doubled. The increase is less for the lower-energy γ rays which show a high absorption within the first 0.5 inch of sodium iodide. For the

364-keV ^{131}I γ rays, the photopeak efficiency increases from 31 to 50%, which is a significant gain when only the pulses in the photopeak are counted.

The sensitivity of any well-counter decreases with increasing sample volume (Fig. 2). This function, which varies with the well dimensions, can be determined easily by diluting a 1-ml sample. The correction also includes any absorption of the γ rays within the larger sample.

TABLE V
3-INCH WELL-COUNTER[a]

γ-Ray energy (MeV)	Quantum-detection efficiency (% per γ ray)	Photofraction (% of total counts)	Photopeak efficiency (% per γ ray)
0.080	95[b]	100	95
0.142	98	98	96
0.279	80	87	69.5
0.321	73	80	58.5
0.364	68	74	50
0.411	66	68	45
0.511	59	61	36
0.662	51	49	25
0.835	47	46	21.5
0.885	46	43	17
1.11	45	37	16.5
1.17	42	36	15
1.27	40	35	14
1.33	39	34	13
2.75	32	23	7.5

[a] Crystal 3 inches in diameter, 3 inches high; well 1 inch in diameter, 2 inches deep; 1-ml samples.

[b] Only at the lowest γ-ray energy has the absorption in the sample and glass test tube been taken into account.

4. CRYSTAL SIZE: 5 INCHES IN DIAMETER, 5 INCHES HIGH

What has been said about the well of 3 × 3-inch crystals also applies to the larger crystals. They permit the accommodation of even bigger sample volumes without reducing the wall thickness, or an increase of wall thickness causing an increased absorption of higher-energy γ rays. Colby and Cobble (*8*) put a small well (5/8 inch in diameter and 2.5 inches deep) into a 5 × 5-inch crystal in order to obtain a high photopeak efficiency by placing a small source at the center of the crystal. The photopeak efficiency for this well-counter is shown in Fig. 7 together with those for the 3 × 3-inch and the standard well-counter. In the case of ^{131}I, about 80% of the emitted 364-keV γ rays contribute to the photopeak, while only 30% are totally absorbed in the standard well. For high-energy γ rays, the photopeak efficiency of the big well-counter is about a factor of 7 greater than that of the standard well, resulting in a marked improvement of the spectral pulse distribution.

By providing practically 4π geometry and high total γ-ray absorption, the pulse-height spectrum of certain γ-ray emitters is markedly altered in comparison with that obtained with a right cylindrical crystal. When two or more γ rays are emitted per disintegration, as in the case of ^{22}Na, ^{24}Na, and ^{60}Co, the light from all γ rays interacting simultaneously with the crystal results in a single scintillation pulse (Chapter 6, Section IV,C,5). For ^{60}Co with increasing crystal size, more and more of the 1.17 and 1.33 MeV γ rays appear in a single peak at 2.50 MeV. This *sum peak* reduces the number of pulses in the individual photopeaks. The photopeak efficiencies of the 5-inch well-counter (Fig. 7) for the 1.17- and 1.33-MeV γ rays are 38.6 and 35.0%. The product of the two photopeak efficiencies yields the efficiency for the sum peak. Therefore, 13.4% of each of the two ^{60}Co γ rays contributes to the sum peak. This reduces the percentage of γ rays that actually contributes to the two photopeaks to 25.1 and 21.5%. For ^{59}Fe, which also emits two γ rays with energies practically identical with those of ^{60}Co, no sum peak is observed. Since only one of the two ^{59}Fe γ rays is emitted per disintegration, the two γ rays do not appear in coincidence, and the values given for the photopeak efficiency in Fig. 7 apply without correction.

If more than one γ-ray peak is observed from a given radioisotope, the presence or absence of a sum peak identifies the emission of two γ rays as in coincidence or as single γ rays, one per disintegration. When there is some doubt whether or not an observed peak is a sum peak, the source should be placed on top of the crystal instead of inside the well. This reduces the count-rate of the sum peak much more than that of single γ-ray peaks.

The 5-inch sodium iodide crystal used by Colby and Cobble (*8*) was mounted on a DuMont 6364 5-inch multiplier phototube. For a ^{137}Cs source at its center, it had a resolution of 11.4%. A 5-inch diameter, 5-inch high crystal* with a well 1.5 inch in diameter and 3.5 inches deep integrally mounted on the same type of multiplier phototube has a 11.1% resolution for ^{137}Cs. These well-counters have a line width that is somewhat wider than that obtainable with right cylindrical crystals (Chapter 6, Section IV,A) but they are still useful for γ-ray spectroscopy.

The quantum-detection efficiency for the 5-inch well-counter can be calculated as has been done for the standard well-counter (Fig. 4), whose

* Radioisotope Service, Veterans Administration Hospital, Boston, Massachusetts.

effective wall thickness was found to be 18% greater than the crystal thickness. Assuming the same increase in effective wall thickness for the 5-inch well-counter, its effective wall thickness was estimated as 5 cm for the 1¾-inch thick wall. The resultant quantum-detection efficiency for a 1-ml sample is shown in Fig. 4. For example, for the 662-keV ^{137}Cs γ rays, the quantum-detection efficiency of the 5-inch well-counter is 74%. Since the ^{137}Cs γ rays are emitted in 82% of the disintegrations, this yields a maximum count-rate of $2.22 \times 10^6 \times 0.74 \times 0.82 = 1{,}350 \times 10^3$ cpm per microcurie of ^{137}Cs.

This value agrees with the one shown in Fig. 8 when all pulses are counted.* The pulses above the high-energy ^{60}Co and ^{24}Na γ-ray lines

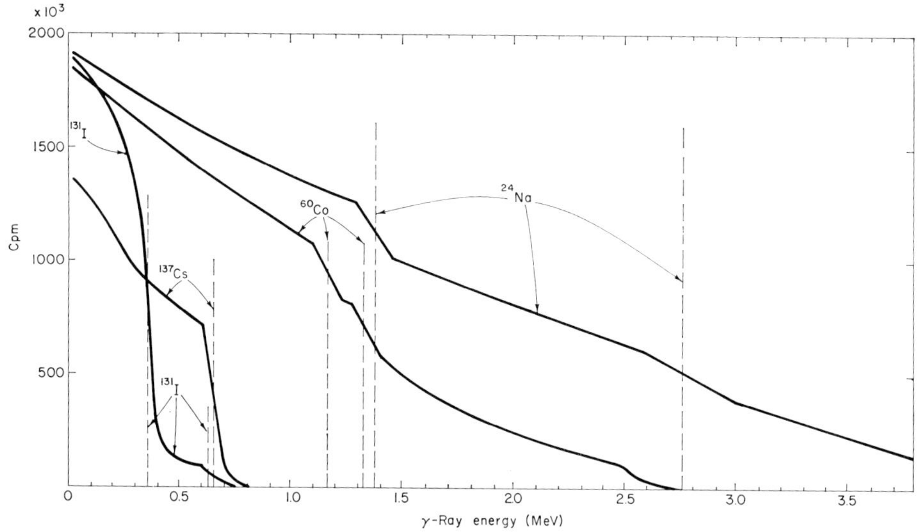

FIG. 8. Counts per minute per microcurie for 1-ml samples in 5 × 5 inch crystal with 1.5-inch diameter well, as function of discriminator setting. The vertical lines represent the main γ-ray energies of the four radioisotopes.

are due to the summing of coincidence pulses. In both cases about one quarter of all pulses appear as sum pulses, though only few pulses contribute to the sum peak representing the full energy of both γ rays.

5. CRYSTAL SIZE: 9⅜ INCHES IN DIAMETER, 8.5 INCHES HIGH

A sodium iodide crystal of this size has been used by Perkins' (*25*) as a well-counter for 500-ml samples. Its counting efficiency is so high that it is possible to measure the natural ^{137}Cs and ^{40}K content of 24-hr

* The 32-keV Ba X rays emitted in 10% of the disintegrations are completely absorbed by the copper container surrounding the sodium iodide crystal.

urine samples. Since such an extreme sensitivity is rarely required, this counter is not discussed here in detail. By using seven 3-inch multiplier phototubes, a resolution of 11.5% was obtained for the ^{137}Cs photopeak. This value is similar to that of the 5-inch well-counters discussed above.

II. COUNTERS FOR LARGE SAMPLE VOLUMES

A number of sodium iodide well-counters presently used for γ-ray sample counting have been described above. Their counting efficiencies are high even for high-energy γ-ray emitters, if the larger-size crystals are used; in addition they all yield good spectral resolution. Large sodium iodide crystals, however, are very expensive. Some important medical radioisotope tests are based on the measurement of the fraction of the administered dose which has been excreted within a given time. These studies require the counting of samples of rather large volume. In the case of vitamin B_{12}, four cobalt radioisotopes are now available for the labeling: ^{56}Co, ^{57}Co, ^{58}Co, and ^{60}Co. The counting efficiencies and geometries of different kinds of well-counters for these radioisotopes have been investigated recently (*2, 14*). For counting large sample volumes with a less expensive γ-ray counter, either the less efficient plastic scintillator or a less efficient geometry with sodium iodide crystals has to be chosen. Better results are often obtained by counting large sample volumes with reduced efficiency than a small sample volume with high efficiency.

A. Organic Scintillator Well-Counters

Several authors (*6, 9, 12, 14, 19*) have investigated the use of organic scintillators, which are less expensive than sodium iodide crystals. Both organic scintillators, plastic and liquid, are used as detectors for large well-counters. Though their construction is quite different, their performance is similar.

For animal or human *in vivo* counting it is more convenient to have the axis of the well in a horizontal plane (Chapter 21). Most counters of this kind employ the liquid scintillator (*12*). For liquid γ-ray samples, however, the horizontal well-counter is not very useful.

Large vertical well-counters for γ-ray samples have been built using plastic scintillators (*6, 9, 14, 19*). The plastic scintillator used by Cook and Valberg (*9*) is 18 inches in diameter and 12 inches high with a well 5 inches in diameter and 6 inches deep. It can accommodate a 1,000-ml sample surrounded by 6 inches of plastic phosphor on all sides. The scintillator is mounted on an 18-inch DuMont multiplier phototube. All surfaces are coated by a reflecting paint and are covered by a light-tight aluminum canister. The scintillator and multiplier phototube are surrounded by a 2-inch lead shielding, weighing 2,200 lb. The complete assembly is 22 inches in diameter and 36 inches high.

The background count-rate is high, as is to be expected for a counter of that size. If an integral spectrum is used, it is 18,000 cpm, which can be reduced to 7,000 cpm by differential counting of a section of the spectrum. For high-energy γ-ray emitters such as ^{60}Co, this introduces no major counting losses, but becomes more serious for the lower γ-ray energies of ^{131}I and ^{51}Cr.

B. Two Opposed Crystals

Placing a sample between two crystals with summed outputs constitutes a partial well-counter (7). A small sample between two large crystals close to each other yields again nearly 4π geometry. As the sample volume increases, the distance between the two crystals becomes larger and more γ rays will escape from the gap between the two opposed crystals. The use of large crystals (8-inch diameter) is expensive and requires a great amount of shielding. When the crystal size is reduced to 3 inches in diameter, the resemblance with a well-counter is practically lost (Fig. 9).

The two crystals facing each other have one definite advantage over most well-counters. The γ-ray absorption in the 3-inch thick crystals is nearly 100% for all γ-ray energies including ^{60}Co (except for the 2.75-MeV ^{24}Na γ rays). Therefore, the counting efficiency is determined only by the sample-to-crystal geometry; however, the absorption of low-energy γ rays within a large sample volume reduces its counting efficiency. The right cylindrical crystals yield good total γ-ray absorption, resulting in a major fraction of the pulses appearing in the photopeak.

The *geometrical efficiency* can be calculated approximately (Table VI), assuming that the effective distance for the volume source between the two crystals is given by the distance from the source center to a 1-inch depth inside the crystals. The 1000- and 2000-ml sample volumes show some additional losses, because the source diameter is larger than the diameter of the crystals resulting in a poorer geometry.

For small sample volumes the counting efficiency is about 20%. This compares favorably with that of well-counters (Fig. 4), since the loss in geometrical efficiency is partially compensated by the increased γ-ray absorption in the 3-inch thick crystals. Though the two vertically opposed crystals would not be used routinely for counting of small samples, they could be used occasionally with good results. A disadvantage is that liquid samples have to be placed in shallow beakers so that the two crystals can be brought close together. Furthermore, owing to the increased size of the two crystals, the background count-rate is higher than that of a well-counter.

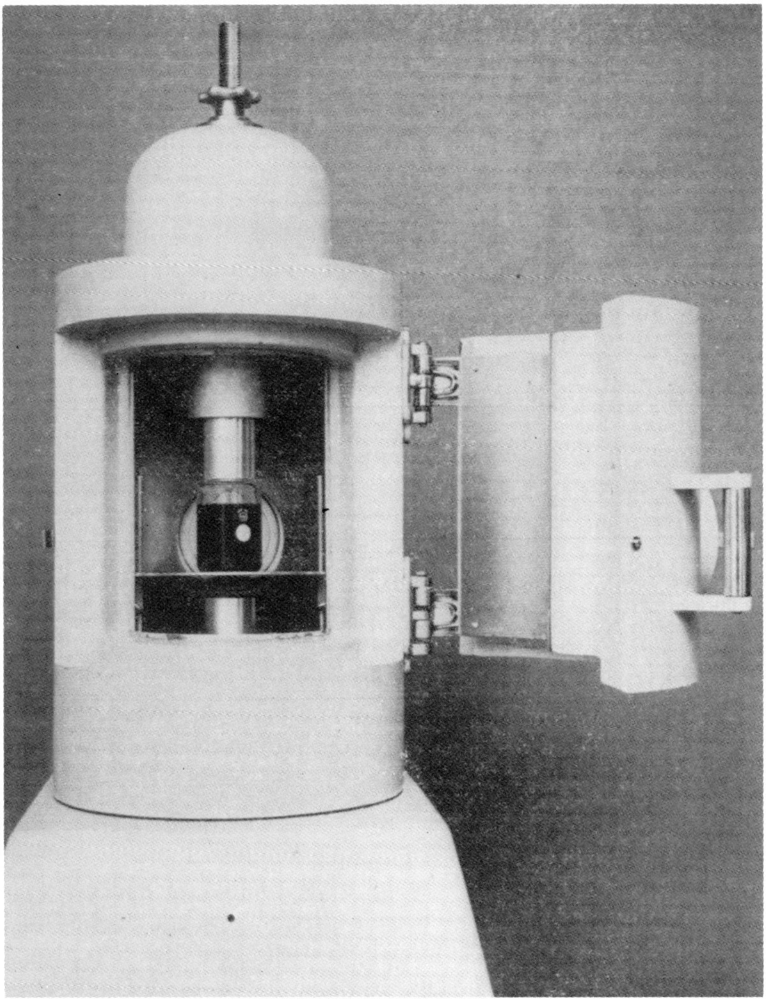

FIG. 9. Two vertically opposed 3 × 3 inch sodium iodide crystals with 1000-ml sample. Distance between crystals is adjustable; maximum sample diameter is 8 inches; maximum height, 6.5 inches. Weight of steel-encased lead shield is 1,500 lb. (Courtesy of Nuclear-Chicago Corp.)

For larger sample volumes the counting efficiency is small. The reduced efficiency, compared with that of well-counters, however, is well compensated by the large increase in usable sample volume. The two-crystal geometry is particularly useful for large samples of high-energy γ-ray emitters (^{60}Co) because good photopeaks are observed with the large crystals.

In a laboratory where samples of different volumes and various γ-ray emitters have to be counted, the two-crystal assembly should be considered before any special-size well-counter is chosen. The distance between the two crystals can be adjusted easily, which secures optimum sensitivity for all sample sizes without preselection of any one sample volume. The counter has a few additional features that are worth mentioning.

Constant background. The two crystals (Fig. 9) are shielded by 1,500 pounds of steel-encased lead with an average thickness of 3 inches. Since the shielding varies neither with sample volume nor position of the crystals inside the shield, the background count-rate and its spectral distribution are the same for all sample sizes. The background count-rate of pulses above 50 keV is about 700 cpm with about 100 cpm in the ^{131}I 364-keV photopeak. This is about twice the background count-rate of a standard well-counter shielded by 2 inches of lead.

TABLE VI
GEOMETRICAL EFFICIENCY (CALCULATED) FOR LARGE SAMPLES BETWEEN TWO 3-INCH DIAMETER OPPOSED SODIUM IODIDE CRYSTALS

Sample volume[a] (ml)	Distance from center of source to 1-inch depth in crystal (inches)	Approximate total counting efficiency[b] (% per γ ray)
100	2.5	18
250	3.0	12
500	3.5	9
1000	4.5	5
2000	5.0	3

[a] Glass beakers are used; their diameter and height vary with the sample volume.
[b] The measured counting efficiency will vary with γ-ray energy; it is reduced by the absorption of the γ rays within the sample. For large sample volumes and low γ-ray energies this reduction will be a large factor.

Independence of sample volume. For a given separation of the two crystals, the summed output count-rate is nearly independent of the sample volume (Fig. 10). As the volume increases, some activity gets further away from the lower crystal, but at the same time gets closer to the upper crystal. This is important for the measurement of excretion samples which vary in volume (*7, 11*). The collection can be made in disposable containers and, using a graph such as given in Fig. 10, a minor correction can be applied for an estimated volume.

Sum peaks and coincidence counting. Two γ rays which are emitted simultaneously can produce a sum peak (Section I,4). However, with increasing distance between the two crystals the probability for coincidence pulses in the two crystals decreases rapidly. With positron emitters, the sum of the two 511-keV annihilation quanta is always present, because the two quanta are emitted in opposite directions. Coincidence counting can be very useful in the case of a mixture of several radioisotopes.

Matching of multiplier phototubes. The pulses from the two crystals can be integrated in a single spectrum only if the outputs of the two

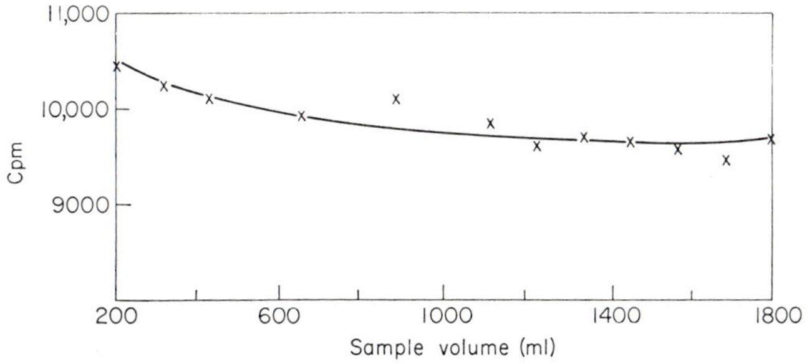

Fig. 10. Variation of count-rate versus sample volume. The two 3 × 3 inch sodium iodide crystals are separated by 4 inches. The count-rate is given per microcurie of ^{131}I, for pulses above 50 keV. (Courtesy of Nuclear-Chicago Corp.)

multiplier phototubes are matched perfectly. This is an adjustment that has to be checked from time to time, while this is not the case for a well-counter using a single multiplier phototube.

An inexpensive version of the two opposed crystals that leads to count-rate independence of sample volume, even in heterogeneously distributed samples, is effected by rotating a source in front of a single crystal partially blinded by a lead aperture (*11*). The reduction in efficiency has to be compensated by an increase in counting time.

C. Marinelli Beaker

With a single crystal a large sample volume can be measured with fairly good sensitivity by placing the sample around the crystal. This geometry was suggested by Marinelli (*17*) for Geiger–Müller counters: "The sample holder is a glass beaker with a hole in its base. A section of glass tubing, long enough to serve as a handle also has been blown into the hole so that the beaker can be slipped over the counter." This type of beaker is often referred to as a Marinelli beaker. It has been modified recently for scintillation counters (*10, 13, 24*).

Figure 11 shows the sample configuration used by Dratz (*10*) for counting dilute ^{60}Co solutions. A 100-ml solution containing 0.005 μCi of ^{60}Co can be counted in 20 min with a 3% standard error. The concentration of this solution is much too low to be counted in a well-counter.

The counting efficiency of the Marinelli beaker geometry depends upon the crystal size, the sample volume, and the γ-ray energy. In addition, the amount of shielding employed determines the background count-rate. Instead of a right cylindrical sodium iodide crystal, a well-

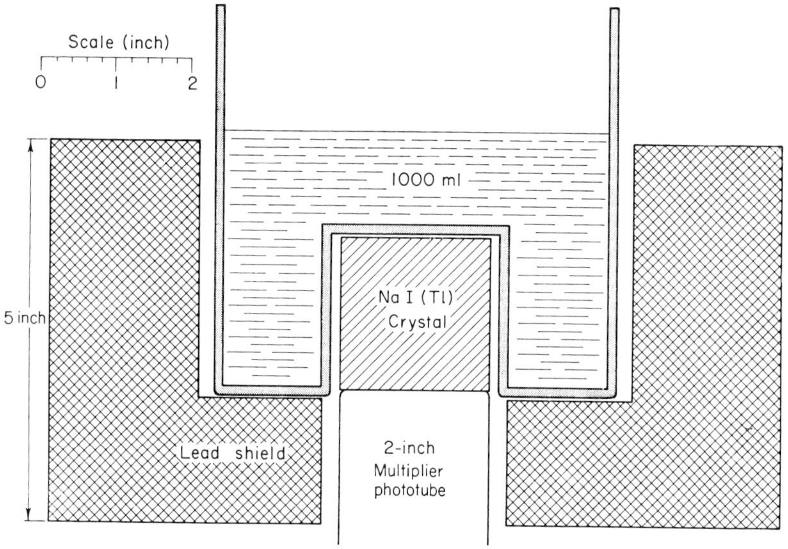

FIG. 11. Improved Marinelli beaker for counting large sample volumes with a single solid sodium iodide crystal (*10*).

counter may be employed with equal efficiency. This gives the choice of placing a small sample inside the well or a large sample around the crystal. Some authors have suggested putting samples simultaneously at both places (*13, 24*).

A 3 $\times$ 3 inch sodium iodide well-counter with provision for insertion of reentrant containers might be regarded as a universal γ-ray sample counter (Fig. 12). It yields a high counting efficiency for small samples inside the well (Section I,3) and also provides good counting geometry for liquid samples up to 1000 ml.

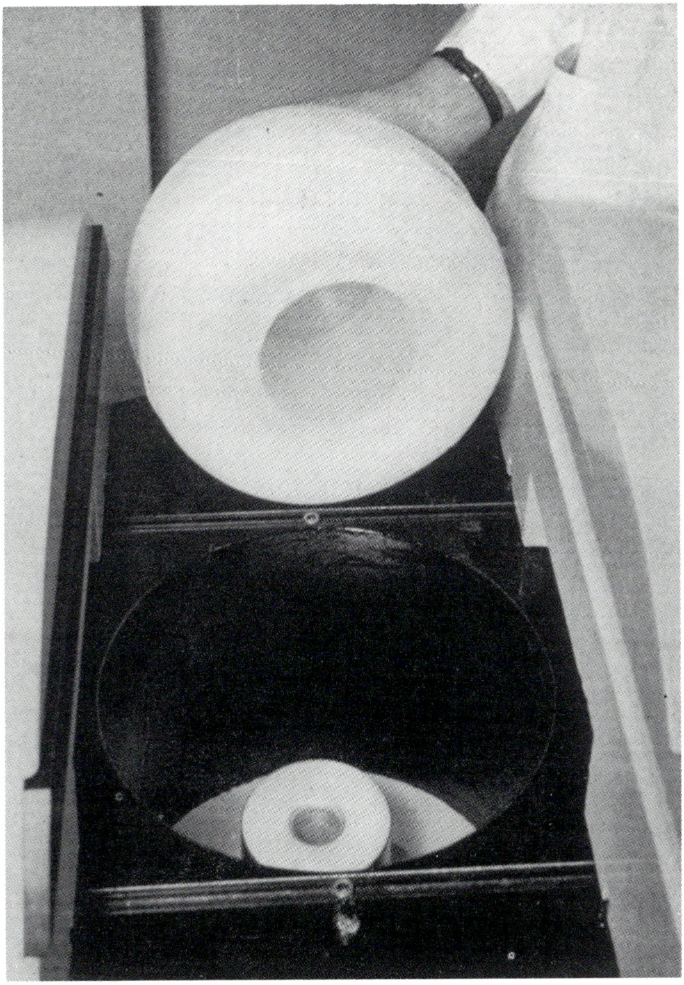

FIG. 12. Polyethylene reentrant container and 3-inch well-crystal in combination steel and lead shielding. The heavy steel-lead shielding is closed by rolling a thick lid over the opening. (Courtesy of Medical Section, International Atomic Energy Agency, Vienna)

III. DOUBLE TRACER TECHNIQUES

Samples containing several γ-ray-emitting radioisotopes are not uncommon. In nuclear activation analysis more than one isotope may become radioactive (Chapter 13). The turnover rates of two elements or labeled compounds might be investigated in a single tracer study. Two pairs of radioisotopes frequently used for diagnostic purposes in man are ^{51}Cr–^{59}Fe and ^{42}K–^{24}Na. A mixture of radioisotopes that cannot be separated according to half-lives may be measured quantitatively by making use of differences in the type or the energy of their emitted radiation.

Before double tracer measurements are described, the detection of β radiation by γ-ray well-counters and special β-ray counters for liquid samples will be discussed.

A. β-Ray Sensitivity of Well-Counters

1. Standard Sodium Iodide Well-Counter

High-energy β rays can escape from a liquid sample, and penetrate the sample container and the aluminum housing of the sodium iodide crystal (Chapter 6, Section IV,C,7). For example, a 5-ml sample of ^{32}P in a glass test tube has a β-ray counting efficiency of 0.2% per disintegration when counted in the standard NaI(Tl) well-counter (*21*). Only few high-energy ^{32}P β rays can reach the crystal. For ^{42}K, with twice the maximum β-ray energy, the β-ray counting efficiency is about 10%.

β-Rays that do not reach the sodium iodide crystal can still contribute to the count-rate. As the β rays are stopped in the source and the surrounding material, electromagnetic radiation is emitted, which is called *Bremsstrahlung*. In the case of ^{32}P, most of the quanta have energies below 100 keV though the continuous spectrum of Bremsstrahlung extends to about 700 keV. With increasing β-ray energy the photon energy as well as the yield for Bremsstrahlung production increases. The counting efficiency for ^{32}P Bremsstrahlung from a 5-ml sample in the standard well-counter is 0.6% (*21*), while that of lower-energy β-ray emitters is insignificant.

The total counting efficiency for ^{32}P is the sum of the contribution of its high-energy β rays and the Bremsstrahlung. For the 5-ml sample in the standard well-counter it is 0.8% per disintegration. Thus the sodium iodide counter can be used to measure some pure β-ray emitters, though with rather low efficiency. On the other hand, in a mixture of β- and γ-ray emitters (^{32}P and ^{131}I), it cannot be assumed that only the γ-ray emitter contributes to the count-rate of a sodium iodide counter.

2. Plastic β-Ray Well-Counters

The counting efficiency of β-ray samples in a well-counter can be increased by using a thin-wall plastic scintillator (*18, 22*). A cylinder of a $\frac{1}{16}$-inch thick plastic phosphor is placed inside a highly reflecting container (Fig. 13). Most of the light produced in the thin-walled scintillator escapes through the narrow circular end of the cylinder. The fraction of the light which escapes from the surface of the cylinder is reflected by the walls of the container, which serves also as a shield against light from the outside.

The thin plastic scintillation counter has a low background requiring little or no lead shielding. Its γ-ray sensitivity is very low compared with that of the standard sodium iodide well-counter. The counting efficiencies for the β and γ rays of a number of radioisotopes are given in Table VII.

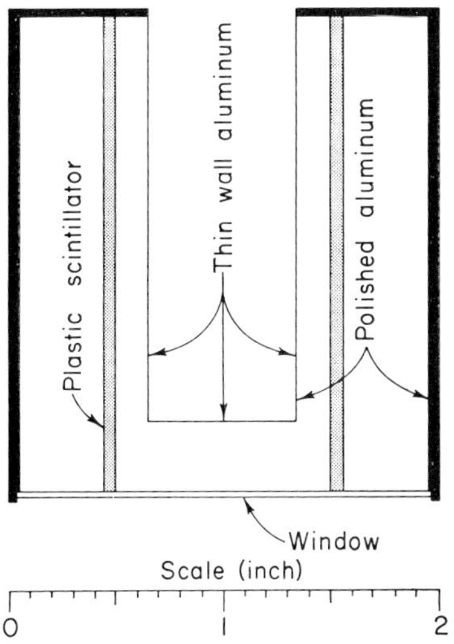

FIG. 13. Thin wall ($\frac{1}{16}$ inch) plastic scintillator for β-ray well-counting in light-tight aluminum container.

The values refer to the counts obtained per disintegration from a 1-ml sample in a plastic test tube, $\frac{1}{2}$ inch in diameter with a wall thickness of 0.01 inch. Only pulses corresponding to an energy of more than 150 keV absorbed in the scintillator were registered. The β-ray efficiency increases with increasing β-ray energy, since fewer β-rays are absorbed in the 1-ml sample. With increasing sample volume, the efficiency decreases rapidly (*22*). The γ-ray efficiency never exceeds a few percent. Therefore, for a mixture of several radioisotopes in a sample, the plastic scintillator strongly favors the high-energy β-ray emitter. However, the plastic test tubes cannot be used for all kinds of samples because the plastic is not chemically inert like glass.

TABLE VII
EFFICIENCIES OF 1/16-INCH THICK PLASTIC WELL-COUNTERS FOR 1-ML SAMPLES IN LUSTEROID TEST TUBE (*22*)

Isotope	Maximum β-ray energies (MeV)	Abundance (%)	Efficiency per disintegration (%) β-Ray	Efficiency per disintegration (%) γ-Ray
^{131}I	0.608	87	1.1	1.5
	0.335	9		
^{198}Au	0.963	99	5.6	1.6
^{24}Na	1.39	100	12	3
^{32}P	1.71	100	16	0
^{86}Rb	1.77	92	17	<0.5
	0.68	8		
^{90}Y	2.26	100	33	0
^{42}K	3.58	82	50	<1
	2.04	18		

3. Two Opposed Plastic Scintillators

A large sample volume placed between two opposed flat pieces of plastic scintillator may yield a high β-ray efficiency (*5*). The sample (80 ml) in a plastic bag is squeezed between two 4-inch diameter, ⅛-inch thick plastic scintillators. This assures a uniform sample thickness (1 cm) and good contact between sample and scintillator. For 80-ml samples of ^{42}K a counting efficiency of 28% per disintegration was observed with good reproducibility.

The light from each flat plastic scintillator was collected by a 5-inch multiplier phototube mounted on the scintillator surfaces opposite the sample (*5*). The scintillator, however, acts like a light pipe and only a fraction of the light escapes through the plane-parallel surfaces. Most of the light is trapped by internal reflections and can escape only through the narrow sides of the scintillator. Recently a method has been developed for collecting the light from the four sides of a thin, square plastic scintillator (Fig. 14). From each side the light passes first through a curved section glued to the scintillator, then through a triangular plate. The narrow ends of the four side pieces join in an area small enough for collecting the light on the photocathode of a 2-inch multiplier phototube.

B. γ-Ray Counting of Two Radioisotopes

Separate counting of two γ-ray emitters in one sample can be done, if the combined γ-ray spectrum of the two radioisotopes has an energy region to which one of the radioisotopes contributes predominantly and another region with a photopeak produced by the other γ-ray emitter (*18*). The relative contribution of each γ-ray emitter to both regions can be determined by means of separate standards of each radioisotope.

A pair of radioisotopes frequently encountered is ^{51}Cr–^{59}Fe. The ^{51}Cr γ rays (0.32 MeV) do not interfere at the energies of the ^{59}Fe γ rays (1.1, 1.3 MeV). However, the Compton electrons produced in the sodium iodide crystal by the ^{59}Fe γ rays yield pulses at the energy of the ^{51}Cr γ rays (Fig. 15). If all pulses above 400 keV including the two ^{59}Fe photopeaks are counted, this results in an increased efficiency for ^{59}Fe

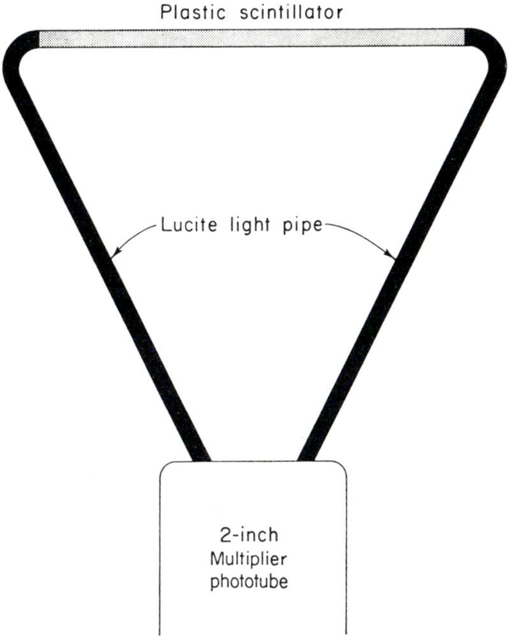

Fig. 14. Method for efficient light collection from the sides of a thin plastic scintillator. (Courtesy of Controls for Radiation, Inc.)

without interference from ^{51}Cr. In the energy interval between 200 and 400 keV, ^{51}Cr is best counted with only some contribution from ^{59}Fe.

Only radioisotopes with γ rays of greatly different energies are easily separated by γ-ray counting. The 320-keV ^{51}Cr and 364-keV ^{131}I γ-ray spectra overlap even when measured in a well-counter with good resolution. Two differential pulse-height analyzers, one for each photopeak, can be used in principle (*1*). This requires an extreme stability in amplifier and multiplier phototube gain, high-voltage supply, and analyzer performance for long periods of time. Therefore, if possible, preference should be given to other counting methods. For another pair of radioisotopes (^{42}K–^{24}Na) which could be measured in a similar way, a better alternative is discussed below.

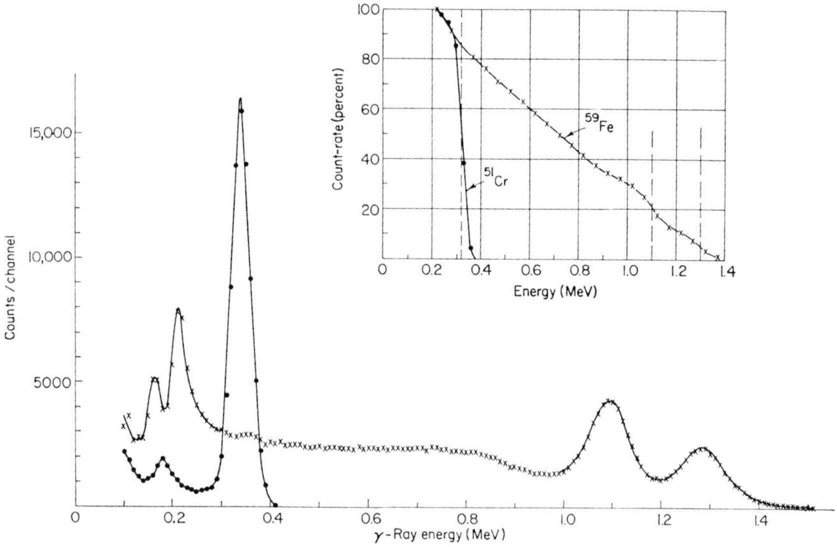

FIG. 15. Pulse-height spectra and discriminator curves for the ^{51}Cr and ^{59}Fe γ rays measured in the standard sodium iodide well-counter.

C. Mixed β-, γ-Ray Counting of Radioisotopes

For a mixture of radioisotopes that cannot be counted adequately by γ-ray spectroscopy, β- as well as γ-ray counting should be considered. For two radioisotopes, best results are obtained if one set of measurements greatly favors one radioisotope and a second type of measurements the other.

In the case of ^{24}Na–^{42}K, ^{24}Na emits the highest-energy γ rays in great abundance, while ^{42}K emits the highest-energy β rays. If equal amounts of ^{24}Na and ^{42}K are counted in a β-ray well-counter (Section III,A,2) 80% of the pulses may be produced by ^{42}K. When the mixture is counted in a standard sodium iodide well-counter, 90% of the pulses result from the ^{24}Na γ rays. Additional measurements of ^{24}Na and ^{42}K standards in both systems permit an accurate determination to be made of the ^{24}Na and ^{42}K content in a mixed sample (*5, 18*).

IV. AUTOMATION OF SAMPLE COUNTING

A. Sample Changers

Samples with high count-rates require only short counting times for both sample and background to achieve a good counting accuracy (Chapter 3, Section I,B). Therefore, 20 or more such samples can be counted manually within an hour. If counting times of 10 min or more per sample are required, or if the daily sample load is high, this procedure becomes cumbersome and time-consuming. Sample changers have been developed that can handle automatically 100 or more samples.

The use of automatic sample changers is not only time saving, but it allows samples to be counted repeatedly. A prolonged counting time

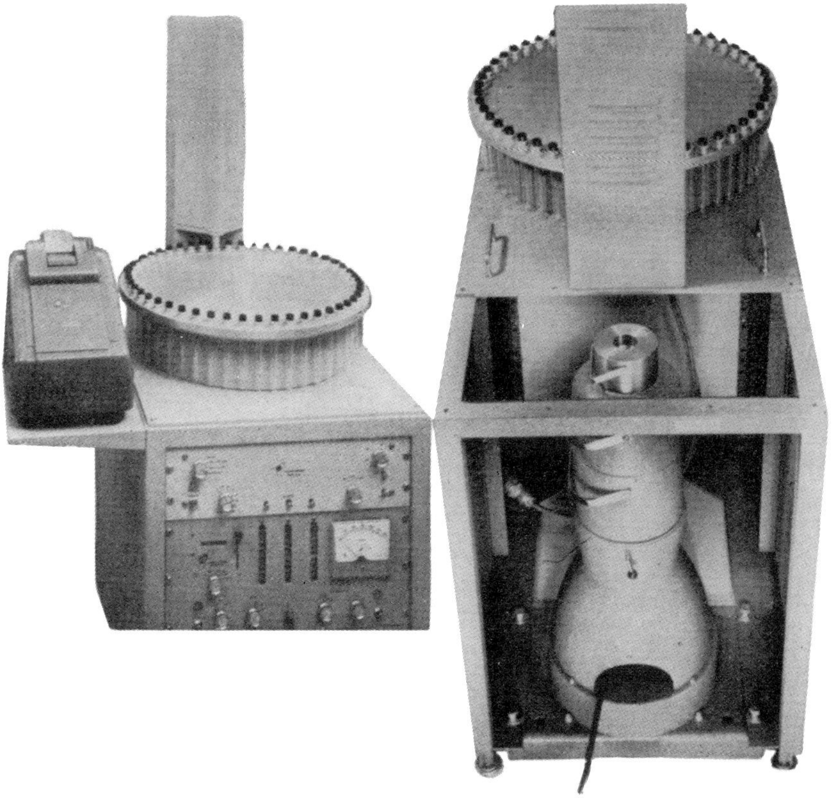

FIG. 16. Front and back view of automatic sample changer for test tubes to be counted in NaI(Tl) well-counter below turntable. (Courtesy of Nuclear-Chicago Corp.)

improves the statistical accuracy of the results, while multiple counting enables the detection of variations in count-rates caused by improper functioning of the counter or electronic equipment, or by a change of the background count-rate.

In automatic sample changers the test tubes are usually placed in a circle around a shielded well-counter. For background measurements, empty test tubes are added to the ones containing samples. The machine inserts one of the test tubes into the well and measures it for the selected time or number of counts, whichever is reached first (Fig. 16). Since the rest of the samples remain at equal distance from the lead shield surrounding the scintillation detector, the background count-rate remains constant for the counting of all samples.

Some automatic sample changers have one minor disadvantage. Because of the mechanism which inserts the test tubes into the well, no lead shielding is placed over the top of the test tube in the counting position. Therefore, the shielding of this well-counter is not as complete as when a lead cover is put in place after insertion of the sample in a manual well-counter (Chapter 3, Fig. 20). This not only causes an increase of the background count-rate, but also makes the counter more susceptible to external radiation sources and scattered radiation from the samples. In practice this is not a serious limitation, but it should be kept in mind, especially for the measurement of low-activity samples.

Either the standard sodium iodide well or a 3×3 inch well-crystal can be used with automatic sample changers. For large sample volumes and other crystal geometries automatic counting equipment has been developed recently (*20*).

B. Computation of Net Count-Rates

For manual counting, different counting times are usually chosen for background, standard, and sample measurements. Their count-rates have to be calculated and the background count-rate has to be subtracted to obtain the net count-rates for standards and samples. All these calculations are simple and therefore no effort has been made until recently to build equipment which gives the results in net counts per minute directly.

An integrated counting system that reads directly in net counts per minute requires only a single readout instead of the usual dual reading of time and counts. Simple and reliable instruments have been developed recently which exclude the possibility of timing errors. The sample may be counted for different lengths of time, but the results are always given in net counts per minute even if the counting time is only a fraction of a minute. The average background count-rate, as determined by counting for a longer period, is automatically subtracted from the sample count-rate, independently of the actual counting time.

C. Computation of Sample Activity as Fraction of Administered Dose

The computation of the net count-rate is only the first step in evaluating the results of a tracer study. The count-rates of the samples must be expressed as percentage of a standard or as fractions of the administered dose. For example, when radioactivity is injected into an unknown volume of fluid, the ratio of the injected to the recovered radioactivity times the sample volume yields the unknown volume.

When this simple principle is applied to *blood volume determinations,* some problems arise concerning the sample measurements (*28*). The dilution is about 1 to 5000 and therefore either the dose has too much or the sample has too little radioactivity to be measured in a well-counter. An aliquot of the injected dose can be diluted and then measured. However, it is not easy to assay the injected dose accurately since a fraction of the dose remains in the syringe after the injection. For a second (postoperative) blood volume determination, the radioactivity remaining in the blood prior to the injection of the second dose has to be taken into account. All steps of this procedure are simple but time-consuming.

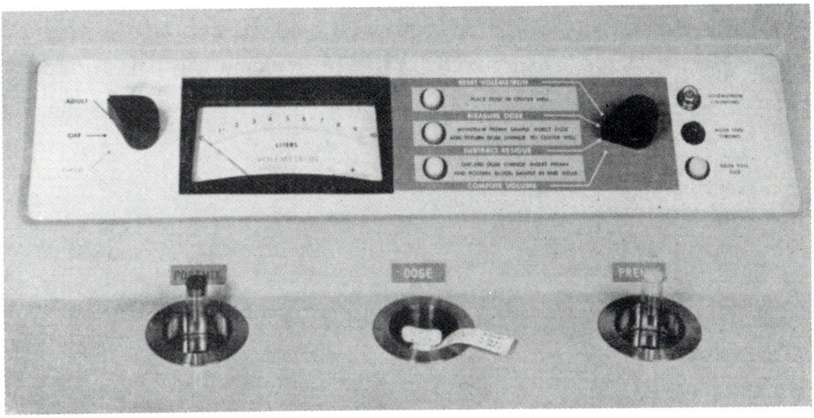

FIG. 17. Control panel of fully automated blood volume counter. The samples are inserted in two well-counters and the dose in a centrally positioned hole as indicated. (Courtesy of Ames Atomium, Inc.)

A programmed well-counter has been developed (*28*) which allows a fast and accurate performance of blood volume determinations without additional dilutions or pipetting. Instead of inserting the dose inside the well, it is placed in a fixed geometry at some distance outside the well-counter (Fig. 17). After injection, the empty syringe is put in the same position and the residual radioactivity is determined. A blood sample is withdrawn before injecting the dose and another one after a mixing period. Both samples are emptied into precalibrated plastic tubes. Since these are inserted into holes traversing the crystal (Fig. 1), the accuracy of the sample measurements depends only upon the diameter of the tubes but not upon the exact sample volume. By following the simple program incorporated into the machine (Fig. 17), the blood volume is computed automatically.

Automation of tracer measurements is not only a convenience and timesaver; the computer-type electronics improves the accuracy of the measurements and excludes human errors. Finally, a test can be carried out and reliable results can be obtained even when personnel without special radioisotope training must be employed.

REFERENCES

1. Adams, R., Woodward, I. C., Crane, M. G., and Holloway, J. E., The simultaneous determination of Cr^{51} and I^{131} activities in double labeled blood. *J. Lab. Clin. Med.* **52,** 754 (1958).
2. Allen, R. A., and Moore, B. T., Comparative counting efficiencies of $Co^{57}B_{12}$ and $Co^{58}B_{12}$ for three counting systems using two detectors. *J. Nucl. Med.* **3,** 300 (1962).
3. Anger, H. O., Scintillation counters for radioactive sample measurements. *Rev. Sci. Instr.* **22,** 912 (1951).
4. Baskin, R., Demorest, H. L., and Sandhaus, S., Gamma counting efficiency of two well-type NaI crystals. *Nucleonics* **12,** No. 8, 46 (1954).
5. Boling, E. A., A vise-configuration β-counter: determination of total exchangeable potassium using a low dose of isotope. *Intern. J. Appl. Radiation Isotopes* **14,** 177 (1963).
6. Brownell, G. L., Ellett, W. H., Rydin, R. A., and Hine, G. J., Large plastic scintillators for radioactivity measurements. *Health Phys.* **5,** 27 (1961).
7. Clapham, W. F., and Hayter, C. J., The measurement of gamma-emitting isotopes in faeces. *Phys. Biol. Med.* **7,** 313 (1962).
8. Colby, L. J., Jr., and Cobble, J. W., Precision calibration of large 4 Pi scintillation crystals for routine gamma counting. *Anal. Chem.* **31,** 798 (1959).
9. Cook, J. D., and Valberg, L. S., The evaluation and use of a large plastic scintillator for gamma counting. *J. Lab. Clin. Med.* **61,** 317 (1963).
10. Dratz, A. F., Well-bottom container improves gamma counting. *Nucleonics* **15,** No. 8, 83 (1957).
11. Dratz, A. F., and Coberly, J. C., The direct determination of I^{131} in heterogeneous fecal specimens. *Gastroenterology* **41,** 380 (1961).
12. Dunavant, B. G., and Christian, J. E., A large-volume 4π liquid scintillation detector. *Intern. J. Appl. Radiation Isotopes* **8,** 223 (1960).
13. Ellenbogen, L., and Williams, W. L., Improved urinary excretion test for assay of intrinsic factor. II. Sensitive counting technic. *Proc. Soc. Exptl. Biol. Med.* **91,** 617 (1956).
14. Ellenbogen, L., Counting efficiency of Co^{56}, Co^{58} and Co^{60} with 2 counters and 3 counting technics. *Proc. Soc. Exptl. Biol. Med.* **102,** 667 (1959).
15. Grodstein, G. W., X-ray attenuation coefficients from 10 kev to 100 Mev. *Natl. Bur. Std. (U.S.) Circ.* **583** (1957).
16. Gunnink, R., and Stoner, A. W., Photopeak counting efficiencies for 3 × 3 inch solid and well-type NaI scintillation crystals. *Anal. Chem.* **33,** 1311 (1961).
17. Hill, R. F., Hine, G. J., and Marinelli, L. D., The quantitative determination of gamma radiation in biological research. *Am. J. Roentgenol., Radium Therapy* **63,** 160 (1950).

18. Hine, G. J., Burrows, B. A., Apt, L., Pollycove, M., Ross, J. F., and Sarkes, L. A., Scintillation counting for multiple-tracer studies. *Nucleonics* **13,** No. 2, 23 (1955).
19. Hine, G. J., and Miller, A., Large plastic well makes efficient gamma counter. *Nucleonics* **14,** No. 10, 78 (1956).
20. Lamson, K. C., Sesko, W. J., and Nicholson, G. C., Automatic sample changer for gamma-ray spectroscopy. *Proc. Symp. Radioisotope Sample Measurement Techniques Med. Biol. Vienna, 1965* p. 127. Intern. At. Energy Agency, Vienna, 1965.
21. Loevinger, R., and Feitelberg, S., Using Bremsstrahlung detection by a scintillator for simplified beta counting. *Nucleonics* **13,** No. 4, 42 (1955).
22. Michel, W. S., Brownell, G. L., and Mealey, J., Jr., Designing sensitive plastic-well counters for beta rays. *Nucleonics* **14,** No. 11, 96 (1956).
23. Nablo, S. V., and Martin, T. C., Efficiencies and photofractions of some commonly used NaI(Tl) well crystals.' *Intern. J. Appl. Radiation Isotopes* **10,** 55 (1961).
24. Pfau, A., and Heinrich, H. C., Eine kombinierte Ringbecher-Bohrloch-Szintillationsdetektor-Messanordnung zur schnellen Bestimmung sehr geringer spezifischer Aktivitäten Gamma-Quanten emittierender Radionukleide. *Atompraxis* **5,** 14, 100, and 160 (1959).
25. Perkins, R. W., A large well crystal for the direct measurement of trace amounts of radioisotopes in environmental samples. *Health Phys.* **7,** 81 (1961).
26. Verheijke, M. L., Calculated efficiencies of a 3×3 in. NaI(Tl) well-type scintillation crystal. *Intern. J. Appl. Radiation Isotopes* **13,** 583 (1962).
27. Wächter, M. H., Ellett, W. H., and Brownell, G. L., Absorption of gamma radiation in NaI well crystals. *Rev. Sci. Instr.* **31,** 626 (1960).
28. Williams, J. A., and Fine, J., Measurement of blood volume with a new apparatus. *New Engl. J. Med.* **264,** 842 (1961).

CHAPTER 13

NUCLEAR ACTIVATION ANALYSIS

JOHN M. A. LENIHAN
REGIONAL PHYSICS DEPARTMENT
WESTERN REGIONAL HOSPITAL BOARD
GLASGOW, SCOTLAND

Activation analysis depends on the observation that almost every element can be converted into a radioactive isotope by bombardment with neutrons or other subatomic particles or radiations. The induced radioactivity is highly specific of the radioisotopes contributing to it. By studying the induced radioactivity, the constituent elements in a sample may be identified and quantitatively estimated. This apparently roundabout procedure is, for more than half of the chemical elements, the most sensitive analytical technique available. The gain in sensitivity by comparison with other methods is often a factor of 10^2, 10^3, or—for a few elements—10^6.

I. SAMPLE PREPARATION

A. Methods of Activation

Any nuclear reaction that produces a radionuclide can be used in activation analysis. Neutrons, protons, deuterons, α particles, tritons, and high-energy photons have all found applications as the activating particles.

Most of the elements of the periodic table with an atomic number Z between 10 and 80 react with thermal and epithermal neutrons. *Thermal neutrons* are commonly used for nuclear activation because they are available from nuclear reactors at high fluxes and at moderate cost. A typical research reactor provides thermal neutron fluxes of 10^{11} to 10^{13} n cm^{-2} sec^{-1}. With thermal neutrons only a single type of nuclear transformation, the (n, γ) reaction is usually induced.

There are many reasons why this type of activation (thermal neutron capture) has been used more than any other. In general, the activation cross sections are relatively high and there are usually no interfering reactions. The four major elements, H, C, N, and O, which constitute approximately 96% of living matter, are either not activated by a (n, γ) reaction, or the induced activity has a short half-life. Otherwise the trace analysis of tissue by thermal neutron activation would be considerably more difficult.

For some elements, especially with Z less than 10, no suitable thermal neutron reactions are available for activation analysis. The use of *fast neutrons,* available from discharge-tube generator sources, should then be considered. By virtue of their relatively large kinetic energy fast neutrons react in a much more complex way than thermal neutrons. Several different types of nuclear transformations are induced by fast neutrons, principally (n, p), (n, α) and (n, 2n). Therefore, the analysis is often not specific, since a nuclide formed from one element may also be formed by another reaction from a second element differing in atomic number by 1 or 2.

Fast neutrons usually yield a much lower sensitivity than thermal neutrons partly because capture cross sections are smaller and partly because of the smaller fluxes available. However, they allow an easy determination of elements such as N, O, and F which are difficult or impossible to detect with thermal neutrons.

Fast neutrons with an energy of 14 MeV are produced by the ^3H (d, n) ^4He reaction. One popular type of generator uses a deuteron beam in a continuously pumped tube to bombard a tritium target. The latter is made by adsorbing tritium gas on titanium, which is then evaporated onto a copper foil of 0.01 inch thickness. The neutron yield from such a target decreases exponentially with time (because of evaporation of the tritium) with a half-life measured in hours, depending on the deuteron beam current. Better performance is obtained from the recently developed sealed-off tubes in which a target composed of erbium deuteride and erbium tritide is bombarded by a mixed beam of

TABLE I
FAST NEUTRON GENERATORS SUITABLE FOR ACTIVATION ANALYSIS

Type of high-voltage generator	Accelerated particles	Particle energy (keV)	Target material	Vacuum system	Useful fast neutron flux (n cm^{-2} sec^{-1})	Useful thermal neutron flux (n cm^{-2} sec^{-1})	Cost ($)
Pulse transformer	Deuterons	120	Tritium on titanium	Sealed tube	10^6	—	7,000
Cockcroft-Walton	Deuterons	200	Tritium on titanium	Pumped continually	3×10^8	2×10^7	20,000
Van de Graaff	Deuterons	500	Beryllium	Pumped continually	4×10^8	4×10^8	70,000
Cyclotron	Deuterons	7500	Beryllium	Pumped continually	2×10^{12}	2×10^{10}	175,000

deuterons and tritons. The tritium lost from the target is replaced from the ion beam. A steady output of 10^{10} n sec^{-1} may be obtained for 100 hr or more.

Fast neutron fluxes of 10^8 to 10^9 n cm^{-2} sec^{-1} are now obtainable from discharge-tube generators and it is likely that further improvements will be made. Specifications of some typical generating equipments are summarized in Table I.

Many of the advantages and disadvantages of fast neutrons are shared by *charged particles*. In general the sensitivity is relatively low and interfering reactions often occur. Their major disadvantages arise from their low power of penetration and the rapid loss of energy in passing through the target material. Nevertheless, for a small number of elements, charged particles, particularly deuterons, have been used successfully for the analysis of biological materials.

A cyclotron or other charged particle accelerator is the source of high-energy charged particles. In contrast to neutrons, positively charged particles have to overcome an electrostatic potential barrier created by the positive charge of the nucleus. This is not a serious obstacle for elements of low atomic number, where charged particles of a few million electron volts energy can penetrate the nucleus, but it becomes a serious obstacle with target elements of high atomic numbers. Cross sections for charged particle reactions become smaller as the atomic number of the target increases.

Irradiation of a standard sample, used in calibrating the subsequent assay, is easy in a reactor, where a uniform neutron flux can be expected over quite a large volume, and where the irradiated sample is reasonably transparent to the bombarding particles. Greater difficulty is experienced with the narrow beam of fluctuating intensity delivered by a charged particle accelerator. A rotating sample holder is often used to ensure that the sample is irradiated in the same flux as the standard.

Heating of the sample is another significant problem. A 1-mA beam of 5-MeV protons will deliver all of its energy in the target, representing a dissipation of 5 kW and necessitating vigorous cooling. Even so, some of the target material may be lost by evaporation or sputtering under intense local heating.

The use of *high-energy photons* in activation analysis has so far received very little attention, principally because of the low values of the activation cross sections and the scarcity of suitable accelerating machines. High-energy photons may be obtained by allowing electrons from a high-energy electron accelerator (linear accelerator or betatron) to impinge on a gold or other high atomic number metal target. Only a small number of useful nuclear transformations has been reported, principally (γ, n) reactions in elements of low atomic number.

B. Sample Handling

When once the sample has been irradiated, there is no danger of contamination from nonradioactive reagents, or from contact with other nonradioactive materials. These hazards are, however, important during the preirradiation stages of the analysis. In rare instances (as, for example, when a seed is irradiated in its pod) handling can be avoided completely; but more usually the sample must go through a number of procedures before it can be placed inside the reactor or in the beam of an accelerator.

Ideally, as soon as it has been obtained, the sample should be transferred to a container that can be sealed and used for the subsequent irradiation. Biological materials, however, present special problems. If animal or plant tissues have to be dissected out or divided, silica knives should be used (a splinter from a broken flask is suitable) in preference to metal blades. Glass vessels should not be employed at any stage, unless a water-repellent coating has been applied, because of the danger of contaminating the sample with trace elements from the glass. Polyethylene is usually satisfactorily free from trace-element contaminants, and therefore may be used in most instances.

Preirradiation chemical treatment is sometimes thought desirable, mainly in order to remove sodium from biological material in which trace elements are to be determined. The danger here is that the materials used in the separation (such as buffer solutions in dialysis) will introduce trace quantities of many elements. The dialysis or other procedure may also partially remove elements other than sodium. With proper precautions the errors associated with preirradiation chemical treatment can be reduced, but some uncertainty is bound to remain.

Samples for irradiation are usually packed in polyethylene, silica, or aluminum. Polyethylene envelopes or tubes are convenient for relatively short irradiations and where elevated temperatures (above 60°C) are avoided. Aluminum tubes with slip-on lids, or aluminum foil, are suitable for many samples, but should not be used when volatile substances are likely to be generated under irradiation. Silica tubes or ampoules can be used for irradiating liquids and are insensitive to temperature or radiation flux. They are, however, relatively costly and are difficult to seal.

Samples packed in one of these ways are usually put into a standard container, depending on the reactor or neutron generator to be used. Sometimes the reactor will accept an aluminum can of up to 30 ml in capacity, allowing a large number of samples (with any necessary standards) to be irradiated simultaneously in the same neutron flux. When charged particles are used for activation, special methods of sample packing and mounting are necessary. Since the particle beam has little penetrating power, the sample should be in the form of a thin layer and in a thin-walled container. A thick specimen may be used only if surface composition is under study.

II. ACTIVATION SENSITIVITY

The sensitivity of activation analysis depends on the amount of the desired activity induced in the sample and the efficiency with which this activity can be assayed. The yield of the induced activity is a function of three parameters, the neutron flux, the irradiation time, and cross section for activation.

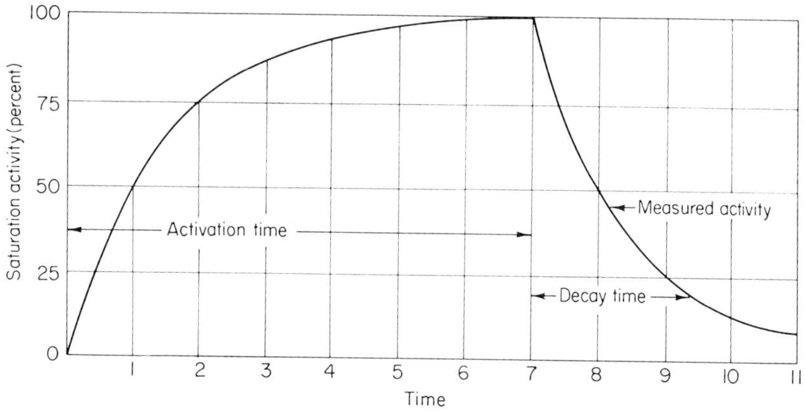

FIG. 1. Activation growth and decay curve. The time is given in units of the half-life of the induced radionuclide.

The *neutron flux* is the number of neutrons crossing an area of 1 cm^2 in 1 sec at the position of the sample. The induced activity will be proportional to the neutron flux, if other factors remain unchanged.

The *irradiation time* should be chosen in relation to the half-life of the desired activity (Fig. 1). The curve illustrates the growth of the induced radioactivity under neutron bombardment in units of the half-life of the activated nuclide. It shows that short-lived activities grow more quickly than long-lived activities. In general, it is not worth while to continue irradiation for more than two half-lives. After this time, the induced activity has reached ¾ of its final saturation value, and further approach to saturation is at an ever slower rate. After completion of the activation, the induced activity decays exponentially.

Interfering activities can sometimes be minimized by suitable choice of irradiation time. Suppose, for example, that it is desired to estimate chlorine in a sample of biological material by the thermal neutron reaction ^{37}Cl (n, γ) ^{38}Cl. The chlorine isotope produced in this way has a half-life of 37 min. Any sample of biological material will probably contain a considerable amount of sodium, giving ^{24}Na ($T = 15$ hr) by the (n, γ) reaction. Often the ^{24}Na will swamp the ^{38}Cl or other less substantial activities. Therefore it is advisable to use a short irradiation time of 30 to 60 min. This will be long enough to produce a reasonable fraction of the saturation activity in chlorine but an activity very much below saturation for the sodium.

Conversely, if it is desired to estimate sodium without interference from shorter-lived activities, a relatively long irradiation time (15 to 30 hr) is chosen. This is then followed by an interval of several hours, during which the ^{38}Cl and other short-lived interferences decay to insignificant levels.

An extreme example of these considerations occurs in the operation of pulsed research reactors, driven to very high power levels for a few milliseconds. In this short time it is possible to deliver a neutron flux a few thousand times greater than for steady state operation. Calculations made for one type of reactor (Triga) where these possibilities have been studied show that the sensitivity for activities with half-lives less than 50 sec is improved by pulsed operation. Elements having short-lived isotopes suitable for this application include O, F, Na, Mg, S, Se, and Au.

The *cross section* of the target element for neutrons, or other bombarding particles, is measured in barns: 1 barn $= 10^{-24}$ cm^2. Other things being equal, the reaction yield is proportional to the cross section. If an adequate yield cannot be obtained by thermal neutron activation, it is sometimes possible to find fast neutron reactions with a higher cross section, though it must be remembered that the available fast neutron flux is lower than the thermal neutron flux from a reactor.

When materials are irradiated for activation analysis, the rate of production is effectively constant, since the number of activated atoms is such a small fraction of the total present. If f is the flux of the bombarding particles (in particles cm^{-2} sec^{-1}), σ the activation cross section for the reaction (in barns), ϕ the fractional abundance of the isotope being activated, W the weight of the element present in the sample, and M its atomic weight, the induced activity A (disintegration rate per second) present at a time t after completion of the activation is given as

$$A = 0.602 f\sigma \frac{W\phi}{M} [1 - \exp(-0.693 t_a/T)] \exp(-0.693 t/T)$$

where T is the half-life of the radioisotope of interest and t_a is the duration of activation.

If the irradiation is carried out for a sufficient number of half-lives, the factor $[1 - \exp(-0.693t_a/T)]$ known as saturation factor (Fig. 1), becomes effectively unity. The decay factor, $\exp(-0.693t/T)$, will be also close to unity, if the activity is determined within a small fraction of a half-life after irradiation ceases. The induced activity is then proportional to the amount of the isotope of interest present in the sample and the reaction cross section of that isotope for a given particle flux.

A. Thermal Neutrons

There are many published compilations showing the sensitivity of thermal neutron activation analysis for various elements. These tables should be used with caution. The experimenter who reads that manganese can be detected at levels of 10^{-11} gm or iodine at 10^{-9} gm will be disappointed if he tries to estimate either of these elements in biological material, where the interference from sodium makes the assay of the trace constituents very difficult. Sensitivities which are attainable for a pure specimen of the element concerned may not be reached when the desired activity must be measured in the presence of other radiations. This difficulty applies both to instrumental and to radiochemical methods of isolation (Section III).

TABLE II
THERMAL NEUTRON ACTIVATION[a]

Minimum sensitivity of detection (micrograms)	Elements
10^{-4}	Ag, As, In, Ir, Mn
10^{-3}	Al, Br, Cu, Ga, I, Na, Sb, Sc, V, W
10^{-2}	Au, Cl, Co, Cs, Ge, Hg, K, Rb, Sr, Ta, U, Y
10^{-1}	Ba, Cd, Cr, Mo, Ni, P, Se, Si, Te, Ti, Zn
1	Bi, Ca, F, Mg, Tl, Sn

[a] 10^{12} n cm^{-2} sec^{-1}.

The published figures of sensitivity are necessarily related to typical, but arbitrary conditions of irradiation flux and time and to specified counting arrangements. Careful study of a particular problem will often show how an improvement of 10 or 100 times may be achieved by the use of higher neutron fluxes or more appropriate methods of assay.

As a general guide, the following sensitivities (Table II) can be expected when a thermal neutron flux of 10^{12} n cm^{-2} sec^{-1} is available (as from a modest research reactor) and when relatively simple counting equipment is used after radiochemical separation of the desired nuclide.

B. Fast Neutrons

Nuclear cross sections for fast neutron reactions are generally lower than for thermal neutron reactions. The analytical sensitivity is, however, dependent on a number of other factors, including the half-life of the activity produced and the available neutron flux. Irradiation times of a day or more are readily obtainable with thermal neutrons, but when fast neutrons are used the life of the target is limited and irradiation times longer than 1 hr are usually not practicable.

Some typical sensitivities, based on a fast neutron flux of 10^9 n cm^{-2} sec^{-1} and an irradiation time of four half-lives, or 1 hr (whichever is shorter), are given in Table III.

TABLE III
FAST NEUTRON ACTIVATION[a]

Minimum sensitivity of detection (micrograms)	Elements
1	Ag, Br, Cu, F, K, P, Sb, Si
10	Al, Cr, Mn, Mo, N, O, V, Zn
100	As, Co, I, Mg, S

[a] 10^9 n cm^{-2} sec^{-1}.

The usefulness of fast neutron activation analysis does not depend wholly on sensitivity, though this is often quite attractive. Advantages of this technique include the compactness, cheapness, and portability of fast-neutron generators in comparison with nuclear reactors. Interference may be from elements which are more easily separated radiochemically or instrumentally than those obtained by thermal neutron activation. Effective analytical techniques may be possible for the light elements ($Z < 10$) where thermal neutron activation is generally not applicable.

C. Charged Particles

Summaries of the kind given above are not easily available for charged particle activation. The main reason for this deficiency is that there are no standard or commonly available sources of charged particles, comparable with the nuclear reactor and the discharge-tube neutron

major or an exclusive function. Consequently, there is no uniformity in such matters as available flux, sample position, or particle energy. The experimenter is therefore obliged to make the necessary predictions and other calculations for each separate investigation.

As already mentioned, a typical sample will withstand a considerable bombardment by neutrons of any energy without suffering appreciable physical damage, though the associated heat, γ-ray flux, and other incidental factors may be troublesome when the highest neutron fluxes are applied to biological materials. When using charged particles, it is necessary to consider carefully the possibility of damage by heating. The penetration of the bombarding particles is very limited and a great amount of energy is liberated, as heat, in a small volume.

The usefulness of charged particle activation analysis is mainly in the study of elements with $Z < 10$. By suitable choice of the bombarding particles and of their energy, sensitivities in the submicrogram region can be obtained.

III. METHODS OF ANALYSIS

Radiochemical separations are often required because the counting equipment is not sufficiently selective to allow the measurement of the radioactivity of one element without interference from the other activities induced in the sample. Biological materials are particularly difficult to analyze, because they contain a very complex mixture of different elements. As an illustration, some of the component activities induced in 0.25 gm of human liver irradiated for 1 week at a flux of about 10^{12} thermal neutrons cm^{-2} sec^{-1} are given in Table IV.

A. Radiochemical Separation

The instrumentation problems in radiochemistry are minor because the various procedures use only the elementary techniques familiar to the analytical chemist. Chemical manipulation of an irradiated sample normally includes the following stages: the addition of carrier, the digestion or other preliminary treatment, and the separation of the desired element.

The addition of carrier serves two purposes. First, it allows a determination of the percentage yield of the chemical processes and a correction for any losses. Second, it avoids excessive loss by adsorption which becomes important when the number of atoms to be handled is relatively small. The chemist operating with milligram amounts of material has about 10^{19} atoms in his sample. A typical glass container may have 10^{15} adsorption sites per square centimeter. Consequently the loss of atoms from the material under analysis is not a serious hazard.

The activation analyst, however, may be concerned with 10^{-10} gm of an element, representing about 10^{12} atoms; the chance of loss by adsorption is clearly very substantial.

The simplest precaution against the danger of a loss by adsorption is the addition of a carrier, containing the element under analysis. A

TABLE IV
ACTIVITIES INDUCED IN 0.25 GM OF HUMAN LIVER BY THERMAL NEUTRON ACTIVATION[a,b]

Element	Weights in 0.25 gm of wet liver (μg)	Radio-nuclide	Half-life	Induced activity (dpm) After irradiation	After 1 week decay
Ag	0.004	^{110}Ag	270 days	1×10^3	1×10^3
Al	0.18	—	—	—	—
As	0.02	^{76}As	27 hr	4×10^4	5×10^2
Br	0.6	^{82}Br	36 hr	4×10^5	2×10^4
Ca	18	^{45}Ca	152 hr	5×10^3	5×10^3
Cd	0.6	^{115}Cd	53 hr	5×10^4	6×10^3
Cl	310	^{38}Cl	37 min	7×10^7	—
Co	0.01	^{60}Co	5.3 years	5×10^2	5×10^2
Cr	0.005	^{51}Cr	28 days	3×10^2	3×10^2
Cs	0.15	^{134}Cs	2.3 years	7×10^3	7×10^3
Cu	2.2	^{64}Cu	13 hr	3×10^6	3×10^2
Fe	46	^{59}Fe	45 days	7×10^3	6×10^3
I	0.3	^{128}I	25 min	5×10^5	—
K	800	^{42}K	13 hr	5×10^7	5×10^3
Mg	41	^{27}Mg	9 min	2×10^5	—
Mn	0.3	^{56}Mn	2.6 hr	3×10^6	—
Mo	0.3	^{99}Mo	67 hr	1×10^4	2×10^3
Na	350	^{24}Na	15 hr	3×10^8	1×10^5
P	675	^{32}P	15 days	4×10^7	3×10^7
Rb	16	^{86}Rb	19.5 days	8×10^5	6×10^5
Sb	0.05	^{122}Sb	2.8 days	5×10^4	9×10^3
Si	6	^{31}Si	2.6 hr	4×10^4	—
Sn	0.1	^{133}Sn	112 days	12	12
Sr	0.008	^{85}Sr	65 days	1	1
Te	270	^{125m}Te	58 days	1×10^6	1×10^6
Zn	12	^{65}Zn	250 days	2×10^4	2×10^4

[a] 10^{12} n cm^{-2} sec^{-1}; duration of irradiation, 1 week.
[b] R. M. Parr, unpublished data.

few milligrams is a suitable amount, the limit being imposed by the risk of self-absorption in the final sample if β-ray counting is necessary and the risk of saturating the resin if ion exchange is used at a later stage in separation. The carrier should be added at the earliest convenient moment in the chemical handling of the irradiated material.

The next problem is to put all of the irradiated atoms and the carrier atoms into the same chemical form. Bombardment with neutrons or other particles can break chemical bonds and alter valency states, producing an accumulation of atoms which, though all of the same element, will not necessarily behave identically in subsequent chemical treatment. A suitable oxidation or reduction process should therefore be undertaken at an early stage in the postirradiation manipulation.

Chemical separation of the desired activity now proceeds by the normal methods, including solvent extraction, chromatography, precipitation, electrodeposition, and volatilization. The choice among these methods is influenced not only by the normal chemical considerations, but by the knowledge of likely interference from unwanted elements in the irradiated specimen and by the necessity for rapid operation in dealing with short-lived nuclides. From this point of view volatilization, precipitation, solvent extraction, and amalgam exchange are rapid techniques, whereas chromatography and electrodeposition are more appropriate for the separation of longer-lived activities.

A typical separation routine will make use of precipitation and coprecipitation before reaching the final step, which is specific for the nuclide under investigation. After the initial preparation of the irradiated sample, carriers are added, corresponding to the element being estimated and to any other elements likely to have been appreciably activated during the irradiation. Suitable reagents are added to precipitate the principal element, leaving the interfering activities still in solution, with their "hold-back" carriers. This process may need to be repeated to obtain reasonably good separation.

The precipitate is then redissolved and a scavenging agent, such as a ferric iron salt, is added. On conversion to the hydroxide, a bulky gelatinous mass is produced. This precipitate has a large surface area which normally has a negative charge. This makes it effective in the adsorption of cations. Other gelatinous precipitates may be formed by metallic sulfides, which usually have a negative charge, or by silver halides, which have a positive charge. The process of removing unwanted ions by adsorption in the manner just outlined is called coprecipitation.

When these techniques have been fully exploited, the desired activity will be effectively separated from the rest of the original sample. Some of it will have been lost in repeated handling, but the necessary correction can be applied by checking the weight recovered against the weight of carrier originally added. The final step may be another precipitation but other methods, such as distillation, ion exchange, solvent extraction, and electrodeposition are also suitable for particular elements. The element to be estimated is eventually delivered in pure form, or in a compound along with the stable carrier. Radioactive assay is then performed.

B. Instrumental Procedures

The assay of induced radioactivity, necessary to complete an activation analysis, uses many of the techniques described in earlier chapters. When a complete chemical separation has been achieved, either β-ray or γ-ray counting may be sufficient to assess the radioactivity of the sample. Often, however, the sample includes a number of induced activities, which must be separated and quantitated by instrumental means.

If the determination of an element by means of γ-ray spectra were of the same simplicity as by optical spectra, these tasks would be relatively easy. In fact, the analysis of γ-ray spectra is difficult, partly because of the poor resolution of the scintillation counter, but also because, beside the photopeak, the γ-ray spectrum includes the Compton continuum with the Compton edge, low-energy γ-ray escape peaks, sum peaks from coincidence γ-rays, and Bremsstrahlung contribution from high-energy β rays (Chapter 6, Section IV).

The issue is further complicated by the fact that the γ-ray spectrum generated by a given amount of activity depends to a marked degree on the characteristics of the detecting system. The activation analyst must therefore prepare his own standards, by irradiating known amounts of the elements of interest and recording their γ-ray spectra under specified conditions that must be maintained for the assay of the unknown specimens.

Geometrical factors, including the sample volume, must be carefully controlled and a high degree of stability in the electronic circuits of the assay equipment is necessary. Sometimes a visual comparison of the unknown spectrum with the library of standard spectra will indicate one or more elements. Quantitative estimation is then made by comparison of the areas under corresponding photopeaks. Often, however, a particular photopeak will include some counts from the spectrum of a different nuclide. Even if several photopeaks are not close enough to overlap, a contribution may occur from the Compton continuum of another element in the sample. It is therefore necessary to resort to spectrum stripping.

Though spectrum stripping is a simple process, it is tedious in actual performance. The first step is to identify the main activity represented in the complex pattern. A γ-ray spectrum of this activity is prepared and the amplitude of its main photopeak is adjusted to equal that of the spectrum under analysis. Subtraction (manual or instrumental) is then performed to remove the single-element spectrum, leaving a residue in which other photopeaks are available for the same treatment. Spectrum matching and stripping can be done automatically with the help of electronic computers. Programs and mechanisms have been developed for the entire process from irradiation to printout of concentrations of selected elements, without human intervention at any stage.

In general, instrumental analysis will be more economical for large numbers of samples, since the capital investment may be substantial. It can be made both fast and accurate though usually without reaching the maximum sensitivity. The ultimate sensitivity will generally be obtained by more time-consuming manual procedures involving radiochemical separation, which, however, can often be carried out with simple and relatively inexpensive equipment. For any particular activation analysis problem, there is an optimum combination of radiochemical and instrumental procedures.

IV. CLINICAL AND BIOLOGICAL APPLICATIONS

The uses of activation analysis in biomedical research are reviewed in a number of recent publications. A few examples will serve to illustrate the scope and potential value of the technique.

A. Arsenic in Hair

The determination of the arsenic content of human hair by standard chemical procedures requires about a gram of hair. For activation analysis, a single hair is sufficient; in some investigations even a 1-mm length of hair has been used successfully. The chemical methods of analysis cannot deal with the arsenic in a single hair, amounting to about 10^{-10} gm. The reagents used in the chemical procedures inevitably contain arsenic as an impurity, at levels comparable with the amounts present in the hair. Furthermore, it is inevitable that tiny amounts of an element will be lost by adsorption onto the surfaces of the containers used for the analysis.

For activation analysis a single hair is weighed and sealed in a plastic container which is placed in a standard irradiation can together with a small, accurately known quantity of arsenic in some convenient chemical form, such as arsenious oxide. The can with the hair and the arsenic standard is put into the reactor for 24 hours. The hair will then have become distinctly radioactive.

Some of the induced activity is due to the presence of sodium, phosphorus, sulfur, and a few other readily activated elements, but an appreciable part of it is associated with arsenic. This element is by no means a major constituent of hair, but it has a large cross section for thermal neutrons as indicated in Table II. The induced radioisotope, ^{76}As, which has a half-life of 26 hours, emits both β and γ rays. It is important to remember that not all of the stable ^{75}As is converted to the radioactive form. In a typical irradiation, about 1 in 10^7 of the arsenic atoms is transformed, but this is enough to produce about 1 curie of ^{76}As per gram as ^{75}As.

The arsenic standard is subjected to the same chemical treatment as the hair sample, the yield is checked, and the eventual product is set aside for assay. The half-life and also the γ-ray spectrum of the ^{76}As from the hair are checked as a means of verifying the integrity of the radiochemical separation. An aliquot of the ^{76}As derived from the arsenic standard is assayed under the same conditions. Then, by simple arithmetic, the mass of the arsenic originally present in the hair is determined.

A notable investigation by thermal neutron activation analysis showed considerable amounts of arsenic in hair samples of the Emperor Napoleon I, which had probably resulted from ingestion of medical preparations containing arsenic.*

B. Determination of ^{127}I

Tracer studies with ^{131}I or ^{132}I give important information about the uptake and turnover of iodine in the thyroid gland. It is desirable also to know the pool of stable iodine with which the radioactive tracer mixes. Chemical methods for the estimation of ^{127}I in blood are effective in skilled hands, but they are subject to error and uncertainty because of contamination problems at the low levels of well under one part per million involved in these determinations.

Activation analysis using thermal neutrons to produce ^{128}I (half-life 25 min) has been attempted in several laboratories. Interference from ^{24}Na is a major difficulty but efficient separation techniques are available. Recently, activation of ^{127}I has been carried out successfully by high-energy photons according to the reaction ^{127}I (γ, n) ^{126}I (half-life 13.3 days). Bremsstrahlung photons produced by 22-MeV electrons from a linear accelerator activate the sample after a chemical separation of the iodide in human plasma by an ion-exchange column. No significant interference from other induced activities is observed. In particular, sodium presents no problem at all in this case.

The possibility of estimating the ^{127}I content of the thyroid gland *in vivo* has recently been discussed. A relatively small dose of thermal neutrons would produce enough ^{128}I to be measured by an external

* S. Forshufvud, H. Smith, and A. Wassen, Napoleon's illness 1818–1821. *Archiv. für Toxicologie* **20**, 210 (1964).

scintillation counter. Calibration might be performed by noting the additional activity produced in a small pellet of NH_4I positioned appropriately in the throat. Interference from ^{24}Na and ^{38}Cl should be minimized by waiting for about 1 min between the end of irradiation and the start of counting; sodium and chlorine are cleared rapidly from the thyroid, while iodine is trapped for slower release.

C. Trace Elements

The trace elements listed in Table V are not present in sufficient amounts to be major constituents of tissues or organs, but each one is

TABLE V
ESSENTIAL TRACE ELEMENTS

Element	Amount in 70-kg man (gm)
Zinc	1.9
Copper	0.2
Manganese	0.02
Molybdenum	0.015
Iodine	0.03
Cobalt	0.003

known to have some essential role as a hormone constituent or a catalyst in an enzyme system. A relatively small number of other elements, including Cd, Cr, F, Ni, Rb, Si, and V, are regularly found in body tissues with some but not conclusive evidence of an essential biological role.

The relation of trace elements to disease may depend on the catalysis of enzyme action. Many metallic elements are involved, at levels near or beyond the limits of conventional chemical estimation. Thermal neutron activation has been applied to the study of zinc metabolism in relation to ureteric calculus, alcoholic cirrhosis of the liver, and hypogonadism. Manganese, molybdenum, vanadium, and other elements have been studied in relation to the mineralization of tooth enamel and the development of dental caries.

There is considerable scope for further work, for example, on the trace element content of drinking water, which in some regions appears to be correlated with the geographical distribution of coronary heart disease.

D. Forensic Applications

A nonbiological application of activation analysis may be of general interest. Circumstantial evidence in criminal cases often depends on the identification of minute amounts of material exchanged between the suspect and the environment. Thermal neutron activation analysis is used in a number of laboratories for the analysis of gunpowder, paint, soil, hair, and other specimens where the presence and relative concentrations of various trace elements often allow reliable judgments to be made on the identity or nonidentity of two submitted samples. A fascinating but inconclusive application of this technique was made during the investigation following the assassination of President Kennedy in 1963. The methods of activation analysis have been used successfully in a number of criminal cases in the United States and are likely to find a useful place in forensic science in other countries before long.

SUPPLEMENTARY READINGS

Albert, P., "L'analyse par Radioactivation." Gauthier-Villars, Paris, 1964.

Bowen, H. J. M., and Gibbons, D., "Radioactivation Analysis." Oxford Univ. Press (Clarendon), London and New York, 1963.

Comar, D. (ed.), "L'analyse par Radioactivation et ses Applications aux Sciences Biologiques." Presses Universitaires de France, Paris, 1964.

Koch, R. C., "Activation Analysis Handbook." Academic Press, New York, 1960.

Lenihan, J. M. A., and Thomson, S. J. (eds.), "Activation Analysis. Proceedings of the 1964 NATO Advanced Study Institute." Academic Press, New York, 1965.

Lyon, W. S. (ed.), "Guide to Activation Analysis." Van Nostrand, Princeton, New Jersey, 1964.

"Modern Trends in Activation Analysis. Proceedings of the 1965 International Conference." McGraw-Hill, New York, 1965.

"Radiochemical Methods of Analysis." *Proceedings of a Symposium. Salzburg, 1965.* Vols. I and II. Intern. At. Energy Agency, Vienna, 1965.

Schulze, W., "Neutronenaktivierung als analytisches Hilfsmittel." Enke, Stuttgart, 1962.

Taylor, D., "Neutron Irradiation and Activation Analysis." G. Newnes, Ltd., London, 1964.

PART IV

RADIOISOTOPE MEASUREMENTS *in Vivo*

CHAPTER 14

THYROID RADIOIODINE UPTAKE MEASUREMENTS

GERALD J. HINE*
RADIOISOTOPE SERVICE
VETERANS ADMINISTRATION HOSPITAL
BOSTON, MASSACHUSETTS
AND
JAMES B. WILLIAMS
AMES ATOMIUM INC.
BILLERICA, MASSACHUSETTS

The determination of the uptake of radioactive iodine by the thyroid gland was the first radioisotope test that required *in vivo* measurements. Innumerable papers have been written concerning the technique and interpretation of thyroidal iodine uptake measurements. All textbooks on the medical use of radioisotopes contain extended discussions on the subject (*11, 13;* see also references of Chapter 2).

A certain amount of radioiodine, usually ^{131}I, is administered to the patient. The test consists of the determination of the fraction of the dose present in the thyroid at a later time, usually at 24 hr. Though this appears to be a simple task, it involves two major problems.

* Present address: International Atomic Energy Agency, Vienna, Austria.

(1) The amount of radioactivity present in an organ has to be determined accurately, though the exact location and size of the organ in the neck varies with different patients.

(2) At the time of measurement only a fraction of the radioactivity present in the patient may be concentrated within the thyroid. Therefore it is of importance to exclude from the measurements as much as possible of the radiation emitted from extrathyroidal tissues without missing any radiation from the thyroid itself.

The instrumentation requirements resulting from those two problems are unique. Because of the wide use of the thyroid radioiodine uptake test, the International Atomic Energy Agency in Vienna in November 1960 invited a number of consultants from seven countries to discuss the standardization of thyroid radioiodine uptake measurements. The group agreed on certain recommendations which are clearly formulated and easy to follow (*7*). To expedite their execution, the consultants added some explanations which are useful for understanding the significance of the recommendations. In addition, the International Atomic Energy Agency is undertaking a project to assist its member states in the calibration and standardization of thyroid radioiodine uptake measurements. It is hoped that in this way confidence in published results will be increased and the comparison of the geographical variation in thyroid function will be provided with a sounder basis (*5a*).

The present discussion of the instrumentation required for thyroid radioiodine uptake measurements will be based on the recommendations from the International Atomic Energy Agency. These recommendations have been widely published and are generally recognized. They will be reproduced here in their entirety. Thereafter, additional points of interest will be discussed and newer developments will be presented.

I. RECOMMENDATIONS AND COMMENTS OF CONSULTANTS FOR THE INTERNATIONAL ATOMIC ENERGY AGENCY*

A. Tracer Dose

1. AMOUNT

1.1. As a general principle, the amount of radioiodine administered to the patient should not be larger than necessary, particularly with children.

In a normal person, administration of 10 μCi of ^{131}I will result in a radiation dose of between 5 and 20 rads, averaged over the whole thyroid

* Comments are given in *italic* type.

gland. The members of the panel recalled that many patients with thyroid disease were correctly diagnosed and adequately treated before ^{131}I became available, implying that the tracer dose can be reduced to zero in cases where the clinical diagnosis is not in doubt.

1.2. The amount to be given will be determined by

(a) the equipment used; and

(b) the nature of other radioiodine tests which it might be desired to perform using the same dose.

Many workers feel that a thyroid uptake measurement should be combined with other radioiodine tests such as, for example, protein-bound ^{131}I plasma levels; this opinion is held particularly strongly in regions with chronic iodine deficiency where thyroid uptake in euthyroid subjects may be frequently higher than in thyrotoxic patients.

1.3. With good equipment and using the procedures suggested below for determining thyroid uptake, not more than 10 μCi of ^{131}I need to be given. However, if other radioiodine tests are considered necessary a dose of 25 μCi may be required.

If it is desired to scan the thyroid gland, a dose of 50 μCi might be necessary to reduce sufficiently the likelihood of overlooking a small "cold" nodule.

1.4. In pediatric work the reduction of the working distance (see Section I,D,1.3) may permit lower doses.

2. Use of Carrier

2.1. The amount of ^{127}I in each individual dose should not exceed 1 μg.

The amount of carrier present in the commercial product should be known, particularly if it is supplied in liquid form; if capsules are used, evaporation and adsorption do not present a problem. If the product is carrier-free, ^{127}I should be added to the stock solution from which individual tracer doses are made up.

3. Administration

3.1. It is recommended below (Section I,D,2) that in routine work thyroid uptake should not be determined before 2 hr after the dose has been given. Intravenous administration will therefore not be required except in experimental work.

3.2. The oral dose should be given in a liquid form; there are no objections on clinical grounds against the use of capsules except for early uptakes (that is, 2 to 6 hr after administration of the dose).

3.3. Ordinarily the dietary state is unimportant, but for early uptakes the patient should be fasting.

B. Standard and Phantom

1. STANDARD

1.1. The amount of radioiodine used as the standard should be the same as the amount given to the patient. The volume of the standard should be comparable to the volume of an average-sized thyroid gland (30 ml). For children the volume should be correspondingly smaller.

Theoretically, it would be preferable to use as the standard an amount of radioiodine which would be comparable to that in the gland. However, the group felt that it would be more practical to use an amount equal to the tracer dose, particularly if a number of patients are given the same amount at the same time; the error resulting from nonlinearity of the counting system should be small compared to other errors inherent in the method. While the average weight of normal thyroid glands is generally taken as 20 gm, it was felt that the volume of the standard should be more representative of the size of the glands for which an uptake test is normally considered necessary.

1.2. The standard vessel should consist of a polyethylene bottle of 30-mm diameter with such height that it will accept a volume of 30 ml of fluid.

The type of bottle suggested is widely available and is cheap. Elaborate vessels simulating the shape of a thyroid gland were not considered necessary.

1.3. So-called "mock" iodine (^{133}Ba–^{137}Cs) is unsuitable for assaying the radioactivity of the ^{131}I dose given to the patient and should therefore not be used for making up the standard.

It should be noted that in the calibration procedure referred to in the introduction above, "mock" iodine in the dummy figure will be compared with "mock" iodine in the standards supplied with it.

2. NECK PHANTOM

2.1. Since some scattered radiation will always be recorded and since comparable geometry for the thyroid gland and the standard in relation to the detector is essential, the use of a neck phantom is recommended.

There was general agreement that the use of a neck phantom is essential, particularly if results of institutions in various parts of the world are to be compared. Note that Geiger–Müller counters are particularly sensitive to scattered radiation.

2.2. This phantom should be a cylinder of 15-cm diameter and of 15-cm height, made preferably of Lucite or Perspex. It should have a hole which would accept the standard vessel described in Section I,B,1.2. The distance from the edge of the phantom to the surface of the hole should be 0.5 cm.

Great care should be taken to avoid contamination of the phantom.

2.3. If it is desired for reasons of greater accuracy to take account of small and large glands and of smaller and greater depths below the skin, it is recommended that correction factors should be determined experimentally by using a water phantom of the same size as the plastic neck phantom. Standards of different sizes will be placed at different depths within this phantom. If large corrections have to be made, both the corrected and uncorrected figures should be reported to facilitate intercomparison.

The use of a water phantom and of standards of different size provides for greater flexibility and consequently for greater accuracy. However, if improperly used this method can lead to further error. Personal judgement as to size and depth of the gland will enter into the calculation of thyroid uptake and reproducibility and intercomparability might suffer.

2.4. If a capsule is used as the standard the neck phantom has to be modified and an additional set of correction factors has to be determined. However, capsules could be dissolved in hot water to prepare a 30-ml liquid standard which could be inserted in the phantom and counted in the usual way.

It was realized that for practical reasons, many workers use commercially available capsules as the standard. While it is entirely feasible to calculate suitable factors to correct for the difference in size, the group felt that intercomparison of results would be facilitated if the use of correction factors were reduced to a minimum.

2.5. A thigh should not be considered as representative of a human athyreotic neck. Nevertheless, measurements of thigh radioactivity may be useful in estimating the contribution of the extrathyroidal neck radioactivity if carefully determined conversion factors are applied; this may be particularly true in early uptake studies when the problem cannot be solved by collimation.

The main objection against the use of a thigh count to correct for extrathyroidal neck radioactivity was that the count-rate over the thigh may differ considerably and unpredictably from that over an athyreotic neck. With exact collimation and positioning the contribution of extrathyroidal activity to the total count-rate should be small, particularly if the uptake is measured 24 hr after the administration of the dose.

C. Equipment

1. DETECTORS

1.1. In order to minimize the quantity of radioiodine to be administered to the patient, a scintillation counter with a crystal size of not less than 2.5 × 2.5 cm should be the instrument normally used.

The group recommended against the use of one (or several) counters symmetrically disposed around the neck of the patient. Although it was realized that such a device facilitates geometrical reproducibility which is important in cases with irregularly shaped goiters, this advantage is more than offset by the lack of a clear definition of the field of vision and by the error resulting from a high contribution by extrathyroidal radioactivity.

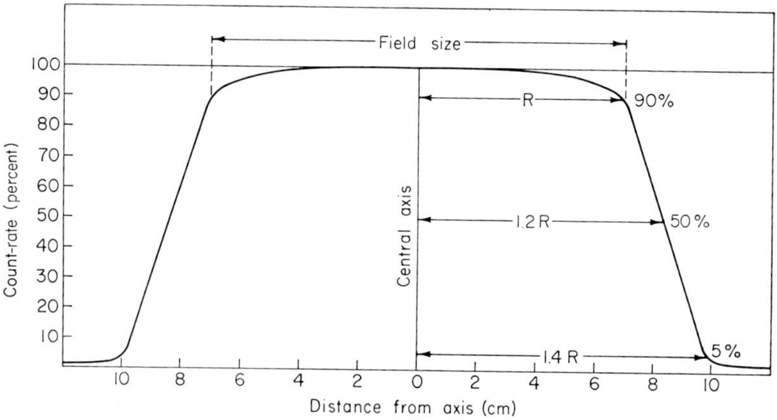

FIG. 1. Definition of size of field of vision in relation to central axis of collimator.

1.2. However, a thick-walled (30–60 mg/cm² of Cu, Bi, or Pb) Geiger–Müller counter can be used effectively where the restrictions as to the administered dose are not stringent (see Section I,A,1.3).

It was felt that a Geiger–Müller counter might still have its place, particularly in situations where the instability of the main voltage supply makes it difficult to operate a scintillation counter properly.

2. SHIELDING AND COLLIMATION

2.1. The visual field at the working distance (see Section I,D,1) should be preferably 12 and certainly not greater than 15 cm in diameter in adults and proportionately smaller in children. This field is defined as the region within which the count-rate from a point source of ^{131}I does not fall below 90% of the value recorded at the center of the field if the point source is moved at the working distance (Fig. 1).

The group stressed the importance of carrying out "once and for all" a series of measurements with a point source (such as a capsule) to ensure that the field of vision is defined precisely and that shielding and collimation are adequate.

2.2. If the source is moved at the working distance beyond the edge of the visual field, the count-rate should fall to 50% or less as the dis-

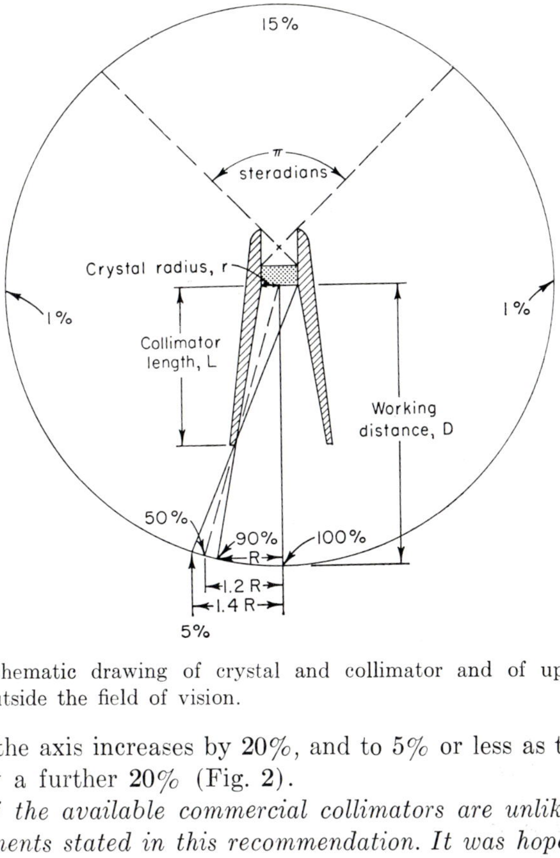

FIG. 2. Schematic drawing of crystal and collimator and of upper limits of count-rates outside the field of vision.

tance from the axis increases by 20%, and to 5% or less as this distance increases by a further 20% (Fig. 2).

Many of the available commercial collimators are unlikely to meet the requirements stated in this recommendation. It was hoped, however, that manufactures might be induced to take up production of collimators specially designed for thyroid uptake measurements which would meet those specifications.

2.3. With a further movement of the point source away from the axis at the working distance, the count-rate should fall rapidly and remain below 1% of the maximum value except in the region behind the crystal which is defined by a solid angle not exceeding 25% (one π). Within this region, the count-rate should not exceed 15% of the maximum value (Fig. 2).

The group emphasized strongly the importance of a rearward shielding. Frequently, measurements of tracer doses are invalidated by the unnoticed presence nearby of large sources such as those carried by patients having received therapeutic amounts of a γ-emitting isotope. In any case, tracer work should be carried out as remotely as possible from X-ray work and radioisotope therapy.

D. Procedure

1. Optimum Distance

1.1. The optimum distance between a single counter and the source will depend on several variables: the size of the field seen by the collimator, the amount of tracer given, the accuracy desired, the size of the gland, and the sensitivity of the detector.

1.2. The distance should be measured from the surface of the sensitive volume of the detector to the skin above the isthmus of the gland and to the surface of the phantom respectively, and should be the same in both situations. In routine work, the distance could also be measured from the front of the collimator.

1.3. In any case the distance should be constant for all patients except in children where it should be shorter and in patients with very large goiters where it could be increased in order to enlarge the field of vision.

It was emphasized that it is essential to "see" the entire gland even if that would result in the inclusion of a larger proportion of extrathyroidal neck tissue in the field of vision.

1.4. Under most conditions encountered in practice a distance of between 20 and 30 cm would appear to be satisfactory.

It should be noted that with an increase in distance the effect of the error in the assumed depth of the gland below the skin will become correspondingly smaller; however, the resulting loss of sensitivity will place a practical limit to such an increase.

2. Optimum Time

The earlier uptake measurements are done after administration of the dose, the more critical the error becomes, owing to the higher body background. Uptake measurements of less than 2 hr are therefore not recommended as a routine procedure.

It was realized that the so-called "early" uptake tests are likely to provide information of greater diagnostic significance than 24-hr or 48-hr uptake measurements; this point should be borne in mind if an uptake measurement is the only test which is carried out on an individual patient.

3. Position of Patient

The patient may be either lying or sitting, provided the working distance is carefully controlled.

Some scintillation counters are sensitive to stray magnetic fields. It is therefore advisable that the counter be kept in the same orientation with respect to the patient and to the standard.

4. Background

4.1. The contribution to the count-rate other than that due to thyroid radioactivity consists of three components:

(a) room background;
(b) leakage from the patient through the shield; and
(c) extrathyroidal neck radioactivity.

4.2. The room background may be measured even with the patient present in the room, provided that shielding of the detector is adequate (see Section I,C,2.3).

4.3. If thyroid uptake is measured 24 hr after administration of the dose, the contribution due to extrathyroidal neck activity is likely to be small compared to that from the thyroid itself. The type of collimation recommended in Section I,C,2 is designed to reduce that contribution further and to eliminate the need for the use of a lead block in front of the thyroid gland. However, if it is desired to measure the uptake earlier, special precautions must be taken.

Some workers use a lead block not so much for eliminating radiation from the gland and thereby assessing the extrathyroidal neck activity but to completely cover the field of vision to test the adequacy of the shielding; this should be superfluous as a routine procedure if the collimator and shield have once been tested as suggested under Section I,C,2. Moreover, if it should be desired to repeat the procedure, the use of a lead block may introduce a variable element because of the difficulty in reproducing exactly its position in front of the gland.

5. Scattered Radiation

5.1. The contribution of scattered radiation from the patient to the total count-rate should be reduced to a minimum. If a Geiger–Müller counter is used this could be done by placing in front of it a lead filter of 1.5-mm thickness; with a scintillation counter this could be accomplished either by using the same type of filter or by properly setting the electrical threshold.

Although it was acknowledged that exclusion of the scattered radiation reduces the sensitivity of the equipment, the fact that the spectrum of the scattered radiation varies from patient to patient would make an intercomparison of results difficult.

5.2. The use of a spectrometer is not essential for an adequate estimation of the thyroid uptake but, if it is available, it may be usefully employed for reducing background and for energy selection.

6. COUNTING STATISTICS

In view of the number and magnitude of other errors involved in thyroid uptake measurements it is not necessary to aim at a less than 3% error in counting statistics.

II. SINGLE-DETECTOR INSTRUMENTS

Though the above recommendations clearly outline all aspects that affect the measurement of ^{131}I uptake by the thyroid, they may not necessarily give the untrained reader a complete picture of the type of instrumentation required for the test. The complexity and therefore the cost for the complete setup can vary considerably and still satisfy the recommendations. In choosing an instrument for thyroid uptake measurements, many aspects have to be considered, some of which are not directly related to the problem on hand (Chapter 2). With respect to the high-voltage supply, the amplifier-spectrometer, and the scaler or ratemeter, required for counting the pulses, any one combination that yields reliable results for other radioisotope counting techniques (Chapter 7) will also suffice for thyroid uptake measurements. Special attention has to be given only to the detector head as described in the recommendations. Since only a few commercially available instruments combine all the desired features, some additional considerations appear appropriate.

A. Crystal Dimensions

The IAEA recommendations suggest the use of a sodium iodide crystal with a diameter of not less than 1 inch and a thickness of 1 inch. The advantages or disadvantages of using a larger crystal are not discussed.

About 70% of the incident 364-keV ^{131}I γ rays are absorbed by 1 inch of sodium iodide. A thicker crystal would increase the counting efficiency less than it would increase the background count-rate. Therefore a crystal thickness greater than 1 inch should be considered only in exceptional cases, for example, when extensive use of the short-life ^{132}I with its higher-energy γ rays is contemplated (*3, 4*).

A larger-diameter crystal increases the counting efficiency and the background count-rate. By going from a 1-inch to a 1.5-inch diameter crystal, both the background and ^{131}I counting efficiency are doubled. For short counting times this yields a sufficiently improved counting accuracy at low count-rates (Chapter 3, Section I,B,3) to justify the increase in cost of crystal and shield. The added weight requires a more rigid support for the whole counter. Therefore, a 1.5- to 2-inch diameter crystal appears to be the optimum size for thyroid ^{131}I uptake measurements. Though a 1-inch diameter crystal yields good results with either prolonged counting times or increased tracer dose, the larger-diameter crystals are definitely preferable.

B. γ-Ray Spectrum

The pulse-height distribution depends on the radiation emitted from the source and the size of the sodium iodide crystal. An increase of the

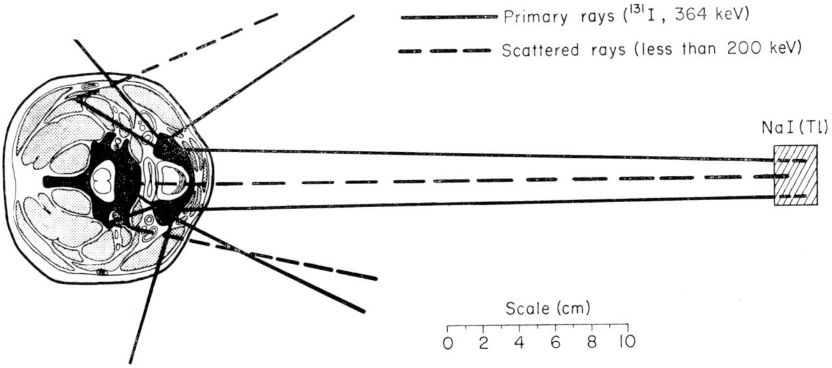

FIG. 3. Cross section of neck containing thyroid gland. γ-Rays backscattered from the tissues surrounding the gland can also reach the detector.

crystal dimensions causes an improved total absorption of the higher-energy γ rays (Chapter 6, Section III,B). The activities in the two sources, the neck phantom and the patient's neck, can be compared only when their pulse-height spectra are identical within the region used for the measurements. The IAEA recommendations only touch on this subject (Section I,D,5).

The ^{131}I γ rays are emitted from the thyroid gland in all directions with only a small fraction reaching the detector (Fig. 3). Of the γ rays entering the neck tissues, a large fraction (about 50%) is absorbed by

Compton interaction, producing scattered radiation. Of this so-called degraded radiation (*12*) or neck scatter (*8*), only the backscattered radiation (scattering angle greater than 90°) has a high probability of reaching the detector (Fig. 3). Since the backscattered radiation has

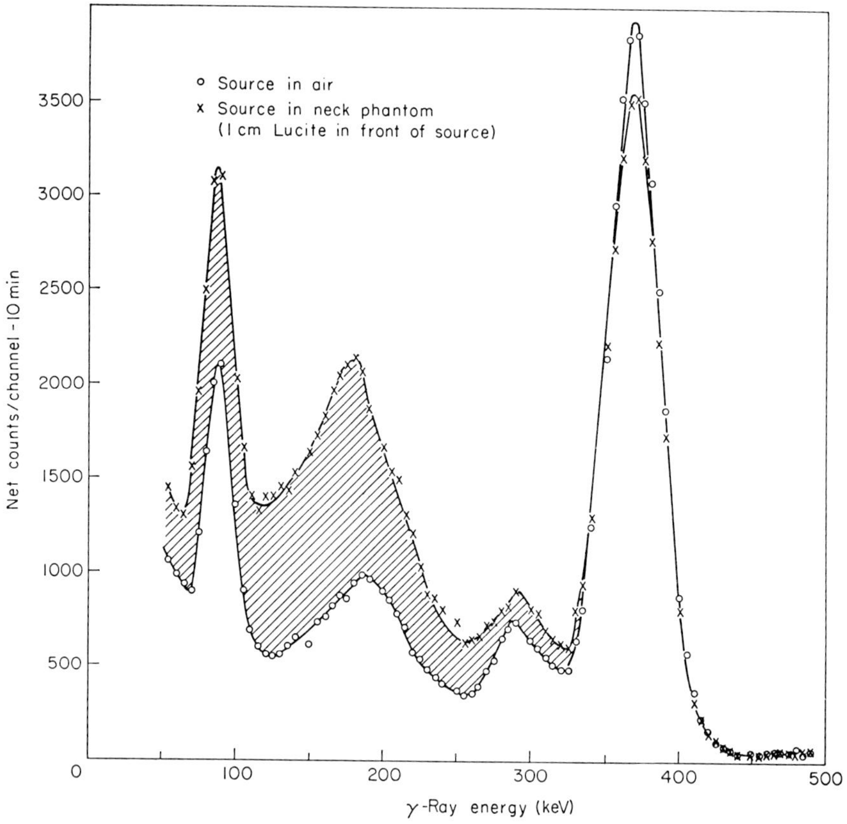

FIG. 4. Pulse-height spectra of 1-ml ^{131}I source (5 μCi) in air and in neck phantom at 30 cm from a 1.5-inch diameter, 1-inch thick sodium iodide crystal. Shaded area shows increase in count-rate due to backscattered γ rays.

about half the energy of the 364-keV ^{131}I γ rays, it is counted with increased efficiency by the sodium iodide detector.

Figure 4 shows the ^{131}I spectra from a 1-ml ^{131}I source in air and in the neck phantom. The shaded area indicates the contribution of the backscattered radiation. Its magnitude relative to the primary ^{131}I γ rays for thyroid uptake measurements depends on many factors such as size of thyroid gland and patient's neck, counter geometry, and dimensions of the sodium iodide crystal (*6, 8, 12, 13*).

There are various ways of dealing with the backscattered radiation. One is the use of a neck phantom (Section I,B,2) which produces a pulse-height spectrum similar to the one observed *in vivo*. This yields not only a maximum counting efficiency since all pulses can be used for the measurements, but also allows a correction for the absorption of the primary γ rays in the tissues between source and detector. However, any one phantom of this kind cannot accurately reproduce the pulse-height distributions obtained from all patients.

For this reason, the pulses of energy below about 300 keV (Fig. 4) are frequently eliminated from the measurements by using a discrimina-

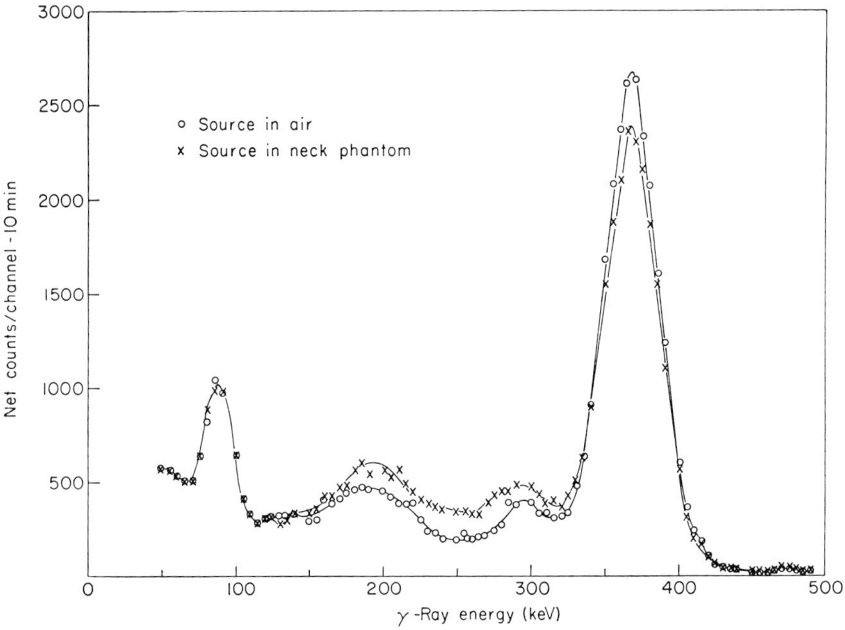

FIG. 5. Pulse-height spectra as in Fig. 4 but with 1.5-mm lead absorber in front of crystal. Contribution of backscattered radiation has been eliminated.

tor or pulse-height analyzer. About half of the useful pulses, produced by Compton absorption of the 364-keV γ rays in the sodium iodide crystal (spectrum in air of Fig. 4), are lost by thus eliminating the backscattered radiation.

An alternative is the use of an absorber in front of the detector. As mentioned in the IAEA recommendations, a 1.5-mm lead absorber is relatively opaque to the backscattered radiation. Figure 5 shows the spectra of the source in air and in the neck phantom as in Fig. 4 but with the 1.5-mm lead absorber in front of the crystal. A comparison of

Figs. 4 and 5 shows that the absorber reduces the detectable 364-keV γ rays by about 30%. The low-energy section of the spectrum is now nearly independent of the scattering conditions within the source (Fig. 5) and therefore all pulses can be included in the measurements. This more than compensates for the counting losses due to absorption of primary radiation and results in simpler and more stable instruments with a lower energy cutoff at about 40 keV. Since only a small fraction of the pulses are so low in energy, a small change in pulse amplification produces a negligible change in counting sensitivity, resulting in an operating plateau. Therefore, the use of a lead absorber instead of an electronic pulse-height selector is preferable whenever the resulting increase in background count-rate can be tolerated.

C. Length of Collimator

After selecting the crystal dimensions and the useful pulse-height spectrum, the counting distance and the dimensions of the collimator have to be chosen.

The counting or working distance, D, is measured from the detector face to the patient's neck (Fig. 2). The effective distance between the center of the radioactivity in the thyroid and the effective center for the ^{131}I γ-ray absorption in the sodium iodide crystal is larger than D by about 3 cm. The location of the thyroid gland within the neck, its size, and the distribution of the ^{131}I within the gland vary from patient to patient causing an uncertainty up to ± 1 cm in the effective distance between source and detector. For a working distance $D = 20$ cm, the variation of the effective distance of 23 cm by ± 1 cm yields an uncertainty of $\pm 8\%$ in the uptake measurements because of the inverse square law. Increasing the counting distance helps to reduce the errors due to variations in the thyroid depth.

For any chosen working distance, D, the desired performance of the collimator is shown in Fig. 1. For adults the field size at the working distance should be less than 15 cm in diameter and therefore the radius $R < 7.5$ cm (Section I,C,2). The sensitivity should drop to 50% or less at $1.2R = 8.4$ cm from the central axis. In order to achieve this, the length of the collimator, L, has to bear a certain relation to the working distance, D (Fig. 2). If the working distance is only a little larger than the collimator length, the lateral cutoff in sensitivity is very sharp. The more the working distance exceeds the collimator length, the less rapid the count-rate will decrease radially (*1*).

It is possible to derive a geometrical relation between the working distance, D, the collimator length, L, and the crystal radius, r, so that the sensitivity at $1.2R$ is about 50% of that at the axis (Figs. 1 and 2).

The dashed line in Fig. 2 at $1.2R$ "sees" only half the crystal by intersecting with the collimator edge and crystal surface center, while the line intersecting at R "sees" practically the whole crystal. Neglecting the fact that some of the γ rays penetrate the collimator edge and that the γ rays are not absorbed at the crystal surface but at various depths within the crystal, the following geometrical relation can be derived:

$$L = D(r/0.2R + r)$$

For a chosen radius, R, of the field at the neck, the length of the collimator, L, becomes a function of the working distance, D, and the crystal radius, r. For $R = 7$ cm and $r = 1$, 2, or 3 cm, $L/D = 0.4$, 0.6, or 0.7, respectively. This shows that for a small crystal the collimator length can be less than half the working distance, while for a large crystal it has to be nearly three quarters of the working distance. If a working distance of $D = 30$ cm is chosen for a 1.5-inch diameter crystal ($r = 2$ cm), the collimator length, L, should be about 18 cm. For a larger working distance of $D = 50$ cm for the same crystal size, the collimator length, L, should be increased to about 30 cm.

D. Detector Shielding

After determining the collimator length, the thickness of the lead required for the collimator and the shielding surrounding the crystal must be established. The IAEA recommendations describe the purpose of the lead shielding (Section I,C,2) without specifying the lead thickness. The mass absorption coefficient of lead for the 364-keV ^{131}I γ rays is 0.26 cm^2/gm. The half-value layer in lead follows as 0.23 cm or about 0.1 inch, and about 2.5% of the incident ^{131}I γ rays can penetrate 0.5 inch of lead (see Appendix, Section I).

As pointed out in the IAEA recommendations, the lead shield must be extended not only in front (collimator), but also in back of the crystal. A lead shield of this kind shown in Fig. 6 has proven to be adequate and practical. The thickness of the lead is greatest close to the crystal and decreases with increasing distance from the crystal. γ Rays emitted from a source in front of the collimator (outside its field of vision) must pass through nearly 1 inch of lead before reaching the crystal. Only γ rays entering the collimator or the multiplier phototube in back of the crystal can reach the crystal without passing through a lead absorber. For a given lead thickness, the weight of the shield and collimator increases with the crystal diameter as the length of the collimator also increases (Section II,C). The assembly shown in Fig. 6 weighs about 35 lb for a 1.5-inch diameter crystal.

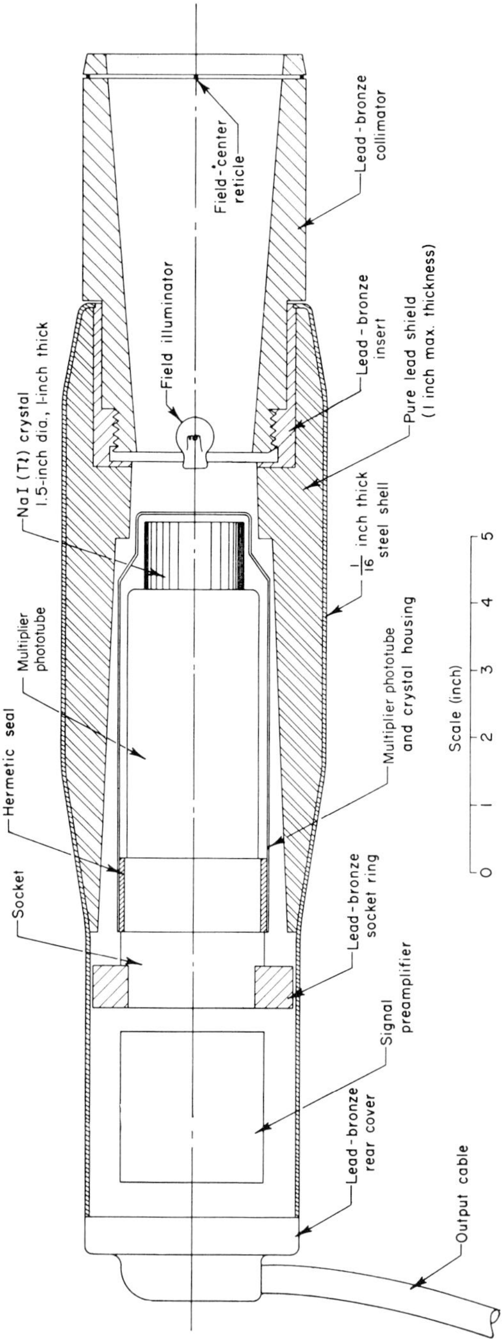

FIG. 6. Schematic of collimator and crystal assembly. The light bulb illuminates an area corresponding to the field of vision. (Courtesy of Picker Nuclear.)

Recently, the constructional details of a thyroid uptake collimator which complies with the IAEA recommendations have been published (*1*). Its design is so simple that a hospital with access to a small workshop could reproduce it at low cost.

E. Complete Instruments

The crystal-multiplier phototube and shield-collimator assembly (Fig. 6) must be suspended so that it can be positioned easily in front of the patient's neck. How this can be accomplished is not mentioned in the IAEA recommendations. At first glance this appears to be a simple mechanical problem which should not require special attention. Experience over the past 15 years however, shows that no solution has yet been found which is satisfactory in every respect.

Most frequently the counter is mounted on an arm which extends from a column (Fig. 7). The detector assembly can travel vertically from about 3 to 6 ft above the floor. It moves easily up and down since it is counter-balanced by weights inside the column. The cables supporting the counterweight must be constructed so that a break is virtually impossible. Furthermore, safety requires a positive locking of all adjustments, when a heavy weight is suspended over the patient's head. The linkages between the arm and the counter bracket allow the counter to be placed in any desired position up to about 3 ft from the column when the patient is lying on a litter.

The disadvantage of such an assembly is its expense. A major fraction of the total equipment cost (perhaps 25%) goes into the support for the counter. Many attempts have been made to reduce its cost, by building simplified stands. They might work well, for counters weighing 10–15 lb, but they all have serious shortcomings for counters of 30–50 lb as required for thyroid uptake measurements. Only stands with a wide, heavy base can offset the eccentric weight of the counter assembly and are safe from tipping over. Because of their wide base, such stands occupy valuable floor space. In hospitals with a heavy patient load for thyroid uptake measurements, this might not be objectionable, but it might be a drawback at places where the instrument finds only occasional use.

Instead of using a floor stand, it is possible to construct a less expensive table model. The end of the collimator can line up with the edge of a table while the patient sits in a chair close to the table. In order to align the patient's neck with the collimator, either the height of the chair or the support of the collimator must have a vertical adjustment. Though a table model is as simple to operate as the floor stand, it is a less flexible arrangement which can be used only for thyroid uptake measurements with the patient in a sitting position. Nevertheless, a simple setup like this should be useful in many places.

The thyroid radioiodine uptake measurements are meaningful only if the patient's thyroid is positioned correctly during the measurements. The IAEA recommendations (Section I,D,3) state: "The patient may be either lying or sitting, provided *the working distance is carefully controlled.*" However, in most instruments presently in use the working

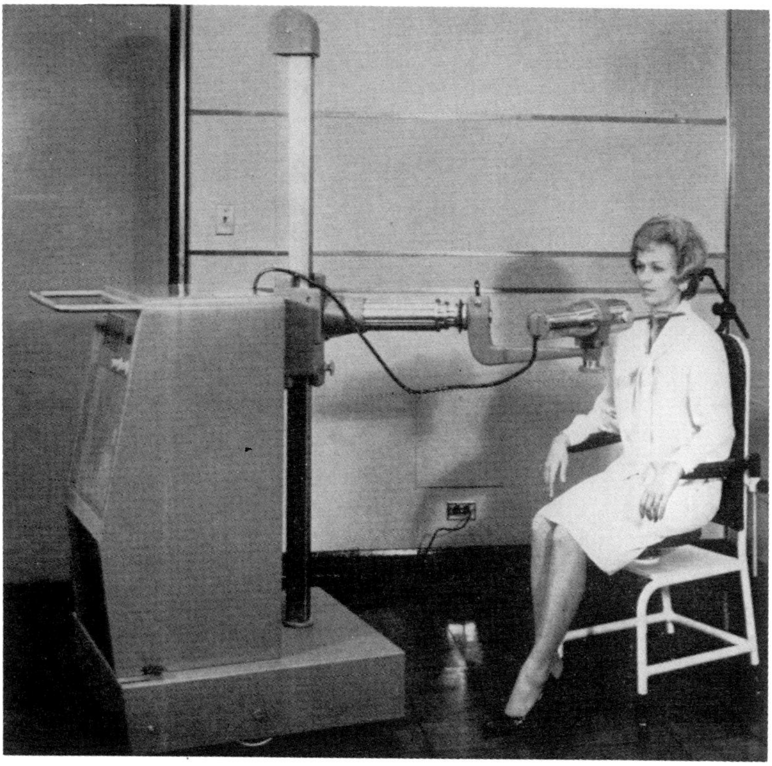

FIG. 7. Complete instrument including electronics and flexible counter mounting. (Courtesy of Picker Nuclear)

distance is not carefully controlled. A typical picture that can be seen in many early as well as recent publications is that of a patient sitting in a chair comfortably leaning backward with the counter somewhere in front of him. Only a mechanical connection between the counter and the patient's neck can secure a fixed distance during the measurements. Some counters have a graduated rod on one side and parallel to the counter axis, which allows a measurement of the working distance. At the end of the rod should be a cross bar which extends to the center of the measuring field (Fig. 8). This cross bar might consist of plastic tubing in order to minimize γ-ray absorption. During the measurements the patient feels the cross bar touching his neck while he remains in the correct position. Without a permanent distance indicator, the patient has a tendency to lean backward or to bend forward during the measurements. Therefore no thyroid iodine uptake measurements should be made without such a positioning device. Finally, it secures an identical position of the neck phantom containing a duplicate of the administered ^{131}I tracer dose. An

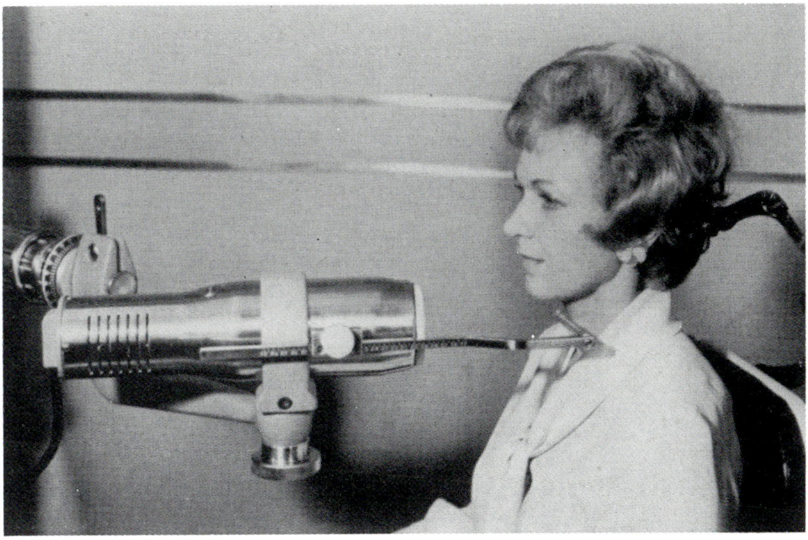

Fig. 8. Collimator of Fig. 6, positioned in front of thyroid. Measuring distance is accurately controlled by positioning device extending from the collimator. (Courtesy of Picker Nuclear)

error in the phantom position introduces as much of an inaccuracy as an error in positioning the patient's thyroid.

III. MULTIPLE-DETECTOR INSTRUMENTS

At present most instruments employ a single γ-ray detector for thyroid iodine uptake measurements. Though the comments to the IAEA recommendations advise against the use of multiple γ-ray detectors (Section I,C,1), an instrument with several unique properties will be described.

In 1950 Freedberg (*5*) suggested the use of four counters placed in a circle around the neck to form a "well-counter" which detects predominantly radiation from the neck region. Though this arrangement seemed to have definite advantages, it never became popular. The ^{131}I γ rays are absorbed in the neck so strongly that the two counters in back of the patient receive very little unattenuated radiation compared with the two counters in front. However, they double the background count-rate and measure mainly extrathyroidal neck radioactivity. Therefore, better results are obtained by using only two counters in front of the neck.

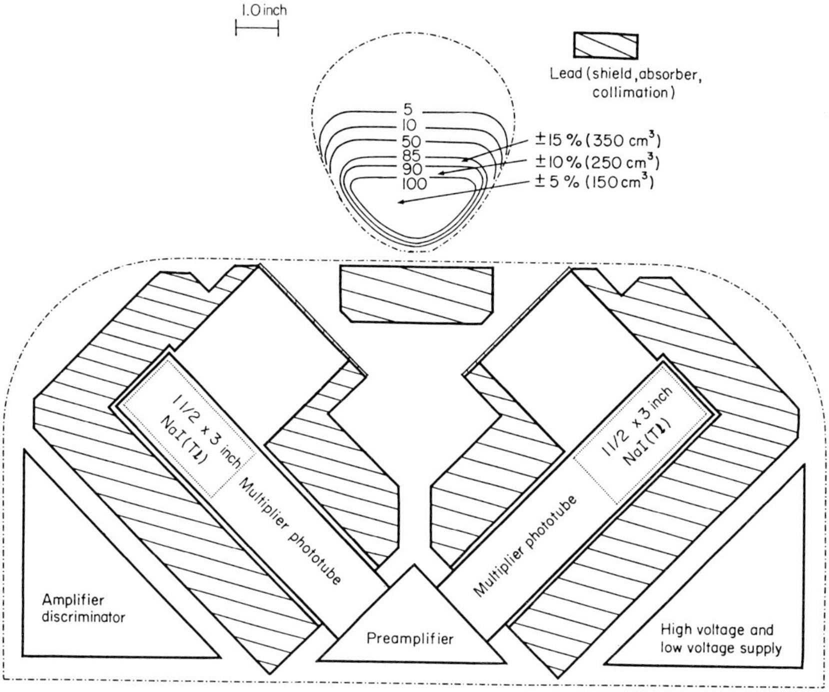

FIG. 9. Duo-detector assembly and isocount curves obtained with point source inside a water container. The maximum sensitivity is observed at a depth corresponding to the position of the thyroid gland. The height of the field is about 10 cm. (Courtesy of Ames Atomium, Inc.)

Figure 9 shows two sodium iodide crystals, each 1.5 inch in diameter by 3 inches long at about 15 cm from the thyroid. This configuration provides a large solid angle for γ-ray detection from the thyroid with a minimum of intervening tissue. The addition of suitable collimation* creates a three-dimensional field which has a response such that the sensitivity initially increases with increasing distance from the detectors (Fig. 9). Furthermore, the cross-collimated fields eliminate lateral varia-

* Thyrimeter, Ames Atomium Inc., Billerica, Massachusetts.

tions in sensitivity within the area of maximum response, and insure a rapid falloff in sensitivity beyond that area. For thyroids positioned within the area of high sensitivity, the counts registered by the duodetectors are practically independent of the actual distribution of the radioactivity within the thyroid area. Therefore, if the front of each patient's neck is maintained at a fixed distance from the detectors, the ^{131}I uptake measurements are affected very little by the size or position of the thyroid gland of an individual patient.

Using two sodium iodide crystals, each viewing the thyroid side-on (area 1.5×3 inches) at close distance, yields a high sensitivity of about 7000 to 8000 cpm per microcurie of ^{131}I in the thyroid. This permits the performance of thyroid iodine uptake measurements with good accuracy using counting times as short as 1 to 2 minutes and tracer doses as low as 1 μCi of ^{131}I.

The IAEA recommendations (Section I,A,1), state correctly that a dose of 25 μCi of ^{131}I may be required if other radioiodine tests are necessary, such as a thyroid scan or ^{131}I PBI. Therefore, full advantage of such a highly sensitive ^{131}I thyroid uptake system can be taken only under restricted conditions applying to certain groups of patients (*2*). These might be children or pregnant women for whom it is especially important to keep the radiation dose to a minimum. It should be remembered that a concentration of 1 μCi of ^{131}I per gram of thyroid delivers about 100 rads to the thyroid gland or an administered activity of 25 μCi of ^{131}I results in a dose of about 40 rads assuming a 30% uptake (Appendix, Table II).

IV. LIMITATIONS OF PRESENT METHODS

The measurement of the radiation emitted from a patient's thyroid does not yet result in a percentage uptake value. A duplicate of the administered dose has to be measured under conditions identical to those existing for the ^{131}I in the patient's thyroid. The IAEA recommendations discuss these conditions in Section I,B. They describe a neck phantom similar to that presently available from many companies (Fig. 10). They suggest the use of a 30-ml container for the duplicate dose recessed 0.5 cm inside the neck phantom.

The neck phantom simulates the conditions for the absorption of the ^{131}I γ rays in the thyroid gland and the overlying tissues for an average patient. However, both the size of the gland and its position inside the patient's neck vary between individuals. An estimate of the effect of this variation using a single detector system can be obtained from Fig. 11. Three volumetric flasks of different volumes containing equal amounts of ^{131}I solution were placed one at a time inside a 2-liter beaker filled with water. The distance between the front of the flask and the wall of the beaker was varied between zero and 3.0 cm. The working distance between the front of the beaker and the face of the crystal was 50 cm. The count-rate obtained with the 25-ml flask with 1 cm of water in front of it was taken as 100%. Figure 11 shows that reducing the water thickness to 0.5 cm increases the count-rate by 4%, and increasing the water thickness to 1.5 cm reduces the count-rate by 4%. Increasing the ^{131}I solution from 25 to 50 ml reduces all count-rates by about 3%. For

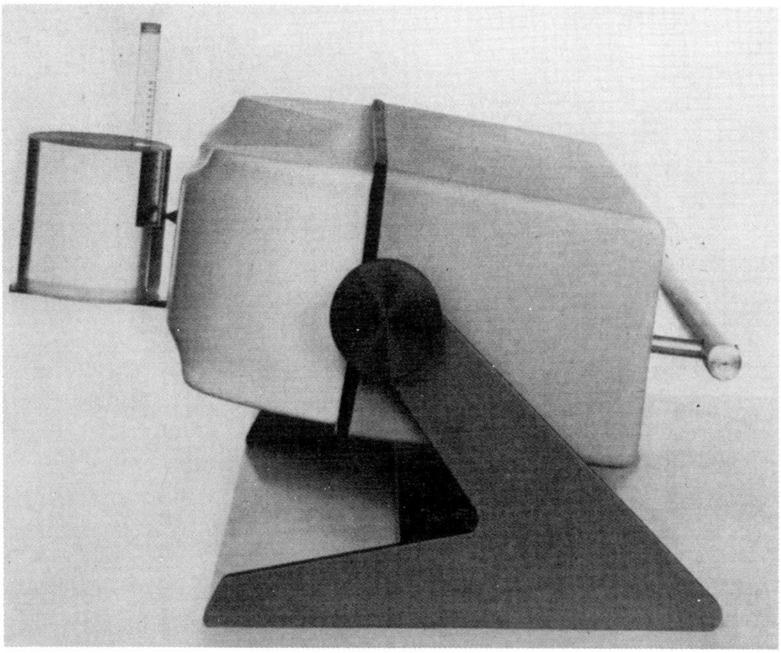

FIG. 10. Lucite neck phantom positioned in front of duo-detectors shown in Fig. 9. (Courtesy of Ames Atomium, Inc.)

practical purposes, the greatest variation that might be encountered to simulate the size and position of thyroids within a population is a 25-ml source with no water in front and a 100-ml source with 2 cm of water in front. Going from one extreme to the other produces a 20% variation in count-rates (Fig. 11). Therefore, the use of an average condition of source size and position for all measurements could cause an error as large as $\pm 10\%$ in exceptional cases. For thyroid iodine uptake measurements performed at a shorter working distance, the error would be enhanced owing to greater inverse square law variations closer to a single γ-ray detector. The duo-detector response (Fig. 9), however, varies much less with source size.

The physical limitations for measuring the percentage of ^{131}I taken up by the thyroid at a certain time after administration of a dose have been outlined in this chapter. Employing presently available instruments, the test can be performed in a few minutes with low to moderately high doses of ^{131}I (0.5–25 μCi). Though the results in general may have an accuracy of ±5%, it should be kept in mind that the fraction of the administered dose of radioiodine present in the thyroid at any one time yields information of only limited value. The percentage of radioactivity retained in the thyroid gland varies with time (*13*), and the rates of uptake and release as well as the maximum percentage uptake depend

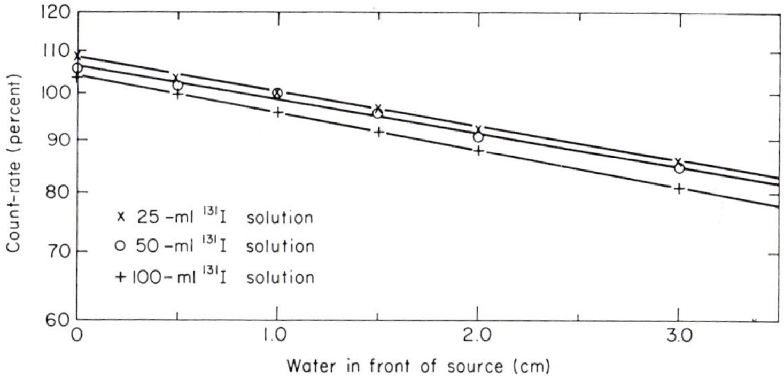

FIG. 11. Variation in count-rate of 25-, 50-, and 100-ml ^{131}I sources with different amounts of water in front of source. Detector-phantom distance is 50 cm.

on many factors. They may be affected by the dietary iodine intake, medication with drugs containing iodine, treatment of the thyroid gland by drugs, surgery, or radiation, stimulation by the pituitary gland, and so forth (*9, 10, 11, 13*).

REFERENCES

1. Belcher, E. H., Gomez-Crespo, G., Trott, N. G., and Vetter, H., A standard collimator for thyroid radioiodine uptake measurements. *Nucl. Med.* **4**, 78 (1964).
2. Cameron, J. R., and Bell, D. B., Thyroid uptake studies with I^{131} in very small doses. *Radiology* **79**, 452 (1962).
3. Cavalieri, R. R., and King, E. R., The use of iodine-132 to study thyroid function following therapy with iodine-131. *J. Nucl. Med.* **3**, 436 (1962).
4. Einhorn, J., and Håstad, K., The prognostic value of early determination of thyroidal radioiodine uptake following I^{131} therapy. *J. Clin. Endocrinol. Metab.* **21**, 1483 (1961).
5. Freedberg, A. S., Chamovitz, D. L., Ureles, A. L., and Van Dilla, M. A., The direct measurement of I^{131} uptake in the thyroid gland; further observations. *J. Clin. Endocrinol.* **10**, 910 (1950).

5a. Gomez-Crespo, G., and Vetter, H., The calibration and standardization of thyroid radioiodine uptake measurements. *Int. J. Appl. Radiation Isotopes* **17,** 531 (1966).
6. Hine, G. J., Burrows, B. A., and Ross, J. F., Thyroid uptake measurements. *Nucleonics* **15,** No. 1, 54 (1957).
7. IAEA consultants meeting on the calibration and standardization of thyroid radioiodine uptake measurements. *Acta Isotopica* **1,** 309 (1961); *Minerva Nucl.* **5,** 4 (1961); *Brit. J. Radiol.* **35,** 205 (1962); *Intern. J. Appl. Radiation Isotopes* **13,** 167 (1962); *Acta Ibér. Radiol.-Cancer* **17,** 183 (1962); *Acta Radiol.* **58,** 233 (1962); *Nucl. Med.* **2,** 300 (1962); *Phys. Med. Biol.* **6,** 533 (1962); *Ann. Radiol.* **5,** 731 (1962); *J. Belge Radiol.* **45,** 511 (1962).
8. Orvis, A. L., Koenig, M. P., and Owen, C. A., Jr., *In vivo* measurement of thyroidal radioiodine: effect of "neck scatter." *J. Clin. Endocrinol. Metab.* **17,** 966 (1957).
9. Pochin, E. E., The examination of thyroid activity with radioiodine. *Brit. J. Radiol.* **33,** 595 (1960).
10. Riggs, D. S., Quantitative aspects of iodine metabolism in man. *Pharmacol. Rev.* **4,** 284 (1952).
11. Silver, S., "Radioactive Isotopes in Medicine and Biology." Vol. 2, Medicine. 2nd ed. Lea & Febiger, Philadelphia, Pennsylvania, 1962.
12. Trombka, J. I., and O'Foghludha, F., The effects of degraded radiation in thyroid uptake measurements. *Phys. Med. Biol.* **1,** 340 (1957).
13. Veall, N., and Vetter, H., "Radioisotope Techniques in Clinical Research and Diagnosis." Butterworth, London and Washington, D.C., 1958.

CHAPTER 15

IN VIVO TRACER STUDIES BY EXTERNAL γ-RAY COUNTING

WILLIAM J. MacINTYRE

DEPARTMENTS OF MEDICINE AND PSYCHIATRY
WESTERN RESERVE UNIVERSITY
CLEVELAND, OHIO

I. FUNDAMENTAL CONCEPTS OF THE TIME-CONCENTRATION CURVE

While numerous radioisotope studies are concerned with the actual localization of the radioisotope depositions, in many cases pertinent information may be obtained by recording the rates of deposition, accumulation, or release of the radioactive material. For example, one of the first applications of external γ-ray counting to *in vivo* tracer studies in medicine was the measurement of the uptake of ^{131}I by the thyroid gland at a specific time following the administration of the dose. Later it was recognized that the accumulation of a tracer dose of radioiodine was an exponentially increasing function and that additional information could possibly be obtained by measuring the rate of uptake rather than the final asymptotic value.

Following this application, the emphasis of *in vivo* tracer studies has been progressively shifted from static measurements to dynamic measurements which are performed over a period of time. The variation of the concentration of radioactivity in any site provides the fundamental relationship to be analyzed.

The concentration to be measured may occur in a number of different sites, organs, dilution volumes, or combinations of such functional entities. In the case of thyroid function, the concentration of interest is the accumulation of the radioiodine in the gland itself which is followed in time. In a study of liver function, a material selectively removed by this organ is administered, and the liver function is evaluated either by measurement of the concentration of the material in the liver or by measurement of the disappearance of the tracer from the circulating blood. In the determination of blood flows of various organs, the concentration which is measured as a function of time is primarily the concentration of the blood flowing to or from the organ. In the evaluation of kidney function by the renogram, however, a more complex system is measured. The time concentration curves in the kidney areas are influenced by the blood flow carrying the radioactivity to the kidneys, the accumulation of this material by the kidney parenchyma, and its later release or excretion.

The purpose of this chapter is to examine the types of analyses which are representative for the various methods in which the time-concentration curve has been used to yield specific parameters. For example, a clearance rate, or the rate of decrease of radioactivity in the circulating blood, may reflect the efficiency of removal of the radioactive material by a specific organ if the blood flow to that organ is known. Conversely, if the efficiency of removal is known, this same time-concentration curve may be analyzed to derive the blood flow to the organ responsible for such removal of the radioactivity. On the other hand, when there is no removal, the principle of conservation of mass may be applied in order to derive the flow-rate to a specific organ from the integral of the time-concentration curve.

Basically, these two parameters of blood flow and organ function represent the primary concern of this type of measurement and analysis. In the following sections the integral expression of the concentration of the injected material in its primary dilution passage is derived in order to obtain a flow value useful in cardiac output determinations. In addition, the differential rates of disappearance of various materials from the circulating blood are analyzed with respect to both organ function and blood flow information, and lastly the accumulation and release curves are examined for functional content alone.

II. RECORDING OF RADIOISOTOPE DILUTION CURVES

One of the primary applications of the recording of the time concentration curve has been the quantification of flow rate by the integration of the dilution curve from injected tracer material. This principle can be applied to any flow system whenever the tracer concentration in the outflow can be sampled; however, the most important physiological adaptation has been the determination of cardiac output (*5, 23, 25*).

Qualitatively it may be seen that if a small volume of radioactive material is injected into the inflow tract leading to the heart, the average dilution of the radioactivity in the large vessels leaving the heart must be a direct indication of the volume of blood passing through the heart and causing this dilution. Quantitatively, it is perhaps best expressed by the principle of conservation of radioactivity in a closed system which requires that the same quantity of injected material must come out of the heart as was injected into the inflow tract. Thus the quantity of injected material, I, must be equal to the product of the flow-rate, F, multiplied by the continuously changing concentration, c, of the tagged material in the blood, integrated over the entire time of the primary circulation. This is represented by the equation

$$I = \int_0^\infty Fc\,dt \tag{1}$$

Such a dilution curve is illustrated by Fig. 1. It shows the sharp rise as the first highly concentrated bolus of radioactivity enters the site of sampling at P_1. This is followed first by the characteristic exponential decrease and then the recirculation at point P_2. The latter occurs since some of the shortest circulatory paths return some radioactivity to the heart before the clearance of the originally injected material has been completed.

If F, the flow rate or cardiac output, may be considered a constant during the time of mixing, Eq. 1 can be reduced to the expression:

$$F = I \Big/ \int_0^\infty c\,dt \tag{2}$$

where $\int_0^\infty c\,dt$ is the area under the primary mixing curve, A, plus portion B under the extrapolation line. Thus,

$$F = \mathrm{I}/(A + B) \tag{3}$$

The area A may be integrated directly while area B must be calculated from the exponential function predicted by the slope of the curve prior to recirculation. If the concentration at a point prior to recirculation is c_b, and λ represents the decay factor of the curve, the area B may be derived by the expression

$$B = \int_0^\infty c_b e^{-\lambda t}\, dt = c_b/\lambda$$

This essentially reduces the measurement to two problems. One is to convert the dilution curve recorded in terms of count-rate to an expres-

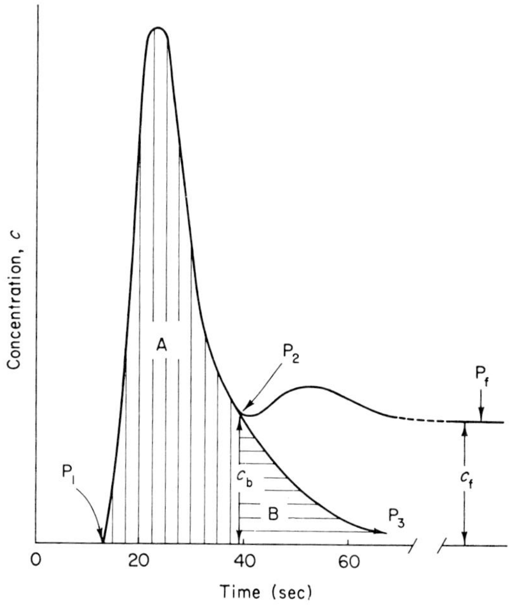

FIG. 1. General form of dilution curve showing the areas to be integrated represented as A and B (*14*). The furthest concentration in time to use as extrapolation for area B is represented by c_b at point P_2. The final concentration, usually taken 5 to 10 min following injection, is shown as c_f.

sion in terms of microcuries per milliliter dilution, and the second is the accurate prediction of the decay factor λ.

A. Relation of Count-Rate to Dilution

The most direct type of blood sampling is to perform an arterial puncture and to lead the blood by external tubing (*14, 22*) adjacent to, or through, the radiation detector. With this system the calibration may be achieved simply by filling the tubing with a known concentration of the radioisotope in terms of microcuries per milliliter and observing the response of the detector in terms of counts per minute. For calibration of the arterial puncture system it has been convenient to withdraw a venous sample of blood sufficiently long after injection for the concentration to be considered as constant over the period of measurement. This concentration, as represented by point c_f of Fig. 1, may then be assayed in a well scintillation counter to yield a value in terms of microcuries per milliliter. Comparing this value to the count-rate recorded on the dilution curve at this point in time by the detector through which the tubing has been passed then produces a calibration of the count-rate of the dilution curve in terms of microcuries per milliliter.

Since the injected dose, I, is equal to the product of the volume of dilution, V_d, and the specific activity of the final dilution, c_f, Eq. 3 may be expressed as

$$F = [c_f/(A + B)]V_d \qquad (4)$$

It must be realized that V_d may not necessarily be identical to the circulating blood volume as usually calculated by dilution methods. V_d is the volume of dilution of the injected material at the time when the sample is withdrawn. If a 10-min mixing time is observed before withdrawal, the observed value of V_d will in most cases clinically approximate the blood volume, but this is not a necessary condition of the formula.

The use of V_d as a calibration factor is valid regardless of when the sample is withdrawn or whether final complete mixing has or has not been reached. Since the first term of the right side of Eq. 4 is a ratio, it is seen that the specific activity at final dilution, c_f, may be expressed in terms of counts per minute and the areas A and B expressed as the product of counts per minute on the ordinate and time on the abscissa. This formulation as expressed by Eq. 4 is not really required in the arterial tap method since the areas A and B can be directly converted to terms of microcuries per unit volume and time. Since a known volume is presented to the detector, the system may be calibrated by presenting a known dilution to the detector in order to relate the count-rate to terms of microcuries per milliliter.

In the *in vivo* or external method, Eq. 4 is a necessary condition for solution, since the external detector focused over an arterial supply cannot define a specific volume. To duplicate the complex geometrical system for calibration would be extremely difficult and even then it would be expected to vary among subjects. The advantage of Eq. 4 for external measurements is that the ratio of count-rate precludes the need for knowledge of the geometric volumes involved and allows calibration merely by measurement of the volume of dilution, V_d.

B. Analysis of Multichamber Techniques

The foregoing discussion has been directed toward the analysis of a single site of dilution. As such it makes little difference whether the flow is externalized and led past a detector or whether a single site of dilution is selected by *in vivo* localization. Since the advantages of the latter method over the earlier techniques of arterial puncture are obvious, considerable effort has been expended on the *in vivo* method. While external focusing on a large artery to record a dilution curve is possible (*15*) the accuracy of placement and the small volume seen by the detector can give rise to many difficulties.

A great number of attempts have been made to view the large chambers of the heart itself. When this is done a single dilution curve is seldom obtained because of the complexity of isolating one of the heart chambers. More commonly a double dilution curve is recorded resulting from the summation of two dilution curves slightly separated in time. Thus if a detector is directed over the precordium so that both right and left chambers of the heart are seen, the first curve will be recorded from the right chamber. After a lag, while the material flows out into the lungs, the second curve will be obtained at the re-entry of the material into the left chamber of the heart.

If two recorders were to record the count-rates individually from the right (r) and left (l) chambers of the heart, Eq. 4 could be written as

$$FA_r = c_{f_r}V_d \tag{5}$$

$$FA_l = c_{f_l}V_d \tag{6}$$

In this case A_r refers to the dilution curve areas A and B, and c_{f_r} to the final concentration of the right heart alone with similar nomenclature for the left heart. Since the same flow, F, goes through both sides of the heart, the sum of Eqs. 5 and 6, or of any number of flow sites, may be consodilated to give the general equation

$$F = [(c_{f_r} + c_{f_l} + \cdots + c_{f_n})/(A_r + A_l + \cdots + A_n)]V_d \tag{7}$$

The importance of Eq. 7 lies in the fact that isolation of one site or sampling of dilution is not necessary in order to calculate the flow output. A dilution curve recorded from two or more sites may be used by measuring the area of the total dilution curve, provided the final calibration value of concentration, c_f, is obtained under identical geometrical relations to these sites as when the dilution curve was recorded. From a practical viewpoint this states that the mixing pools observed by the detector should not have an appreciable component that appears after the primary circulation curve has been recorded. An example of such an undesirable factor would be the appearance of radioactivity in the capillary volume, which would tend to make the value of c_f too large, since it would occur after the primary curve.

It is this restriction which makes it difficult to obtain valid results from external viewing of a large artery. In the example of focusing a detector over the femoral artery, the primary dilution curve may be satisfactory. In the measurement of c_f, however, the volume seen includes not only the artery but also the volume of the femoral vein adjacent to the artery as well as associated capillary circulation.

Of course additional contribution from capillary and venous circulation will always be present in any technique. The success of cardiac out-

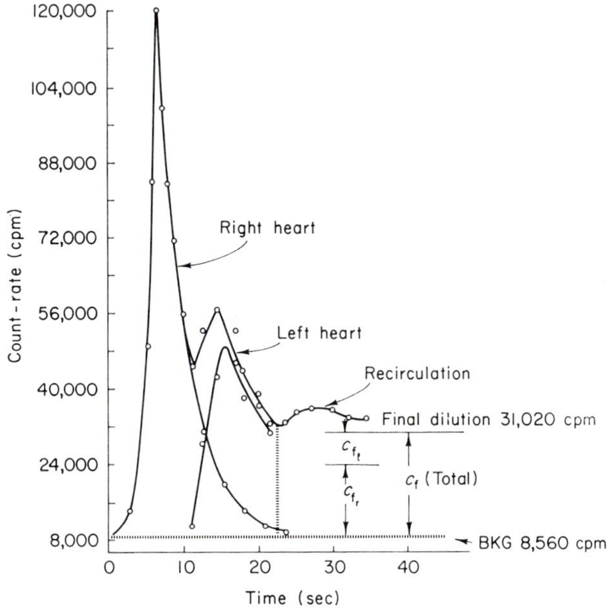

FIG. 2. Dilution curve obtained by counter receiving contribution from both heart chambers (dominant right heart). Ratios of final dilutions represent the ratio of measured areas of right and left heart (*15*). In this and the following figures the dotted vertical intercept from the descending line to the time axis separates the measured areas from the extrapolated areas of the dilution curve. This point is arbitrarily chosen to be reasonably far down on the descending line so as to minimize the contribution of the extrapolated area while still being unaffected by the effects of recirculation.

puts calculated from the selection of the large chambers of the heart is due mainly to the procedure of minimizing the capillary contribution with respect to the primary site.

A dilution curve recorded from more than one chamber of the heart is shown in Fig. 2. The extrapolation of the right heart descending line allows the dilution of the left heart to be separated into components of right and left heart dilution areas shown by the ratio of final dilutions. For cardiac output calculations, however, this separation is not necessary and for practical measurements the area of the dilution curve is treated as a single unit corresponding to the single value of the final dilution c_f.

For some dilution curves the prediction of the extrapolation line may be difficult. While it is generally assumed that each chamber is clearing by an exponential process, the summation of two or more time-phase curves is not exponential and can exhibit a considerable departure from a semilogarithmic straight line. Such a departure is illustrated by a curve recorded by a counter placed directly over the precordium (Fig. 3). The

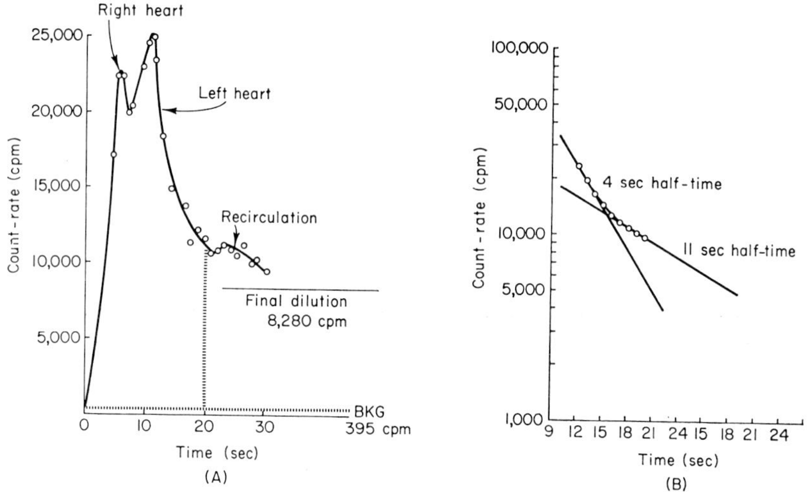

FIG. 3. (A) Dilution curve obtained by counter focused directly over mid-precordium. (B) Descending line shows two components of 4 and 11 sec due to right and left heart clearance. Extrapolation area corresponds to 35% of total area (*15*).

descending line in this case is affected by the clearance of both the right and left chambers. With this dual clearance, different values of the clearance constant would be obtained, depending on which points are emphasized. Since the extrapolated area is commonly 20 to 40% of the total area, a few seconds' variation in clearance time may double the observed cardiac output. It is advisable, therefore, to avoid any precordial site that might exhibit equal contributions from both chambers.

One approach has been to select preferentially either one of the two heart chambers to obtain a reasonably long period of single phase extrapolation. In Fig. 4 a predominantly left heart curve and in Fig. 5 a

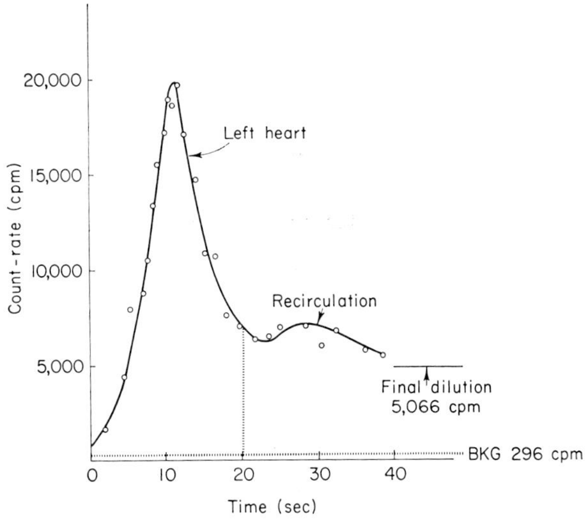

FIG. 4. Predominantly left heart curve *(15)*. Calculated cardiac output of 6.9 liters/min. Ratio of extrapolated area to total area is 30%. Half-time of extrapolated line is 6.5 sec.

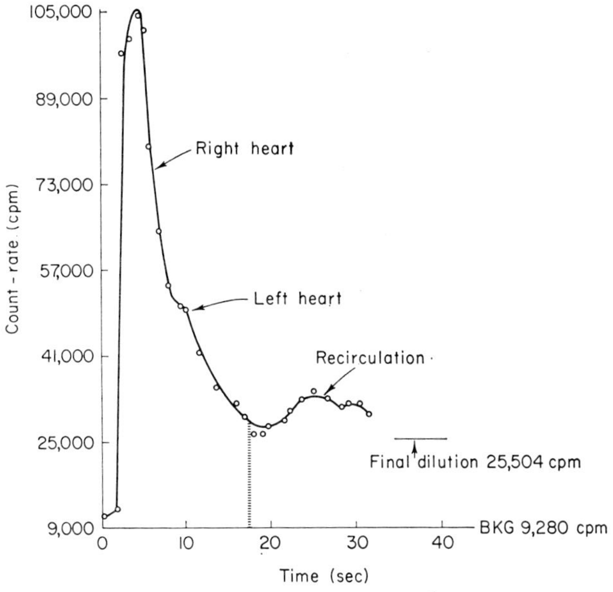

FIG. 5. Predominantly right heart curve *(15)*. Calculated cardiac output of 6.5 liters/min. Ratio of extrapolated area to total area is 22%. Half-time of clearance is 5.5 sec.

predominantly right heart curve are illustrated. In both cases the line of extrapolation is sufficiently long for accurate prediction. Thus, two criteria have been followed. The first is to maximize a single chamber clearance so as to keep the extrapolated area at a minimum and the second is to obtain as many points on the descending portion of the final dilution curve as possible. If these conditions are observed, the choice of placement of the radiation detector is secondary and may be made to fit the specific geometric configuration at hand (*19*).

C. Detector Collimation

From the above considerations it has been indicated that the external counting method requires minimizing the capillary contribution and at the same time restricting the field of view to the large chambers. For this reason most investigators have selected a cylindrical aperture in the range of 2.5 to 4.0 cm in diameter with the crystal recessed 5 to 10 cm from the surface. The recession from the surface reduces the effect of inverse square geometry so that the capillary volume at the chest wall will not be detected with a much greater efficiency than the radioactive material in the heart chambers. The diameter of the collimator should be sufficiently large to obtain a high counting efficiency while at the same time restricting the field of view to the region of one heart chamber.

Too wide collimation results in a volume other than the mixing chamber to be observed and thus a falsely high final concentration is recorded. Too narrow collimation results in lower counting efficiency and requires a more exact placement of the collimator (*15*) but makes it easier to concentrate on a single chamber. Typical collimators used for cardiac output measurements are shown in Fig. 6. It should be emphasized that a fairly wide variety of collimators has been used for these studies. Each variation exhibits differences in terms of depth dependence, in volumes seen other than the heart chambers, and in multiple contributions from the two chambers.

Differences in collimation allow variations in counting techniques. Areas of the heart that have exhibited suitable curves with the collimator of Fig. 6A are shown in Fig. 7. For the technique of maximizing the contribution from a single chamber, the single lined areas indicate satisfactory sites while the cross-shaded area appears unsatisfactory. The latter area could be satisfactory, however, with higher resolution which would be capable of resolving the two components of the curve as shown in Fig. 2.

The resolution can also be increased by delivering the dose to the chamber of the heart in a highly concentrated volume. Various cardiac curves recorded from the same site but with different injection techniques are shown in Fig. 8. In Fig. 8A the injection of a 3-ml volume of radio-

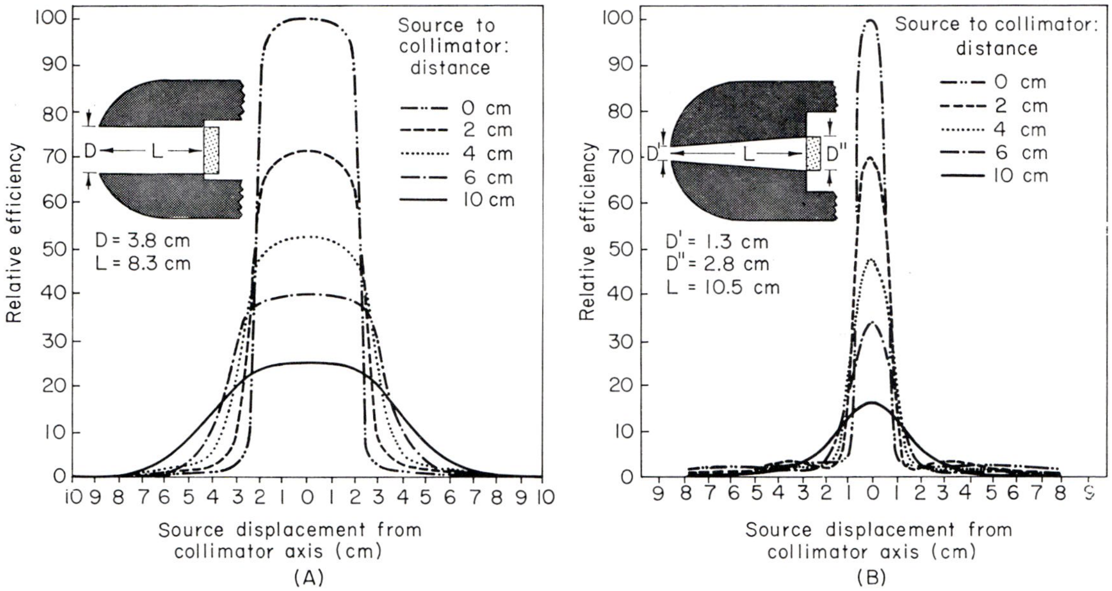

FIG. 6. Dimension and depth response of two types of collimators (*19*). (A) Cylindrical collimator of moderate collimation and (B) tapered collimator of high collimation. While the high collimation of B allows greater isolation of one heart chamber the efficiency is less than $\frac{1}{20}$ of that of collimator A. Collimator A has been used for all dilution curves in Fig. 2-5.

isotope dilution was followed by a 10-ml saline flush to hasten the inflow into the heart. A predominantly left heart curve was obtained with this particular placement of the collimator with a resolved small peak from the right chamber of the heart. In Fig. 8B the same 3-ml volume injected with no flush resulted in a less discrete curve. The peak of the curve is not displaced appreciably in time but the final slope of clearance is slower. In Fig. 8C an 8-ml injection without a flush resulted in a slower rise, a displacement of the peak later in time, and a much delayed final clearance. Although flushing compresses the trailing end of the volume injected into a smaller volume, theoretically it affects the quantification of the cardiac curve only little. However, the slope and length of the clearance curve determine the accuracy of the extrapolation as well as the percentage of the extrapolated area to the total area. For example, in Fig. 8A, 8B, and 8C the percentages of the extrapolated areas to the total

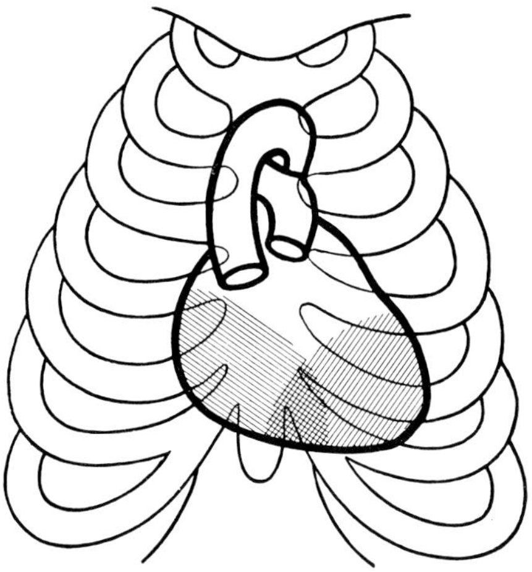

FIG. 7. Diagram of precordium (*19*). Single lined areas indicate regions from which satisfactory cardiac output curves were recorded with either predominant right or left contributions using high or moderate collimation. The cross-shaded areas are regions giving rise to double peaked curves which were difficult to extrapolate with high collimation techniques.

area are respectively 17%, 34%, and 39%. The larger the extrapolated area becomes the greater is the potential error of the method.

D. Recording Equipment

In addition to the selection of a suitable collimator to insure consistency of the final mixing volume with the volume of the dilution curve, the only other critical factor is the preservation of the fidelity of the cardiac curve. In the recorded decay rates, clearance half-times as short as 2 sec are commonly observed.

These clearance curves are recorded by a count ratemeter (Chapter 7,

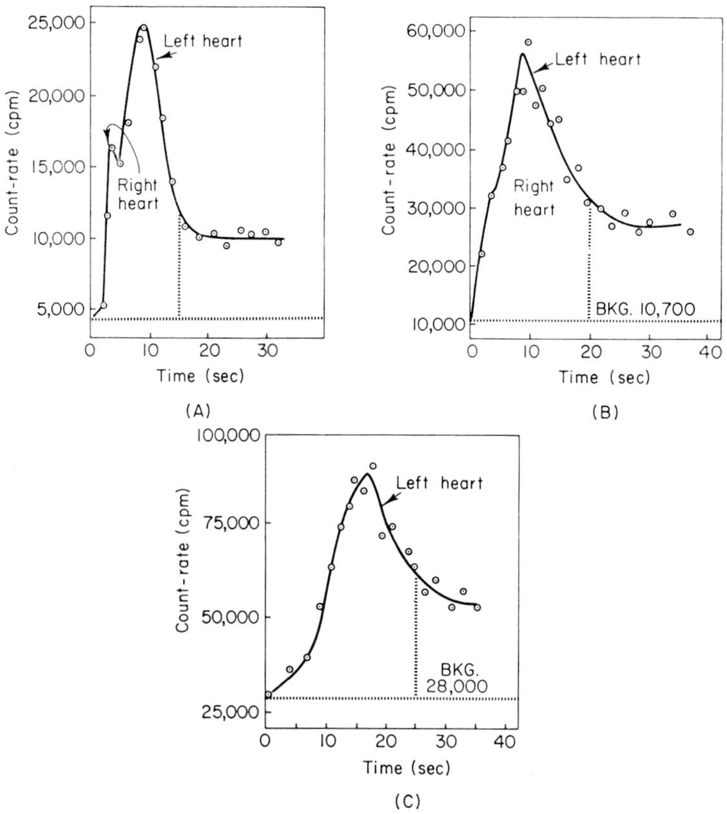

FIG. 8. Curves from same patient recorded at same precordial site with decreasing rates of injection (*19*). Calculated cardiac output from curve A, 7.4 liters/min; from curve B, 6.7 liters/min; and from curve C, 6.1 liters/min. Half-time clearances of the above curves, 3.5, 9.3, and 10 sec, respectively.

Section VI,B) with the basic circuit shown in Fig. 9. Although at equilibrium the voltage, V, is in direct relationship to the steady state current, i, this relationship is not maintained when i represents a varying function with respect to time. If we consider the case where the imposed current is an exponential function of the form $(i = i_0e^{-\lambda t})$, the differential equation describing the voltage V is then

$$(dV/dt) + (V/RC) = (i_0e^{-\lambda t}/C) \tag{8}$$

If it may be assumed that the readout voltage $V = V_0$ at time zero, the expression for the voltage as a function of time is then

$$V = [V_0/(1 - RC\lambda)][e^{-\lambda t} - RC\lambda e^{-t/RC}] \tag{9}$$

Only in the case where the time constant of the count ratemeter is very much smaller than the inverse of the decay constant λ $(RC \ll 1/\lambda)$ does the readout voltage have an exact relationship with the imposed exponential, since Eq. 9 reduces to

$$V = V_0 e^{-\lambda t} \tag{10}$$

Even in the case where the ratemeter time constant is as small as one fifth of the inverse of the decay constant ($RC = 1/5\lambda$) a considerable error in the observed readout voltage can arise. Substitution of this term in Eq. 9 gives the expression

$$V = V_0[\tfrac{5}{4}e^{-\lambda t} - \tfrac{1}{4}e^{-5\lambda t}] \tag{11}$$

The choice of the RC time constant affects the integration of the function under the exponential decay. Integration of Eq. 11 with time from

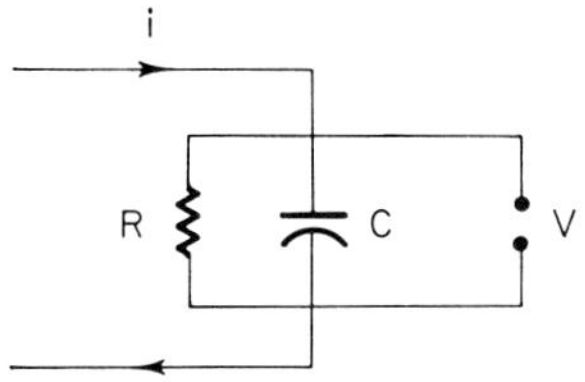

FIG. 9. Basic circuit of count ratemeter.

zero to infinity yields a value $\%_5$ as large as the corresponding integration of Eq. 10. Thus even with the common practice of using a ratemeter time constant five times as fast as the variation of the phenomenon observed, an error of 16% in area can be introduced.

In view of the mechanism of the basic RC circuit of the conventional ratemeter such an error is not unexpected. What has been largely neglected, however, is the utilization of such expressions as Eq. 11 as correction factors in this type of recording.

The time lag of the readout voltage with respect to the imposed current is an inherent property of the RC current and is commonly referred to as the memory effect of the ratemeter. It is primarily to reduce this memory effect that many other devices have been designed. In general these devices are digital in nature and involve the measurement of the time required to collect a specified number of counts or the measurement of the number of counts collected in a specified period of time. This has been accomplished by the use of scalers with printing timers (*11*), strip chart recorders with a side marking pen which records the time between successive collections of counts (*7*), and digital ratemeters (*8*).

III. DETERMINATION OF ORGAN BLOOD FLOW BY THE CLEARANCE OF RADIOACTIVE TRACERS FROM CIRCULATING BLOOD

The previous description of the tracer dilution method of determining blood flow may be viewed as a *direct* method, wherein the injected radioisotope does not interact with the organ itself but merely provides a convenient index of dilution. The data required thus involve both the measurement of the amount of the material flowing into an organ and the concentration of this material as it leaves the organ.

From a similar rationale, the clearance method may be thought of as an *indirect* system, since the concentrations of the flow into and out of a specific organ must not necessarily be known. Instead, all that is needed for this type of analysis is the rate of removal of the injected material from the circulating blood as a whole. This type of measurement is based on the selection of a material for which only one site or organ is responsible for its removal. Thus the rate of change in the concentration of the radioisotope in the circulating blood must be an indication of the blood flow through the organ resulting in its removal.

Such a method postulates that the mass, dm, removed from the bloodstream per unit time must be proportional to the efficiency of removal, a, the concentration of material in the circulating blood, c, and the flow rate, F, through the organ. This relationship yields the equation:

$$dm = -aFc\,dt \tag{12}$$

Utilizing the additional relationship that the mass removed, dm, must be equal to the volume of dilution, V, multiplied by the change in concentration, dc,

$$dm = V dc \tag{13}$$

Eq. 12 may be integrated into the usual exponential form:

$$c = c_0 \exp\left[-a(F/V)t\right] \tag{14}$$

where c_0 represents the concentration after the initial injection. The integration may be accomplished, of course, only if the quantities a, F, V may be considered constant during the time of measurement.

Since Eq. 14 represents an exponentially declining curve, its slope, λ, may be determined by a semilogarithmic plot of the concentration versus time curve. Then

$$\lambda = a(F/V) \qquad \text{or} \qquad F = V(\lambda/a) \tag{15}$$

To apply this method to a specific blood flow measurement, all that is required is a substance which is removed only by the organ whose blood flow is to be measured, a determination of the volume of dilution for the injected substance, and a known efficiency of its removal.

A. Hepatic Blood Flow Measurements

One obvious application of the clearance method has been the measurement of hepatic blood flow based on the rate of removal of colloidal particles from the peripheral blood by the reticuloendothelial (Kupffer) cells. Since the primary sites of reticuloendothelial cells are the liver and spleen, the rate of clearance of colloidal material must depend mainly on the blood flow to these organs.

Since colloids do not readily diffuse out of the circulating blood, the volume of dilution, V, in Eq. 15 is equal to the circulating blood volume. Some difficulty has been encountered with the evaluation of the efficiency of removal, a. The usual preparation of radiocolloids results in a spectrum of particle sizes, not all of which are cleared with the same efficiency. Depending upon this spectrum of sizes, probabilities of aggregation, or variable combining factors, the concentration, c, in Eq. 14 may be thought of as a summation of initial concentrations with different efficiencies of removal (*13*). Thus,

$$c = \sum_i c_i$$

and

$$c = c_1 \exp\left(-a_1 \frac{F}{V} t\right) + c_2 \exp\left(-a_2 \frac{F}{V} t\right) + \cdots \qquad (16)$$

The first colloid used for such determinations was colloidal chromic phosphate tagged with ^{32}P (*4*). While this material was satisfactory in animal studies it was not considered as useful in man (*20*). With the introduction of colloidal ^{198}Au (*31*) the advantages of γ-ray emission and subsequently the application of external counting techniques could be utilized.

Because of variations in particle size, the extraction of colloidal gold has not been constant and has differed considerably from the theoretical 100% (*10, 17*). In most cases, however, the disappearance curve may be adequately described as a two-component system (*10, 16*). If it is assumed that the most rapidly clearing component exhibits a clearance efficiency, a, approaching 100%, the decay constant may be determined graphically (Fig. 10) and liver blood flow can be calculated by Eq. 15.

Various methods have been employed for the measurement of this disappearance curve. While the early measurements were performed with withdrawn samples, the number of samples required, especially for the slow component, becomes restrictive. External counting methods have been employed (*3, 28*) by directing a counter over large blood pools. While the most obvious pool to be selected is the large chamber of the heart, the proximity of the liver complicates the placement of the counter in that area. With the accumulation of the colloid by the liver, the background is continually changing even for a well-shielded detector. For that reason a more common placement has been laterally over the temporal region of the head using wide collimators as illustrated in Fig. 6A.

The instrumentation requirements are in general less stringent than those for the cardiac output techniques. Conventional ratemeters are acceptable since the half-times of clearances are seldom less than 3 min in man or under 1 min in animal studies. Again caution must be exercised so as to be sure the time constant of the ratemeter does not cause a distortion of the actual data.

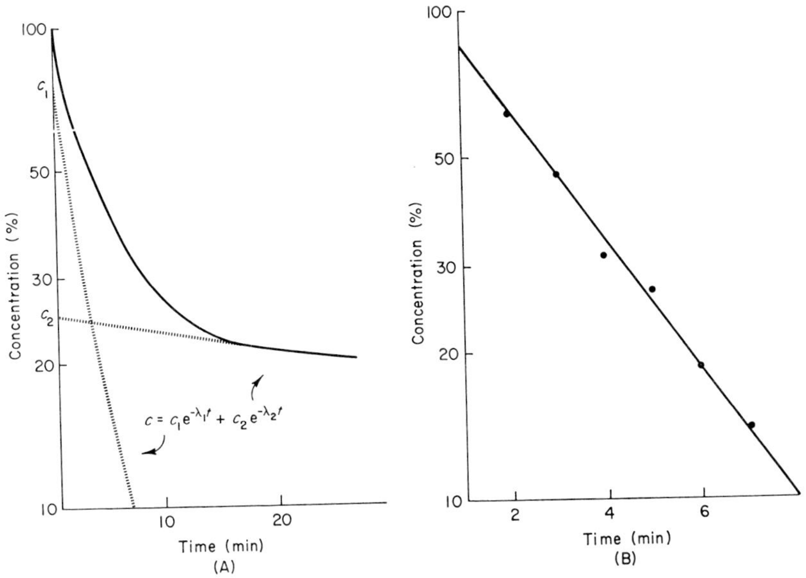

FIG. 10. Typical disappearance curve of colloidal ^{198}Au from external recording over the right temporal region of the head (*12*). The dotted line of the fast component in A is shown plotted on a time-expanded scale in B.

It must be emphasized that any clearance method must be a measurement of effective flow, not actual flow. Thus in the case of arteriovenous shunting, the actual flow may stay in the normal range even though the removal of the tracer material is drastically reduced and the effective flow drops subsequently. In this case the slower clearance is indicative of a reduced functional flow to the liver, or a decrease in the perfusion of functioning sinusoids.

In a similar sense, it is possible to use a colloid that has a reduced clearance by the reticuloendothelial cells in the liver but has an increased clearance by the cells in bone marrow. Techniques are now available for producing some colloids with a wide range in particle size, such as heat-denatured human serum albumin labeled with radioiodine (*1, 24*). By administration of the same colloid in various particle sizes and measurement of its removal by the liver, it may be determined what particle sizes are primarily removed by hepatic extraction and what particle sizes should be used for measurements of extra hepatic extraction.

B. Renal Blood Flow Measurements

An analysis similar to hepatic blood flow has been applied to the calculation of renal blood flow following the administration of ^{131}I-tagged *o*-iodohippurate (Hippuran). This measurement is somewhat more complicated than the colloid techniques since the *o*-iodohippurate is not confined to the circulating blood but diffuses out into a larger volume of dilution. Figure 11 illustrates the decrease in concentration of *o*-iodohippurate in the blood as a function of time.

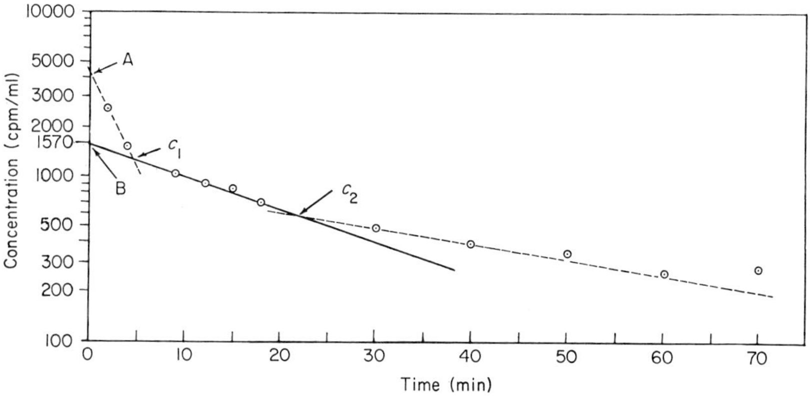

FIG. 11. Disappearance of radioactive Hippuran from the circulating blood of a dog as measured by withdrawn blood samples (*18*). Note the three phases present. Simplified calculation of renal blood flow is based on the measurement of slope between c_1 and c_2 and the volume of dilution calculated from intercept B and the injected dose. Primary mixing occurs between intercept A and point c_1.

Various models have been proposed for the interpretation of this disappearance. Some investigators (*2, 33*) have assumed a two-compartment model as shown in Fig. 12. In this model V_1 represents the vascular space, V_2 the extravascular space of the *o*-iodohippurate dilution, and F is the blood flow rate into the kidney. This analysis thus predicts a double exponential decay of the form

$$c = A \exp(-\lambda_1 t) + B \exp(-\lambda_2 t) \qquad (17)$$

where A is the intercept of the fast component on the concentration ordinate, B is the intercept of the slow component on the concentration ordinate, and λ_1 and λ_2 are the disappearance constants or slopes of the semilogarithmic lines. From this expression, the equation for renal blood flow F in milliliters per minute may be derived as

$$F = I\lambda_1\lambda_2/(A\lambda_2 + B\lambda_1) \tag{18}$$

where I equals the injected dose. In this model it is assumed that the fast component is influenced by the diffusion out of the vascular system into a secondary space and that the same diffusion constant α (Fig. 12) is present in the reverse direction to delay the re-entry into the vascular component. In addition the boundary condition assumed for the solution is based on instantaneous mixing in the vascular space.

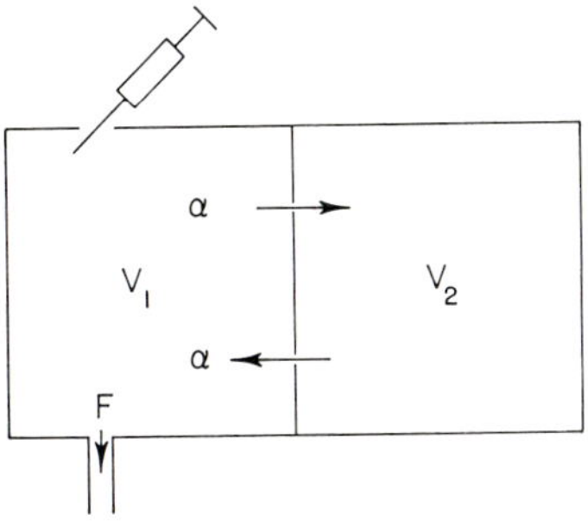

FIG. 12. Two-compartment model of *o*-iodohippurate mixing and excretion. See text for explanation.

Other investigators (*18, 26*) have attributed the early portion of the disappearance curve to mixing and dilution phases and have assumed that once equilibrium is reached the clearance of the slower phase serves as a close approximation for the clearance due to extraction from renal blood flow alone. With this approximation, the equation for renal blood flow may be expressed as

$$F = (I/B)\lambda_2 \tag{19}$$

where again I is the injected dose, B the intercept at time zero of the slow phase on the concentration ordinate, and λ_2 the semilogarithmic slope of the second phase of the curve. Since the term I/B represents the total dilution volume, V, the expression for renal flow then is similar to Eq. 15.

The discrepancy between calculations based on the two different models will be no greater than the ratio of $A\lambda_2$ to $B\lambda_1$. What is more important are the assumptions that both models imply. That the model may be considerably more complicated has been demonstrated by long-term monitoring (*6*) showing four resolvable components for the Hippuran disappearance as illustrated in Fig. 13.

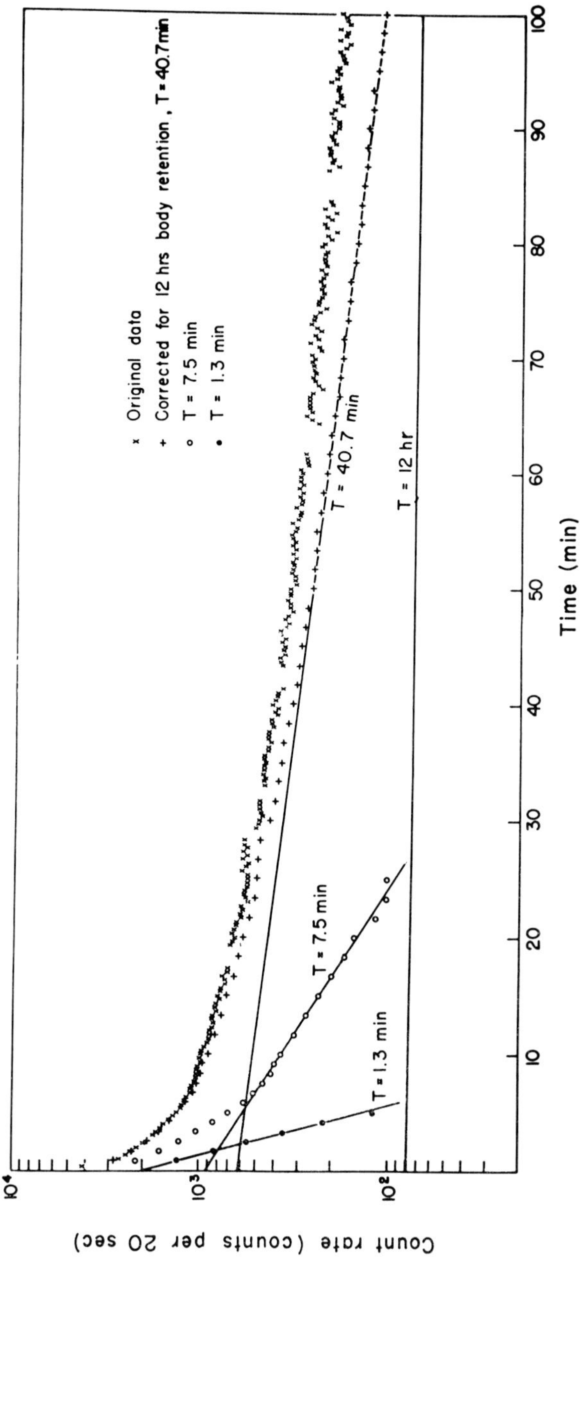

FIG. 13. Disappearance of radioactive Hippuran as recorded by precordial monitoring *(6)*. Counts were integrated for 20 sec from a 100-min magnetic tape recording of all pulses. The 12-hour half-time was derived from body retention data and contains about 5% of the original dose.

The data of Fig. 13 were obtained from a magnetic tape recording of the disappearance curve. This has the advantage that the various time phases may be examined without preselection of time constants and without loss of the original data. While most of the renal blood flow measurements have been obtained by withdrawn samples of peripheral blood, Fig. 13 demonstrates that external methods similar to hepatic flow measurements may be possible. While empirical correlations have been successful, further elucidation of the compartmental model of the Hippuran dilution is still needed before renal blood flow alone can be identified.

C. Applications to Other Organs

The above methods have been characterized by the injection of radioactive materials whose removal is confined to a specific body site. Somewhat similar principles may be applied to materials that are not metabolized by a specific organ but that may be injected directly into a selected organ. The flow of the tracer material may be expressed by Eq. 20.

$$Fc_a = Fc_v + V(\Delta c_t/\Delta t) \tag{20}$$

This equation merely represents the conservation of the tracer material. The rate of input of tracer brought to an organ is equal to the flow rate, F, to that organ, multiplied by the arterial concentration, c_a. This in turn must be equal to the rate of tracer leaving the organ, Fc_v, where c_v is the venous concentration, in addition to the rate of tracer deposition in the tissue. This accumulation may be expressed as the volume of the organ or region, V, multiplied by the change of concentration in the tissue per unit time, $\Delta c_t/\Delta t$. Solving for flow rate, F, per unit mass then results in the expression

$$F/V = \frac{dc_t/dt}{c_a - c_v} \tag{21}$$

This equation may be expressed in the integral form as

$$F/V = c_t \bigg/ \int_0^t [c_a - c_v]\, dt \tag{22}$$

which is the Kety–Schmidt formula for blood flow rate per unit mass of tissue (*9*).

If we express the concentration of the tracer in the tissue, c_t, as the product of venous concentration, c_v, multiplied by a partition coefficient, S, Eq. 21 may then be expressed as

$$dc_t/dt = (F/VS)(c_aS - c_t) \tag{23}$$

which may be integrated into the expression

$$c_t = c_{t_0} \exp(-(F/VS)t) \tag{24}$$

While originally applied to cerebral blood flow *(9)* it is obvious that this procedure can be applied wherever a direct injection into the arterial supply of an organ can be made. This method has been postulated for the use of substances that are not metabolized, such as the noble gases ^{85}Kr and ^{133}Xe. The measurement consists then primarily of determining the rate of washout of the injected tracer, as obtained by semilogarithmic plotting. As before, the disappearance constant λ of the

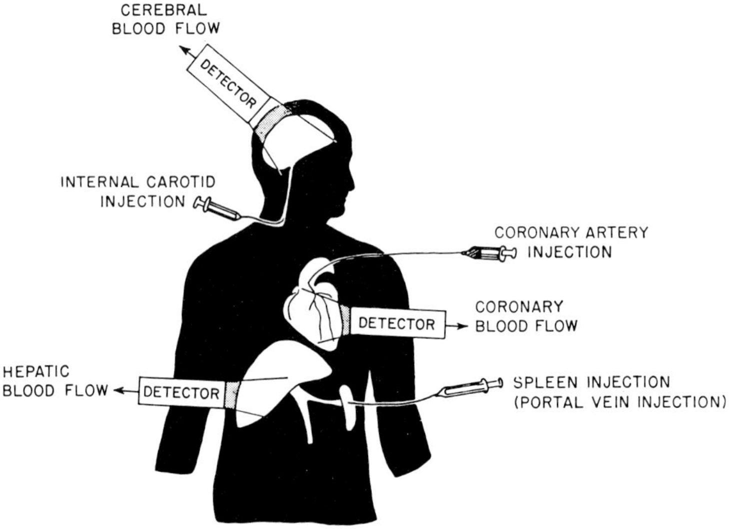

FIG. 14. Schematic presentation of various sites of injection and monitoring techniques for measuring regional blood flow by determining the rate of clearance of a radioactive gas injected into the blood supply of this region *(32)*.

curve, is equal to the exponent F/VS. Some of the many possible variations of this type of measurement are illustrated schematically by Fig. 14.

The instrumentation techniques for these types of measurement are no different from those described above. In each case the collimation must be adapted so as to subtend a large segment of the organ but without overlapping into adjacent areas. As always, shielding from other sites is mandatory and since the entire measurement is based on a rate determination, no distortion by the ratemeter time constant can be permitted.

IV. MEASUREMENT OF ORGAN FUNCTION BY ACCUMULATION OR DISAPPEARANCE MEASUREMENTS

The process of obtaining information as to the function of an organ or physiological system by means of following the accumulation, uptake, or metabolism of a radioisotope is represented by perhaps the oldest and best established application of radioactivity to a clinical, diagnostic measurement. This application is, of course, the use of radioiodine to measure the function of the thyroid gland (Chapter 14).

In view of the success of this test it is surprising that only few similar applications have been established with external counting techniques. The reason may be found by examining the three requirements of the method. First, the substance must be concentrated primarily in one site or organ. Second, the accumulation or release of the substance must be sufficiently rapid so as to make a continuous recording clinically feasible. Third, a separation of the measured parameters must be readily established between the normal and the abnormal state.

It is the combination of the last two requirements that has been responsible for so few tests being established. While many substances exhibit a difference in metabolism in the normal and abnormal states, most of these variations are manifested in terms of hours or days rather than in minutes. In this category can be listed such well-known tests as radiocobalt-tagged vitamin B_{12}, tagged protein, tagged fats, electrolyte distribution, iron metabolism, and many others. Since few continuous external measurements are practical beyond an hour, except for whole-body measurements (Chapters 20, 21), the above differentials have been established primarily through withdrawn peripheral samples and fall into the category of *in vitro* measurements.

Two measurements have met the above requirements of site selectivity and rapid accumulation and release. These tests are the use of ^{131}I-tagged rose bengal for liver function and the I^{131} Hippuran renal function test.

A. Liver Function Tests by External Hepatogram

Following the discovery of the affinity of various halogenated phenolphthaleins for the liver, the clearance of bromsulfalein (BSP) from the blood has become a widely used clinical test for liver function. While as a substitution, a radioactive dye such as radioiodine-tagged rose bengal could be used in a similar clearance test, more attention has been directed to the accumulation and release of this material by direct measurement with an external γ-ray detector.

As originally proposed (*29, 34*), this test was concerned primarily with such parameters as time of maximum liver uptake, half-time of accumulation, and rate of release. These measurements made over the liver were often supplemented by external measurements of blood clearance by a detector placed over the head, and by a detector focused over the midabdominal area below the liver edge in order to detect the presence of radioactivity released by the common duct into the bowel. An illustration of these three types of measurement is shown in Fig. 15.

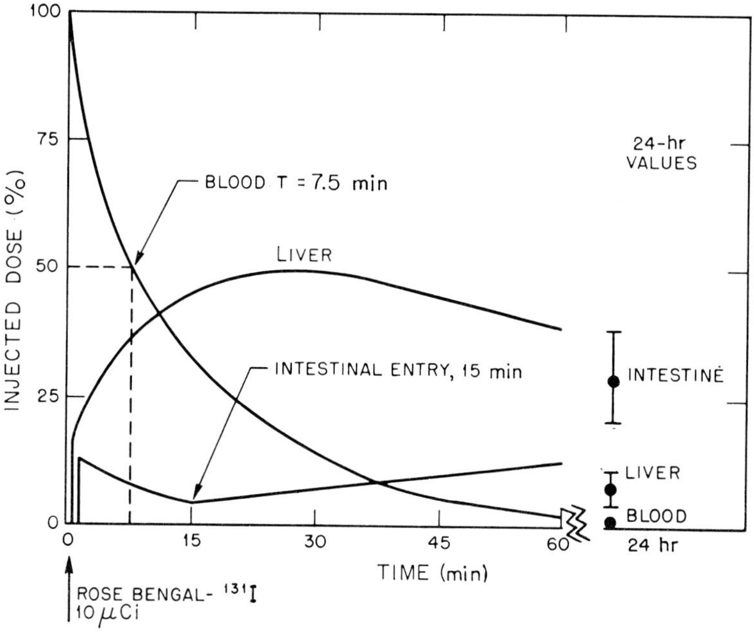

FIG. 15. Concentrations of ^{131}I rose bengal in the blood, liver, and intestine as a function of time (*27*).

Many parameters have been suggested in order to differentiate various abnormal aspects of the curve. While the most direct determination would be that of the clearance constant, measured either by disappearance of the material from the blood or by the accumulation in the liver, many other values have been utilized. Ratios of count-rates at various times, half-times of release, and time of appearance of activity in the bowel have all been considered. The direct measurement over the liver has the advantage of determining an ever increasing specific radioactivity as compared to the difficult problem of the external clearance methods, where the concentration is progressively less and the counts are more and more subject to statistical fluctuations. Thus a smaller amount of radioactive material may be used while still a well-defined curve can be obtained. The exponential curves of accumulation and clearance theoretically should be reciprocals of each other. However, it must be realized that the curve recorded over the liver represents both the accumulation of the tagged dye by the liver cells and the decrease of radioactivity through the clearance of the dye from the vascular supply of the liver. Even so, some investigators (*21*) have found the accumulation curves more indicative of various disease states with liver blood flow alterations than the disappearance curves.

With the advent of the heat-denatured serum albumin aggregates, interest has been revived in the general techniques of accumulation and release of this material in the liver. While this technique has not yet attained the status of a routine laboratory test, it is possible that eventual standardization of some type of measurement will permit more accessible correlation with clinical diagnosis.

B. Kidney Function Tests by the Renogram

Qualitatively, the radioisotope renogram measures the same basic parameters as the liver function test, namely the concentration of radioactivity in the vascular region of the kidney, the accumulation of the material by the kidney, and the subsequent release in the urine. As shown by a typical Hippuran renogram of Fig. 16, all of these times are somewhat faster than the liver curve with rose bengal.

In terms of complexity of interpretation, the kidney has provided even more difficulty than the liver. To begin with, the liver is a large organ that is relatively homogeneous, so that a well-shielded collimator such as shown in Fig. 6A can sample a characteristic segment of the liver in most cases without receiving appreciable counts from adjacent areas. Thus choice of aperture, crystal size, and distance from the liver are all relatively unimportant.

This is not so in the case of kidney measurements. Since each kidney is smaller and does not concentrate the kidney function material uniformly throughout its parenchyma, the slope of the renogram may be greatly influenced by the choice of the detector, its aperture, and its placement. These factors still vary greatly as applied by present investigators. Some investigators (*6, 29*) have adopted collimator apertures of 4–5 cm in diameter, with the crystal recessed 4–5 cm from the opening. Placement of these detectors has been flush with the skin over the renal areas, usually the area of greatest radioactivity. Other investigators (*30*) feel it is more important for the detector to subtend the entire kidney and have gone to 3-inch diameter crystals placed as far away as 18–23 cm from the skin. With such variations in the field of view, the configuration of the renogram curve is qualitatively but not quantitatively the same. One must exercise great caution when attempting to correlate the specific values determined by one investigator with those obtained by others using widely different measurement techniques.

In addition, various physiological conditions cause variations of the renogram. The degree of hydration of the patient, the amount of carrier Hippuran, and the urinary flow rate greatly affect the character of the curve. Even differences in position of the subject during the

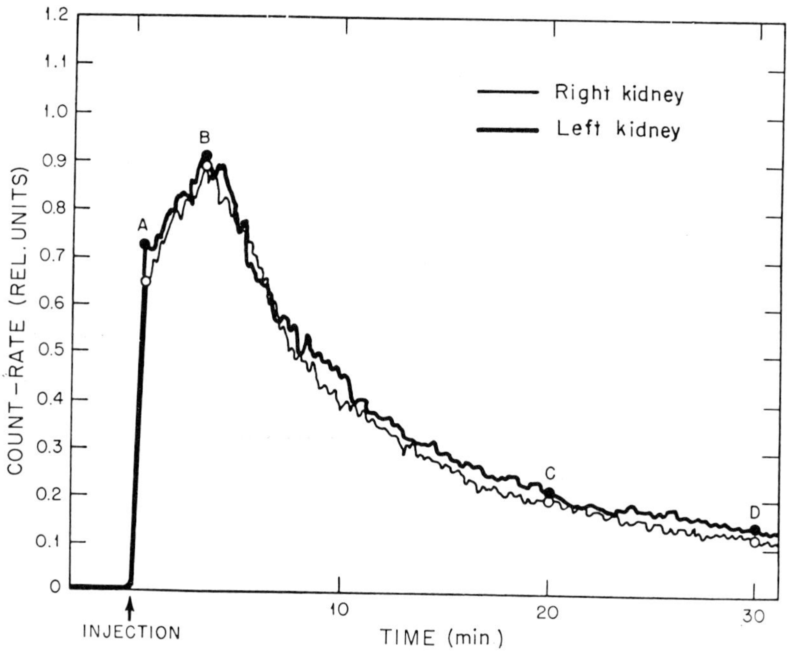

FIG. 16. Typical normal renogram obtained with one detector over each renal area (*30*). Curves from the two kidneys are superimposed. Point *A*, primarily an index of size of the renal vascular bed, occurs 15 to 30 sec after injection of the Hippuran. Point *B* is the point of highest accumulation and the segment *BCD* is indicative of Hippuran release.

measurements, either in a sitting or prone position, cause some variation in the recorded curve.

The type of kidney function material chosen also influences the appearance of the curve. In the early investigations, tagged Diodrast, Miokon, Urokon, and other contrast materials were used. At the present time most renograms are obtained with some form of *o*-iodohippurate (Hippuran).

Though the renogram curve is influenced by all of the variables mentioned above, there is general agreement that the renogram consists primarily of three phases (Fig. 16). The first segment, consisting of the primary sharp rise, reflects the appearance of the radioactivity in the vascular segment of the kidney as well as the surrounding tissues subtended by the detector. The second phase represents primarily the accumulation of the material in the kidney with secondary effects due to clearance of the material from the circulating blood and possible early excretion from the kidney. The third segment represents excretion from the kidney as well as further clearance from the blood. It is obvious that the volume and specific areas of the kidney seen by the detector as well as the surrounding regions will cause variations in all three segments. Especially important are the contributions from extrarenal areas which may reflect blood clearance throughout and urine drainage from the upper urinary passages in the third segment of the curve.

Similar to the liver function studies, many investigators have considered the third portion of the curve most significant for evaluating kidney function. This is reasonable, since whether this segment of the curve reflects blood clearance or kidney excretion it must be closely correlated with the ability of the kidney to remove the radioactive material. Since a considerable amount of interest in the renogram has centered on the hypertensive patient, attention has also been directed to the earlier parts of the curve that may reflect renal blood flow.

Much effort has been directed to the correlation of various characteristics of the curve with other physiological or clinical parameters. Slopes of the segments, half-times of rise and clearance, and ratios of count-rate levels at specific times after injection have all been utilized to determine empirical indices for differentiation of normal or abnormal values with respect to renal blood flow and renal function in various categories of patients. The many variations of both techniques of analysis as well as measurement have made correlations between various laboratories quite difficult.

It is the unique advantage of the radioisotope method of external measurement over an organ that a full time course of the incorporation and release of a tracer material can be measured. At the same time, this advantage has perhaps been the greatest handicap to the progression of these measurements into accepted routine tests. The reason for this delay is that routine tests cannot be accepted without standardization. The arbitrary approach to standardize both the counting method and data analysis has handicapped both the liver and kidney function applications.

REFERENCES

1. Benacerraf, B., Biozzi, G., Halpern, B. N., Stiffel, C., and Mouton, D., Phagocytosis of heat-denatured human serum albumin labelled with I^{131} and its use as a means of investigating liver blood flow. *Brit. J. Exptl. Pathol.* **38,** 35 (1957).
2. Bianchi, C., and Toni, P., Possibilita di impiego dello o-iodo-ippurato di sodio (Hippuran) marcato con I^{131} per la valutazione della portata renale plasmatica. *Minerva Nucl.* **6,** 34 (1962).
3. Burkle, J. S., and Gliedman, M. L., External recording method for estimating hepatic blood flow with the use of radiogold. *Gastroenterology* **36,** 112 (1959).
4. Dobson, E. L., and Jones, H. B., The behavior of intravenously injected particulate material; its rate of disappearance from the bloodstream as measure of liver blood flow. *Acta Med. Scand.* **144,** Suppl. 273, 1 (1952).
5. Hamilton, W. F., Moore, J. W., Kinsman, J. M., and Spurling, R. G., Simultaneous determination of the pulmonary and systemic circulation times in man and of a figure related to the cardiac output. *Am. J. Physiol.* **84,** 338 (1928).
6. Hine, G. J., Farmelant, M. H., Cardarelli, J. A., and Burrows, B. A., Four channel magnetic tape recording and digital analysis of radio-Hippuran renal function tests in normal subjects. *J. Nucl. Med.* **4,** 371 (1963).
7. Huff, R. L., Feller, D. D., Judd, O. J., and Bogardus, G. M., Cardiac output of men and dogs measured by *in vivo* analysis of iodinated (I^{131}) human serum albumin. *Circulation Res.* **3,** 564 (1955).
8. Kaess, K., Gammacardiography. *In* "Clinical Applications of Nuclear Medicine," p. 44, Renner Clinic Foundation, Cleveland, Ohio, 1965.
9. Kety, S. S., and Schmidt, C. F., The nitrous oxide method for the quantitative determination of cerebral blood flow in man: theory, procedure, and normal values. *J. Clin. Invest.* **27,** 476 (1948).
10. Krook, H., Circulatory studies in liver cirrhosis. *Acta Med. Scand.* **156,** Suppl. 318, 1 (1956).
11. Love, W. D., O'Meallie, L. P., and Burch, G. E., Assessment of cerebral circulation by an external isotope technique. *J. Lab. Clin. Med.* **58,** 445 (1961).
12. MacIntyre, W. J., Christie, J. H., Koch-Weser, D., and Gomez-Crespo, G., The ratio of colloidal gold—Rose bengal clearance as a differential measurement of impaired hepatic function. *In* "Radioaktive Isotope in Klinik und Forschung" (K. Fellinger and R. Höfer, eds.), Vol. 5, p. 378, 1963.
13. MacIntyre, W. J., Moses, J. M., Schapiro, R. L., Koch-Weser, D., and Christie, J. H., Factors affecting the measurement of liver blood flow with radioactive colloids. *Proc. 7th Congr. Nucl.,* p. 30, Comitato Nazionale Energia Nucleare, Rome (1962).
14. MacIntyre, W. J., Pritchard, W. H., Eckstein, R. W., and Friedell, H. L., The determination of cardiac output by a continuous recording system utilizing iodinated (I^{131}) human serum albumin. Animal studies. *Circulation* **4,** 552 (1951).
15. MacIntyre, W. J., Pritchard, W. H., and Moir, T. W., The determination of cardiac output by the dilution method without arterial sampling. 1. Analytical concepts. *Circulation* **18,** 1139 (1958).
16. Meredith, O. M., Jr., Coffman, W., Post, J., and Holmes, J., Measurement of liver blood flow with radioactive colloidal gold. *Am. J. Physiol.* **202,** 1 (1962).
17. Playoust, M. R., McRae, J., and Boden, R. W., Inefficient hepatic extraction of colloidal gold: Resulting inaccuracies in determination of hepatic blood flow. *J. Lab. Clin. Med.* **54,** 728 (1959).

18. Pritchard, W. H., Eckstein, R. W., MacIntyre, W. J., and Dabaj, E., Correlation of renal blood flow determined by the single injection of Hippuran I^{131} with direct flow measurements. *Am. Heart. J.* **70,** 789 (1965).
19. Pritchard, W. H., MacIntyre, W. J., and Moir, T. W., The determination of cardiac output by the dilution method without arterial sampling. II. Validation of precordial recording. *Circulation* **18,** 1147 (1958).
20. Rankin, J. G., Playoust, M. R., and Beal, R. W., Significance of alterations in extraction and distribution of colloidal chromic phosphate in patients with liver disease. *J. Lab. Clin. Med.* **58,** 920 (1961).
21. Razzak, M. A., The use of radioactive isotopes to study the hemodynamic pattern, function and morphology of the liver in hepato-splenic bilharziasis (schistosomiasis). *J. Nucl. Med.* **5,** 125 (1964).
22. Rossi, H. H., Powers, S. H., and Dwork, B., Measurement of flow in straight tubes by means of the dilution technique. *Am. J. Physiol.* **173,** 103 (1953).
23. Sevelius, G. (ed.), "Radioisotopes and Circulation." Little, Brown, Boston, Massachusetts, 1965.
24. Shaldon, S., Chiandussi, L., Guevara, L., Caesar, J., and Sherlock, S., The estimation of hepatic blood flow and intrahepatic shunted blood flow by colloidal heat-denatured human serum albumin labeled with I^{131}. *J. Clin. Invest.* **40,** 1346 (1961).
25. Stewart, G. N., The output of the heart in dogs. *Am. J. Physiol.* **57,** 27 (1921).
26. Stokes, J. M., and Ter-Pogossian, M. M., Double isotope technique to measure renal function, single injection technique without urine collection. *J. Am. Med. Assoc.* **187,** 20 (1964).
27. Taplin, G. V., Dore, E. K., and Johnson, D. E., Hepatic blood-flow and reticuloendothelial-system studies with radiocolloids. *In* "Dynamic Clinical Studies with Radioisotopes" (R. M. Kniseley and W. N. Tauxe, eds.), TID-7678, p. 285. U.S. At. Energy Comm., Washington, D.C., 1964.
28. Taplin, G. V., Hayashi, J., Johnson, D. E., and Dore, E. K., Liver blood flow and cellular function in hepatobiliary disease. Tracer studies with radiogold and rose bengal. *J. Nucl. Med.* **2,** 204 (1961).
29. Taplin, G. V., Meredith, O. M., Jr., Kade, H., and Winter, C. C., The radioisotope renogram. An external test for individual kidney function and upper urinary tract patency. *J. Lab. Clin. Med.* **48,** 886 (1956).
30. Tauxe, W. N., Maher, F. T., and Hunt, J. C., The isotope renogram as a test of renal function. *In* "Dynamic Clinical Studies with Radioisotopes" (R. M. Kniseley and W. N. Tauxe, eds.), TID-7678, p. 383. U.S. At. Energy Comm., Washington, D.C., 1964.
31. Vetter, H., Falkner, R., and Neumayr, A., The disappearance rate of colloidal radio-gold from the circulation and its application to the estimation of liver blood flow in normal and cirrhotic subjects. *J. Clin. Invest.* **33,** 1594 (1954).
32. Wagner, H. N., Jr., Regional blood flow measurements with krypton-85 and xenon-133. *In* "Dynamic Clinical Studies with Radioisotopes" (R. M. Kniseley and W. N. Tauxe, eds.), TID-7678, p. 189. U.S. At. Energy Comm., Washington, D.C., 1964.
33. Wagoner, R. D., Tauxe, W. N., Maher, F. T., and Hunt, J. C., Measurement of effective renal plasma flow with sodium iodohippurate I^{131}. *J. Am. Med. Assoc.* **187,** 811 (1964).
34. Winter, C. C., A clinical study of a new renal function test: the radioactive diodrast renogram. *J. Urol.* **76,** 182 (1956).

CHAPTER 16

RADIOISOTOPE SCANNING

GORDON L. BROWNELL, SAUL ARONOW
PHYSICS RESEARCH LABORATORY
MASSACHUSETTS GENERAL HOSPITAL
BOSTON, MASSACHUSETTS
AND
GERALD J. HINE
INTERNATIONAL ATOMIC ENERGY AGENCY
VIENNA, AUSTRIA

I. SCANNING INSTRUMENTATION

Radioisotope scanning has found an important role in many diagnostic procedures. It was used first to delineate the thyroid gland and to determine hot or cold nodules in the gland. As ^{131}I was the isotope primarily used in these studies, most scanners were designed for use with that radioisotope. Even today this historical development is reflected in the fact that most scanners and collimators are designed for ^{131}I and for a focal distance of 3 inches. However, radioisotope scanning soon found other fields of use; particularly in localization of brain tumors, searching for metastases in the liver, delineation of kidneys, lungs, and heart, determination of position and size of the placenta, and other clinical applications (*21, 26, 34*).

Two major problems confront the designer of radioisotope scanners. First, it is necessary to achieve sufficient sensitivity so that the distribution of the radioactivity can be determined with adequate statistical precision. Second, it is necessary that the detecting device be capable of sufficient resolution so that the distribution of radioactivity can be reproduced with adequate detail. As in the design of most instruments these two requirements are in conflict, some compromise between the two must be reached.

The scintillation counter, with sodium iodide crystals, is a very sensitive detector which may record virtually all the radiation striking the crystal. The principal loss in sensitivity occurs in the collimating system, which is necessary to produce the desired resolution. In general, the higher the resolution, the lower the sensitivity. With most collimators this relationship is quite marked.

Although analogies can be carried only so far, there are many similarities between radioisotope scanners and devices that produce photographic images or that record X-ray pictures. In all cases, the object is to obtain a visually interpretable representation of the phenomena under consideration. In the case of photography, this is the intensity of light emitted at various points from a surface. In the case of diagnostic X-ray pictures, it is the variation in absorption of the X rays from point to point. In the case of radioisotope scanning, the original information lies in the distribution of a radioisotope throughout an organ or the body. The success of the technique is measured by the ability of the final picture to accurately reproduce the original distribution.

The radioisotope scanner described here is only one of several devices designed to delineate a radioisotope distribution in visual form. Other devices, such as positron scanners (Chapter 18), and various forms of stationary visualizing devices such as the scintillation camera (Chapter 19), differ considerably in construction but have many basic features in common with the conventional scanner. In particular, the choice of optimum resolution depends on the same parameters and the analysis proceeds in the same manner.

A. Components of Scanners

A radioisotope scanner consists of a number of components, which are illustrated schematically in Fig. 1. The focusing collimator scans the distribution of radioactivity, usually in two dimensions. The detector converts the γ radiation transmitted by the collimator into pulses, which can be further amplified and treated by the electronic components of the scanner. The readout system presents the processed information in a form suitable for visual interpretation. In the conventional mechanical scanner, a system of motors and controls moves the detection system with respect to the patient and synchronizes the readout with the position of

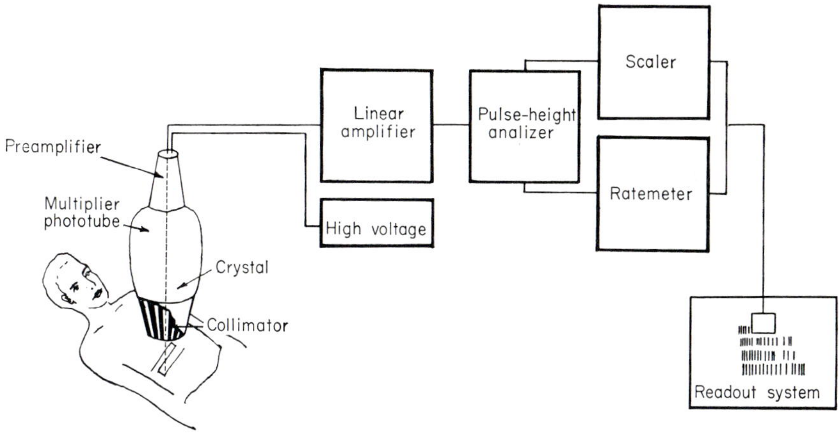

FIG. 1. Block diagram of radioisotope scanner.

the detector. Each of these components will be discussed in some detail in the following sections.

The radioactivity and its distribution are important in that they impose requirements on the scanner components. In general, the shape of the source is that of the organ to be visualized. The choice of the radioisotope determines the radiation viewed by the scanner and most important the flux of radiation emerging from the source which is available to the collimator. Some of the radiopharmaceuticals frequently used for scanning, the amounts required, and the time the scan is started after administration of the dose are listed in Table I.

The thyroid, which concentrates a large fraction of all iodine entering the body, presents a rather special scanning situation. The small size of the organ coupled with the high iodine uptake results in a high concentration of the radioactivity. Consequently, high-resolution scans can be readily obtained. The radiation background is usually not an important problem because of the low concentration of activity in the surrounding tissues.

TABLE I

EXAMPLES OF γ-RAY EMITTING RADIOPHARMACEUTICALS USED FOR SCANNING

Organ	Agent	Physical half-life (days)	Administered radioactivity (μCi)	Time of scanning after adminis-tration (hr)
Brain	Chlormerodrin-^{203}Hg	47	500–700	2–4
	Chlormerodrin-^{197}Hg	2.7	700–1,500	2–6
	Pertechnetate-^{99m}Tc	0.25	10,000–15,000	0.2–1
	Serum albumin-^{131}I	8	300–500	0.1–1
Bone	Strontium nitrate-^{85}Sr	65	50–100	48–72
Kidney	Chlormerodrin-^{203}Hg	47	100–150	1–5
	Chlormerodrin-^{197}Hg	2.7	200–400	1–5
Liver	Rose bengal-^{131}I	8	100–200	0.2–0.5
	Colloidal gold-^{198}Au	2.7	100–300	0.5–4
	Aggregated albumin-^{131}I	8	300–500	0.2–0.8
	Technetium sulfide-^{99m}Tc	0.25	2,000	0.2–1
Lung	Macro-aggregated serum albumin-^{131}I	8	250–350	0.1–2
	Macro-aggregated serum albumin-^{51}Cr	27.8	800–1,000	0.1–2
Pancreas	Selenomethionine-^{75}Se	120	200–300	0.2–0.5
Placenta	Serum albumin-^{99m}Tc	0.25	500–1,000	0.1–1
	Serum albumin-^{131}I	8	1–5	0.1–1
Pericardial effusion	Cholografin-^{131}I	8	250–500	0.1–0.5
	Serum albumin-^{99m}Tc	0.25	2,000	0.1–0.5
Spleen	Heated red cells-^{51}Cr	27.8	300–1,000	1–24
	BMHP-^{197}Hg	2.7	300–500	0.5–2
Thyroid	Sodium iodide-^{131}I	8	30–80	24–48
	Sodium iodide-^{125}I	60	50–100	24–48

The earliest scanners employed a single cylindrical bore collimator often in conjunction with a calcium tungstate crystal as radiation detector. Although these scanners had a very low sensitivity, they could delineate high levels of radioactivity in the thyroid gland. The development of the focusing collimator, consisting of a cluster of tapered apertures focused at a fixed point, led to considerably higher sensitivity (Chapter 17). This development was parallel with the advent of large sodium iodide crystals. Most scanners presently employ sodium iodide crystals of 3-inch diameter and 2-inch height.

The circuits used for pulse amplification, scaling, and obtaining average count-rates were developed early in scanning history. The incorporation of a pulse-height analyzer provided a substantial step forward in radioisotope scanning (Fig. 1). With a radioisotope that emits γ rays of essentially one energy, pulse-height analysis (that is, the use of the photopeak only) permits the exclusion of radiation which has been scattered in the source. As this scattered radiation will have originated away from the area of focus, the suppression of this radiation results in sharper scans.

The scanning speed and line spacing are variable in all scanners. Scanning speeds between 20 to 400 cm/min are commonly employed depending on the concentration of radioactivity within the organ and the time available for completing the scan. Obviously, the slower the scanning speed the better will be the statistical accuracy of the scan. On the other hand, large organs like the liver usually require scanning times of about 40 min at relatively fast scanning speeds. The choice of the line spacing is related to that of the scanning speed. If the scanner advances as little as 3 mm for each successive line, a scan readout with no empty space between the lines can be obtained. However, the more lines appear per unit area the faster must be the scanning speed for a given scanning time. The total information contained in a scan is proportional to scanning time independently of the actual number of lines as long as they are not spaced further apart than the resolution distance of the collimator (Section II,A).

A variety of readout systems offers several choices depending on personal preference and on the scanning problem. The earliest and simplest method of scan presentation and one which is still used is the dot record. In this method, a stylus moving over a piece of paper stamps a dot or bar for every fixed number of input pulses. The resultant scan shows a pictorial density variation proportional to the dot density and consequently to the count-rate at that position.

Photographic recording is now widely employed as a scanning readout system. A light which is moved over photographic film is focused to a point or a line. The light flashes once for a fixed number of input counts. The intensity of the light may be varied in proportion to the count-rate to give a nonlinear presentation of the variation of the radiation intensity in the source.

An electronic method, termed background suppression, eliminates all information from areas in the scan where the count-rate falls below a preselected value. The remainder of the scan is presented usually in a linear fashion. Color scanning has the effect of presenting on one scan contour levels corresponding to different erase levels without loss of any information. The various readout systems are discussed in detail in Section IV.

B. General Purpose Scanners

A general purpose scanner is shown in Fig. 2. The focusing collimator is located at the lower end of the shielded detector assembly, which includes a sodium iodide crystal, the multiplier phototube, and a preamplifier. The detection head is mounted on an arm which permits the

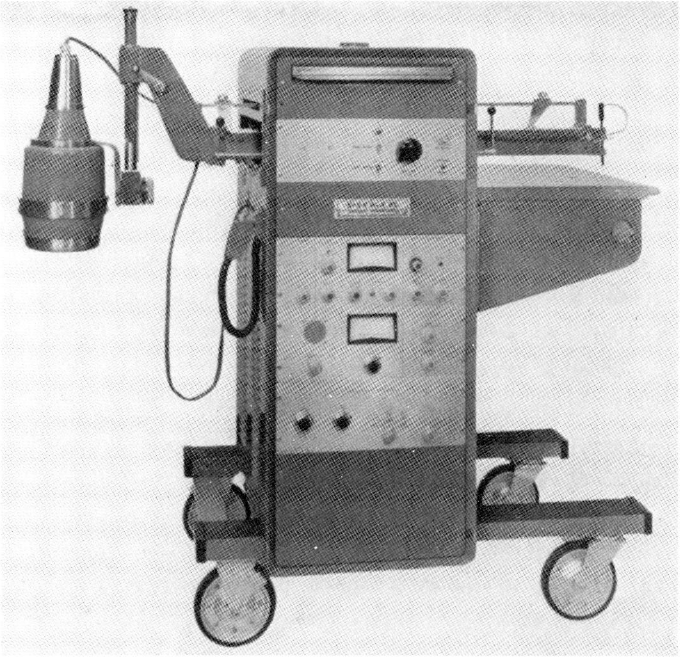

FIG. 2. A general purpose scanner with a focusing collimator detector. Readout provides both mechanical and photographic prints. (Courtesy of Picker Nuclear)

detector to be moved over the area to be scanned. This motion is usually continuous in one axis and stepwise in the perpendicular direction.

Scanners usually move in a horizontal plane with the patient lying on a bed. This is a matter of convenience, and some scanners have rotatable arms, allowing scanning in a vertical plane as well in order to scan a patient in a sitting position.

The electronic components, consisting of an amplifier, pulse-height analyzer, scaler, and count ratemeter, are located in the main console. In addition controls for scanning speed, line spacing, selection of background erase, and the various readout methods are required. Finally, the size of the scan area can be preselected by adjustment of limiting switches. Valuable time would be lost by scanning too large an area which contains no useful information.

Large-crystal scanners may be roughly grouped into those with 5- or 8-inch diameter crystals, all usually 2 inches thick. The object of using larger crystals is primarily an increase of sensitivity or to allow the use of higher-energy γ rays. Sometimes both factors are important. Figure 3

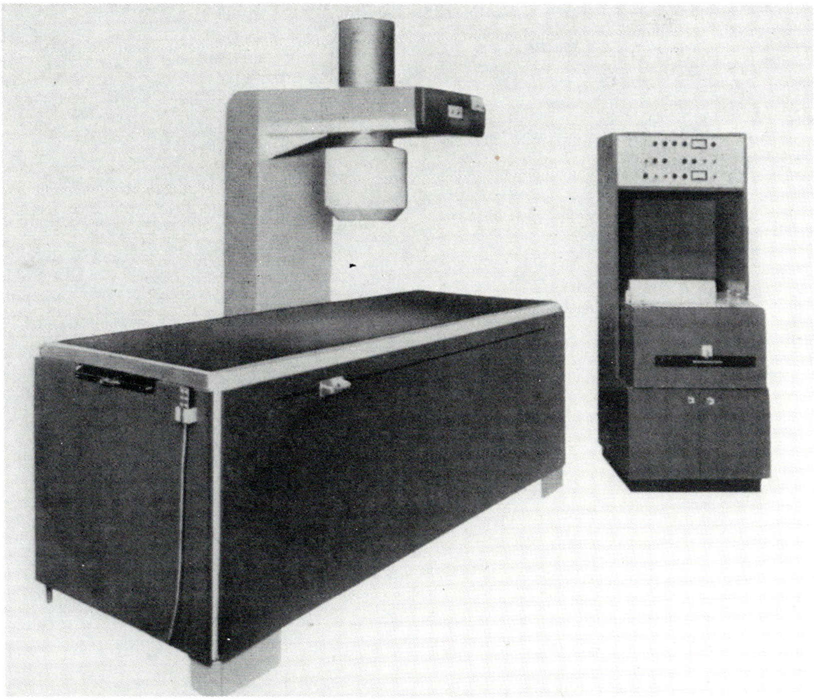

Fig. 3. A large-crystal scanner. This instrument has a 5-inch crystal above the patient and an 8-inch crystal mounted under the table. Both have focusing collimators. (Courtesy of Ohio-Nuclear, Inc.)

shows a scanner where a large-diameter crystal and shield move below the support for the patient. In other designs the detector assembly is fixed and the patient's bed moves. The increased sensitivity of large-crystal detectors is obtained at the price of greater criticality of the focusing properties of the collimator (Chapter 17, Section II,A).

C. Three-Dimensional Visualization of Scans

At the present time no practical technique for true three-dimensional visualization of radioisotope sources has been developed. Both a single crystal with collimation and positron detection determine the location of the emitted quanta roughly along a line providing essentially planar two-dimensional information. To determine the third dimension, another observation must be made. A number of possibilities for such measurements could be proposed, although they are not readily feasible with present instrumentation. In the case of positron detection, the difference in arrival time of the annihilation quanta at the two detectors would yield information as to the location of the source in the third dimension. In the case of γ-ray emitters, if the disintegration yields two or more cascaded photons, two collimators might be used in orthogonal planes to pin-point the location of the source in three dimensions.

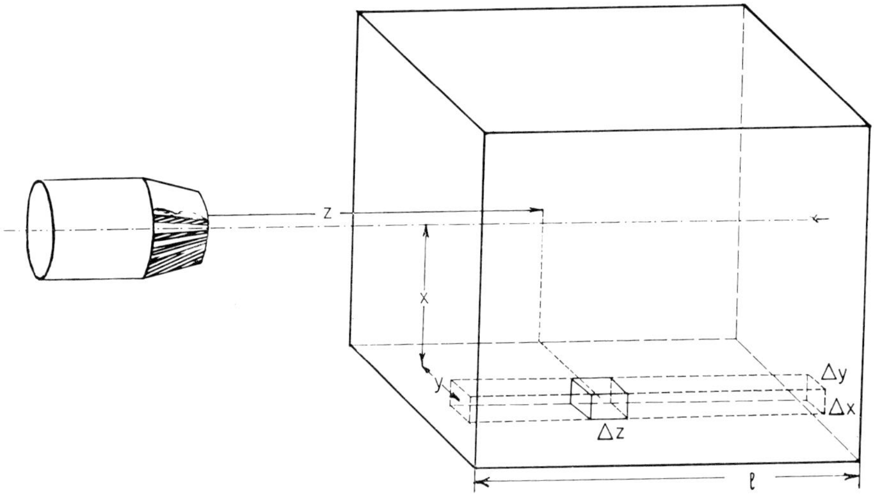

FIG. 4. Idealized object to be scanned. The activity concentration, ρ, is a function of (x, y, z), where the spatial parameters are referred to the collimator axis. See text for explanation.

Over and above practical problems of radiation detection, a basic statistical limitation poses itself in three-dimensional scanning. Figure 4 shows schematically an object to be visualized in three dimensions. Each volume element, $(\Delta x, \Delta y, \Delta z)$ must be assayed for its radioisotope content. If ρ is the radioactivity per unit volume, then $\rho\ \Delta x\ \Delta y\ \Delta z$ is the activity in the volume element. If the radioactivity is to be determined to a certain statistical accuracy in a fixed time, this activity must be compared to that of a two-dimensional scanning volume element of length l, whose activity is $\rho l\ \Delta x\ \Delta y$. For equal concentration the ratio is $\Delta z/l \ll 1$. Hence, considerably more activity or a much longer scanning time must be used for equivalent statistical accuracy. This difference becomes greater as the resolution, Δz, is made smaller.

Most suggestions for three-dimensional visualization utilize multiple two-dimensional localizations. Perhaps the most obvious technique is obtaining two two-dimensional scans in orthogonal planes. However, other techniques have been suggested and are of interest to examine if only from a theoretical point of view. For example, Rankowitz *et al.* (*35*), have proposed a technique employing a ring of 32 scintillation detectors surrounding an object containing a positron emitter. Figure 5

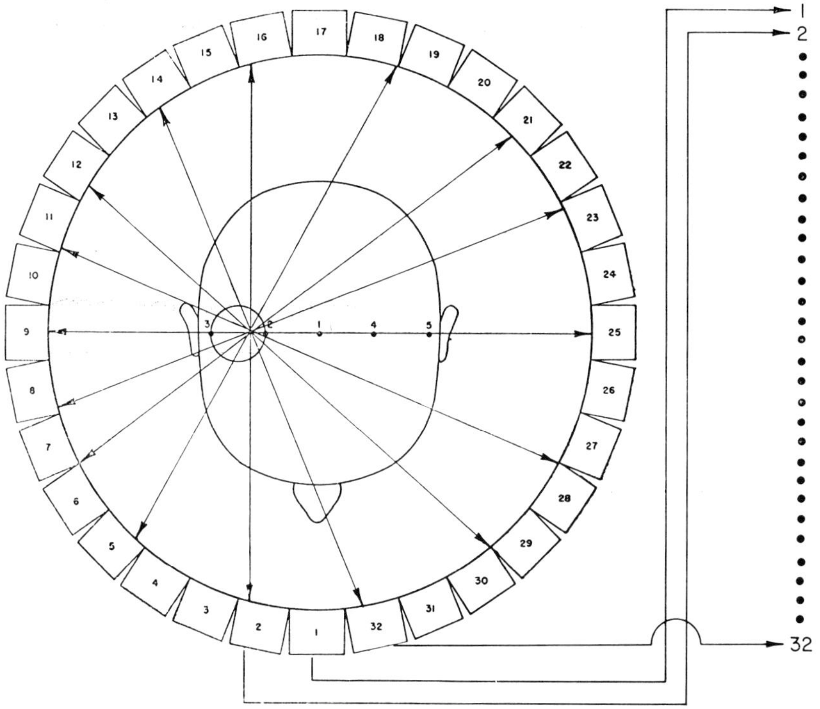

FIG. 5. Schematic diagram of multiple coincidence device for brain tumor localization in three dimensions (*35*). Coincidences between each pair of detectors are observed and recorded in a magnetic memory.

shows a schematic diagram of this device, as proposed for brain tumor localization. Coincidences are recorded between any pair of detectors. As only the line of flight of the two annihilation quanta resulting from the positron emission is recorded, a point source in the final scan (Fig. 6) is presented as a line. In Fig. 6, X and Y refer to the numbers of the detector pairs recording coincident events. In principle it would be possible to interpret the information on such a resultant display in terms of abnormalities in the object being visualized. However, attempts are under way to program a computer matix inversion system to extract the original radioisotope distribution from these data. In this technique the radioisotope distribution in one plane is observed. The ring of detectors could be raised to determine the distribution in other planes.

Kuhl and Edwards (*28*) have discussed a number of possible techniques involving rectilinear scanning with focused collimators to yield three-dimensional information. In general, these techniques involve procedures whereby radioactivity on a desired plane is observed in focus, whereas radioactivity on other planes appears out of focus. The technique of section scanning, similar to tomography in radiology, appears promising. In this procedure scans are obtained with the detector viewing the object at different angles. Superimposing the resultant pictures after shifting their relative positions sideways provides information in focus of the radioisotope distribution at a particular depth. Activity at other depths is defocused into a background blur (Fig. 7). In Fig. 7A scans

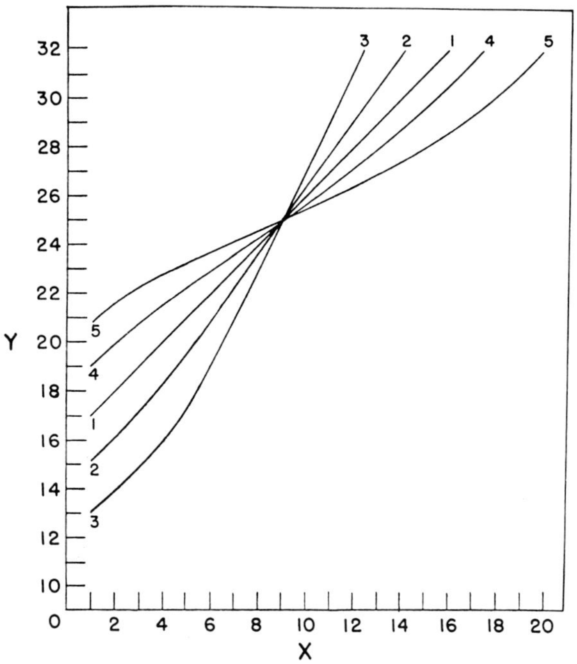

FIG. 6. Track of coincidence pairs for point sources shown in Fig. 5 (*35*). Note that each of the point sources is transformed into a line. A computer program may be used to reconstruct the original isotope distribution in the scanned plane from the set of coincidences.

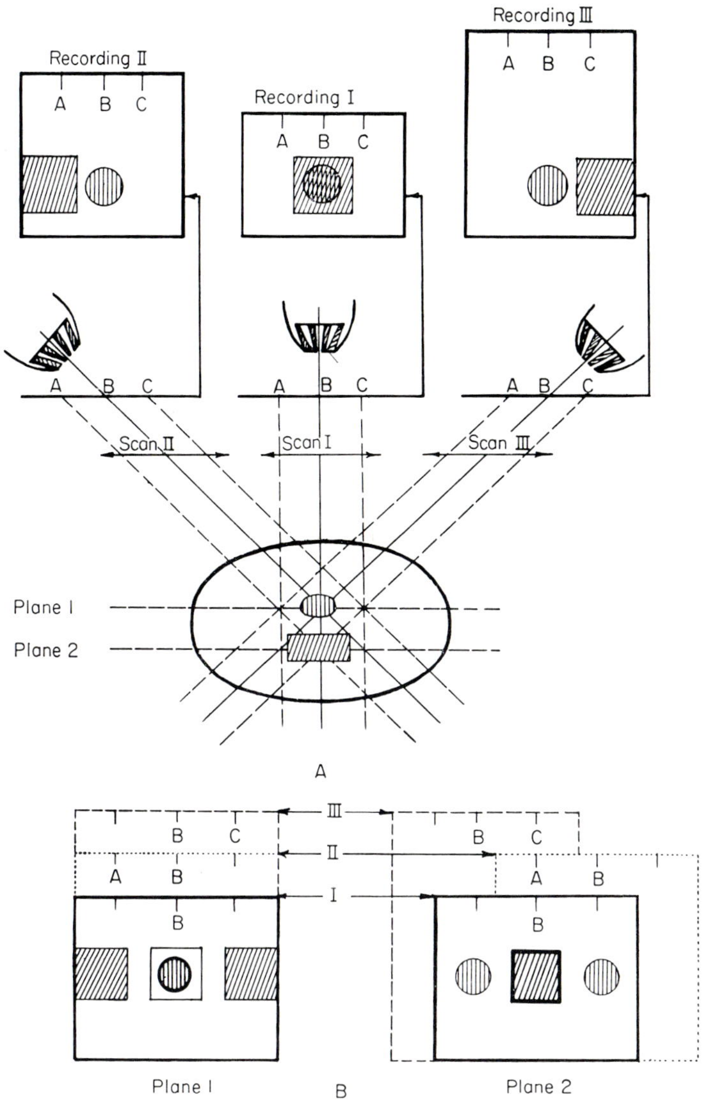

FIG. 7. Illustration of longitudinal section scanning (*28*). (A) Three separate scans are made with the detector inclined at different angles. The resultant scans are superimposed with different amounts of translation. (B) The three transparent film recordings are superimposed in two ways, first, so that the circle is enhanced and second, so that the square is enhanced.

are obtained at three different viewing angles. The resultant scans individually contain little apparent information. However, when superimposed and translated at appropriate distances, as shown in Fig. 7B, the scans do portray the radioisotope distribution on various planes.

These and other techniques for three-dimensional visualization involve summation and subtraction of count-rates and hence require a high degree of statistical accuracy. Further, in most cases a high-contrast

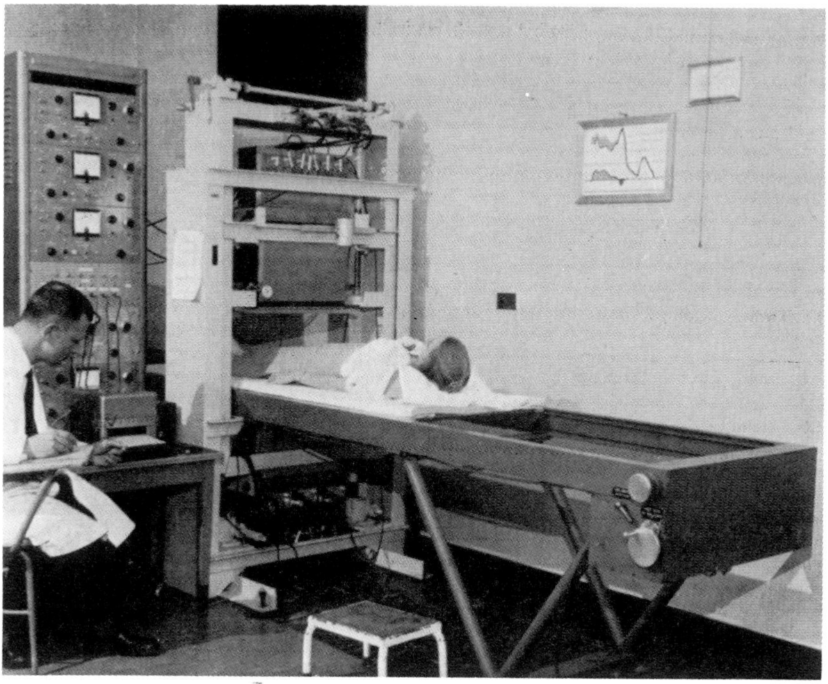

FIG. 8. A linear scanner consisting of two rows of six crystals each, one row above and one row beneath the patient (*36*). Each row of crystals is shielded by a common slit collimator. The cot with the patient moves longitudinally between the upper and lower detector assemblies.

recording system must be employed. Areas of only slightly increased radioactivity may be missed and consequently careful adjustment of the contrast control is required.

D. Linear Scanning

Another variation from conventional planar scanning is linear or one-dimensional scanning (Fig. 8). The detector may be a rectangular crystal or an assembly of crystals wide in the transverse direction and narrow in the longitudinal direction, with a slit-shaped collimator in front of it (*36*). The assembly sweeps the length of the patient counting the sum of all the radioactivity in a narrow transverse slice. The record, usually a count-rate curve on a strip chart recorder, is often called a profile scan (*33*).

This form of scanning is useful for rapid surveys of the whole body, for example, to locate distributed metastases. For the same reason that planar scanning is an order of magnitude more sensitive than three-dimensional scanning, linear scanning is an order of magnitude more sensitive than planar scanning. Thus a linear scan can be made very rapidly to find an approximate target area for a planar scan which, at slower speeds, will yield finer two-dimensional details.

II. COLLIMATOR PERFORMANCE

The purpose of the collimator is to limit the field of view of the detector. Only in this way can the scanner achieve spatial resolution, that is, resolve two point sources of radioactivity lying in proximity to each other. The collimator performs a function somewhat analogous to a lens in a camera. However, as γ rays cannot be easily refracted, the collimator can limit the detection volume only by absorbing radiation from unwanted areas. This procedure inevitably results in a marked decrease in the amount of detected radiation, or a loss of sensitivity.

A. Point Source Response

The performance of a collimator is often described in terms of its response to a point source. Since any distribution of radioactivity can be considered as a collection of point sources, the response to such a distribution may be obtained by summing the responses to each of the point sources. With appropriate interpretation almost all the desired information on collimator performance can be obtained from the point source response curves.

A typical focusing collimator of the Oak Ridge design (*15*) is shown in Fig. 9. The collimator consists of 37 tapered apertures with lead septa between them. The collimator and crystal are in a lead shield to reduce the background count-rate. The axes of the tapered apertures intersect at a point, which is called the focus of the collimator. Figure 10 shows the point source response curve for this collimator at the focal point in a plane perpendicular to the collimator axis. The bell-shaped response adjacent to the axis of the collimator is typical of the geometrical response of tapered apertures. At large distances from the axis, deviations from this smooth curve are observed, reflecting septa and side wall penetration. The theoretical derivation of such curves and the influence of various parameters are discussed in Chapter 17.

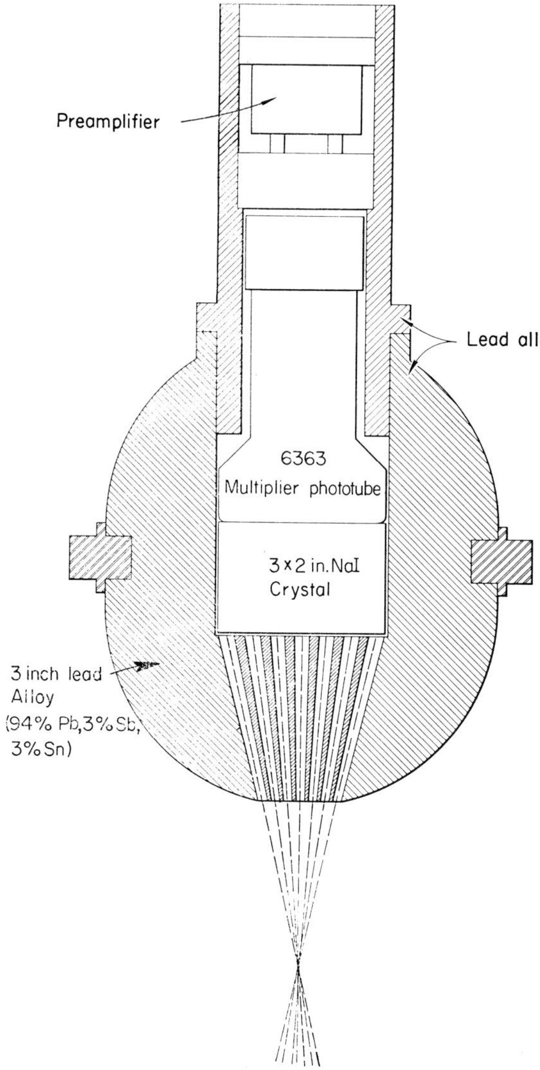

FIG. 9. 37-Hole focusing collimator of honeycomb design with lead septa and lead shielding (*15*).

From point source response curves at different depths, a point source response pattern may be constructed as shown in Fig. 11 for a different collimator. This pattern permits the determination of the collimator response to point sources in air at any point on a plane containing the axis of the collimator. If the response is symmetrical about the axis, this completely determines the spatial collimator response. For honeycomb collimators consisting of circular or hexagonal holes in a hexagonal array, this nearly applies, although the exact orientation of the hexagonal array may cause a slight angular variation. However, for other designs such as square collimators the orientation will be quite important and it may be necessary to construct a family of response patterns for different orientations.

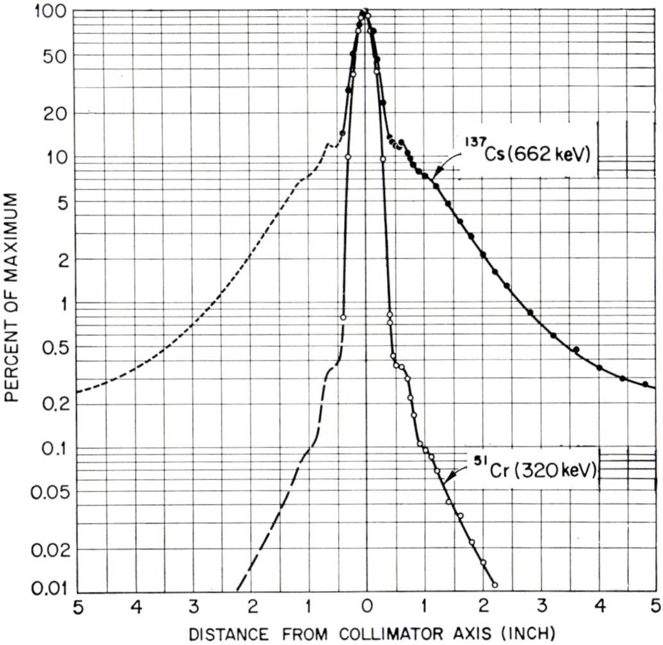

FIG. 10. Point source response curve at the focal plane of collimator shown in Fig. 9 (*15*). Responses to ^{51}Cr (320 keV) and ^{137}Cs (662 keV) are similar over the central region corresponding to the geometrical transmission but differ markedly in wings of curve indicating different degrees of septa and side wall penetration.

To determine the response of a collimator to radiation from an extended source, one should know the response pattern of the collimator, the distribution of the radioisotope within the source being scanned, the attenuation of the radiation within the object containing the source and the absolute sensitivity of the detector (Chapter 17, Section I). In practice, one usually attempts to simplify the analysis. It is often convenient to represent the central portion of the point source response curve shown in Fig. 10 by a Gaussian distribution. This has the advantage that it can be completely characterized by two parameters. The effects of septa and side wall penetration cannot be included in such a simplification, but these may be considered separately. Indeed, the septa

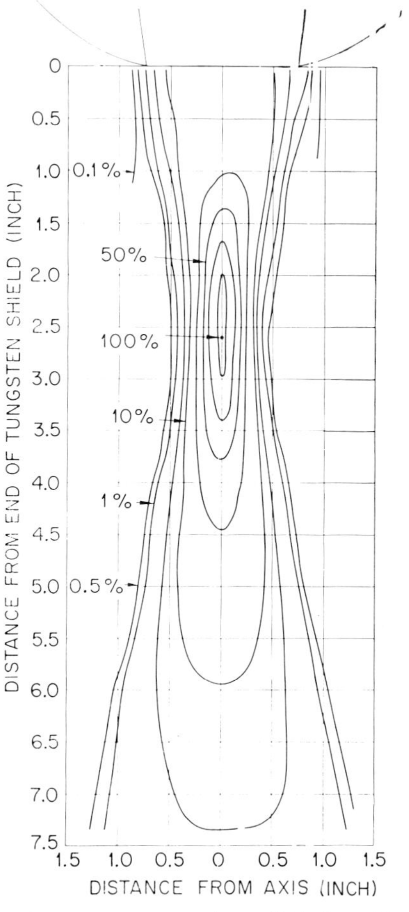

FIG. 11. Point source isoresponse curves for a 37-hole gold collimator in tungsten shield to ^{131}I γ rays in air (*15*).

and side wall penetration tend to increase the background level of the radioisotope scan, reducing the target-to-off-target contrast ratio, whereas an increase in the width of the central portion of the point source response curve has the effect of diminishing the detail that may be observed in a radioisotope scan. Although these two effects are not completely separable, they may be treated independently as a first approximation.

Figure 12 shows the calculated point source response function for two source geometries (7). Curve A represents the response of a focusing collimator consisting of round tapered apertures to a point source moving in the focal plane. The focal plane is defined as the plane containing the point of convergence of the apertures in the focusing collimator. Curve B represents the response of the focusing collimator to the point source in a plane 0.4 of the distance from the collimator face to the focal plane. Curve C shows a theoretical Gaussian distribution.

The curves in Fig. 12 are plotted as the ratio of $g(x)$, the count-rate of a point source located a distance x (cm) radially from the axis of the

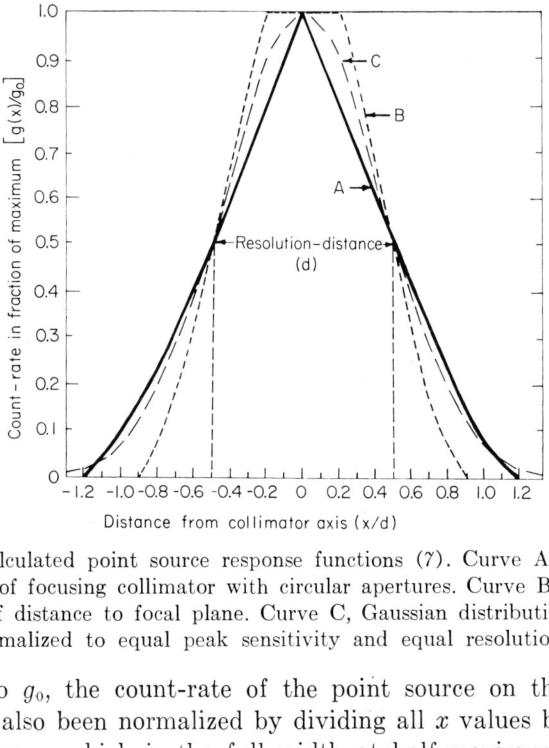

FIG. 12. Calculated point source response functions (7). Curve A, point source in focal plane of focusing collimator with circular apertures. Curve B, point source on plane 0.4 of distance to focal plane. Curve C, Gaussian distribution. All curves have been normalized to equal peak sensitivity and equal resolution distance, d.

collimator, to g_0, the count-rate of the point source on the axis. The abscissa has also been normalized by dividing all x values by d, the resolution distance, which is the full width at half-maximum (FWHM) of the response function. Consequently all three curves will be equal at $x/d = 0.5$, that is, the FWHM. These are the logical two points at which a Gaussian curve with its two adjustable parameters would be fitted to the actual distributions. The similarity of the Gaussian curve C to the calculated response curves A and B over the rest of the range of x/d is an indication of how well a fitted Gaussian distribution can be used to approximate an actual point source response curve. Although the agreement is far from perfect, the Gaussian curve does provide a fair approximation to the calculated curves. Furthermore, it is usually observed that the experimental point source response curves, such as shown in Fig. 10, more nearly resemble a Gaussian distribution than the calculated curves. This results from the summation of a number of effects such as small-angle γ-ray scattering and penetration of the edge of the septa in multichannel collimators.

If the Gaussian approximation is made, the point source response in a given plane may be characterized completely by two parameters, first, the peak sensitivity when the point source is directly on the axis of the collimator, and second, the full width at half-maximum (FWHM), the distance between the two positions of a point source at which the response is one-half the maximum. In the focal plane, these two parameters are generally referred to as the *focal geometrical efficiency,* g_0, and the *resolution distance,* d. Similar parameters may be obtained in other planes although, of course, the numerical values will differ. The definition of resolution of a collimator as the full width at half-maximum in the focal plane is an arbitrary one. However, it is a reasonable choice and in conformity with the definition of resolution in other fields.

If x and y are orthogonal dimensions in a plane perpendicular to the axis of the collimator and r is the radial distance ($r^2 = x^2 + y^2$), and if the collimator response is symmetrical about the axis, the radial point source response, assuming a Gaussian distribution in each dimension, can be expressed as

$$\begin{aligned} g(r) &= g(x)g(y) \\ &= g_0 \exp(-2.78x^2/d^2) \exp(-2.78y^2/d^2) \\ &= g_0 \exp(-2.78r^2/d^2) \end{aligned} \tag{1}$$

The radial response may also be considered as the product of an x and y response for any other experimental or theoretical curve.

B. Plane Source Response

In the previous section, it was shown that the response of a collimator could be evaluated by integrating, point by point over the complete source volume, the product of the collimator point source response and the radioisotope concentration, taking account of γ-ray attenuation and absolute detector efficiency. As a three-dimensional source distribution may be considered to be composed of thin slabs of radioactivity, the use of the collimator plane source response may simplify this evaluation. It requires only one integration of the radioactivity concentration as a function of depth. Again, the γ-ray attenuation and absolute detector efficiency must be considered.

Neglecting attenuation in the source, it can be shown that the response of a given focusing collimator to a large thin uniform slab of radioactivity is nearly independent of the distance of the slab from the collimator (7). The plane source geometrical response, G_s, can be found by integrating the point source geometrical response, $g(r)$, over a plane:

$$G_s = \int_0^\infty g(r) 2\pi r \, dr \tag{2}$$

The concept also holds for nonradially symmetrical response distributions although integration over two dimensions is required.

As the plane source response, G_s, is independent of the plane distance from the collimator, it is often convenient to calculate this quantity for a plane located at the surface of the collimator. At this plane the multihole collimator is merely an array of separate tapered apertures. The response of each of these to a thin layer of uniform radioactivity at its open end is simply summed to give the total plane source response.

The point source response may be approximated by a Gaussian distribution with two parameters, the resolution distance, d, and the point source response, g_0 (Section II,A). As the plane source response can be obtained by integrating over the point source distribution, it is logical that the plane source response may be expressed in terms of the same two parameters. Table II gives the ratio of the plane source response,

TABLE II
Ratio of Plane Source Response, G_s, to g_0d^2

	G_s/g_0d^2
Focusing collimator with round apertures and point source response in focal plane	1.03
Focusing collimator with round apertures and point source response in plane at 0.4 of distance to focal plane	0.93
Focusing collimator with square apertures and point source response in focal plane	1.05
Gaussian distribution	1.18

G_s, to the quantity g_0d^2, calculated for the three curves shown in Fig. 12, as well as for a focusing collimator with square apertures. The fact that this ratio is nearly constant confirms the assumption that G_s can be expressed in terms of g_0 and d. Indeed, as the ratio of G_s/g_0d^2 is very nearly equal to unity, the plane source response, G_s, may be closely approximated by g_0d^2.

C. Line Source Response

Another useful test pattern for the performance of a collimator is its response to a line source in a plane perpendicular to the axis of the collimator (Fig. 13). The collimator scans on the x axis across the line source, yielding a bell-shaped response curve as with the point source. The line source response function may readily be found from the point source response. If $g(x, y)$ is the two-dimensional point source function, the line source response, $G_l(x)$, will be

$$G_l(x) = \int_{-\infty}^{\infty} g(x, y)\, dy \tag{3}$$

If the Gaussian approximation is assumed for the x and y dependence, the line source response becomes

$$G_l(x) = 0.423 g_0 d \exp(-2.78x^2/d^2) \tag{4}$$

Therefore, the shape of the line source function is identical to that of the point source function. Measurements of the resolution distance, d, obtained with the line source will be the same as those obtained with the point source. It should be noted that Eq. 1 for the point source gives a response per unit amount of radioactivity at the point—counts per disintegration for instance. However, Eq. 4 for the line source gives the response per unit amount of radioactivity per unit source length—counts per disintegration per centimeter of length of the line source, for example.

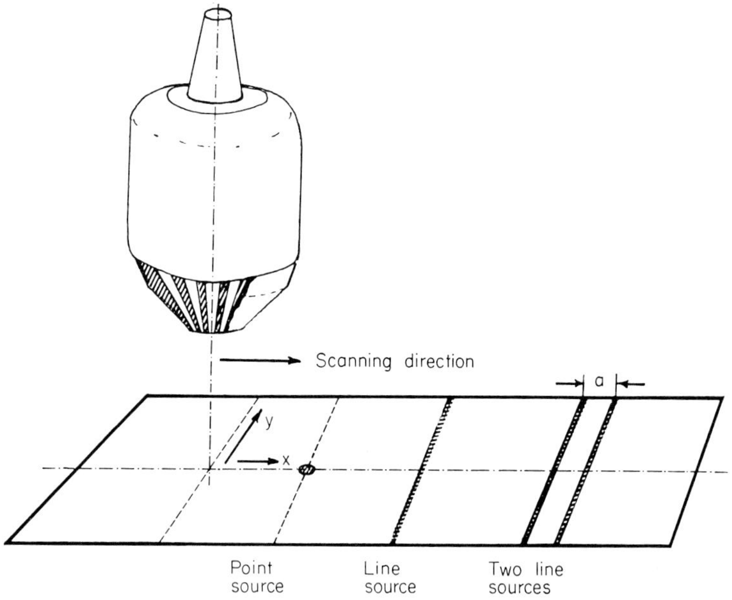

FIG. 13. Schematic diagram of scanner viewing point source, single line source, and two line sources, separated by a distance a.

Resolution is often defined as the distance between two points or lines which are barely distinguishable. Although such a definition is qualitative, it is of interest to examine the collimator response to two point or line sources as a function of their separation, assuming a Gaussian response curve for each source. Figure 14 shows the calculated response patterns for two point or line sources. The first point or line source is located at the position $x = 0$, while the second is located at the distance $x = +a$ (as in Fig. 13). All dimensions are given in units of d, the resolution distance, and the response is in units of g_0 for the point sources or $0.423 g_0 d$ for the line sources. It is assumed that both point sources

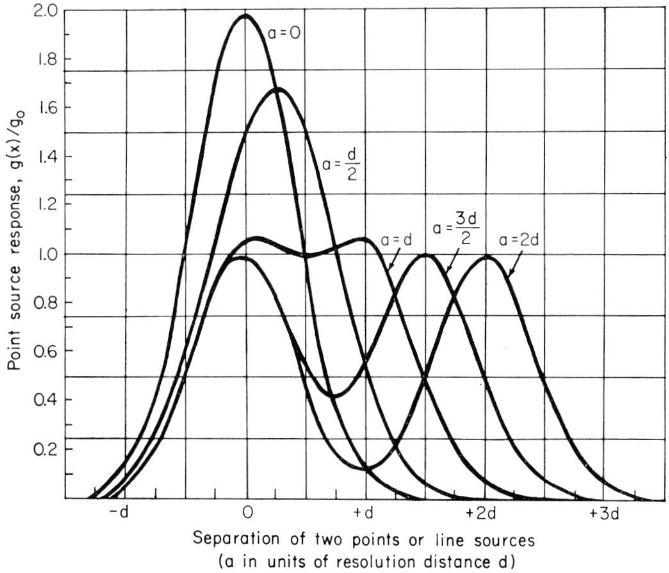

FIG. 14. Response of scanner to two point or line sources as a function of their separation a. Scanning of sources as shown in Fig. 13.

have unit radioactivity or that both line sources have unit radioactivity per centimeter of length.

It is seen from Fig. 14 that the two sources can barely be resolved if they are separated by a distance $a = d$. However, they can be clearly resolved at a distance $a = 2d$. This observation adds further weight to the use of d as a resolution parameter since it corresponds to that distance at which two point or line sources can barely be resolved.

III. COLLIMATOR-DETECTOR SENSITIVITY

Essentially all scanners and scintillation cameras at the present time use NaI(Tl) crystals as radiation detectors. For several reasons selection of only those pulses falling within the photopeak region is advantageous in radioisotope scanning. The background count-rate is markedly reduced since all background pulses except those within the photopeak region are excluded. Of equal importance is the fact that scattered γ rays, which have a lower energy, are not registered. Hence, only those γ rays which reach the detector in a straight line without undergoing a deflection by Compton interaction in the source are recorded. This has the effect of reducing the general background level and of preventing the degradation of the target-to-nontarget contrast ratio.

On the basis of the collimator response discussed in the previous section, the collimator-detector sensitivity may be determined. An idealized object containing radioactivity scanned by a multiaperture collimator and detector is shown in Fig. 4. If all measurements are referred to the axis of the collimator, the collimator-detector sensitivity, S, follows as

$$S = \int_V g(x, y, z)\rho(x, y, z)e^{-\mu z}\eta s \, dx \, dy \, dz \tag{5}$$

The function $g(x, y, z)$ is the point source response, $\rho(x, y, z)$ the concentration of radioactivity at the point (x, y, z), and $e^{-\mu z}$ corrects for the attenuation of radiation emerging from a depth z in the object. The fraction of disintegrations giving rise to detectable radiation is η and the absolute detector sensitivity is s. The latter two factors, which depend on the radioisotope decay, the γ-ray energy, and the detector dimensions are independent of collimator design.

If the volume source can be approximated by a series of uniform plane sources the collimator-detector sensitivity of Eq. 5 can be reduced to

$$S = G_s s\eta \int_0^l \rho(z)e^{-\mu z} \, dz \tag{6}$$

Here G_s is the plane source response and $\rho(z)$ represents the z variation of the radioactivity concentration along the axis of the collimator, that is, $x = y = 0$. In most cases the variation of ρ with x and y will be small compared to the resolution distance, d, and consequently the assumption of a series of plane sources of uniform surface concentration can be made. Even in cases where ρ varies rapidly with x or y, the value $\rho(z)$ may be considered as the average value on the axis, weighted over the x and y sensitivity distributions of the collimator.

It is convenient to assign a single term, F, to the distribution of radiation emerging from the source. This is called the source flux, and in terms of Eq. 6,

$$F = \eta \int_0^{\cdot} \rho(z)e^{-\mu z} \, dz \tag{7}$$

The collimator-detector sensitivity can now be written as

$$S = G_s s F \tag{8}$$

The source flux, F, characterizes the source and its self-attenuation; the plane source response, G_s, is determined by the collimator properties, and the detector sensitivity, s, by the size of the detector.

A. Variation in Source Flux

The source flux, F, may be considered as a flux of radiation emerging from the object being scanned. Its local variations represent differences in radioisotope content in the object and consequently comprise the information content of the radioisotope distribution. For two-dimensional scanning, F varies over a plane and may be considered as being composed of an average radiation level, $\bar{F}$, and a term $\delta F(x, y)$, representing deviations from the average level, at each point (x, y).

$$F = \bar{F} + \delta F(x, y) \tag{9}$$

The analysis of variations in δF with respect to the spatial coordinates x and y may be expressed in terms of spatial frequencies, expressed as cycles per centimeter. At first glance, this may appear as an unusual terminology. However, the analysis of variations in space in terms of spatial frequencies is entirely analogous to the analysis of variations with time in terms of temporal frequency, that is, cycles per second. Indeed it is usually possible to convert spatial frequencies into temporal frequencies and vice versa; actually, this is what a scanner does.

The Fourier transform is a method of analysis of time-varying phenomena and can equally well be applied to quantities varying from point to point in space. This transformation yields a spectrum in terms of either temporal or spatial frequencies. For example, the Fourier transform of a pure sine wave is a single line at the frequency of the sine wave. A mixture of sine waves of different frequencies yields a transform having a series of lines. The analysis, furthermore, is perfectly general as any pattern of variation in time or space can be represented as a summation of many sine waves varying in frequency and phase. The Fourier transform of nonrepetitive patterns will appear as a continuous frequency spectrum indicating the fact that many frequencies are present.

The two-dimensional Fourier transform, $F_s(k_x, k_y)$, of $\delta F(x, y)$ yields the frequency spectrum of the radiation distribution emerging from the source.

$$F_s(k_x, k_y) = \int\int_A \delta F(x, y) \exp[2\pi i(xk_x + yk_y)]\, dx\, dy \tag{10}$$

It is common to use the square of the absolute value of F_s expressed per unit area. Such a function is called the Wiener spectrum, W_s, of the radiation distribution (7) and is analogous to the power spectrum encountered in the analysis of electrical circuits.

$$W_s(k_x, k_y) = A^{-1}|F_s(k_x, k_y)|^2 \tag{11}$$

where A is the area of the scan. This spectrum represents the pattern of the radiation distribution which is presented to the scanner.

The output of the scanner will differ from the input and this difference will be reflected in the frequency distribution of the output pattern, $F_0(k_x, k_y)$, and the Wiener spectrum of the output pattern, $W_0(k_x, k_y)$. These two quantities are defined in the same manner as in Eqs. 10 and

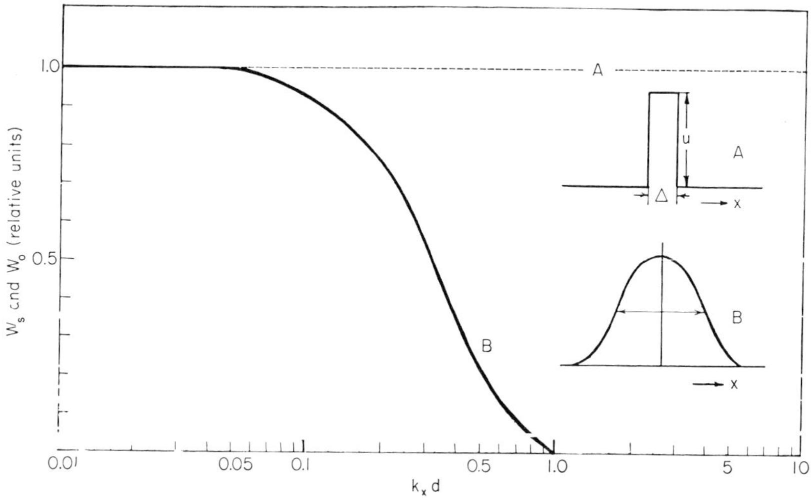

FIG. 15. Wiener spectra of line source. Spatial distribution A represents radioactivity of line source; curve A, Wiener spectrum of source. Spatial distribution B shows collimator response to line source; curve B, corresponding Wiener spectrum.

11 except that δF, the variation in the source distribution, is replaced by δN, the variation in the scanner output.

For example, the spatial frequency analysis may be applied to the line source. In this case, the analysis can be reduced to one dimension, that is, the variation with x, as the activity is assumed to be uniform with respect to y. A line source, therefore, will be represented as a narrow wedge of increased activity as shown in diagram A of Fig. 15. It can be shown that the Fourier spectrum of this distribution is

$$\begin{aligned} F_s(k_x) &= \int_{-\Delta/2}^{\Delta/2} u(\cos 2\pi k_x x + j \sin 2\pi k_x x)\, dx \\ &= u\Delta \end{aligned} \tag{12}$$

where u is the height of the activity step and Δ is its width. The Wiener spectrum of this distribution is

$$W_s(k_x) = \frac{1}{l}(u\Delta)^2 \tag{13}$$

This spectrum is shown in Fig. 15 as the horizontal line (A). This indicates that all frequencies are present at equal intensities in the pattern.

A scanner will record the line source as a distribution resembling a Gaussian distribution as shown in diagram B of Fig. 15. The effect of the collimator is to remove the higher spatial frequencies from the original pattern. The spectrum is plotted against the dimensionless parameter, k_xd, which is frequency times resolution distance. For example, if d is 1 cm, the scale will read k_x directly in lines per centimeter. From curve B, it can be seen that line sources spaced at one line in 10 cm, or 0.1 line per centimeter, will be clearly resolved, whereas line sources spaced at one line per centimeter or closer will not.

The effect of the collimator on spatial frequencies is quite analogous to that of a low-pass filter on temporal frequencies. Further, $1/d$ may be compared to the cutoff frequency of such a filter. Clearly, the smaller the value of d, the higher the value of the spatial frequency that can be resolved and the sharper the resultant picture.

The transmission, $T(k_x, k_y)$, of the collimator may be defined as the ratio of the output spectrum to the input spectrum (*22*).
Therefore,

$$\begin{aligned} T(k_x, k_y) &= F_0(k_x, k_y)/F_s(k_x, k_y) \\ &= [W_0(k_x, k_y)/W_s(k_x, k_y)]^{1/2} \end{aligned} \tag{14}$$

The absolute value of the quantity, $T(k_x, k_y)$, is called the *modulation transfer function* (MTF). The MTF will decrease at higher spatial frequencies, becoming negligible at frequencies above $1/d$. For a point or line source pattern, the MTF will have a shape similar to Curve B of Fig. 15.

B. Choice of γ-Ray Energy

The variation in the source flux, F, reflects variations in isotope content of the source. The magnitude of these variations will determine the probability of detecting a region of abnormally high or low concentration in the source. In particular, the ratio of F over an abnormal area to the value of F over a normal area is often called the *target-to-nontarget ratio*. This ratio is an important factor for the detection of the abnormal area. However, it should be realized that its value depends also on other factors such as collimator resolution.

The determination of the target-to-nontarget ratio may serve as a useful criterion for the selection of radioisotopes having an appropriate γ-ray energy. If all other factors are equal, the isotope yielding the highest ratio will offer the greatest possibility of detecting the abnormal area. The γ-ray energy affects the target-to-nontarget ratio through the attenuation term, $e^{-\mu z}$, in Eq. 5. Since the attenuation coefficient is larger for lower-energy γ rays, the flux is reduced more for deep-seated targets.

The detector sensitivity, s, in Eq. 5 is increased for lower-energy γ rays. However, the target-to-nontarget ratio is more important than the

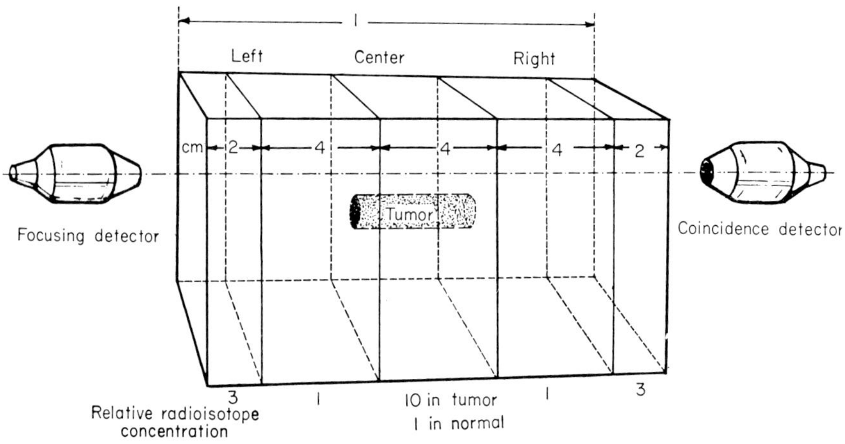

FIG. 16. Model for comparison of γ-ray and positron detection for brain tumor localization. Focusing collimator and detector view object from left side. Dimensions and relative radioisotope concentrations are shown. A tumor-to-normal-brain concentration ratio of 10 to 1 is assumed.

detector sensitivity since the latter can be compensated by administering a greater amount of radioisotope or using a longer scanning time.

For example, with the model shown in Fig. 16 the optimum energy of γ-ray emitters for brain tumor localization may be determined, and the use of γ-ray and positron emitters may be compared. The greater radioactivity concentration at the surface of the model corresponds to increased radioactivity in parts of the head, such as scalp, skull, and dura, relative to that in normal brain tissue. A tumor with an area that is large compared to the resolution distance of the scanning device is indicated in the center location. It may also be located in the left or right section.

The responses of focusing collimators and positron detectors of equal resolution for tumor relative to normal regions as calculated by Eqs. 6 and 7 are shown in Fig. 17. For positron emitters the response is independent of tumor location because the sum of the distances traversed by the two annihilation quanta is constant (Chapter 18). In the case of γ-ray detection the ratio of tumor to normal brain response depends strongly on the tumor location as well as on the γ-ray energy. As would be expected, a tumor adjacent to the surface (left side) is detected with a high efficiency and consequently the tumor-to-normal-brain ratio is

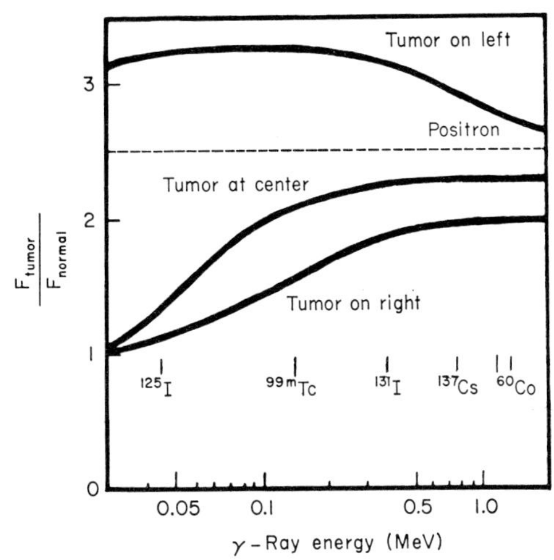

FIG. 17. Ratio of radiation flux, F, over tumor and over normal area of model shown in Fig. 16 for γ-ray emitters of various energies. The relative response of a detector over these two areas will equal the flux ratio. Curves are shown for the tumor in three locations, left, center, and right.

increased. However, if the tumor is at the center or back (right) location, the ratio is decreased. The center location is perhaps the most important one for brain tumor scanning as superficial tumors are relatively easy to detect. In this case positron detection offers a small, but distinct advantage over even high-energy γ rays. Low-energy γ rays, that is, with energies below 100 keV, would yield poor results (Fig. 17).

C. Relation between Sensitivity and Resolution

If the sensitivity of a collimator were not a function of its resolution, obviously all collimators would be designed for the highest possible resolution, that is, the smallest value of the resolution distance, d. Using the detector response given in Eq. 8 for an average radiation flux, $\bar{F}$, together with a scanning time, T, the total number of quanta, N, recorded with a detector of sensitivity s will be

$$N = G_s\bar{F}sT = g_0d^2\bar{F}sT \tag{15}$$

since $G_s/g_0d^2 \sim 1$ (Table II). Different kinds of collimators and scanners can be categorized by the dependence of N on d, the resolution distance. In general, they can be considered as d^4 scanners if N varies as d^4, d^2 scanners if N varies as d^2, and resolution-independent scanners, or d^0 scanners, if N is independent of d.

The dependence of N on d is derived below for a number of scanning systems (7). In each case the length of the collimator was assumed to be equal to the geometrical focal distance, both designated as a. The radius of the crystal is R and the large radius of the aperture close to the crystal is r_0.

1. d^4 SCANNERS

Single cylindrical and single tapered aperture collimators and also single pair positron detectors fall into this first category. For a single hole cylindrical collimator the point source response $g_0 = r_0^2/16a^2$ and the resolution distance $d = 4r_0$ (Table III). Consequently, $g_0 = d^2/256a^2$,

TABLE III

COLLIMATOR EFFICIENCY AND RESOLUTION[a]

Collimator	Point source geometrical response (g_0)	Resolution distance (d)	Plane source geometrical response ($G_s = g_0d^2$)	G_s (relative) normalized to equal d
Cylinder	$r_0^2/16a^2$	$4.0r_0$	(r_0^4/a^2)	1
Taper	$r_0^2/16a^2$	$1.75r_0$	$0.19(r_0^4/a^2)$	5.15
Focus (n apertures)	$nr_0^2/16a^2$	$1.75r_0$	$0.1n(r_0^4/a^2)$	$5.15n$
Coincidences	$r_0^2/4a^2$	$0.82r_0$	$0.17(r_0^4/a^2)$	96.5

[a] a is length of collimator and collimator to focal plane distance for cylinder, taper, and focus collimator and is the crystal-to-source distance for coincidence detectors. r_0 is radius of cylindrical collimator, radius of large end of taper in single taper or focus collimator, and radius of crystal in coincidence detectors.

and the number of recorded quanta, N, follows from Eq. 15 as

$$N = K(d^4/A^2) \tag{16}$$

where

$$K = 3.90 \times 10^{-3} \frac{\bar{F}sTA^2}{a^2} \quad \text{cylindrical aperture}$$

$$K = 2.04 \times 10^{-2} \frac{\bar{F}sTA^2}{a^2} \quad \text{tapered aperture}$$

$$K = 3.72 \times 10^{-1} \frac{\bar{F}sTA^2}{a^2} \quad \text{positron detection}$$

and A is the scanned area. The quantity K is proportional to the average radiation flux, $\bar{F}$, the scanning time, T, as well as some detector-collimator parameters. Thus, the level of radioactivity and the scanning time may be traded for each other. Furthermore, either or both may be decreased without affecting the scan if it is possible to increase the collimator-detector efficiency without decreasing the resolution.

A radioisotope scan may be considered as a series of observations of radioactivity in resolution areas or cells of area d^2. This area is arbitrarily defined, as the resolution distance, d, was arbitrarily defined. The number of observations is A/d^2 and the number of recorded quanta per resolution area, m, for a d^4 scanner will be

$$m = N(d^2/A) = K(d^6/A^3) \tag{17}$$

where K may assume any of the values given in Eq. 16.

2. d^2 SCANNER

A focusing collimator can, under certain assumptions, be considered a d^2 scanner. In particular, it is assumed that the crystal size is constant but that the number and size of the collimator holes can vary. If it is assumed that one half of the area of a detector of radius R is exposed to apertures, the number of apertures, n, will be $n = R^2/2r_0^2$, and N, the total number of recorded quanta, will be

$$N = K(d^2/A) \tag{18}$$

where

$$K = 3.18 \times 10^{-2} \frac{\bar{F}sTR^2A}{a^2}$$

The number of recorded quanta per resolution area will be

$$m = K(d^4/A^2) \tag{19}$$

3. d^2 CAMERAS

The pinhole camera and the multiaperture camera (Chapter 19) fall in the d^2 category and may be analyzed by entirely analogous means. Some care must, however, be taken in the definition of resolution. In the case of the pinhole camera, the definition is illustrated in Fig. 18, where two points, a distance d apart, project on the detector circular images whose area of overlap is one-half the area of the circle. This definition is analogous to the definition of resolution as full width at half maximum as used for focusing collimators.

The resolution of the camera for an object at a distance a from the pinhole, which is, in turn, at a distance a from the detector, is $d = 0.84b$ where $b/2$ is the pinhole radius or the effective radius if γ-ray penetration is appreciable. The point source response is $g_0 = b^2/16a^2$. The number of recorded quanta will be

$$N = K(d^2/A) \tag{20}$$

where

$$K = 8.86 \times 10^{-2} \frac{\bar{F}sTA^2}{a^2}$$

The relation for m will be the same as in Eq. 19.

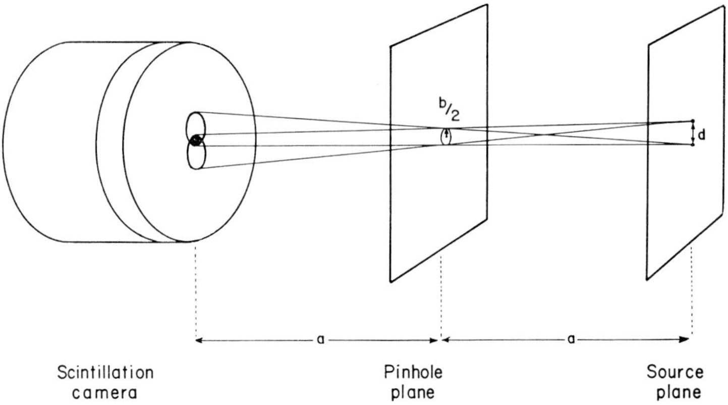

FIG. 18. Illustration of definition of resolution for pinhole camera.

The multiaperture camera can consist of a matrix of tapered apertures in front of a large area camera detector. If the apertures have a length a and the distance from the front of the aperture to the source plane is also a, and if one half of the area of a detector of radius R is exposed to tapers, the number of recorded quanta will be

$$N = K(d^2/A) \tag{21}$$

where

$$K = 3.12 \times 10^{-2} \frac{\bar{F}sTR^2A}{a^2}$$

and the relation for m will be the same as in Eq. 19.

4. RESOLUTION-INDEPENDENT CAMERA—POSITRON CAMERA

A number of devices have been proposed or built to combine the camera concept with use of positron-emitting radioisotopes. The positron camera (*2*) (Chapter 19, Section IV) shown in Fig. 19 uses a large crystal in a scintillation camera and in addition a matrix of small crystals. Pulses from a small crystal gate the camera to select annihilation radiation. A sectional plane is brought into focus by displacing the position of the observed scintillation on the oscilloscope screen according to the location of the particular small crystal from which a pulse was obtained. If it is assumed that the radius of the small crystals, b, can be

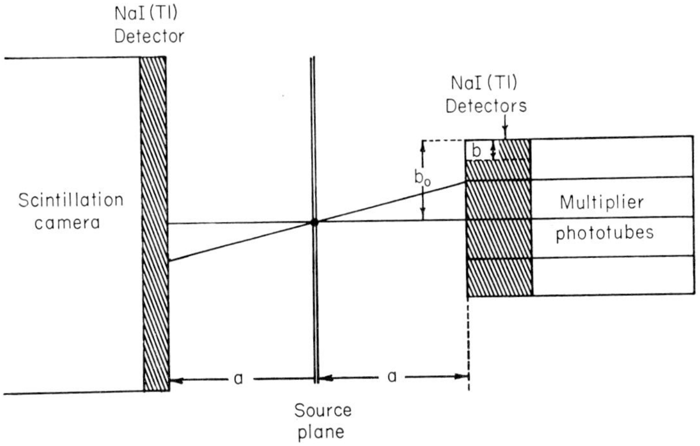

FIG. 19. Positron scintillation camera (*2*).

varied while the radius of the cluster, b_0, is kept constant, it can be shown that

$$N = K \tag{22}$$

where

$$K = \frac{\bar{F}sTb_0^2}{4a^2}$$

and

$$m = K(d^2/A) \tag{23}$$

In the case of the scintillation camera, other factors than geometrical considerations can limit the resolution. In particular, statistical variations in the number of emitted photoelectrons impose a resolution limit in the multiple multiplier phototube imaging device. This will not affect N but will make the positioning of the pulses less precise. If d_g is the geometrical resolution distance and d_0 is a resolution distance imposed by other conditions, the effective resolution d follows as

$$d^2 = d_g^2 + d_0^2 \tag{24}$$

This effect will also be observed with scanners where it is usually less important.

D. Choice of Optimum Resolution

Though each particular scanning application has an optimum resolution, its determination is perhaps the most difficult task facing the designers of radioisotope scanners. There may be two general approaches to this problem. The first involves the concept of maximizing a "figure of merit." This quantity has been differently defined by various authors but is based on the probability of detecting a region of given target-to-nontarget ratio. The result of such an approach is that the resolution distance is optimized to be approximately equal to the dimension of the object being detected (*3, 13*).

An alternative approach is to consider the problem as one in information transfer (*7, 8*). First some assumption as to the information content of the original radioisotope distribution must be made, expressed in terms of its spatial frequency spectrum. The scanner loses some information in producing the resultant scan, the amount being transferred depending on the scanner sensitivity and resolution. The smaller the value of the resolution distance, d, the higher the cutoff frequency. The minimum value of d is determined by the size of the smallest objects that must be seen. This, translated into spatial frequency, dictates how much filtering can be tolerated. The solution to this problem will indicate if the requisite resolution can be obtained with reasonable amounts of radioactivity and sufficient statistical accuracy.

IV. READOUT SYSTEMS

In regard to their information content, all recording methods are equivalent provided they do not sacrifice information by use of a background erase method, scaling factors, or other preprocessing of the data. For interpretation of scans, however, different methods of data display show various virtues based on the information communicated by the scan. These differences are to some extent subjective, or matters of taste, but to some extent they are subject to analysis. For example, the eye does not seem to be able to judge small variations in dot spacing or film density as easily as it does changes in color. Readout methods which record information in the form of spots per unit area communicate their information content as pattern fluctuations.

Statistical fluctuations always are the limiting factor in interpreting a scan. The statistical uncertainty of each small area of the scan pattern could be computed by conventional statistical formulas, but in practice this is not appropriate. The eye does not see point by point, but rather in terms of patterns and areas. The clinician judges the scan in terms of regularities and patterns which are known or meaningful to him, and the presence or absence of such patterns is statistically much less uncertain than the analysis of each elementary area would indicate.

In general, the quality of a scan is primarily dependent upon the information available during the time of measurement but the interpretation of this may be affected by the readout system. This section examines the practical compromises and data manipulation techniques that are employed to obtain maximum useful information from a scan.

A. Point-by-Point Counting

For all radiation measurements the counts per unit time* are an indicator of the detected radiation intensity. Therefore, recording

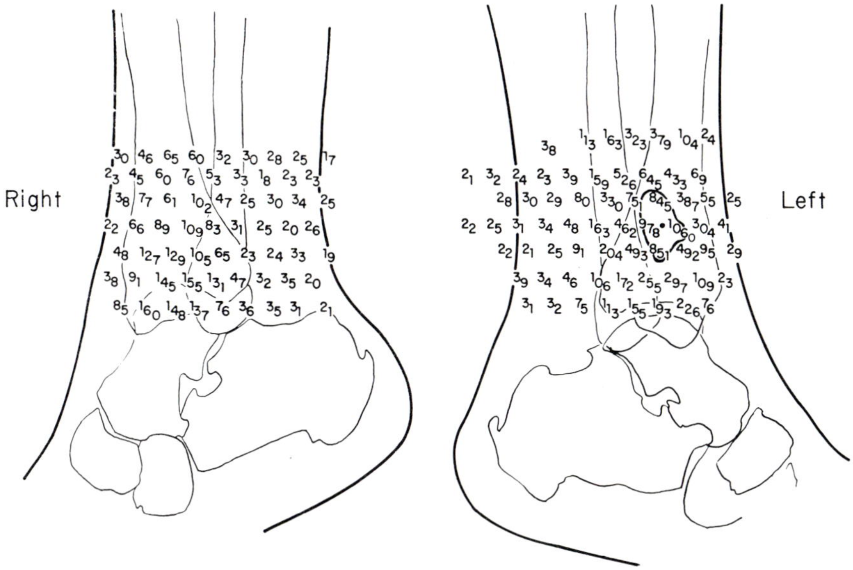

FIG. 20. Stepwise scans of ankles (*12*). Preset time 25 sec; scanning steps 3/8 inch in both horizontal directions. Area of high uptake on left ankle (16 days after a dose of 300 μCi of ^{85}Sr) corresponds to osteoblastic lesion.

of the counts per unit time at each point of a radiation field yields a true representation of the field (Fig. 20). Knowing the actual counts registered also helps to evaluate statistical fluctuations (Chapter 3, Section I,A). To determine the counts per unit time at any one point, the position of the counter must remain fixed for some length of time (*12*,

* There is no difference between the count-rate and the counts per unit time. We use the latter here to indicate that the counts are registered in digital form.

32). Furthermore, a special printout system must correlate the observed counts with the actual position of the detector during the measurements.

If a sufficient number of points were taken, the point-by-point readout would be ideal for demonstrating the presence or absence of a tumor or abnormality that concentrates or rejects the administered radioisotope. However, even if all the information were present, it would be difficult to visualize the size and shape of an organ (thyroid, kidney, liver) by looking at the counts per unit time as printed in Fig. 20. A more coherent picture is obtained by drawing contour or isocount lines around areas of approximately equal counts per unit time, as shown in Fig. 21.

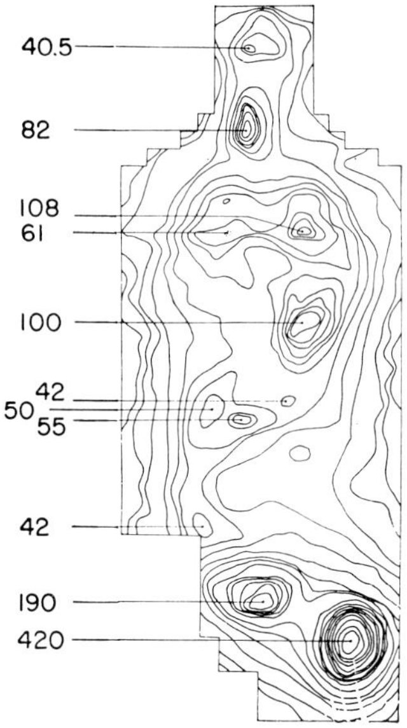

FIG. 21. Isocount curves of patient with metastatic carcinoma of thyroid, two days after tracer dose of ^{131}I (*32*).

All scanning readout systems are modifications of the basic point-by-point counting. To some degree, the ability to interpret the statistical significance of the data is reduced when a pictorial form of display is employed. However, the greater ease of comprehending the information content makes a picture preferable.

B. Count-Rate Profiles

Instead of a digital recording of counts obtained in a stepwise movement of the detector, the latter may travel in a continuous line with the observed count-rate measured by a count ratemeter and displayed in analog form on a strip chart recorder. This results in a count-rate profile for each traverse of the scanning area (*10, 30, 33*). A composite of juxtaposed profiles yields a three-dimensional representation of the radioactivity distribution (Fig. 22).

This method of data display has certain advantages and disadvantages. There are no arbitrarily preselected points for which information is obtained, since continuous measurements are taken over the whole area. The observed count-rates can be analyzed for changes in the radioisotope distribution pattern as well as for statistical variations and accuracy of the results (*10*).

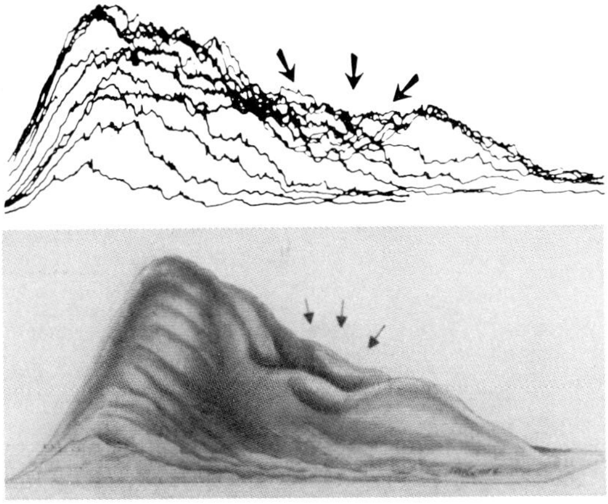

Fig. 22. Composite series of juxtaposed profiles over the liver recorded at 0.5-inch intervals (*10*). In the laboratory these profiles are displayed on transparent sheets with 0.5-inch spaced holders to obtain the three-dimensional representation. An artist's drawing is shown below.

The time constant of the ratemeter must be short to minimize distortion of significant count-rate variations due to lag of response relative to the scanning speed. Since the actual measuring time is short, for low count-rates a short time constant causes wide statistical fluctuations which make the interpretation of the scan uncertain.

The count-rate profile display yields very useful results. Its major disadvantage is that only one line at a time is immediately available, and a three-dimensional representation of the radioisotope distribution is obtained only after assembling a number of two-dimensional profiles.

C. Symbol Printing

The next obvious approach is to use a tapper or symbol printer. A solenoid is coupled to follow the movements of the detector. The pulses from the detector are fed into a scaler which activates the solenoid each time a preselected number of pulses has been accumulated. The solenoid carries a marker which prints on a piece of paper, either through a typewriter ribbon or carbon paper, symbols in the form of dots, lines, bars, or crosses.

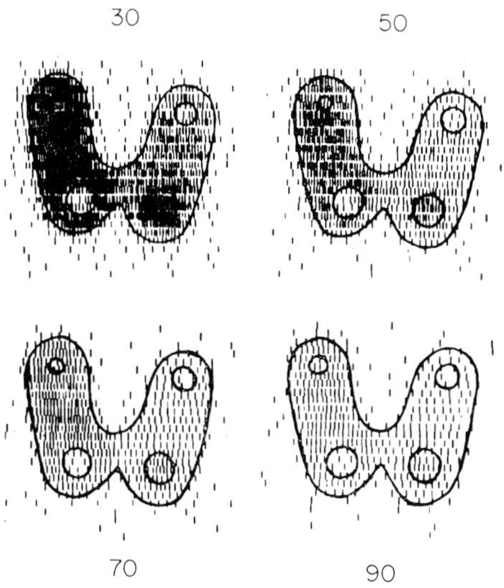

FIG. 23. Scans of thyroid phantom (Picker). In order to demonstrate the effect of different print factors for symbol printouts, unusually high count-rates are employed to minimize statistical fluctuations. The scaling factors are 30, 50, 70, and 90 as indicated. The depth of the ^{131}I solution on the left side is twice that on the right side. On the lower right side there is an area with also twice the solution depth. The other three marked areas of various sizes do not contain any radioactivity. Depending on the choice of the scaling factor, these variations in radioisotope distribution become more or less apparent.

Symbol printing has several advantages. The method is simple and inexpensive; it is reliable and the results become immediately apparent during the scanning operation. The resulting pattern (Fig. 23) indicates the areas of variation of radioisotope distribution and the density of the printed symbol is proportional to the count-rate.

In contrast to the first two methods (Sections IV,A and IV,B), it is more difficult to retrieve quantitative information concerning variations in count-rate from a symbol printout. If a low scaling factor is used, large areas might appear black though the count-rate may vary significantly within the area. Furthermore, the printer may jam at high count-rates even though a specially designed fast tapper is employed (*16*). Too high a scaling factor is also undesirable since the low density of the printed symbols makes it difficult to recognize the resulting pattern and it is even more difficult to judge small variations in the printing frequency (Fig. 23). Furthermore, the printed pattern can be geometrically distorted by a high scaling factor since at low count-rates the

FIG. 24. Multidot printout of liver scan with rose bengal-^{131}I (*16*). The tappers are fired in the order 1-3-2-4.

scanner has to travel a larger distance until the preselected number of counts is reached. The printout, therefore, appears displaced relative to the location of the radioactivity. The extent of the dislocation varies with the count-rate and the scan speed and is in the direction of the scanning motion. As a result of this effect, a bidirectional scan can produce a scalloped picture as shown in Fig. 23 with scaling factors of 30 and 50.

A variety of technical modifications have been tried to improve symbol printouts (*1, 16*). Most printing scanners use a *bar* which is thin in the direction of the scanning motion and long enough to join consecutive scan sweeps (Fig. 23). Mechanical printers with large symbols are necessarily noisy in operation.

A fast *four-stylus tapper* which increases the dynamic range of the mechanical tapper has been developed (*16*). Employing a selected scaling factor, a simple switching circuit activates each of the four strikers in sequence. This results in a more diffuse printing pattern (Fig. 24) allowing various shades of gray to be recognized.

A *dot* pattern type of scan is obtained by use of electrosensitive Teledeltos paper. A conducting stylus is moved over the surface of the

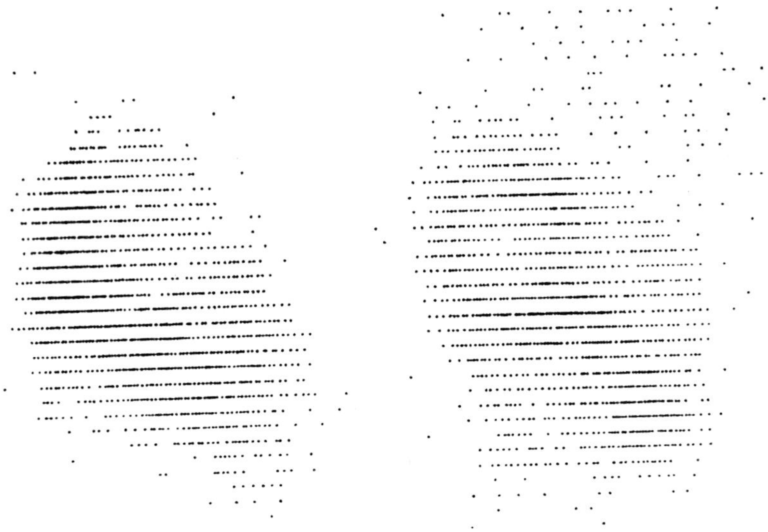

FIG. 25. Dot printout on electrosensitive Teledeltos paper of kidney scan. Patient with surgically proven bilateral polycystic kidneys; largest cyst on lower pole of left kidney. Scan started 1.5 hr after a dose of 60 μCi of Neohydrin-^{203}Hg. Compare dot printout with simultaneously obtained photoscan in Fig. 28.

electrosensitive paper and a dot is made on the paper by an electrical impulse sent through the stylus to the paper. This recording method is relatively fast and noiseless and employs no fast moving mechanical parts. However, the dot pattern, consisting of lines of small dots (Fig. 25) is hard to interpret and variations in dot density are difficult to recognize. Furthermore, this type of recording paper gives only a single copy while with a mechanical tapper, several carbon copies can be obtained.

D. Data Processing, Background Erase

Each scan includes areas where the counts result from the natural background and radioactivity in portions of the patient's body beyond the region of primary interest. This background count-rate contains little useful information. The registered background counts show large statistical variations and they may be dislocated owing to the scaling factor employed for the printing. As they visually disturb the scan picture

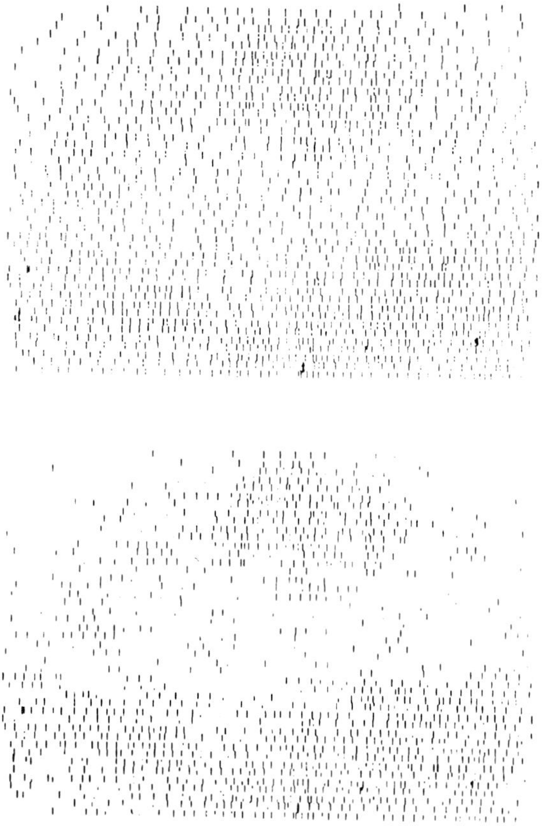

FIG. 26. Right lateral brain tumor scan with Neohydrin-^{203}Hg (*20*). The upper printout (carbon copy of color scan) contains all counts printed with a scale of 8. In the lower printout (color scan) no visible lines are printed at low count-rates. This has the effect of a background erase which makes the tumor on top of the head more clearly visible.

(Fig. 26), a count-rate cutoff circuit is often employed which prevents any data recording at count-rates below a preselected level (*10, 29*).

The cutoff technique may be extended beyond mere background removal by selecting higher cutoff levels (*10, 11, 29, 37*). It is thus possible to record only the regions encompassing a known percentage of the maximum count-rate (Fig. 27). This allows reconstructing the different levels of radioactivity contained within a scan, particularly if all the data are stored initially, as discussed in Section IV,G.

Background erase or selection of various levels of count-rate cutoff requires the use of a count ratemeter, which must determine if the count-rate at any moment is above or below the preselected level. When its time constant is too long, the command to start or stop the printout is

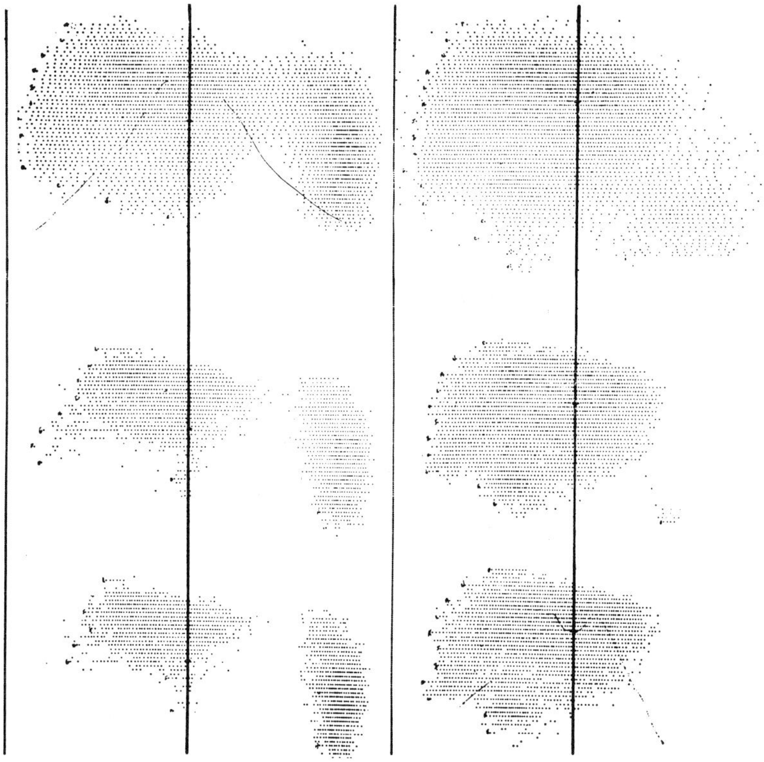

FIG. 27. Two liver scans with 25, 60, and 75% cutoff from top to bottom (*11*). The scan on the left side shows the shape of the spleen more clearly at higher cutoff levels. The more uniform distribution of radioactivity in the liver on the right side is less affected by higher cutoff levels.

delayed. At low count-rates the instantaneous count-rate varies constantly and the accuracy of the background erase is limited by statistical fluctuations. Areas of increased radioactivity can be well delineated at higher cutoff levels.

If for a scan only a single printout employing a preset count-rate cutoff is available, important data may be lost by improper choice of the cutoff level. It is frequently difficult to prejudge the correct erase level because the distribution of the radioactivity and the statistical fluctuations are unknown. Several simultaneous printouts at different cutoff levels are possible but require elaborate equipment.

E. Color Scanning

Instead of discarding counts below a selected cutoff, all the information can be preserved if the mode of printing is altered according to the count-rate. By changing the printing color, this is readily accomplished and the results are easy to interpret (*19, 20, 31*). The tapper strikes one of several colors of a typewriter ribbon; the color is selected by a count ratemeter according to the instantaneous count-rate. Before starting a color scan, the area yielding the highest count-rate is located and the output of the ratemeter is adjusted so that the color designed as the highest intensity is chosen. From there on each color is selected automatically by dividing all count-rates up to the maximum into as many equal intervals (usually 6 to 8) as there are colors employed. The result is a color coded digital printout of all the informations contained in the scan.

When a colorless ribbon is employed for the lowest count-rate interval, this has the effect of a background erase for the color printout. However, on the carbon copies obtained simultaneously with the color printout, all pulses are preserved. The color cutoff at low count-rates yields an improved visualization of areas such as brain lesions, which are difficult to localize because of high tissue background (Fig. 26).

The interpretation of the color scan is not based on the color distribution alone. The density of the print varies with the count-rate as in any symbol printout. The color serves as a code for a digital evaluation of the scan, delineating areas of different count-rates.

F. Photoscanning

The mechanical readout systems described above, including color printout, have some disadvantages. One objective disadvantage is that a scaling factor must be used, causing some degree of distortion depending upon the scan speed and direction (Fig. 23). A subjective factor is that the clinician who reads the scan is often more familiar with the shadings of photographic presentations than with the digital form of symbol prints. To achieve the former, photographic film is frequently used for the recording of light flashes corresponding to individual detector pulses (*4, 5, 27*). Owing to the wide dynamic range of photographic emulsions, it is possible to record every pulse and remain in the useful film density range between 0.3 and 2.0. This method of data recording is generally known as photoscanning. Its greatest disadvantages are that the results are not immediately available and that nonlinearity of emulsions makes the numerical significance of the prints much less evident. Therefore, all commercial photoscanners provide an additional, direct mechanical readout system.

As light source, a cathode-ray tube with a screen phosphor of extremely short persistence is frequently employed (*18*). In a light-tight housing X-ray film is exposed to the light source, which is moved in synchronism with the radiation detector. The amount of film darkening produced by each light flash can be controlled by varying the brightness

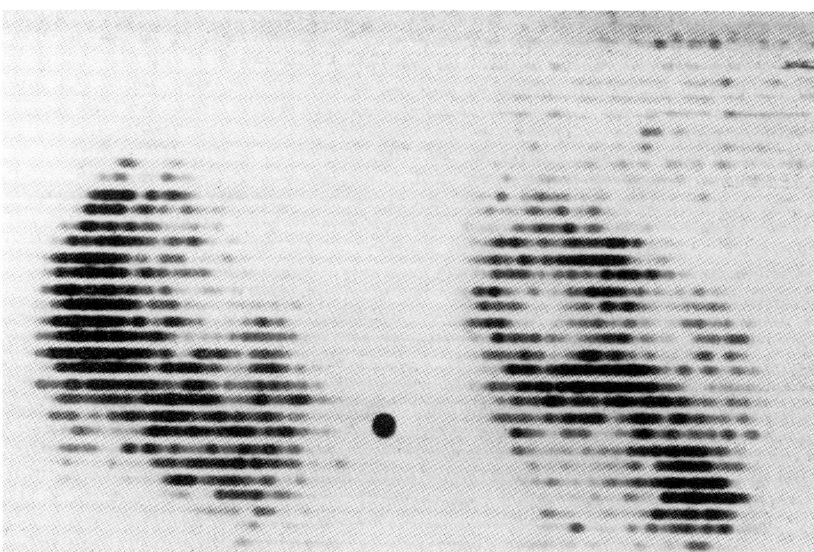

FIG. 28. Photoscan of polycystic kidneys obtained simultaneously with dot readout of Fig. 25. Owing to contrast enhancement, the areas of high radioactivity concentration are prominent and the defects (cysts) in both kidneys can be better recognized.

of the light flash or its duration, or sometimes both. For a selected scan speed, the light intensity can be adjusted so that maximum film darkening is achieved at a specified count-rate.

A combination of digital and analog methods (*4, 18, 27*) can further increase the effectiveness of photoscanning. This is done by controlling the brightness of each light flash by the output of a count ratemeter (Fig. 28). The control may be adjusted so that practically no film darkening occurs over areas where the count-rate is below a preselected level. When the count-rate increases above that level, the brightness of each light pulse is rapidly increased. A count-rate differential can be selected which covers the full film density scale from white to black. This nonlinear method of recording, a form of contrast enhancement, can be very effective, when applied with discretion in emphasizing small variations in count-rate. It has the hazard, however, that it requires an *a priori* decision of the low-level information to be rejected, similarly to the count-rate cutoff method (Section IV,D). Also significant information of high-level variations may be lost.

It is possible to produce color photoscans (*24*) by using color film and exposing it to colored light. Like color scanning (Section IV,E), the colors are chosen according to the count-rate. This again enhances differences in count-rate without preselection of a cutoff level. The use of color film has the same advantage as photoscanning, that is, no scaling factor has to be employed.

G. Data Storage and Reprocessing

In all readout systems described so far, the objective was to produce a finished picture at the conclusion of the scan. In each case this required some compromise in the readout system with the possible loss of valuable information. The ideal solution would be to preserve all the data accumulated by the detector in an accessible form so that it may be reevaluated numerically or subjected to nonlinear transformations for emphasizing the desirable information. Such data storage systems allow maximum flexibility of data handling, which is often desirable for research applications. For routine clinical scanning, on the other hand, any one or a combination of several of the readout methods described above has the distinct advantage of simplicity.

1. RESCANNING

The wide dynamic range of photographic film is excellent for preserving the full range of information accumulated during a scan. It can be recovered by means of a densitometer which measures variations in film density (*17*). The processed and illuminated film is rescanned in the same manner as the γ-ray detector had scanned the patient in making the original record. Any of the readout systems described above can be employed for displaying the rescan data. Rescanning can be performed repeatedly with modification of various parameters to search out the pertinent information. However, it is time consuming and requires additional equipment beside the scanner.

2. CLOSED CIRCUIT TELEVISION

The contrast of a photoscan can be controlled by viewing the scan through a closed circuit television system. The processed film illuminated by an X-ray viewing box is surveyed by the television camera and displayed on the television monitor. Contrast and brightness controls are adjusted for high contrast and the video gain control is increased until only the maximum density of the scan appears black (Fig. 29A). When the video gain is decreased, areas of lesser film density become successively darker (Fig. 29B and 29C) until the background of the scanning area may darken the whole field of vision. In this manner the televised image of the scan can be examined with adjustable high differential contrast (*5, 14*).

Depending on the selected contrast, a smaller or larger section of the complete scan becomes visible. The various pictures must be viewed repeatedly or a series of new photographs of the pictures on the monitor must be taken. The amplification of small variations in film density may result in a series of confusing pictures, especially in the presence of large statistical count-rate fluctuations. Therefore, this powerful method should be used only by an experienced interpreter.

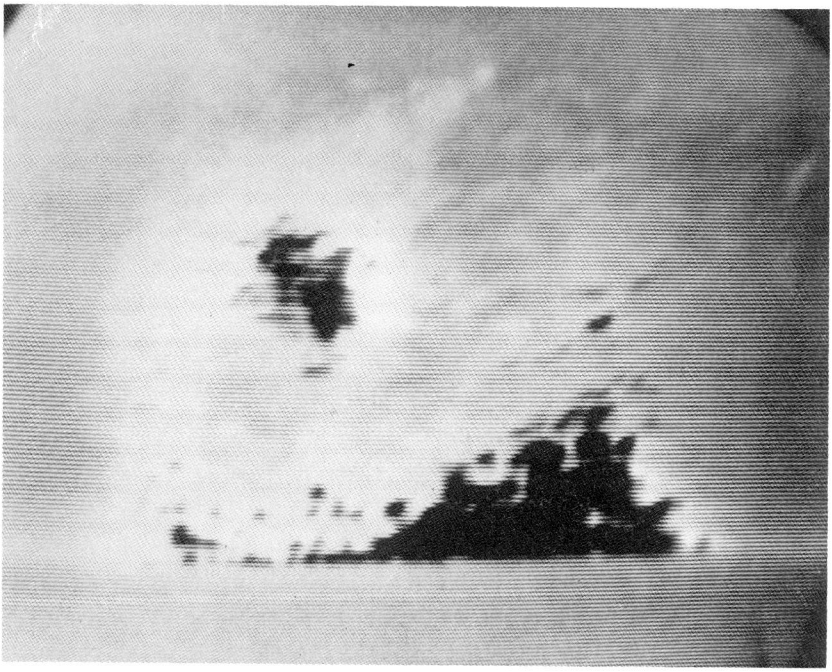

FIG. 29(A).

FIG. 29. Series of photographs of television monitor screen with various degrees of contrast of anterior-posterior brain tumor scan (*14*). (A) High contrast, showing only areas of highest radioactivity concentration. (B) Medium contrast; brain tumor as well as facial muscles are well recognizable. (C) Low contrast; picture quality is reduced by background counts.

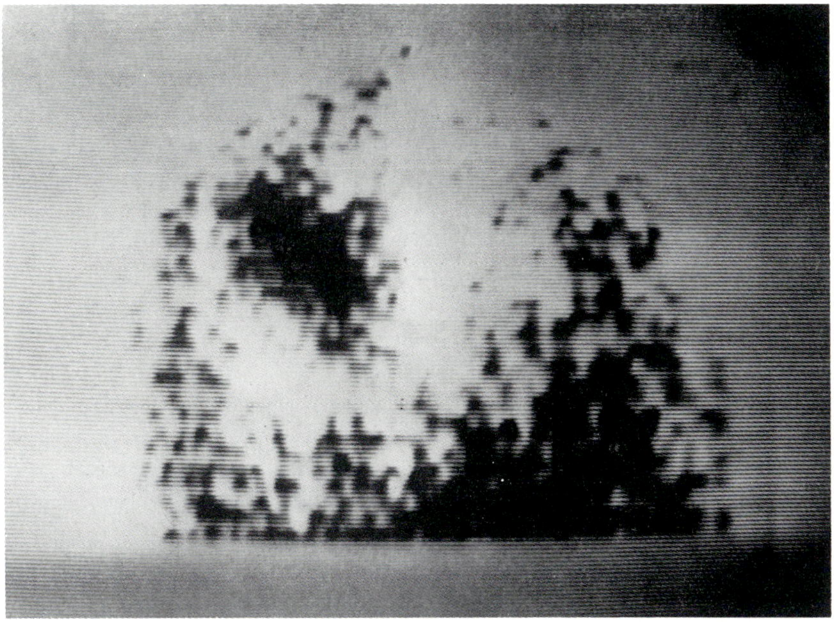

FIG. 29(B).

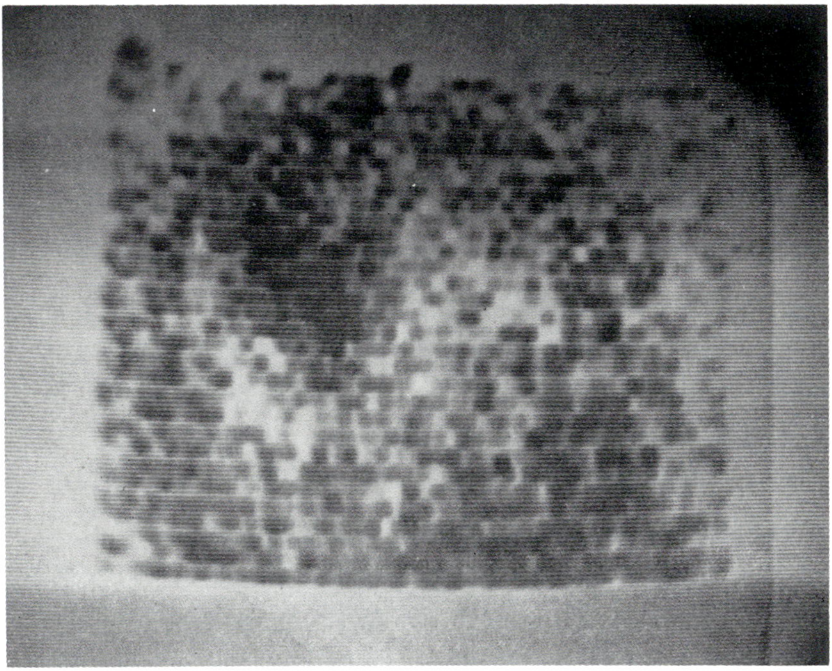

FIG. 29(C).

When, instead of a black and white closed circuit television system, a color television is employed, the various degrees of contrast can be transposed into different colors (*9*). This allows a simultaneous display of all pictures representing different count-rate ranges. However, it requires a rather complex electronic system and the appearance of the different colors depends on the technique used by the operator.

Unlike the simpler, direct method of colorscanning (Section IV,E), where the colors represent known fractions of the maximum count-rate, the television contrast enhancement techniques are highly qualitative. The unknown degree of nonlinearity of the original photoscan is further distorted by the complexities of the electronic system.

3. Magnetic Tape and Foil Storage

While direct mechanical printing and photographic recording are the most commonly used means of data storage, a rapidly growing technique is the magnetic tape or foil system. Each pulse may be recorded as a small magnetized region of the material. As for photographic recording, no scaling factor is needed, and as for mechanical printout, the recording is linear. Once the recording is made, it may be read back immediately in a nondestructive manner. It may be processed into a mechanical or photographic printout, or directly into an oscilloscope picture by interspersing suitable electronic controls. Magnetic recording has the great advantage that the signal comes out in electrical form ideally suited for processing in a high-speed digital computer (*25*). While these techniques are still in the research stage, they show great promise for future evaluation of scanning data.

The use of magnetic tape for the recording of scanning data (*6*) requires that synchronizing signals be recorded as well as counting information so that the motion of the detector can be communicated to the playback system. Depending on the particular types of mechanical movements and readout devices, fairly complicated recording and control systems are needed.

The use of magnetic foil (*23*) eliminates some of these difficulties. These foils are large sheets of magnetically sensitive material over which the recording head moves in a manner similar to a direct symbol printer. Thus, the line structure of the original scan is preserved on the foil. Although little experience has yet been obtained with this system, it seems the most suitable medium for storage of scanning data.

REFERENCES

1. Ackerman, N. B., McFee, A. S., Miller, W. D., and Marvin, J. F., Improved mechanical printer for liver scanning. *J. Am. Med. Assoc.* **179,** 134 (1962).

2. Anger, H. O., and Rosenthal, D. J., Scintillation camera and positron camera. *Proc. Seminar Med. Radioisotope Scanning, Vienna, 1959* p. 59. Intern. At. Energy Agency, Vienna, 1959.
3. Beck, R. N., A theoretical evaluation of brain scanning systems. *J. Nucl. Med.* **2,** 314 (1961).
4. Bender, M. A., and Blau, M., A versatile, high-contrast photoscanner for the localization of human tumors with radioisotopes. *Intern. J. Appl. Radiation Isotopes* **4,** 154 (1959).
5. Bender, M. A., and Blau, M., Photoscanning. *Proc. Seminar Med. Radioisotope Scanning, Vienna, 1959* p. 31. Intern. At. Energy Agency, Vienna, 1959.
6. Bonte, F. J., Krohmer, J. S., and Romans, W. E., Magnetic tape recording of scintillation scan data. *Intern. J. Appl. Radiation Isotopes* **14,** 273 (1963).
7. Brownell, G. L., Theory of radioisotope scanning. *Proc. Symp. Med. Radioisotope Scanning, Athens, 1964* Vol. 1, p. 3. Intern. At. Energy Agency, Vienna, 1964.
8. Cederlund, J., Information theory and radioisotope scanning. *Proc. Symp. Med. Radioisotope Scanning, Athens, 1964* Vol. 1, p. 57. Intern. At. Energy Agency, Vienna, 1964.
9. Charkes, N. D., and Gershon-Cohen, J., Color television contrast expansion of photoscans. *Am. J. Roentgenol. Radium Therapy Nucl. Med.* **90,** 406 (1963).
10. Christie, J. H., and MacIntyre, W. J., Information limitations of radioisotope scanning. *Radiology* **79,** 472 (1962).
11. Christie, J. H., MacIntyre, W. J., Gomez-Crespo, G., and Koch-Weser, D., Radioisotope scanning in hepatic cirrhosis. *Radiology* **81,** 455 (1963).
12. Corey, K. R., Kenny, P., Greenberg, E., and Laughlin, J. S., Detection of bone metastases in scanning studies with calcium-47 and strontium-85. *J. Nucl. Med.* **3,** 454 (1962).
13. Dewey, W. C., and Sinclair, W. K., Criteria for evaluating collimators used in *in vivo* distribution studies with radioisotopes. *Intern. J. Appl. Radiation Isotopes* **10,** 1 (1961).
14. Fleming, W. H., McIlraith, J. D., and King, E. R., Medical scintillation scanning utilizing closed circuit TV contrast enhancement. *Am. J. Roentgenol. Radium Therapy Nucl. Med.* **87,** 128 (1962).
15. Harris, C. C., Bell, P. R., Francis, J. E., Jr., Satterfield, M. M., Jordan, J. C., and Murray, J. P., Collimators for radioisotope scanning. *In* "Progress in Medical Radioisotope Scanning" (R. M. Kniseley, G. A. Andrews, and C. C. Harris, eds.), TID-7673, p. 25. U.S. At. Energy Comm., Washington, D.C., 1963.
16. Harris, C. C., Bell, P. R., Francis, J. E., Jr., Jordan, J. C., and Satterfield, M. M., Data recording for radioisotope scanning. *In* "Progress in Medical Radioisotope Scanning" (R. M. Kniseley, G. A. Andrews, and C. C. Harris, eds.), TID-7673, p. 66. U.S. At. Energy Comm., Washington, D.C., 1963.
17. Harris, C. C., Bell, P. R., Satterfield, M. M., Ross, D. A., and Jordan, J. C., Analysis of scan records with a recording densitometer—the "re-scanner." *Proc. Symp. Med. Radioisotope Scanning, Athens, 1964* Vol. 1, p. 529. Intern. At. Energy Agency, Vienna, 1964.
18. Herring, C. E., A universal photorecording system for radioisotope area scanners. *J. Nucl. Med.* **1,** 83 (1960).
19. Hine, G. J., Color-coded digital print-out for radioisotope scanning. *J. Nucl. Med.* **4,** 439 (1963).

20. Hine, G. J., Patten, D. H., and Burrows, B. A., Contrast enhancement by multi-colour print-out of thyroid, kidney, liver and brain scans. *Proc. Symp. Med. Radioisotope Scanning, Athens, 1964* Vol. 1, p. 465. Intern. At. Energy Agency, Vienna, 1964.
21. *IAEA, Proc. Symp. Med. Radioisotope Scanning, Athens, 1964* Vol. 1 and 2. Intern. At. Energy Agency, Vienna, 1964.
22. Jones, R. C., Information capacity of photographic film. *J. Opt. Soc.* **51,** 1159 (1961).
23. Jordan, K., and Winkler, C., Elektrotechnische und elektromagnetische Verfahren zur Aufnahme und Auswertung von Szintillogrammen. *In* "Radioaktive Isotope in Klinik und Forschung" (K. Fellinger and R. Höfer, eds.), Vol. 5, p. 67. Urban & Schwarzenberg, Munich, 1963.
24. Kakehi, H., Arimizu, N., and Uchiyama, G., A new method for colour scanning. *Proc. Symp. Med. Radioisotope Scanning, Athens, 1964* Vol. 1, p. 451. International Atomic Energy Agency, Vienna, 1964.
25. Karvin, B., and Huston, F. V., Dataphone computer system for radioisotope scan display. *Proc. 16th Conf. Eng. Med. Biol., Baltimore, 1963.* Institute of Electrical and Electronics Engineers, New York, 1963.
26. Kniseley, R. M., Andrews, G. A., and Harris, C. C. (eds.), "Progress in Medical Radioisotope Scanning," TID-7673. U.S. At. Energy Comm., Washington, D.C., 1963.
27. Kuhl, D. E., Chamberlain, R. H., Hale, J., and Gorson, R. O., A high-contrast photographic recorder for scintillation counter scanning. *Radiology* **66,** 730 (1956).
28. Kuhl, D. E., and Edwards, R. Q., Image separation radioisotope scanning. *Radiology* **80,** 653 (1963).
29. MacIntyre, W. J., and Houser, T. S., A method for the visualization of the configuration and structure of the liver. Part B. A counting rate cut-off circuit for increased contrast in automatic scanning. *Am. J. Roentgenol. Radium Therapy Nucl. Med.* **77,** 471 (1957).
30. MacIntyre, W. J., Gomez-Crespo, G., and Christie, J. H., The use of the counting rate profile in radioisotope scanning techniques. *J. Nucl. Med.* **1,** 262 (1960).
31. Mallard, J. R., Fowler, J. F., and Sutton, M., Brain tumour detection using radioactive arsenic. *Brit. J. Radiol.* **34,** 562 (1961).
32. Mehl, H. G., Grundlagen und Ergebnisse der in-vivo-Messung radioaktiver Substanzen im menschlichen Organismus. *In* "Medizinische Grundlagen Forschung" (K. F. Bauer, ed.), Vol. 3, p. 97. Georg Thieme Verlag, Stuttgart, 1960.
33. Pochin, E. E., Profile counting. *Proc. Seminar Med. Radioisotope Scanning, Vienna, 1959* p. 143. Intern. At. Energy Agency, Vienna, 1959.
34. Quinn, J. L. (ed.), "Scintillation Scanning in Clinical Medicine." Saunders, Philadelphia, Pennsylvania, 1964.
35. Rankowitz, S., Robertson, J. S., Higinbotham, W. A., and Rosenblum, M. J., Positron scanner for locating brain tumors. *IRE Intern. Conv. Record* **9,** 49 (1961).
36. Ross, D. A., Linear scanning. *In* "Progress in Medical Radioisotope Scanning" (R. M. Kniseley, G. A. Andrews, and C. C. Harris, eds.), TID-7673, p. 190. U.S. At. Energy Comm., Washington, D.C., 1963.
37. Yagan, R., MacIntyre, W. J., and Christie, J. H., Estimation of liver size by the multiple cut-off scintillation scanning technique. *Am. J. Roentgenol. Radium Therapy Nucl. Med.* **88,** 289 (1962).

CHAPTER 17

MULTIHOLE COLLIMATORS FOR SCANNING

JOHN MYHILL

UNIVERSITY OF SYDNEY AND
INSTITUTE OF MEDICAL RESEARCH
ROYAL NORTH SHORE HOSPITAL OF SYDNEY
SIDNEY, AUSTRALIA

AND

GERALD J. HINE

INTERNATIONAL ATOMIC ENERGY AGENCY
VIENNA, AUSTRIA

I. COLLIMATOR PROPERTIES

A multihole collimator, often called multichannel, honeycomb, or focusing collimator, is constructed of shielding material placed between the radiation detector and a γ-ray emitting radioisotope source. Several holes through the shielding allow radiation to reach the detector from a specified spatial location only (Chapter 3, Fig. 11). The field of view of a multihole collimator is simply the superposition of the fields of view of each of the several holes. At the focal plane, they superimpose quite exactly. Everywhere else the superposition is only partial, depending on the distance from the focal plane. Tapered holes must be used to make the maximum amount of crystal area available to the incident radiation.

The main properties of multihole collimators, their resolution, sensitivity, and depth response, have been discussed in Chapter 16. They will be summarized here only briefly.

Resolution refers to the ability of a collimated detector to distinguish between two radioisotope sources placed close together (Chapter 16, Section II,C). A collimator which allows two point sources 5 mm apart to be recognized as two distinct sources has a better spatial resolution than one which requires the sources to be 10 mm apart for recognition as distinct sources. Although any definition of resolution is somewhat arbitrary, for many purposes the spatial resolution of a collimator may be quantitatively defined as the distance on a point source response curve between the two points where the response is half of the maximum (Chapter 16, Section II,A). This is the familiar full width at half maximum (FWHM) of the response curve. In the case of a multihole collimator, the response curve referred to in this definition is that plotted in a plane perpendicular to the collimator axis which contains the point of maximum response of the collimator (focal point). In any other plane, either closer or further away from the collimator, the resolution is usually reduced, that is, FWHM is larger.

Depth response of a collimator depends on its focal distance. Multihole collimators are usually designed so that the axes of all holes meet at a point in front of the collimator. This point is called the geometrical focus. The count-rate for a point source at the experimental focus (which usually lies a little toward the collimator from the geometrical focus) is greater than at any point located some distance in any direction from the focus. As a point source is moved from the collimator face along the axis of the collimator, the count-rate at first increases to a maximum at the focus and then decreases as the point source is moved farther along the axis of the collimator.

Sensitivity of a collimator refers to its ability to detect radiation from a radioisotope source. Sensitivity is difficult to define, but for many purposes the sensitivity may be expressed as that fraction of all γ rays emitted by a point source, placed at the focal point of the collimator, which reaches the detector. This is a point source definition of sensitivity (Chapter 16, Section II,A).

An important plane source sensitivity may also be defined (Chapter 16, Section II,B). For a large plane source perpendicular to the collimator axis, the focusing collimator sensitivity is practically independent of source-to-collimator distance, if the γ-ray energy is low enough to avoid septa penetration. The area of the field of view of the collimator increases as the square of the distance, offsetting the inverse square law of the decreasing fraction of γ rays reaching the detector as the source-to-detector distance increases (see Figs. 6 and 7).

Based on this fact, a simple method for the determination of the collimator plane source sensitivity is shown schematically in Fig. 1. The results obtained with a 19-hole collimator are given in Fig. 2. The curve on top is the observed count-rate as a function of source-to-collimator distance for a large plane source of ^{131}I. The graph at the bottom shows the same curve with the decreasing count-rate given in percent, to-

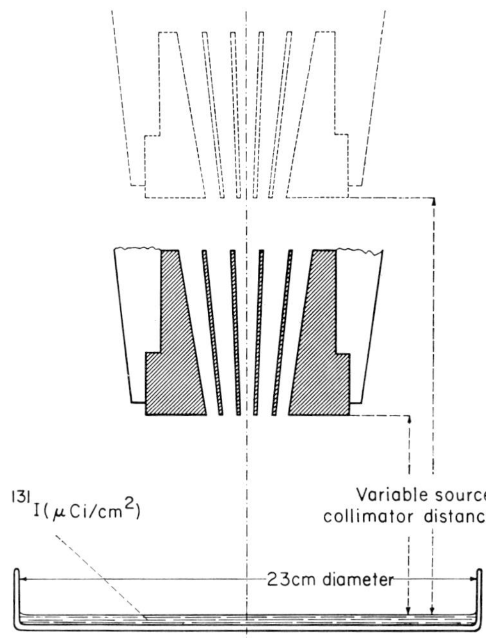

FIG. 1. Determination of the plane source sensitivity of a focusing collimator. A large plane source is positioned perpendicular to the collimator axis at various distances from the collimator.

gether with the corresponding values for a plane source of ^{57}Co (122-keV γ rays). The faster increase in count-rate with the higher-energy ^{131}I γ rays is caused by an increase of septa penetration at closer source-to-collimator distances. Since the count-rate decreases slowly in either case, any value may be chosen as sensitivity. However, for simplicity the sensitivity of a collimator may be given as the count-rate of the plane source at its focal distance.

γ-Ray detectors of high spatial resolution and high sensitivity are required for the accurate delineation of a radioisotope distribution. While single-hole collimated detectors (*10, 11, 26–28*) can achieve high resolution with a sufficiently narrow hole, their sensitivity is low (Chapter 16, Section III,C,1). The resolution of a single-hole collimator is proportional to the diameter of the hole, but the sensitivity is proportional to the square of the hole diameter. Thus, halving the hole diameter improves the resolution by a factor of 2, while the sensitivity is reduced by a factor of 4. In most clinical applications the amount of radioisotope necessary to achieve a good scan in a reasonable length of time with a single-hole collimator is too great. For example, with a multihole

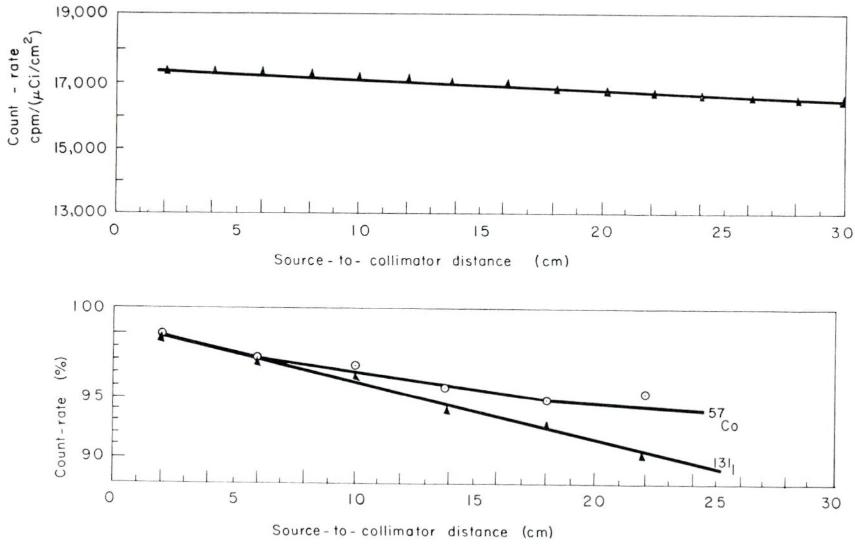

FIG. 2. Sensitivity measurements with a plane source of ^{131}I and a 19-hole Picker collimator. *Top:* count-rate as a function of source-to-collimator distance. *Bottom:* Percentage decrease of count-rate with source-to-collimator distance for the ^{131}I and a ^{57}Co source.

collimator a dose of 50 μCi of ^{131}I-labeled rose bengal yields a satisfactory liver scan (*4*). With a single-hole collimator of the same resolution one would need about 2.5 mCi.

Multihole collimators provide both high spatial resolution and adequate sensitivity. The resolution is improved by narrowing the holes, and the sensitivity is maintained by placing more of the narrower holes in front of the radiation detector. The properties a collimator must have for its successful use depend upon the γ-ray energy of the isotope being scanned, the size of the source, the strength (μCi) of the source, the detail to be resolved (required resolution) and the time available for the scan. Multihole collimators used for purposes other than radioisotope scanning will not be considered in this chapter.

The parameters which may be varied to achieve the desired collimator properties are size of holes, distribution of holes, shape of holes, focal length of collimator, and septa thickness. The septa are the portions of shielding material between the holes in the collimator.

II. COLLIMATOR STRUCTURE

The general outline of collimator structure given below is not meant to represent an optimum design for any scanning situation. The reader is referred to the literature for mathematical design principles (*1, 2, 5–7, 9, 13, 16, 30, 32, 34, 35, 37*) and for details of the major types of collimators (*14, 18, 19, 20, 21, 23, 29, 31, 33*).

A. Crystal Size

The choice of the crystal size depends on a number of factors. With increasing diameter of the sodium iodide crystal it is possible to design a more sensitive multihole collimator. The depth responses of two collimators with about equal resolution at their focal plane, at about 6 cm from the collimator, are shown in Fig. 3. The 31-hole collimator on the right for a 5-inch diameter crystal has about 2.5 times the sensitivity of the 19-hole collimator for a 3-inch diameter crystal on the left. This increase in sensitivity will be a distinct advantage for many scanning applications.

The large-diameter crystal not only allows for a greater number of holes, but gives also an improved photopeak efficiency (Chapter 6, Section III,B). On the other hand, its outer holes are at a larger angle with respect to the collimator axis. Therefore, the resolution of the larger-diameter crystal collimator varies more with distance, on both sides of the focal plane, than is the case for the resolution of the smaller crystal collimator. This loss of resolution outside the focal plane will decrease the overall resolution of this collimator for most scanning applications, except in those cases where the radioactivity is confined to a shallow region close to the focal plane (Fig. 3).

Economic considerations also limit the size of the sodium iodide crystal. The larger crystal requires more side shielding in addition to the larger collimator. This adds considerably to the weight that has to be moved by the scanner. It requires a very sturdy construction of the scanner, which older and less expensive designs are lacking.

At present, sodium iodide crystals of 3-inch diameter are generally used for multihole collimators. The crystals are mostly 2 inches thick, though 3-inch thick crystals have been tried. For very low-energy γ- or X-ray emitters, such as ^{125}I (27 to 35 keV), a crystal of 2-mm thickness is adequate; but it must be encased in a can with a beryllium window (0.005-inch thick) rather than the usual 0.03 inch of aluminum.

B. Collimator Material

Lead is the cheapest and generally the best collimator material. It is easy to work with and collimators can be made simply by casting. Be-

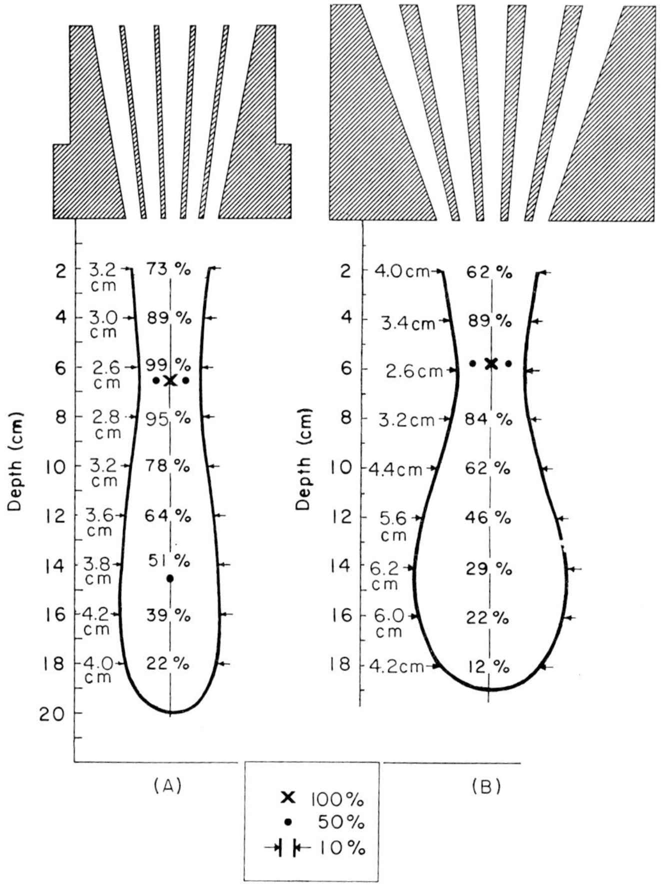

FIG. 3. Depth response of two focusing collimators. (A) Picker 19-hole collimator for a 3-inch diameter crystal. (B) Picker 31-hole collimator for a 5-inch diameter crystal. Percentage depth response along the collimator axis and the 10% response are shown. Measurements were made with an ^{131}I line source in air (*21*).

cause pure lead is too soft, lead containing a few percent of antimony and bismuth is preferred. For the casting of the collimator, the holes of the collimator are occupied in the mold by steel or aluminum pins. carefully machined to the correct size and shape.

Materials with a greater absorption than lead for high-energy γ rays are mercury, tungsten, gold, and some other precious metals of prohibitive cost. A mercury multihole collimator has been fabricated by making the collimator holes of a low-density wood and pouring mercury into the spaces between the assembly of holes (*17*). When used as a collimator the wooden holes present little obstruction to the γ rays while the mercury septa are nearly opaque.

Tungsten itself is so difficult to work that it is not used in collimators made of a single piece of metal. Tungsten powder mixtures (alloys) have nearly the same γ-ray absorption as pure tungsten and are easier to work. Casting or even pressure molding is not a technologically feasible procedure for objects of the size and shape of multihole collimators. If round tapered holes are acceptable then these may be reamed in tungsten powder mixtures at a reasonable cost and with good accuracy, yielding a very good collimator (*14*).

Gold has a greater absorption for high-energy γ rays than mercury or tungsten and is theoretically a better material for collimators. Since the gold in the collimator has the same value as it had before manufacture, it may be possible to obtain it on a long-term loan. Gold may be cast, and if the septa are thick, $\frac{1}{4}$ inch, for example, this presents no problem. If the holes are round tapered they may be reamed from a block of metal without difficulty. If the holes are not round, and the design dictates thin septa, about $\frac{1}{16}$ inch, for instance, then the collimator may be cast but the manufacture is difficult.

The transmissions of different collimator materials are shown in Table I. For lead collimators with the usual septa thickness (about $\frac{1}{8}$ inch), geometrical considerations (*7, 37*) are satisfactory for γ rays with energies up to about 150 keV. For 150 to 400 keV radiation septa penetration has to be considered while for radiation with energies over 400 keV septa penetration dominates. For equal septa thickness, little septa penetration is observed with tungsten for γ rays in the energy range up to 300–450 keV and with gold up to 450–700 keV γ rays. Above 700 keV thick septa must be used, with concurrent loss of sensitivity.

In general, a large-diameter collimator made of a material of lower γ-ray absorption will be as efficient as a smaller one made of superior material. For example, a lead collimator 6 inches thick in front of a 6-inch diameter crystal can be designed to have the same resolution and sensitivity as a gold collimator 3 inches thick in front of a 3-inch diameter crystal. This can be done by having about the same number and size of holes in each collimator, but making the septa in the lead collimator thicker and distributing the holes over the 6-inch diameter crystal

TABLE I

NARROW BEAM TRANSMISSIONS, IN PERCENTAGE OF INCIDENT RADIATION, THROUGH 1, 2.5, AND 5 CM OF LEAD, TUNGSTEN, AND GOLD FOR VARIOUS γ-RAY ENERGIES (*19*)

	1 cm			2.5 cm			5 cm		
γ-Ray energy (keV)	Pb	W	Au	Pb	W	Au	Pb	W	Au
160 (^{199}Au)	0.01	*	*	*	*	*	*	*	*
279 (^{203}Hg)	0.7	0.09	0.045	2×10^{-4}	*	*	*	*	*
320 (^{51}Cr)	2.2	0.5	0.25	8×10^{-3}	2×10^{-4}	*	*	*	*
411 (^{198}Au)	9	3.5	2	0.24	0.025	0.02	1.4×10^{-4}	*	*
662 (^{137}Cs)	30	17	14	4.8	1.2	0.7	0.23	0.014	0.005
1310 (^{47}Ca)	53	37	35	19.5	7.6	6.5	3.9	0.58	0.46

NOTE: Asterisks indicate a value of less than 10^{-4}%.

face. The thicker lead septa will offer the same absorption to γ rays as the thinner gold septa.

The larger collimator has the disadvantage that it will be heavier owing to more shielding around the larger crystal, and this requires a more robust scanning machine. It has the advantage that the major expense is in the crystal assembly and not in the collimator material or cost of manufacture. Thus different inexpensive lead collimators can be made to be used with the one crystal for different scanning applications. Furthermore the larger crystal yields a higher photopeak efficiency. On the other hand, as pointed out above, the resolution of large-diameter collimators is apt to vary more with distance from the focal plane than that of smaller-diameter collimators.

Since the response of a collimator at points some distance from the collimator axis should be low for obtaining a good scan, collimators constructed for ^{131}I are generally unsuitable for energies above 400 keV. They are unsuitable whenever high resolution is required or when the target-to-nontarget radioisotope concentration difference is small. For a 37-hole 3-inch diameter lead collimator (*19*) the resolutions for 320- and 662-keV γ rays are nearly the same, but at 1 inch (about three times the resolution distance) from the axis of the collimator, the response to the 662-keV γ rays is about 70 times greater than that to 320-keV γ radiation (Chapter 16, Fig. 10).

Even with the Oak Ridge 37-hole 3-inch diameter gold collimator with tungsten side shielding (*19*) the off-axis response to 662-keV or 1.1-MeV γ rays is not entirely satisfactory. At 2 inches off axis in the plane containing the point of maximum response it is about 0.5% and 3%, respectively, while for 364-keV γ rays it is less than 0.01%.

C. Size, Shape, Distribution, and Number of Holes

The number of holes, their size, shape, and distribution, the thickness of the septa between the holes, the thickness (length) of the collimator itself, and the taper of the holes cannot be determined separately. They are really always, and for higher γ-ray energies most obviously, one complex of parameters, which must be optimized as a group. This largely comprises the subject of theoretical multihole collimator research (*2, 25, 30, 32, 36*).

To a first approximation the hole size may be calculated to give the desired spatial resolution, according to the geometrical response (Section II,F). The hole shape which is less important is discussed below. The distribution of the holes depends on their shape and the cross section (round or square) of the crystal. The number of holes is determined by the crystal size and the required septa thickness (Section II,D).

If a square crystal is used, the holes are placed in a square array in front of the crystal and are of square cross section. Some advantage is derived from this design, as in rectilinear scanning a higher sensitivity can be achieved for a given resolution in the direction of scanning. However, the relative merits of square and round holes in real scanning situations with extended sources of varying activity have not yet been evaluated.

Circular cylinders of crystal are generally easier to use and they are also cheaper. The holes are placed in front of the crystal in such a pattern as to maximize the use of the crystal face. Usually the hexagon formed by the outer holes of a hexagonal array inscribes the circular crystal face (Fig. 4A). The holes themselves may be of hexagonal or

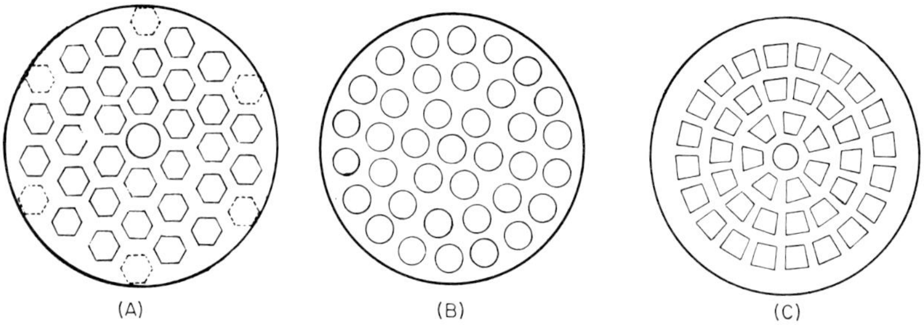

FIG. 4. Three different kinds of hole distributions. (A) Hexagonal holes in an hexagonal array. (B) Round holes in a circular pattern. (C) Trapezoidal holes in a circular pattern (*17*).

round cross section. A hexagonal cross section ensures that the thickness of the septa between holes is uniform around the holes and is constant in any plane parallel to the crystal face. If the holes have a round cross section equal in area to that of the hexagonal holes discussed above, then the minimum septa thickness is less than the septa thickness for hexagonal holes. Since γ-ray penetration varies exponentially with absorber thickness, in this design more γ rays penetrate the septa if round holes are used. However, since γ rays from an extended clinical source are incident on the septa from all angles, the effect is somewhat reduced. Accurate experimental data on this aspect of design are not available.

If the round holes of one collimator are of such size that they inscribe the hexagonal holes of another collimator of otherwise identical design, then the septa penetration in the collimator with the round holes is certainly a little less but also the area of the crystal exposed to unobstructed radiation is 8.5% smaller. This causes a reduction of the collimator sensitivity by about the same amount. Such a decrease in sensitivity may be significant in some applications where the radioisotope concentration is so low that the information to be obtained from the scan is at the threshold of visibility. In general, it is unimportant in most clinical investigations.

Other design patterns (*33*) place the holes (usually of circular cross section) in two or three circles around a central hole (Fig. 4B). For a given crystal size the average septa thickness is often made much larger in these collimators and thus septa penetration is small, usually so small as to allow an accurate calculation of the collimator's resolution by simple geometrical considerations (Section II,F). However, sensitivity is sacrificed to achieve this. Another design (*17, 22*) uses septa in the form of a series of concentric conical surfaces intersecting with radial septa to form the collimator holes (Fig. 4C).

D. Thickness of Septa

Septa thicknesses have largely been assigned empirically, and the result is checked after the collimator has been built. One criterion for collimator design is to cover about half of the crystal face with holes and the other half with septa (Table II). Since the hole sizes are determined mainly by the resolution that is desired, it follows that this criterion fixes the septa thickness.

A better criterion may be to make the septa of such thickness that only a few percent of the radiation incident on them from all feasible directions will penetrate to the crystal. This criterion, however, may be too stringent in that some penetrating radiation may be allowable for achieving the optimum compromise between spatial resolution and sensitivity. This would mean thinner septa and thus more holes in front of the same crystal.

The thickness (length) of a collimator is determined by two considerations. First, the spatial resolution of a collimator depends on the length of holes as well as their diameter. Second, septa penetration should be small to provide adequate shielding in front of the crystal. For example, if a thyroid scan is performed 24 hr after the administration of a tracer dose of ^{131}I, most of the background counts come from the thyroid itself. Thus, when a collimator with a 6-mm resolution (FWHM) is accumulating counts from a 50-mm^2 region of the thyroid, the remaining region of the gland, which is about 50 times larger, contributes to the background. These background counts must be reduced to much less than the counts from the region being counted. To reduce their contribution to 1% requires a lead thickness of about 1.5 cm if pulse-height analysis of the 364-keV ^{131}I peak is being used (see Appendix, Fig. 4).

The septa thickness of many collimators varies between 0.2 and 0.3 cm and the length of the collimator between 8 and 10 cm (Table II).

TABLE II

SPECIFICATIONS OF COLLIMATORS FOR ^{131}I WITH 3- AND 5-INCH DIAMETER NaI(Tl) CRYSTALS[a]

Type of collimator	Number of holes (n)	Radius of crystal (R) (cm)	Radius of holes on top (r_0) (cm)	Radius of holes at base (r_1) (cm)	Crystal opening $(r_0^2 n)/R^2$ (%)	Collimator length (l) (cm)	Septa thickness on top (s_0) (cm)	Septa thickness at base (s_1) (cm)
3-Inch crystal, 3-inch fine focus, No. 2102	31	3.81	0.4	0.15	34.2	10.2	0.30	0.14
3-Inch crystal, 3-inch broad focus, No. 2107	19	3.81	0.6	0.30	47.2	7.8	0.31	0.2
5-Inch crystal, 3-inch fine focus, No. 2112A	163	6.35	0.35	0.15	49.1	8.7	0.30	0.12
5-Inch crystal, 3-inch broad focus, No. 2112	31	6.35	0.8	0.40	49.2	8.7	0.65	0.30
5-Inch crystal, 5-inch fine focus, No. 2111A	265	6.35	0.25	0.15	41.2	8.7	0.20	0.12
5-Inch crystal, 5-inch broad focus, No. 2111	85	6.35	0.45	0.29	42.7	8.7	0.50	0.24

[a] Courtesy of Picker Nuclear.

The response of the 19-hole collimator (Fig. 3A) at the focal plane to ^{131}I and ^{57}Co point sources in air is shown in Fig. 5. At the 1 percent level the full width of the response curve, compared with the resolution

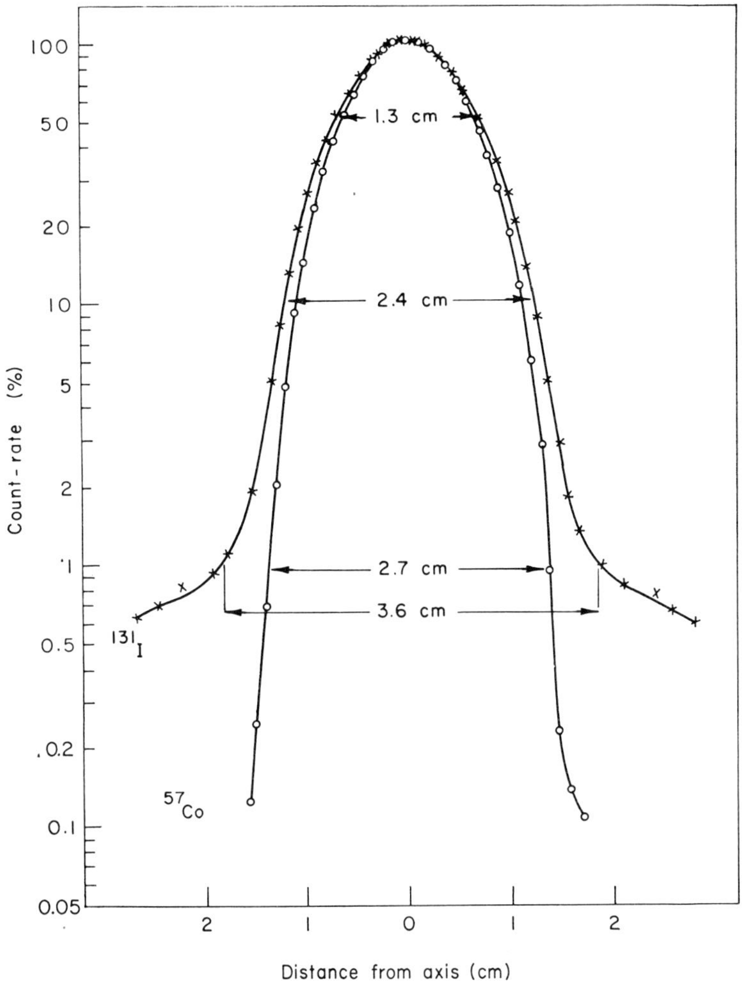

FIG. 5. Response of 19-hole collimator (Fig. 3A) at focal plane determined with ^{131}I (364 keV) and ^{57}Co (122 keV) point sources in air.

at 50%, is about 3 times greater for the 364-keV ^{131}I γ rays but only 2 times greater for the 122-keV ^{57}Co γ rays. The ^{57}Co response curve follows the geometrical response of the collimator, while for the higher-energy γ rays the curve is broadened because of septa penetration.

The number of septa a γ ray has to penetrate in order to reach the crystal and its path length within each of the septa both depend on its angle of incidence with respect to the collimator axis (*30*). For the 19-hole collimator γ rays from outside the 10% response region must penetrate at least 2 septa at about a 30° angle. For an average septa thickness of 0.25 cm this yields a total path length of about 1 cm of lead. As shown in Fig. 5, this is not quite sufficient for the ^{131}I γ rays, which yield a point source response curve with a definite break at about the 1% level.

Empirically, it has been determined that a collimator is good enough for most clinical scanning if the departure from the geometrical response occurs at a response level of 1% of the maximum or lower. For difficult scanning procedures where the target-to-nontarget ratio is small, it is desirable to have a collimator with a departure from the geometrical response occurring at an even lower level, may be at 0.1%. This is

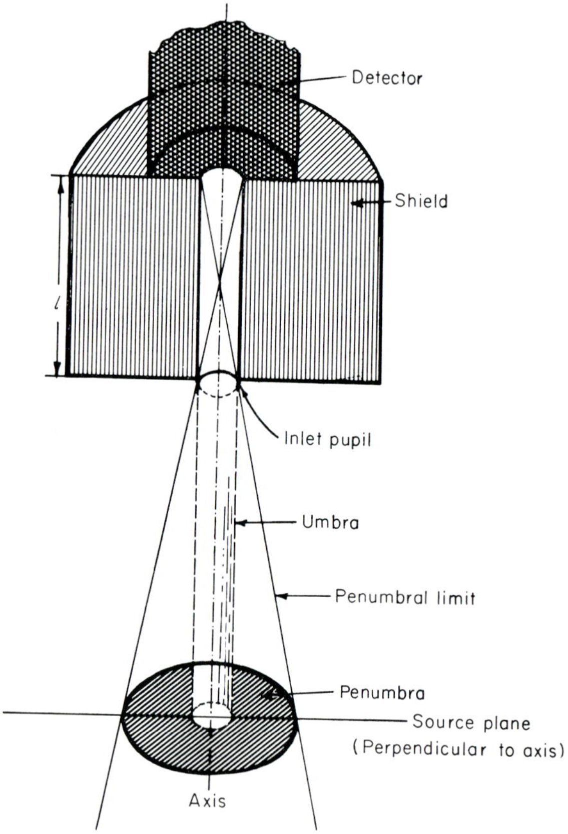

FIG. 6. Cylindrical hole collimator and its field of vision (*19*).

frequently the case for brain tumor scanning. By using a γ-ray emitter with an energy lower than that of the ^{131}I γ rays the collimator performance can be improved. On the other hand, with γ rays of higher energy, the break in the response curve may occur even at the 10% level. Under these conditions the resulting scan will yield a poor reproduction of radioactivity distribution in the patient.

E. Taper of an Individual Hole and of the Array of Holes

A single cylindrical hole collimator is shown in Fig. 6 and the tapered hole of a focusing collimator in Fig. 7. In the source plane there are three regions for each of the two collimators. The central region (umbra) is one in which γ rays from a point source can reach all of the area of the crystal at the top of the hole. Within this region the count-rate of a point source at a distance f, or closer to the collimator, is approximately constant at a fixed distance and follows the inverse square law with

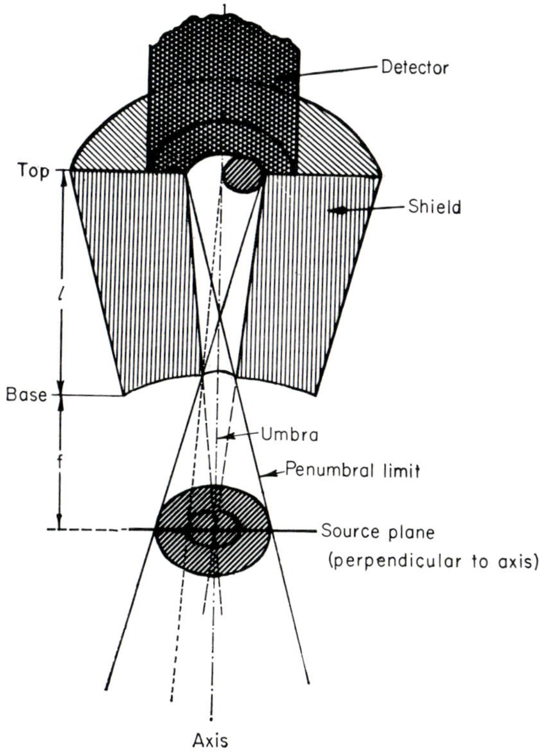

FIG. 7. Tapered hole collimator and its field of vision (*19*).

varying distance. The same applies to the extension of the umbra beyond the distance f, only that now a fraction of the detector area can be reached by the γ rays which is limited by the size of the hole at the base of the collimator.

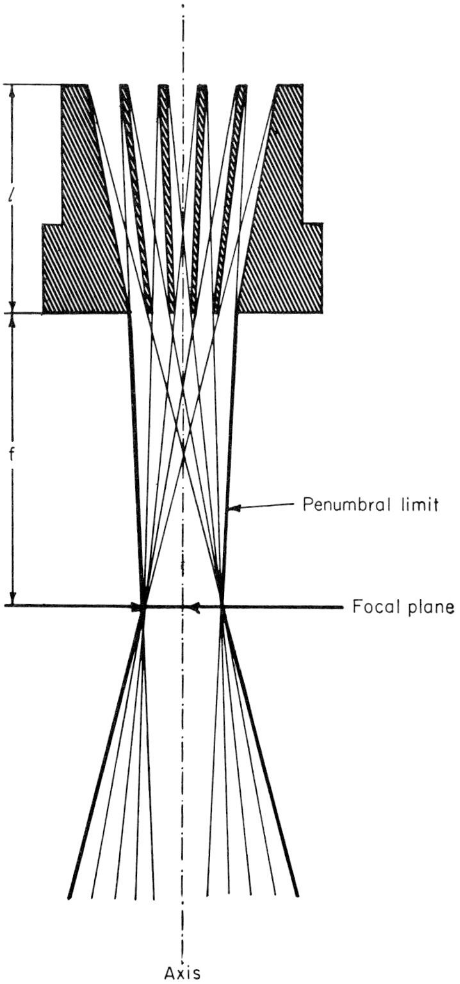

FIG. 8. Penumbra of multihole collimator. The fields of view of the individual holes superimpose only in the focal plane.

Surrounding the umbra there is an annular region called penumbra from which γ rays can reach only a section of the holes at the top. Thus for a source in this region of partial response, the count-rate ranges from zero to close to the maximum obtained within the umbra. γ Rays from a point source outside of the penumbra cannot reach the crystal without penetrating the collimator material at the base of the hole. This is true for both the cylindrical and tapered hole collimators.

However, the ratio of the areas in the two regions (umbra to penumbra) must be considered for the two collimators. This is much greater for the cylindrical hole collimator than for the tapered hole collimator, where the umbra is only a point on the collimator axis at the focal plane. Thus in the case of a cylindrical hole collimator a much greater fraction of all γ rays reaching the crystal comes from the region of maximum response. If the tapered hole is so designed that the spatial resolution in the source plane is equal to the resolution in the same plane of the cylindrical hole collimator, then the maximum sensitivity can be made much greater for a tapered hole collimator.

The taper of the array of holes, that is, the inclination of the hole axes to each other, determines the geometrical focal length of the collimator (Fig. 8). The penumbra of the individual holes superimpose in the focal plane and the field of view of a multihole collimator is about the same as that of a single hole. Therefore, the count-rate from a point source in the focal plane is approximately n times that for a single hole, where n is the number of holes.

At distances closer to and further than the focal plane, the fields of view of the individual holes do not superimpose. In order to keep the resolution nearly constant between the collimator face and the focal plane and some distance beyond, the taper of the array should be matched with the taper of the individual holes. This puts the surface of zero geometrical response (penumbral limit) of the collimator nearly parallel to the collimator axis (Fig. 8). Generally, a multihole collimator has along its axis a broad region of relatively high response about its focus (Fig. 3 and Chapter 16, Fig. 11). Few collimators have a genuine point focus effect, that is, very high maximum response near the focus and almost zero response elsewhere. However, in most situations the extended volume of high response near the focus is indeed desirable.

Some workers (*33*) have found it advantageous to stagger the focusing of the holes, that is, to divide the holes into three or four classes. Each class has a common focus, but the geometrical focal distance of each class is different. Thus the holes close to the axis of the collimator may be made to focus nearer to the collimator face and the holes in successive rings away from the center of the crystal may be made to focus at successively greater distances from the collimator face. This broadens the region of volume response of the collimator and may have the effect of increasing the distance along the collimator axis over which the response is relatively constant. For many applications, such as brain scanning, this is considered a desirable feature (*7*).

F. Geometrical Response

The dimensions of the individual holes of a multihole collimator define the geometrical response of the collimator. As mentioned above, the observed collimator performance will be described by its geometrical response if the energy of the γ rays is sufficiently low to avoid septa penetration.

As an example we shall consider round holes of a multihole collimator with a tapered aperture as shown in Fig. 7. The geometrical sensitivity for a single aperture is calculated by finding the solid angle subtended by the shaded area at the crystal. The shaded area is the area of overlap of the projection of the hole area at the collimator face on the hole area at the crystal face. A point source on any plane perpendicular to the collimator axis may be within the umbral region where the geometrical response is constant as the area of overlap is constant. Furthermore, as described above, the source may be within the penumbral region where the response decreases as the area of overlap decreases. Finally, outside the penumbra, the geometrical response is zero.

The calculated geometrical response curves for a tapered aperture are shown in Fig. 9. In this case, the length, l, of the hole is equal to the focal distance, f. This means the radius, r_1, of the opening at the front of the aperture is exactly one-half the radius, r_0, at the crystal end of the aperture. In this nondimensional plot, the radial distance, r, is expressed in units of r_0 and the distance, x, from the face of the collimator in units of the collimator length, l.

On this plot of the calculated geometrical response three areas can be distinguished. The area outside the zero isoresponse line is the region outside the penumbra (Fig. 7); the umbra is the region where the isoresponse curves are straight lines perpendicular to the axis of the collimator. Between these two regions is the area of varying geometrical response, the penumbra.

The point source geometrical response of a multihole collimator may then be determined by superimposing the sensitivities of the individual tapers by simple addition (*5*). For a crystal of radius R, and holes of radius r_0 in the collimator at the side next to the crystal, where $r_0 = R/5$, the isoresponse curves are given in Fig. 10; the conical apertures are focused on a plane at $f = l$, the length of the collimator. If it is assumed that one half of the area of the detector is available to the apertures, this would correspond to about 12 conical holes. The geometrical response curves have been normalized to 100 at the geometrical focal point

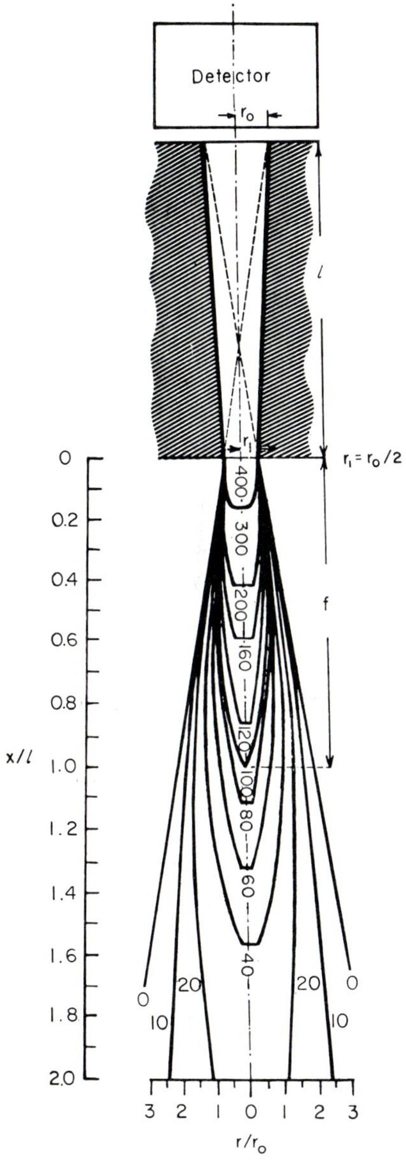

FIG. 9. Calculated point source response for a conical hole (5). The efficiency decreases rapidly with increasing distance from the hole.

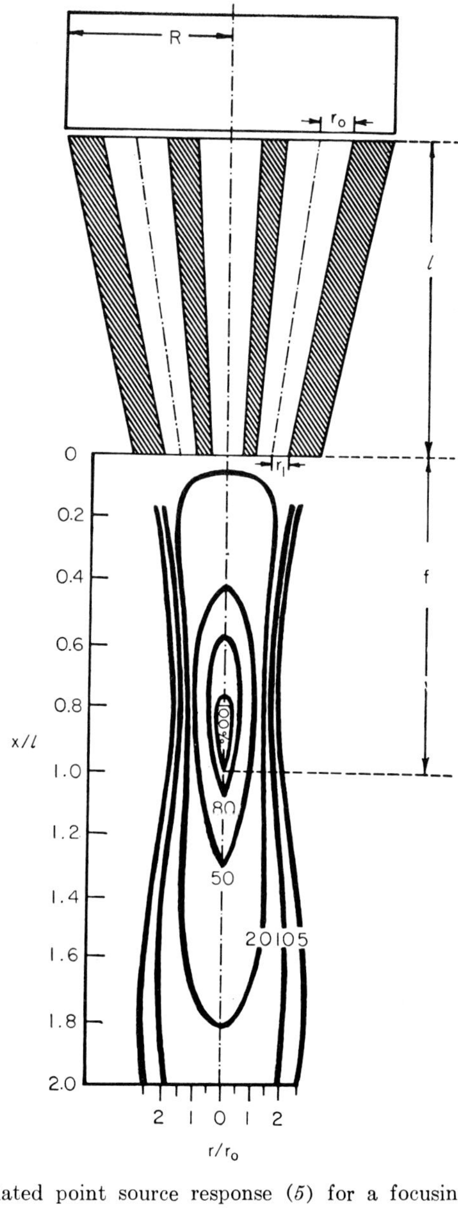

FIG. 10. Calculated point source response (*5*) for a focusing collimator with a focal point at $f = l$, for $r_0 = 0.2R$. The efficiency of the multihole collimator is highest close to the focal point.

($x/l = 1.0$ and $r/r_0 = 0$). It is seen that a focal area for point sources does exist and that the point of maximum response occurs at a point ($x/l = 0.85$, and $r/r_0 = 0$) somewhat closer to the detector than the geometrical focal point. The 50% surface approximates to a certain degree a cylinder within the object being scanned. Thus, not only is the efficiency increased but the resolution is maintained over a greater range of depths within the object than with a single aperture collimator.

If the point of convergence of the individual tapers coincides with that of the focusing array, the sensitivity of the point source at the geometrical focal point can be seen to be simply the area of exposed crystal divided by $4\pi(l+f)^2$ where $(l+f)$ is the total distance from the point source to the crystal.

III. EVALUATION AND COMPARISON OF COLLIMATORS

The evaluation of collimator performance is a difficult problem and there are several ways of approaching it. The first involves obtaining the point source isoresponse curves and using them to deduce the response of the collimator in any given clinical situation. This is possible in principle, but difficult in practice.

A second method would be to place extended sources (*21, 26*) in various experimental positions and use these results to predict the response of a collimator in a clinical situation. This extrapolation from the experimental to the clinical case is easier though the data obtained by this method do not intrinsically contain any more information than that inherent in the point source isoresponse curves.

Phantom experiments may be performed with phantoms especially designed to simulate a precise clinical situation, for example, several cold metastases in the liver. The results of these experiments are more easily related to the clinical usefulness of the collimator but even here certain effects observed in human radioisotope scanning, such as the variation in anatomy from patient to patient and the time dynamics of radioisotope distribution, are not accurately simulated.

Ultimately one would like to compare scans of clinical situations made with different collimators. However, the presentation of the radioisotope distribution, which is obtained with a collimated detector, is distorted by various factors inherent in the treatment of the data. Thus, a poor data presentation may mask the true excellence of a collimator, and conversely it is possible that an improved method of data presentation may hide the lack of merit of a collimator. However, if a sufficiently large number of patients were scanned by several different collimators with a constant procedure of evaluating the scans, useful information might be obtained.

A. Point Source Response Curves

The size of the point source is important. If the point source response curves change rapidly over a distance less than the dimension of the point source, then these changes will not be seen. In Chapter 16, Fig. 11, a point source isoresponse pattern is shown in which small variations in response are clearly visible. This was obtained with a point source of 0.012 inch in diameter. Since the response at rather large distances from the axis of the collimator may be important, the isoresponse curves must be plotted out to the region where the response is something like 0.5% of the maximum response.

Scans obtained with point sources can be of value in assessing the effects of γ-ray penetration of the septa in a collimator and of the side

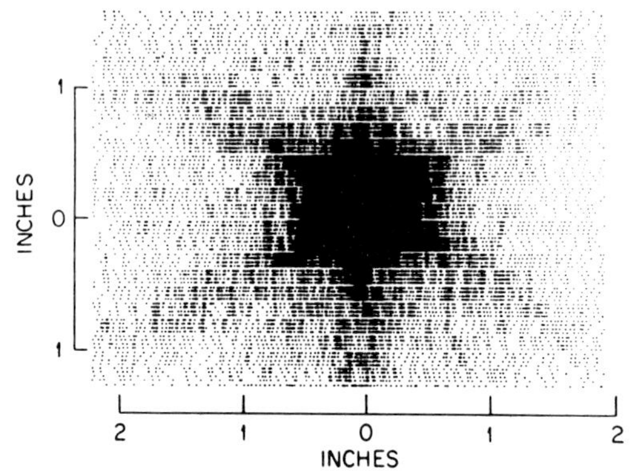

FIG. 11. Scan of circular point source (^{137}Cs γ rays) $\frac{1}{16}$ inch in diameter (*19*). The edges of the star pattern represent between 0.1 and 5% of the maximum response over the center of the source.

shielding around a collimator (*19*). A greatly distorted scan of a point source, $\frac{1}{16}$-inch in diameter, is shown in Fig. 11. The scan has a six-pointed starlike appearance, because the 662-keV γ rays penetrate the septa unevenly. With the holes placed in a hexagonal array, the collimator does not possess complete circular symmetry.

Point source response curves should strictly be determined in some tissue-equivalent medium. However, it has been shown that these curves in water may be deduced from the curves obtained in air. The effect of an absorbing medium is simply to move the response curves toward the collimator. The sensitivity at the point of maximum response is reduced by the γ-ray attenuation in the medium between this point and the collimator face. The resolution in a direction perpendicular to the collimator axis remains unchanged (*15, 16*). Isoresponse curves for some region, which is partly in air and partly in tissue or bone, may be plotted under experimental conditions using tissue- and bone-equivalent materials, or they may be derived by calculations from the response curves obtained in air.

Approximate isoresponse curves may be obtained quickly by reversing the position of source and detector. For example, if a uniform plane source of ^{125}I (27 to 35 keV) is placed against the back surface of the collimator (where the crystal usually is located) and a photographic film is placed along the collimator axis, then a pattern as shown in Fig. 12 is obtained (*2*). The density of the film at any point is a measure of the collimator's response at that point. Isodensity lines approximate the isoresponse curves. It has been shown that the film does not detect scattered radiation in this case. The method can be extended by using any radioisotope, or by using X rays incident on the rear surface of the collimator.

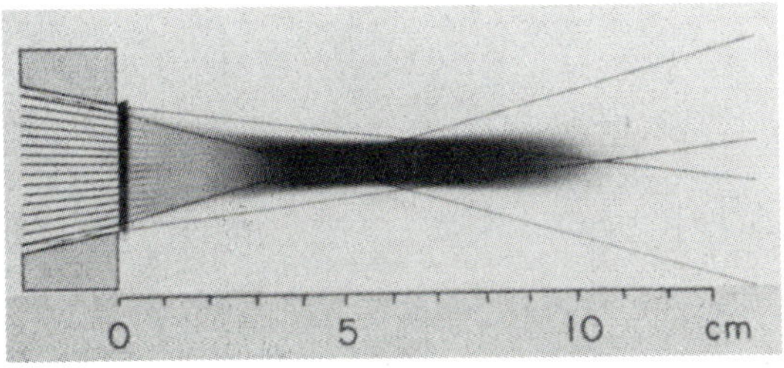

Fig. 12. A quick method of assessing isoresponse curves (*2*). A plane radioisotope source of low-energy γ rays is placed at the collimator surface where the crystal usually is located. A photographic film in front of the collimator, placed along its axis, is darkened in proportion to the collimator response.

At the usual γ-ray energies (100 to 500 keV) the effects of radiation scattered from the collimator would have to be taken into account.

B. Response to Extended Sources

Collimators may also be evaluated by determining their response to volume sources of varying size and shape in different positions in front of the collimator.

A source may be located on the axis of the collimator at some depth. The effect of source size on the collimator response may be measured by increasing the size of the source serially. This may be done for plane circular or for spherical sources extending in size radially. If the dimensions of an extended source are much larger than the point source resolution of the collimator, then the collimator's focusing effect will be lost. As stated above (Section I), for a large plane source perpendicular to the collimator axis, the sensitivity of a multihole collimator is practically constant, that is, the count-rate does not vary with source-to-collimator distance.

A collimator of focal length 8.4 cm and resolution 0.5 cm possesses no focusing property (no region of maximal response along the collimator axis) for a circular plane source 3 cm in diameter (6 times the resolution) as the source is moved away from the collimator along its axis with the

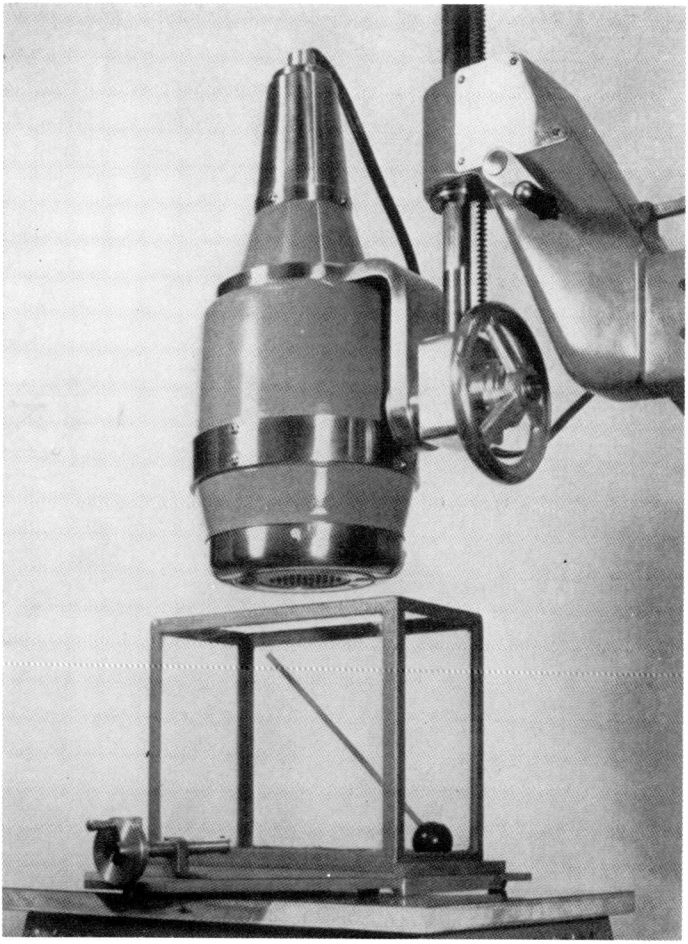

FIG. 13. Water tank with line source at 45° (*21*) and multihole collimator in horizontal plane above.

plane of the source parallel to the collimator face (*16*). However, a collimator of focal length 7.6 cm and resolution 0.64 cm possesses a focusing effect for a right cylindrical source of 1.9-cm diameter (3 times the resolution) and height 2.5 cm (*33*). Thus, it is not possible to evaluate the performance of a collimator with any one extended source, since the results depend on the source dimensions relative to the collimator resolution at the focal plane.

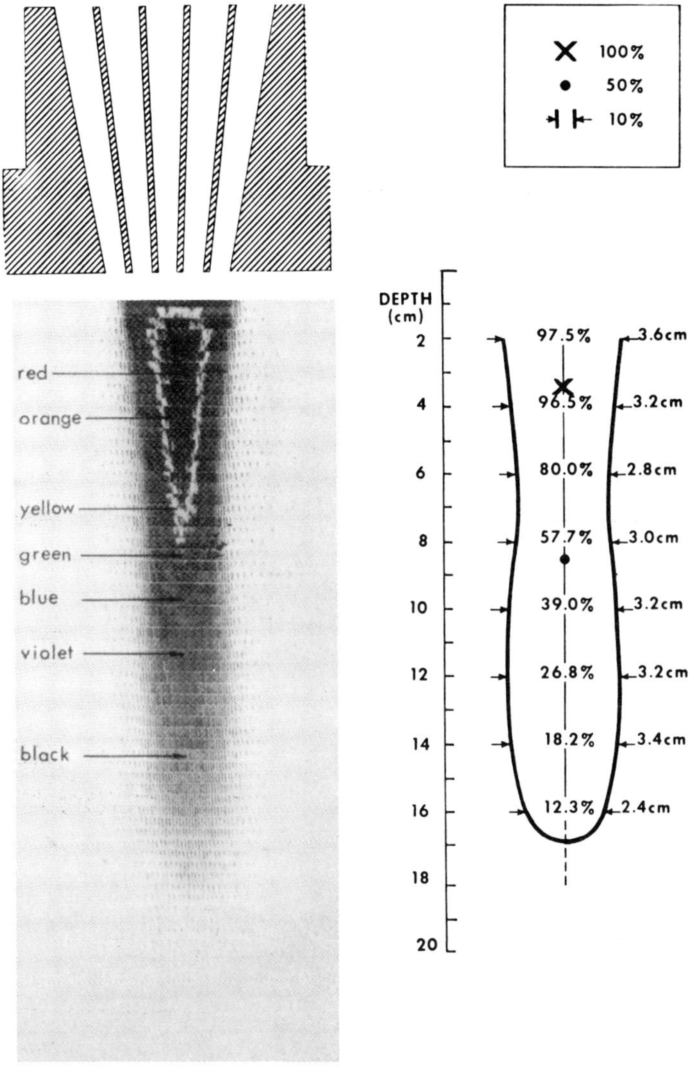

FIG. 14. Black and white print of color scan of ^{131}I line source in water with Picker 19-hole collimator, and depth response in percentage of maximum as obtained from color scan.

Any clinical scanning problem can be simulated only by the use of extended sources. A good compromise to satisfy the contradicting requirements for an "extended point source" is the use of a line source, which is small in one dimension and large in the other. By placing such a source at 45° to the axis of the collimator (Fig. 13), a simple method for the evaluation of collimator performance was obtained (*21*). A displacement of the collimator along the source causes an equal change of source distance from the collimator in a horizontal plane. By placing the line source in a tank with water, the change in collimator response caused by absorption and scattering of the γ rays can be investigated.

At each depth, the collimator views a length of the line source which depends on the resolution of the collimator at that depth. Therefore, even with the source in air, the resulting response curves will not be identical with those obtained with a point source. However, the line source simulates to a first approximation the collimator response to an extended source. Figure 14 shows the black and white print of a color scan of the line source in water and the corresponding response curve obtained with a Picker 19-hole collimator. The resolution of the collimator as shown

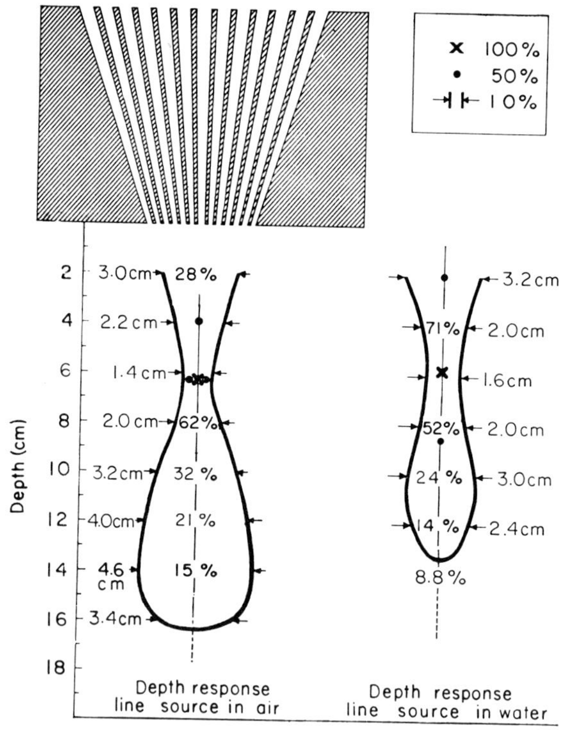

FIG. 15. Response of Picker 163-hole collimator for 5-inch diameter crystal to line source in air and in water.

in Fig. 3A can be well recognized. The depth response of the 19-hole collimator is modified by the absorption of the ^{131}I γ rays in the water. An organ which has some width, in addition to the depth of the source, will yield a scan which is extended perpendicularly to the source axis of the line source shown in Fig. 14.

The absorption of the γ rays appears to improve the performance of a focusing collimator (Fig. 15). Close to the collimator the effect of γ-ray absorption is minimal because of the small thickness of the absorbing medium. At some distance beyond the focal plane at 6 cm the path lengths have increased sufficiently to make γ-ray absorption significant. Regions around the collimator axis which yielded in air a 10% response relative to the maximum show a reduced relative sensitivity in water. This improves the resolution of the collimator in depth.

C. Experiments with Phantoms

Collimators may also be evaluated by scanning of phantoms. They may be made to simulate a clinical situation, or they may be purely of an experimental design (*24*).

A phantom containing a thyroid and metastases and also blood vessels has been used to evaluate thyroid scanning collimators (*8*). A thyroid phantom containing hot and cold nodules of various sizes (Fig. 16A) is commercially available. It consists of a Lucite container with the shape of a thyroid that can be filled with a radioisotope solution. This phantom is very useful for evaluating the performance of a scanner. With a high-resolution collimator and a good readout system it is possible to recognize all four defects under favorable conditions, that is, with 30–50 μCi of ^{131}I in the phantom, a low scanning speed, and the phantom centered at the focal plane (Fig. 16B).

Beside checking the overall performance of a scanner, the thyroid phantom can also be used to study the response of collimators. For example, by rescanning the thyroid phantom at different collimator-to-phantom distances, the variation of collimator resolution off the focal plane can be investigated. Or, for a constant scanning distance, the effect of choosing a narrow or wide window for the photopeak can be determined. Of course, in order to obtain maximum sensitivity for any collimator, the widest window should be used that still gives adequate resolution. The thyroid phantom can also be used for comparing different readout systems and for estimating the minimum radioisotope concentration that still yields an interpretable scan.

Since the requirements for brain tumor scanning are somewhat different than for organ scanning, a special phantom must be used for the study of brain tumor localization (*26*). Spherical containers of different

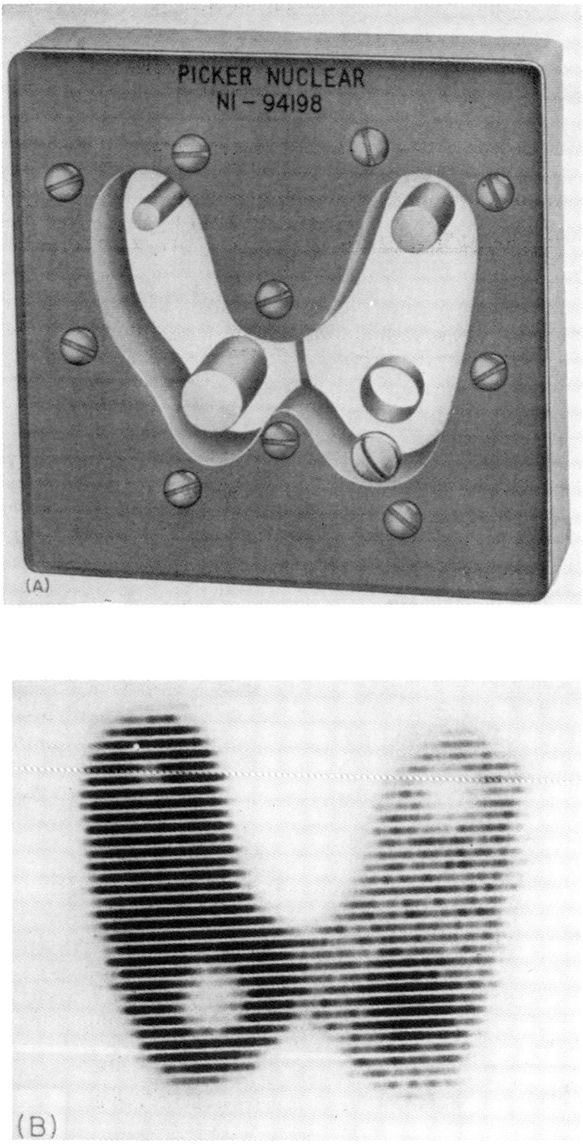

FIG. 16. (A) Lucite thyroid phantom (Picker) with one hot and three cold defects. (B) Photoscan of thyroid phantom with a high-resolution collimator. (Courtesy of Picker Nuclear.)

sizes are placed at various positions in a tank approximating the size of a human head. With any one collimator, the observed results depend on the absolute and relative amounts of a chosen radioisotope inside the spherical container and in the tank surrounding it. Furthermore the size and position of the sources in the tank as well as the energy of the γ rays affect the results. For brain tumor scanning the resolution of a collimator is less important than its sensitivity and depth response. However, a collimator with a poor resolution will detect a lot of the γ rays from a low concentration of the radioisotope in the normal brain. This decreases the probability of brain tumor detection if the target-to-nontarget ratio is low. Owing to the great number of interrelated variables it is difficult to determine the best conditions for brain tumor scanning (*1, 26, 29*) (Chapter 16, Section III,B).

TABLE III
SPATIAL RESOLUTION AND RELATIVE COUNT-RATES OF VARIOUS COLLIMATORS[a]

Collimator	Length of collimator (inch)	Crystal diameter and height (inch)	Drop from peak (%)	50% width (mm)	Count-rate compared with ½-inch bore
Single hole ¼-inch diameter	3	¾ × ¾	35.0	23	0.1
Single hole ⅜-inch diameter	3	¾ × ¾	34.0	23	0.4
Single hole ½-inch diameter	3	¾ × ¾	31.0	23	1.0
19-Hole lead (Picker)	3	3 × 1	28.5	23	5.0
Center hole of 19-hole lead	3	3 × 1	35.0	23	0.2
37-Hole gold septa with tungsten shielding (Oak Ridge National Laboratory)	3	3 × 2	37.5	23	5.0

[a] Measurements of a 3-cm cube defect in a 5-cm deep solution of radioactivity (*12*).

A number of nonanatomical phantoms have been suggested for testing collimator and scanner performance. A simple phantom consisting of a six-pointed star with point sources ranged along the legs at different distances from each other has been suggested to evaluate the resolution of collimators (*7*). This design was chosen so that the direction of scanning would not influence the assessment of the collimator's resolution.

In one study a number of collimators were compared (Table III) by means of a homogeneous phantom, consisting of a 5-cm deep radioactive solution, and a simulated tumor at its center (*12, 23*). The latter consists of a solid 3-cm cube which was placed at the bottom of the dish containing the radioactive solution. The surface of the solution was 5 cm from the face of the collimator. In this study resolution was expressed in two ways. First, as the percentage drop over the "tumor" from the peak count-rate over the solution and second, as the width at 50% of the total drop, the latter being the same for all collimators (Table III). The drop from the peak count-rate which is a measure of the spatial resolution of the collimator varied by 24% from the worst to the best collimator tested, but the two multihole collimators had a greatly increased sensitivity.

A scanning phantom proposed by the International Atomic Energy Agency can be used to evaluate collimators. This phantom simulates a clinical situation with control of conditions of target depth, target size, target-to-nontarget isotope concentration ratio, and absolute concentration of the radioisotope. Four 3-inch multihole collimators have been evaluated with isotopes ranging in γ-ray energy from 0.027 to 1.3 MeV. The targets were spheres varying from 1 to 3 cm in diameter, and were situated at depths from 0 to 15 cm from the surface. The radioisotope concentration in the spheres varied from zero to 10 times the concentration in the phantom. The scans were made with a commercial scanning machine and photoscan recording was used (*3*).

Such phantom studies are valuable in guiding a clinician in the following ways. They can establish limits for the minimum concentration ratio that must exist between a tumor and a nontumor region for a tumor of given size to be seen at various depths by a collimator of given design using a certain radioisotope. In a real clinical situation other factors, not taken into account when scanning a phantom, will supervene to make the situation in general somewhat less favorable. However, these experimental determinations are valuable for they clearly establish what cannot be done with a collimator.

REFERENCES

1. Beck, R. N., A theoretical evaluation of brain scanning systems. *J. Nucl. Med.* **2,** 314 (1961).
2. Beck, R. N., Collimators for radioisotope scanning systems. *Proc. Symp. Med. Radioisotope Scanning, Athens, 1964* Vol. 1, p. 211. Intern. At. Energy Agency, Vienna, 1964.
3. Bender, M. A., and Blau, M., Collimator evaluation with the IAEA scanning phantom. *Proc. Symp. Med. Radioisotope Scanning, Athens, 1964* Vol. 1, p. 175. Intern. At. Energy Agency, Vienna, 1964.
4. Bender, M. A., and Blau, M., Detection of liver tumors with I^{131} rose bengal. *Proc. Seminar, Med. Radioisotope Scanning, Vienna, 1959* p. 83. Intern. At. Energy Agency, Vienna, 1959.
5. Brownell, G. L., Theory of radioisotope scanning. *Intern. J. Appl. Radiation Isotopes* **3,** 181 (1958).
6. Brownell, G. L., Theory of radioisotope scanning. *Proc. Symp. Med. Radioisotope Scanning, Athens, 1964* Vol. 1, p. 3. Intern. At. Energy Agency, Vienna, 1964.

7. Brownell, G. L., Theory of isotope scanning. *Proc. Seminar, Med. Radioisotope Scanning, Vienna, 1959* p. 1. Intern. At. Energy, Vienna, 1959.
8. Brucer, M., "Radioisotope Scanning. An Introduction to the Use of the Area Scan in Medical Diagnosis." Oak Ridge Institute of Nuclear Studies, Oak Ridge, Tennessee, 1958.
9. Cassen, B., Theory of scanning and imaging of radioisotope distributions. *Proc. Symp. Med. Radioisotope Scanning, Athens, 1964* Vol. 1, p. 77. Intern. At. Energy Agency, Vienna, 1964.
10. Cassen, B., Curtis, L., and Reed, C., A sensitive directional gamma-ray detector. *Nucleonics* **6**, No. 2, 78 (1950).
11. Cassen, B., Curtis, L., Reed, C., and Libby, R., Instrumentation for I-131 use in medical studies. *Nucleonics* **9**, No. 2, 46 (1951).
12. Christie, J. H., and MacIntyre, W. J., Information limitations of radioisotope scanning. *Radiology* **79**, 472 (1962).
13. Courtial, J., and Gandy, A., Note sur la sensibilité et le pouvoir de résolution en scintigraphie. *Proc. Symp. Med. Radioisotope Scannings, Athens, 1964* Vol. 1, p. 91. Intern. At. Energy Agency, Vienna, 1964.
14. Corey, K. R., Kenny, P., Greenberg, E., Pazianos, A., Pearson, O. H., and Laughlin, J. S., The use of calcium-47 in diagnostic studies of patients with bone lesions. *Am. J. Roentgenol. Radium Therapy Nucl. Med.* **85**, 955 (1961).
15. Cradduck, T. D., and Fedoruk, S. O., A study of collimators for use in radioisotope scanning techniques. *J. Can. Assoc. Radiol.* **13**, 9 (1962).
16. Dewey, W. C., and Sinclair, W. K., Criteria for evaluating collimators used in *in vivo* distribution studies with radioisotopes. *Intern. J. Appl. Radiation Isotopes* **10**, 1 (1961).
17. Dias-Neto, A. L., A honeycomb collimator of variable focus for use in radioisotope scanning. *Nucl. Med.* **3**, 221 (1963).
18. Francis, J. E., Jr., Bell, P. R., and Harris, C. C., Medical scintillation spectrometry. *Nucleonics* **13**, No. 11, 82 (1955).
19. Harris, C. C., Bell, P. R., Francis, J. E., Jr., Satterfield, M. M., Jordan, J. C., and Murray, J. P., Collimators for radioisotope scanning. *In* "Progress in Medical Radioisotope Scanning" (R. M. Kniseley, G. A. Andrews, and C. C. Harris, eds.), TID-7673, p. 25. U.S. At. Energy Comm., Washington, D.C., 1963.
20. Harris, C. C., Bell, P. R., Satterfield, M. M., Ross, D. A., and Jordan, J. C., The design and performance of a large high-resolution focusing collimator. *Proc. Symp. Med. Radioisotope Scanning, Athens, 1964* Vol. 1, p. 193. Intern. At. Energy Agency, Vienna, 1964.
21. Hine, G. J., and Vetter, H., Evaluation of focusing collimator performance. *Nucl. Med.* **4**, 333 (1965).
22. Jensen, P. G., *Proc. Seminar Med. Radioisotope Scanning, Athens, 1959* p. 29. Intern. At. Energy Agency, Vienna, 1959; and unpublished data.
23. MacIntyre, W. J., Christie, J. H., and Tatsuno, I., The evaluation of straight-bore, tapered and focusing collimators as a function of gamma-ray energy. *Proc. Symp. Med. Radioisotope Scanning, Athens, 1964* Vol. 1, p. 153. Intern. At. Energy Agency, Vienna, 1964.
24. Mallard, J. R., Medical radioisotope scanning. *Phys. Med. Biol.* **10**, 309 (1965).
25. Mather, R. L., Gamma-ray collimator penetration and scattering effects. *J. Appl. Phys.* **28**, 1200 (1957).
26. Matthews, C. M. E., Comparison of coincidence counting and focusing collimators with various isotopes in brain tumor detection. *Brit. J. Radiol.* **37**, 531 (1964).

27. Mayneord, W. V., and Newberry, S. P., An automatic method of studying the distribution of activity in a source of ionizing radiation. *Brit. J. Radiol.* **25,** 589 (1952).
28. Miller, E. R., and Scofield, N. E., Studies with radioiodine. IV. Collimating cones for crystal counters. *Radiology* **65,** 96 (1955).
29. Myers, M. J., and Mallard, J. R., Some long-focusing "depth-independent" collimators for *in-vivo* radioisotope scanning. *Intern. J. Appl. Radiation Isotopes* **15,** 725 (1964).
30. Myhill, J., Theory of multichannel collimated scintillation detectors. *Intern. J. Appl. Radiation Isotopes* **12,** 10 (1961).
31. Newell, R. R., Saunders, W., and Miller, E., Multichannel collimators for gamma-ray scanning with scintillation counters. *Nucleonics* **10,** No. 7, 36 (1952).
32. Rotenberg, A. D., and Johns, H. E., Collimator efficiency and design. I. Collimator efficiency. *Phys. Med. Biol.* **10,** 51 (1965).
33. Shy, G. M., Bradley, R. B., and Matthews, W. B., Jr., "External Collimation Detection of Intracranial Neoplasia with Unstable Nuclides." Livingstone, Edinburgh and London, 1958.
34. Simons, H. A. B., and Chomet, S., A study of the external gamma-ray field arising from a radioactive source situated in air and in a scattering medium. *Phys. Med. Biol.* **3,** 233 (1959).
35. Simons, H. A. B., A comparison between collimator theory, extended to allow for the effect of wall penetration, and experiment. *Proc. Symp. Med. Radioisotope Scanning, Athens, 1964* Vol. 1, p. 115. Intern. At. Energy Agency, Vienna, 1964.
36. Tomnovec, F. M., and Mather, R. L., Experimental gamma-ray collimator sensitivity patterns. *J. Appl. Phys.* **28,** 1208 (1957).
37. Van der Dose de Bye, J. A. W., Analysis of the scintiscanning problem. *Nucleonics* **14,** No. 11, 128 (1956).

CHAPTER 18

POSITRON SCANNING

SAUL ARONOW
PHYSICS RESEARCH LABORATORY
MASSACHUSETTS GENERAL HOSPITAL
BOSTON, MASSACHUSETTS

I. POSITRON EMISSION AND ANNIHILATION

A positron is a particle of the same size and mass as an electron, but with a positive rather than a negative electrical charge. Its discovery in 1932 opened the door to the explosively rapid development of nuclear physics because this confirmed the apparently meaningless requirement of mathematical theory that electrons exist in negative as well as positive energy levels (*8*). Two properties of positrons that are of interest to applications in nuclear medicine will be discussed briefly.

A. Positron Emission

Many unstable neutron-deficient radionuclides achieve stability by converting a proton into a neutron. The excess energy and charge may be carried off by a positron. Alternatively, the nucleus may capture an orbital electron in a competing process called electron capture. In the lighter elements and in the more neutron-deficient radioisotopes, positron emission tends to predominate. In the heavier elements electron capture, and later α-ray emission, tend to become the sole decay process.

As an example, the decay scheme of ^{64}Cu is shown in Fig. 1. This nuclide ($Z = 29$, $A = 64$) in 39% of its decays emits a β^- particle and goes to zinc ($Z = 30$, $A = 64$); in 19% it emits a β^+ particle and becomes nickel ($Z = 29$, $A = 64$); and in 42%, it captures an electron and goes also to nickel.

The positron is emitted with high kinetic energy and in almost all

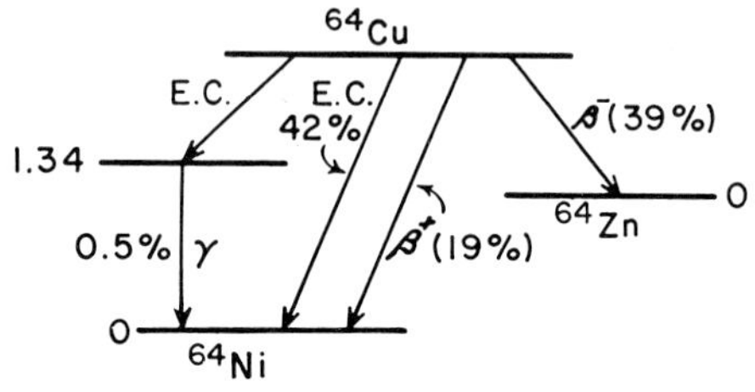

FIG. 1. Decay scheme of ^{64}Cu.

respects is the same as a β ray until its kinetic energy is absorbed, mainly by ionization.

Some positron emitters useful in nuclear medicine are listed in Table I. Their rather short half-lives and the fact that neutron-deficient

TABLE I
POSITRON-EMITTING RADIOISOTOPES USEFUL FOR SCANNING

Isotope	Half-life	Chemical form	Production
^{11}C	20.4 min	CO_2	Cyclotron
^{13}N	10 min	N_2	Cyclotron
^{15}O	118 sec	CO_2	Cyclotron
^{18}F	122 min	KBF_4	Reactor
^{22}Na	2.6 years	NaCl	Reactor
^{47}V	33 min	Na_3VO_4	Cyclotron
^{62}Zn	9.3 hr	ZnCl	Cyclotron
^{64}Cu	12.8 hr	Cu-DTPA	Reactor
^{68}Ga	68 min	Ga-DTPA	Cyclotron
^{72}As	26 hr	Na_3AsO_3	Cyclotron
^{74}As	17.5 days	Na_3AsO_4	Cyclotron
^{89}Zr	80 hr	Citrate	Cyclotron
^{124}I	4.5 days	Gamma globulin	Cyclotron

radioisotopes are not readily made in a reactor have restricted their exploitation at present.

B. Annihilation Radiation

For scanning purposes it is not the positron but rather the γ rays resulting from its annihilation that are of interest. In dense matter (water and tissue) the positron is slowed down to thermal velocities within a few millimeters whereupon it interacts with a negative electron. The two particles disappear as mass, and in their place two γ rays, called annihilation radiation, appear. Their energies are equivalent to the masses of the two particles, each 9.11×10^{-28} gm. According to the mass-energy relation each γ ray has therefore an energy of 0.511 MeV. Since the interaction takes place at thermal velocities the momenta of the particles are practically zero. The net momenta of the resulting γ rays must also be zero, requiring that the two γ rays proceed in precisely opposite directions, that is, 180° apart.

It is this property, the generation of the two annihilation γ rays precisely related in time and direction, that allows the instrumental technique of coincidence detection to be effectively utilized.

II. INSTRUMENT DESIGN

Scanners have been developed for localizing the distribution of a positron-emitting isotope *in vivo,* on the basis of the detection of the annihilation radiation. Although similar in overall performance to scanners using focusing collimators, there are some basic differences.

A. Coincidence Detection

The annihilation radiation from positron emission is detected by a coincidence system, illustrated in Fig. 2. Two detectors, X_1 and X_2, are placed on opposite sides of the radiation source. Fast electronic systems determine the time of arrival of the γ rays at each detector and feed suitable signals to a coincidence circuit. This generates an output pulse only when the two input signals arrive simultaneously in time. The circuitry can be made quite fast so that the time interval in which a coincidence is detectable, the resolving time, is of the order of a tenth of a microsecond.

In addition to the time coincidence, there is the geometric limitation that the γ rays travel 180° apart. If the annihilation takes place at point a of Fig. 2 along the axis of the two detectors, this pair of γ rays has a high probability of being detected. However, a pair of γ rays starting from point b, near the edge of the sensitive volume, has only a small probability of being detected. If the line of the γ rays is at a small angle to the axis of the detectors, one of the γ rays will miss its detector. An annihilation occurring at a point just beyond the edge of the crystals cannot be detected at all. If one γ ray hits a crystal, its mate must miss the other one.

Utilizing these relations of time and geometry it is possible to achieve a high degree of resolution in the region between the two detectors without the use of absorbing collimators. This property gives the positron annihilation detection technique high sensitivity with sharp spatial resolution.

Another property which follows from the geometry of this system, is that the sensitive region between the two detectors is symmetric and relatively unaffected by the lateral position of the source between the two detectors. For as the source moves away from one detector and its sensitivity decreases, it moves closer to the other.

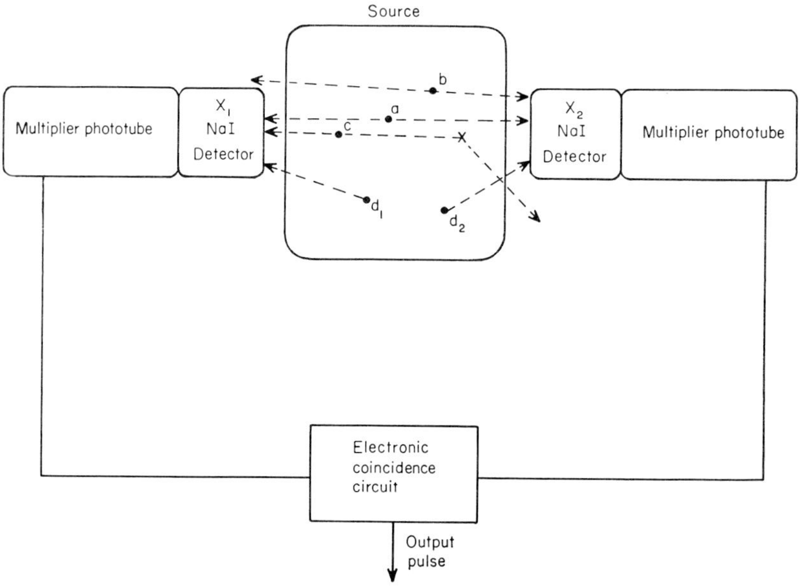

FIG. 2. Principle of coincidence detection of annihilation radiation. Annihilation pair (a) is detected by coincidence. Pair (b) is not detected because of geometry. Pair (c) is not detected because of scatter. The γ rays d_1, d_2, cause a random coincidence.

Because of the lateral symmetry, the isoresponse curves for this system are approximately cylinders between the two detectors, as shown in Fig. 3. The resolution may be defined as the distance across the 50% contour lines. It is seen in the diagram to be about half the diameter of the crystals and to extend effectively from one side to the other.

If, as is usually the case, there is an absorbing medium, rather than air, between the two detectors, the sensitivity is decreased, but the resolution remains the same. The absorption of the γ rays decreases as the source approaches one detector but the absorption to the other detector increases. This is shown by experimental curves in Fig. 4, where a thin

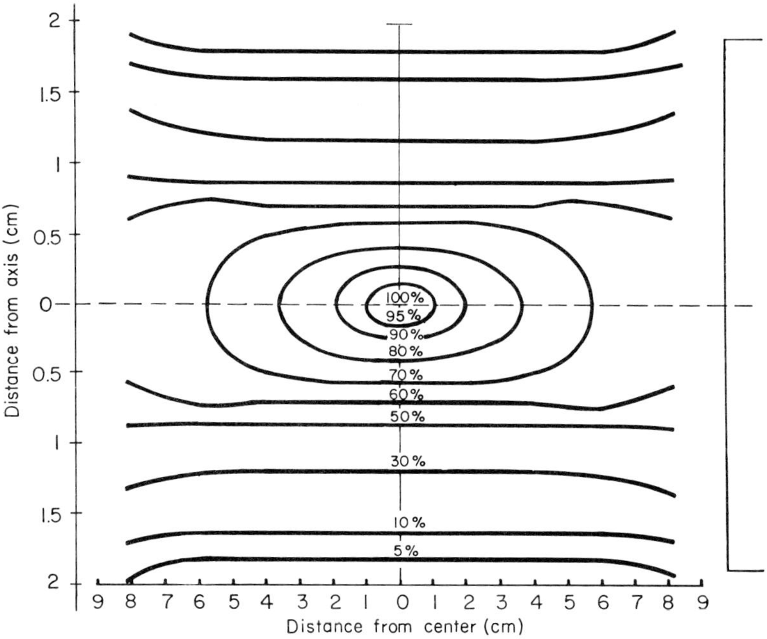

Fig. 3. Isoresponse curves for coincidence detection crystal pair. Measured response in axial plane for 4-cm diameter crystals.

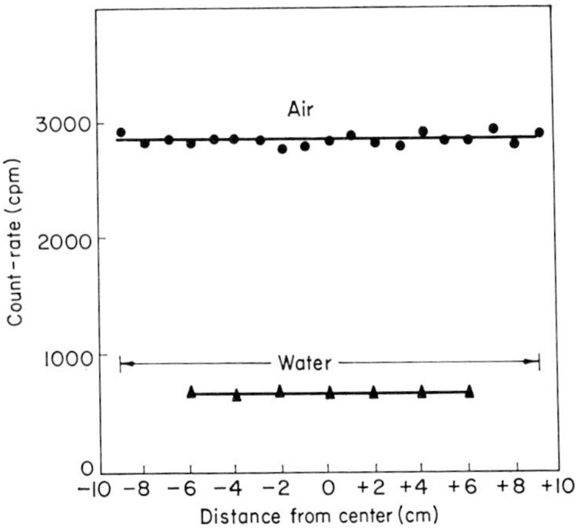

Fig. 4. Response of coincidence detector to thin plane source of positron-emitting ^{74}As between the crystals in air and in a water phantom.

plane source of a positron emitter is moved between the two detectors in air and in a water phantom. Having two half thicknesses of absorber between the detectors cuts the sensitivity by a factor of 4, but the relative response remains independent of source positions. This uniform cylindrical response pattern of the annihilation radiation detection system is particularly useful for problems, such as brain tumor localization, where a thick, symmetrical organ is examined and the radioisotope distribution is at an unknown depth.

The absolute sensitivity for a coincidence detection system can be calculated from the geometry, crystal efficiency, and radioisotope source data. For a point source centrally located between the two detectors, the coincidence count-rate N_c is

$$N_c = 2.2 \times 10^6\ Cf\eta_g(\eta_a)^2(\eta_d)^2 \quad \text{cpm} \tag{1}$$

where C is the amount of radioactivity of the source (μCi); f the fraction of disintegrations yielding positrons; η_g the geometric efficiency, to one detector, $r^2/4\ w^2$; η_a the transmission in medium to one detector; and η_d the detection efficiency of one detector.

As example, $C = 1$ μCi of ^{64}Cu with $f = 0.19$; the radius of the crystals is $r = 1.5$ cm and their center distance $w = 10$ cm, so that $\eta_g = 5.6 \times 10^{-3}$; one half-thickness of absorber $\eta_a = 0.5$ and a detection efficiency $\eta_d = 0.8$. The coincidence count-rate follows then as $N_c = 380$ cpm.

For a pure positron emitter, such as ^{18}F, $f = 1$ and $N_c = 2000$ cpm. This sensitivity corresponds to a resolution of 1.5 cm.

B. Unbalance Detection

The coincidence system described above counts all the radioactivity lying between the two detectors as if it were on a single plane located anywhere between the detectors. However, having two detectors viewing the same radioisotope concentration can provide additional information, as indicated in Fig. 5. Each individual detector is counting the total number of γ rays impinging on it, as any single channel detector. If the source is midway between the two detectors, each detector counts at the same rate; but if the source is closer to one side, as at point S, its count-rate increases rapidly because of the inverse square law, while the count-rate of the opposite side decreases. The signals from each side, suitably amplified and scaled down, may be fed to a difference scaler. It calculates continuously which side has the higher count-rate and actuates a recording device. The system thus provides a sensitive indication of any net asymmetry in the source position to the right or to the left side.

If the crystals are uncollimated, as assumed in the previous discussion, the resolution of the unbalance system is very poor. This is not important, however, since the fine resolution is provided by the coinci-

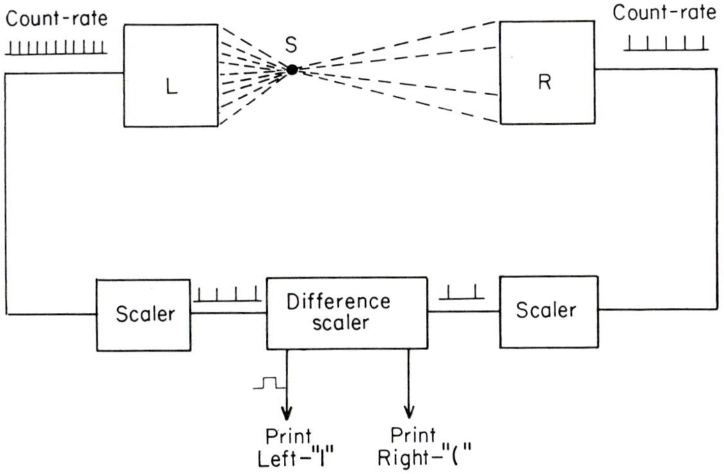

FIG. 5. Asymmetry of measuring system. If source is closer to left detector, its count-rate is higher. Difference scaler activates printer with straight marks indicating an unbalance to the left and with curved marks for right unbalance.

dence system. Simultaneous printing of the coincidence and unbalance pictures provides a three-dimensional portrayal of the radioisotope distribution within the scanned area.

C. Background Counts

1. RANDOM COINCIDENCES

In the preceding sections the ideal situation was assumed where all the detected pulses are due to γ rays from the target source. However, in practice all detection systems are limited in their ability to distinguish desired signals from undesired ones. The latter may come from natural background radiation, from electrical noise generated in the detection system, or γ rays emitted from other parts of the body than the organ being viewed. Together they constitute the informational "noise." Most of these noise signals occur randomly in time and since the probability of two random pulses occurring at exactly the same time is very low (γ-ray pair d_1, d_2 in Fig. 2), the coincidence detection system helps to discriminate against them and thereby improves the signal-to-noise ratio.

It is, of course, not possible to determine exact time coincidence. Any system requires a finite resolving time τ in which to decide whether one or two events have occurred. In Fig. 6A, if a γ ray hits detector 1 and another hits detector 2, more than τ seconds later, no coincidence is recorded. In any two random sequences of events, there is some probability that a γ ray will hit detector 2 within τ seconds of another γ ray hitting detector 1 as in Fig. 6B. This will be recorded as a coincidence. Since either detector may be hit first, the total time within which the pulses may overlap is 2τ.

If the count-rate of the first detector is N_1, and that of the second is N_2, then the number of random coincidence counts per unit time Nr is

$$Nr = 2\tau N_1 N_2 \tag{2}$$

The random coincidence count-rate varies essentially as the square

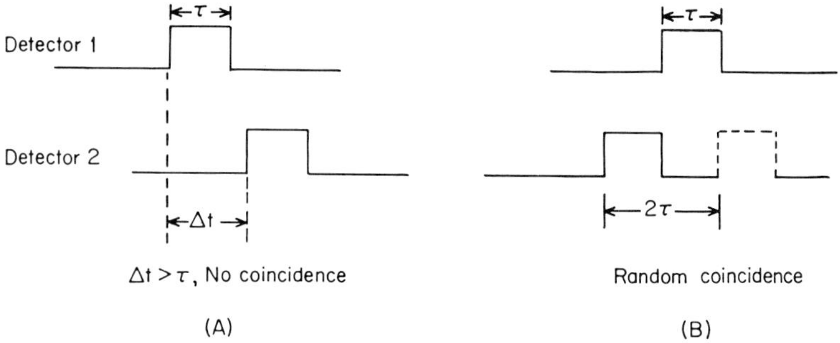

FIG. 6. Coincidence resolving time. (A) Random pulse separated by $\Delta t > \tau$, no coincidence output. (B) Time interval for observing random coincidence is 2τ, where τ is the pulse width.

of the total γ-ray count-rate. This places a constraint on the total radioactivity that can be used in a coincidence counting system. Increasing the amount of radioactivity raises the random background count-rate as the square of the true coincidence rate.

Some typical numbers will illustrate this effect. Assume we are viewing a radioisotope, such as ^{74}As, which emits other γ rays in addition to the annihilation radiation, and that the coincidence system has a resolving time of $\tau = 0.1$ μsec. If two true coincidences per second are observed for each 1000 counts at each detector, there would be 0.2 random coincidences per second, yielding a signal-to-noise ratio of $2/0.2 = 10/1$. If the amount of radioactivity is doubled, the ratio of true to random coincidences decreases to $4/0.8 = 5/1$, whereas if the activity is halved, the signal-to-noise ratio increases to $1/0.05 = 20/1$.

Such signal-to-noise variation is unusual but very desirable for a scanning system, since it improves rapidly as the source becomes less intense. This is quite the reverse with conventional γ-ray detection systems where the signal-to-noise ratio remains the same or gets worse as the radioactivity decreases.

2. NONRANDOM COINCIDENCES

Coincidence detection systems are subject to two peculiar sources of background counts. One occurs with vertically placed detectors. Cosmic rays, having essentially vertical paths, can traverse both detectors and yield truly coincident pulses. Therefore, in vertically mounted coincidence systems, it must be expected that a background count-rate of several pulses per minute will be encountered.

Additional background coincidences occur if the radioisotope emits γ rays in cascade with a positron or another γ ray. The cascade γ rays are emitted simultaneously in time but are randomly oriented in space. If the probability of a γ ray hitting one of the detectors is η_g (<1) the probability of the two random γ rays hitting the two detectors is η_g^2 ($\ll 1$). In contrast, because of their geometric alignment, the probability of two annihilation γ rays hitting two detectors remains η_g. Although the efficiency of detection of cascade γ-ray pairs is low compared to annihilation γ rays, this source of background counts may become serious if the total activity is large. It can be reduced by appropriate shielding.

A similar effect occurs with annihilation γ rays if one of the pair undergoes Compton scattering in the source. The scattering angle is random and geometric alignment is lost (γ-ray pair c of Fig. 2). The two γ rays act like a pair of cascade γ rays rather than annihilation radiation. Fortunately, as the scattering angle becomes larger the energy is reduced. This makes the shielding more effective.

3. SHIELDING

An annihilation detection system provides spatial resolution without collimators. Its resolution is determined entirely by the size of the crystals. However, some shielding is required to reduce the background counts. This is particularly true in brain scanning, where the small amount of radioactivity in the head might be masked by the greater activity in the rest of the body.

Shielding would be a more serious problem with the high-energy, 0.51-MeV γ rays of the annihilation radiation were it not that the random coincidence count-rate (Eq. 2) depends on the product of the individual γ-ray count-rates. For example, if the shielding at each detector cuts the γ-ray count-rate by a factor of $\frac{1}{2}$, the random coincidence rate is cut to $\frac{1}{4}$. Therefore, only half as thick shielding on each detector is needed to achieve the same background reduction as would be necessary for single 0.51-MeV γ-ray attenuation. This more than compensates for the fact that there are two detectors. Wide-angle Compton scattered γ rays, being of low energy, are even more drastically reduced.

The unbalance system which uses the total γ ray counts, and not coincidences, is more seriously affected by lack of shielding and collimation. Even for its modest resolution requirements, some collimation is necessary. Moving the crystals back from the patient's head to allow for this collimation reduces the coincidence count sensitivity. Therefore a compromise must be reached. A single bore collimator, with a depth equal to its diameter, is quite satisfactory.

The amount of shielding around the crystal is also not critical. A convenient thickness is about 2 inches of lead. For 0.51-MeV γ rays, this is about 12 half-thicknesses ($d_{1/2} = 0.4$ cm). According to Eq. 2, this

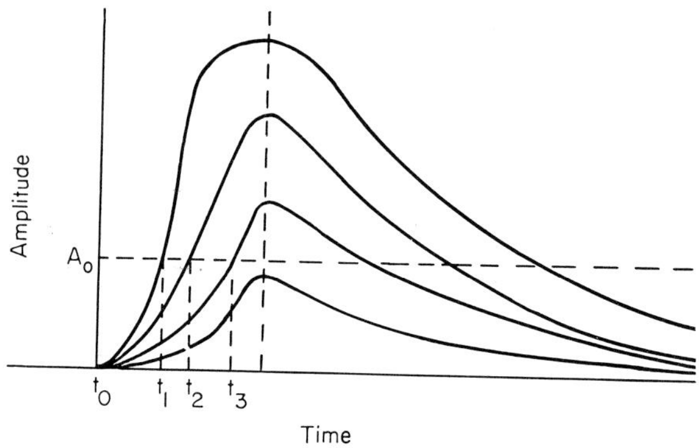

FIG. 7. Time jitter. Apparent difference in arrival times (t_1, t_2, t_3) of pulses differing in amplitude, if fixed threshold A_0 is used as trigger of pulses starting at time t_0.

shielding would reduce the random background counts by a factor of $2^{24} \sim 10^7$ from the unshielded value.

D. Electronics

1. Coincidence System

Successful operation of a coincidence system requires a fast pulse resolving time, of the order of 0.1 μsec. Since the most common radiation detector, NaI(Tl), has a pulse decay time constant of 0.25 μsec, even with a fast preamplifier its output pulses would be too long to be used directly. It is therefore necessary to use electronic methods to time accurately the advent of a pulse and generate a very fast signal pulse as a time reference.

It would not be difficult to time the pulses precisely if they were uniform in size. Unfortunately, while successive pulses from the crystal–multiplier phototube combination are similar in shape, they differ in size even with single-energy γ rays. As a result, an uncertainty or time

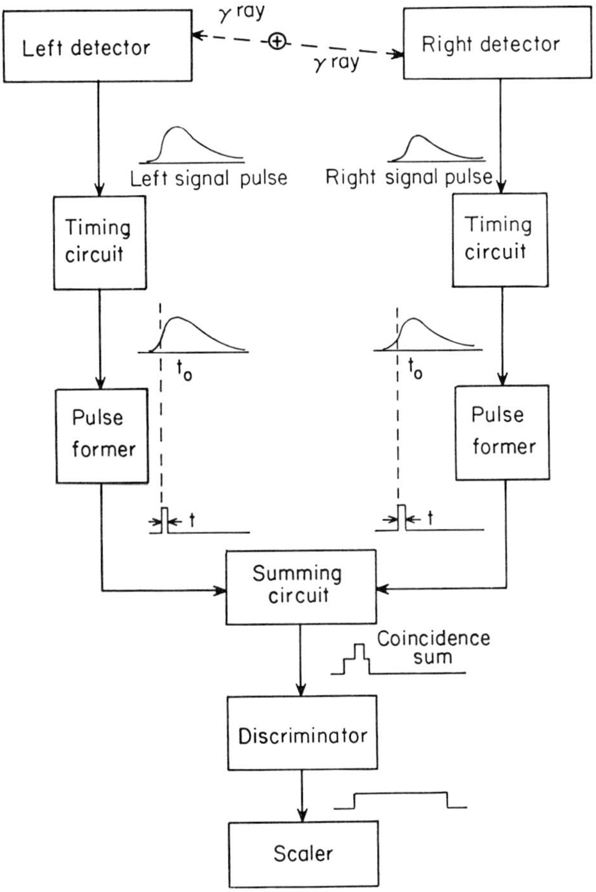

FIG. 8. Block diagram of coincidence circuit. Timing circuit establishes a fiducial time mark t_0. Pulse former generates a narrow comparison pulse of width τ. Summing circuit adds pulses if they are in coincidence.

jitter is introduced into the measurement. This is illustrated in Fig. 7, where four pulses differing in amplitude are shown. If one defines the time of arrival as the time the pulse crosses a fixed threshold A_0 (a low-level discriminator), the pulses appear to occur at three different times. Similarly, if the time of very start of the pulse, t_0, is the criterion, the statistical fluctuations of the multiplier phototube became significant.

Many electronic systems have been designed to reduce the limitations of jitter and to obtain fast timing even with slow pulses. A basic block diagram is shown in Fig. 8. The timing circuit is the critical element. It operates on the detector pulse to define t_0, and transmits a trigger to the pulse former. This generates a standard pulse of fixed, narrow width, τ. The coincidence circuit proper is some form of summing circuit which decides when it has received pulses from the two channels at the same time.

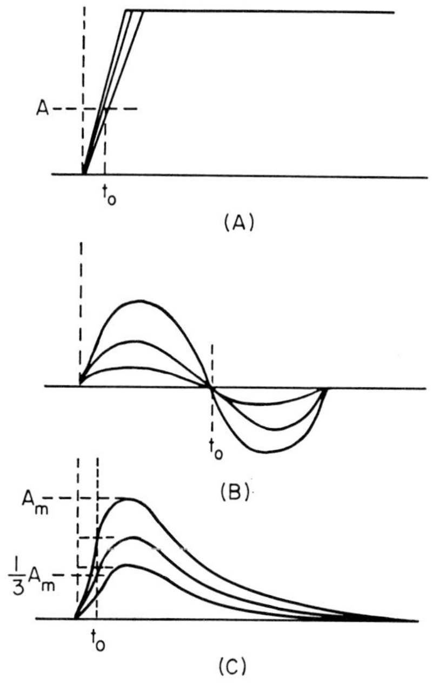

FIG. 9. Techniques for precise timing of slow pulses. (A) Leading edge detector. (B) Zero cross-over detector. (C) Discriminator set at fixed ratio of maximum amplitude.

The characteristic wave forms for three types of timers are shown in Fig. 9. The first (Fig. 9A) is typical of many variations of leading edge detection (*5*). Each channel has a very high-gain amplifier which accurately amplifies the region of the pulse close to t_0, and may discard the rest of the pulse. When the amplified pulse crosses a fixed threshold, A_0, the pulse timing circuit is triggered. The resolving time is limited by the width of the timing pulse, which may be reduced until it is limited by the uncertainty of input pulse amplitude. This in turn can be reduced by increased amplification until the signal is blurred by statistical noise. Using only the front edge of the pulse wastes timing information contained in the rest of the pulse. However, tunnel diodes, current-fed from the multiplier phototube, can be a reliable trigger on very small signals. These can utilize the very fast initial light pulse. Coincidence times in the order of tens of nanoseconds can be achieved. At these speeds limitations are imposed by the statistics of the multiplier phototube and the collection of light photons.

The other two systems overcome this limitation by effectively integrating over the entire pulse, at the expense of increased circuit complexity. The zero crossing technique (*9*) is illustrated in Fig. 9B. The signal pulses are amplified in a linear, double-differentiating amplifier. All the pulses, though differing in amplitude, have the same shape, and cross through zero at the same time t_0. A Schmitt discriminator may be set to trigger at this zero crossing, generating the timing trigger pulse. The second zero crossing may be determined much more reliably than the beginning of the leading edge.

The third system (Fig. 9C) takes advantage of the full rise time of the signal pulse by automatically adjusting the triggering level to a fixed ratio of the peak amplitude (*7*). Since the relative amplitudes of points on the pulse are fixed in time independent of the pulse size, a fixed ratio of the peak occurs at a fixed time t_0 after true zero. To change the triggering level the incoming signal pulse is held in a delay line while its peak is measured and a fast discriminator is set to the desired ratio of this peak. This method has the advantage of reducing the amount of jitter and still retaining pulse height information on a fast time scale. This is particularly useful if pulse-height selection is used, as well as time coincidence, to select only the 0.51-MeV annihilation radiation.

2. PULSE-HEIGHT ANALYSIS

Since the annihilation radiation always has a fixed energy of 0.51 MeV it might seem advantageous to use pulse-height selection to discard scattered radiation and reduce the background random coincidences. However, this would cause too great a loss of true coincidences. Many of the γ rays, because of scattering in the crystal, do not give a photopeak light pulse. To exclude them would greatly reduce the number of true coincidences detected, particularly since the use of two detectors per coincidence squares any reduction in detection efficiency. Time resolution is usually sufficient to cut the random coincidence count-rate low enough so that pulses as small as 10% of the photopeak can be used.

3. Data Processing and Readout

The output pulse of the coincidence circuit is transmitted to a scaler and is then registered by a printer or other readout system. This is similar to other scanners except that the count-rate is usually much lower, hundreds rather than thousands of counts per minute.

The unbalance circuit may, in its simplest form, print out marks corresponding to a difference between the two detectors of a fixed number of counts. More elaborate data processing could be used for special emphasis of count-rate variations. The difference scaler could require a minimum count-rate to remove background prints. It could provide a higher than linear power of the difference, emphasizing large differences in count-rate, or it could operate on the logarithm of the difference, emphasizing small differences in count-rate.

E. Positron Brain Scanner

Since a positron scanner requires two detecting heads and utilizes high-energy γ rays, it might appear at first that the amount of mass to be moved would be great, with consequent severe mechanical requirements on the design. Actually, as discussed above (Section II,C,3) relatively little shielding is needed. The principal mechanical requirement is that the two detecting heads be rigidly mounted so that they are accurately aligned facing each other at all times.

A positron scanning apparatus specifically designed for brain lesion localization is shown in Fig. 10. The patient lies supine with his head between the pair of horizontally positioned detectors. The motors, the drive mechanism and printers are beneath the patient's head. The detector heads are mounted on a carriage which is moved automatically by the horizontal and vertical drive motors. Two sets of printing solenoids are mounted on the same carriage. They are located inside the large side doors in the machine frame (Fig. 10). Thus precise alignment is maintained between the detectors and the printers. The readout consists of direct mechanical printing on paper attached to two printing boards which are fastened to the frame of the machine. The coincidence counts printed on one board are scaled down by an appropriate factor, usually 10. The unbalance scan is printed on the other board which is mounted on the other side of the machine. Two printing solenoids, one with a curve mark and one with a straight mark, indicate a right unbalance and a left unbalance, respectively. The coincidence and unbalance scans are obtained simultaneously. Usually the line spacing is 9 mm and the type bars just fill this space. The coincidence type bar has the form of a very narrow "O" to allow the maximum apparent gray scale as prints overlap.

The electronic circuitry is contained in the separate console shown in Fig. 10. The leading edge system described in Section II,D,1 is employed. The pulses that go to the coincidence tube are also transmitted to an upper chassis where they are scaled down for the differencing circuit.

The detectors are 3-cm square NaI(Tl) crystals, 4 cm long. They are surrounded by about 4.5 cm of lead shielding and set back 3 cm from the shield face. This crude collimator provides enough resolution for

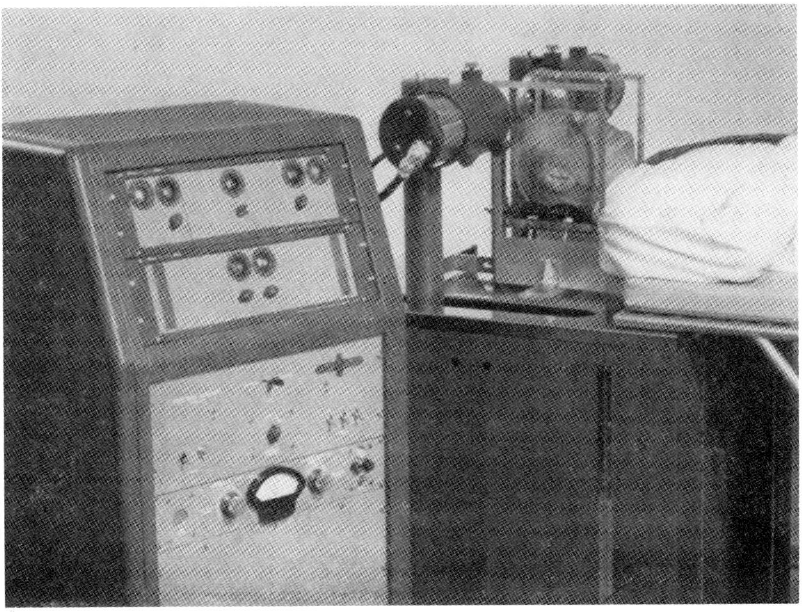

FIG. 10. Commercial version of a positron brain scanner.

the unbalance circuit without excessively increasing the total distance between the pair of detectors.

The 3-cm wide sodium iodide crystals yield a spatial resolution of the coincidence system of 1.5 cm. For a pure positron-emitting point source midway between the two detectors, the sensitivity is about 2000 cpm/μCi. In a typical scan, where a 70-kg patient had received 1.5 mCi of ^{74}As, the coincidence count-rate over a normal area of brain might be about 200 cpm. With a normal scanning speed of 10 cm/min, this corresponds to 1 print (10 counts) in 0.5 cm (3 sec). Over a tumor area, the count-rate might increase to 1000 cpm. The single-channel count-rate would be 50,000 cpm over the normal brain area and 300,000 cpm over a large tumor.

A primary design objective in this machine was simplicity of operation. The operator has almost no parameters to adjust and is chiefly concerned with the comfort of the patient. This particular machine does not have photographic recording or other nonlinear contrast enhancement. Again, this is in the interest of simplicity, since these devices have not seemed necessary.

III. APPLICATION TO BRAIN SCANNING

Positron scanning is particularly appropriate for the difficult diagnostic problem of localizing focal abnormalities in the brain (*14*). As noted above, the cylindrical isocount contours are ideal when the source may be at any point from one side of the brain to the other. The symmetry of the head also makes the interpretation of an unbalance scan simple and significant.

The brain has, besides its physical location, another unique property, the blood-brain barrier. With exception of a few metabolically important chemicals, most trace materials are excluded from the normal brain. When the brain is disturbed by growth of a tumor, a vascular accident, or other more subtle disturbances, this barrier mechanism breaks down in some manner and allows previously excluded chemicals to enter into the tissue. In addition, in some tumors, there appears to be a definite affinity of the tumor tissue for certain chemicals.

A number of positron emitters have been studied as localizing agents. These are listed in Table II together with typical administered doses,

TABLE II
POSITRON-EMITTING RADIOISOTOPES USED FOR BRAIN SCANNING[a]

Isotopes	Chemical form	Dose (mCi/70 kg)	Begin scan after injection (hr)	Time for lateral scan (min)	Number of patients scanned (1966)	Comments
^{74}As	$As_3O_4^-$	1.5	$1\frac{1}{2}$	45	4,600	Standard isotope, excellent for tumor and vascular lesions
^{72}As	$As_3O_4^-$	0.8	1	45	200	Equivalent to ^{74}As
^{64}Cu	DTPA	2	1	45	1,850	Good for tumors, less effective for vascular lesions
^{68}Ga	EDTA	1	$\frac{3}{4}$	20	12	Similar to ^{64}Cu
^{18}F	BF_4^-	3	$\frac{1}{2}$	20	10	Similar to ^{64}Cu

[a] Massachusetts General Hospital, unpublished data.

their chemical form, and some applications. The most extensively used positron emitter has been ^{74}As though it has a number of disadvantages. It is cyclotron produced and therefore difficult to obtain. It has a long half-life (18 days). Its spectrum includes β rays as well as positrons and a number of other γ rays (*11*). Still its localizing properties are superior compared with other positron emitters. The action of the arsenate appears to be more specific than general protein linkage and parallels in some respects the action of phosphate. For physical reasons, ^{72}As would be preferable to ^{74}As but it is more difficult to obtain. Reactor-produced ^{64}Cu has also been extensively used (*4*). In chelated form it localizes in tumor almost as well as arsenate, but not as well in vascular lesions.

Other positron emitters have been used in a smaller number of cases. Fluoride ions are taken up too readily in bone to be useful for brain scanning, but fluoroborate, $B\,^{18}F_4$, has been shown to provide excellent visualization of tumors (*3*). Another short-lived radioisotope that has been found useful is ^{68}Ga (*13*). It has a great advantage in that it is easily milked from long-lived ^{68}Ge (*1*).

For brain scanning the tracer is injected intravenously ½ to 2 hr prior to scanning. With ^{74}As in particular, the time of scanning is not at all critical, and the scan is frequently repeated on the second day to observe a transient process. With the standard tracer dosage, the patient is scanned in the supine position in about 45 min. An A-P scan, with the patient on his side, is usually performed as well. This takes about 30 min. The scanning time may be lengthened or shortened depending on the amount of radioactivity used. With the short-lived radioisotopes, the dose may be doubled and the time halved.

The patient's head outline is recorded manually by noting its position on ruled lines on the Lucite side supports. Since the scan picture is immediately available, the patient may be rescanned if there were technical problems, or if a better position appears desirable.

A. Normal Scan

The pattern of a normal scan depends on the radioisotope as well as the mode of pictorial representation. One views a composite structure consisting of different tissues, all of which contribute to the observed count-rates. Each tissue may have a different uptake and depending upon its physical position it may contribute different amounts to the total count-rate.

An ^{74}As scan of a normal subject is shown in Fig. 11. In the coincidence picture (Fig. 11A) below the level of the line from the tragus of the ear to the orbit of the eye, there is a dense region corresponding to the temporal musculature. This extends down to the inferior occipital re-

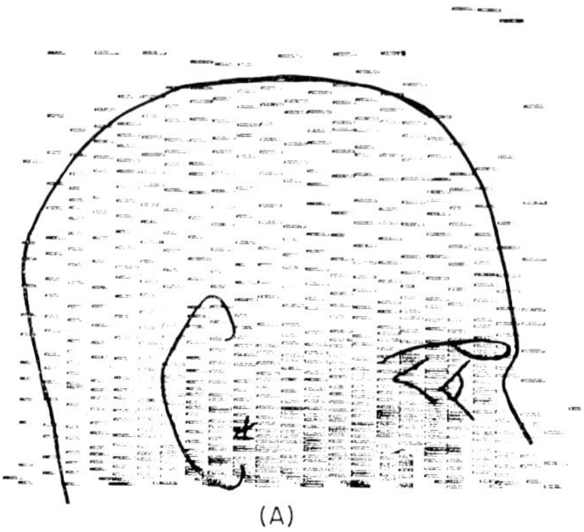

(A)

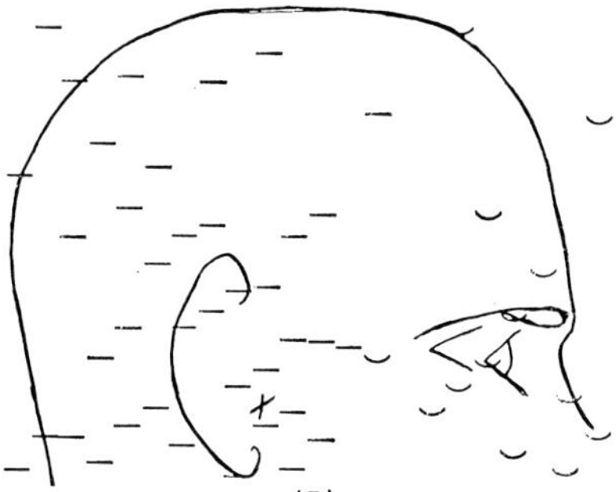

(B)

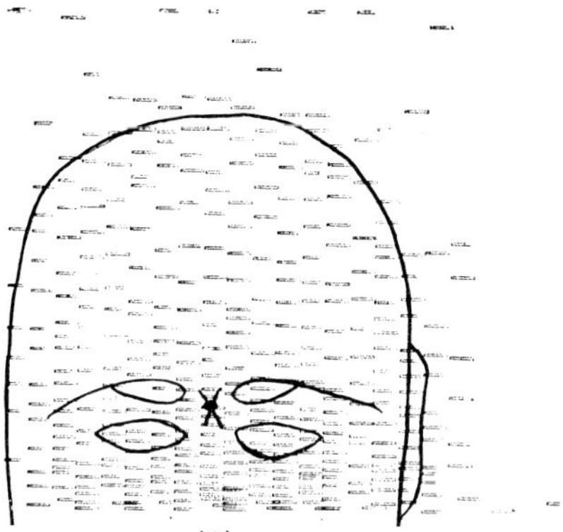

(C)

FIG. 11. Positron scan of normal subject with ^{74}As. (A) Coincidence scan, lateral view. (B) Unbalance scan, lateral view. Shift from left to right unbalance indicates slight tilt of head. (C) Coincidence scan, A-P view.

gion. The periphery of the head is denser than the central region because the detectors are viewing the scalp and skull on edge where the radioactivity levels are higher than in the brain proper. With copper the periphery appears relatively denser than with arsenic because there is higher uptake in the skin and less uptake in the brain proper. Compounds which remain in the blood for a long time, such as RISA, tend to accentuate the vascular pattern and, in particular, the large venous sinuses. This may be a very useful property if one wishes to observe anatomical structures in the brain (*6*).

The unbalance picture of a normal brain (Fig. 11B) is blank, or shows uniform markings indicating a small residual asymmetry of the patient's position. The normal A-P coincidence scan (Fig. 11C) also shows the periphery and an inferior increased density due to musculature.

B. Abnormal Scans

A set of scan pictures taken with ^{74}As for a patient with a meningioma is shown in Fig. 12. The lateral coincidence scan (Fig. 12A) indicates a clearly defined concentration in the frontal-parietal region. The higher density over the tumor compared to the temporal muscle area would indicate a specific uptake of the trace material by the tumor. In the unbalance view (Fig. 12B) the dense concentration of curve marks indicates that the tumor is strongly to the right. The straight marks on the other parts of the head are not significant; they are a geometric artefact because of the marked unbalance. The third view (Fig. 12C) is an A-P coincidence scan taken with the patient resting on her right side and shows that the concentration is in the upper right part of the head.

The primary brain tumors, glioblastoma multiforma and meningioma, are most readily visualized. Metastatic tumors often tend to be multinodular and dispersed and are frequently missed. Tumors in the sella and in the brain stem tend to produce serious neurological deficits while still small and also tend to be masked by the overlying musculature. They are therefore less readily seen.

A summary of the scan results in a series of 969 patients with tumors verified at operation or pathological examination (*2*) is given in Table III. Checking many scans against operative results has shown that the scans are dimensionally accurate as well as qualitatively indicative. Scanning thus provides an invaluable complement to other neurosurgical diagnostic procedures.

Since increased tracer uptake is primarily due to breakdown of the blood brain barrier, other focal lesions, such as those caused by vascular disease, should also be visualized. Animal experiments on brain lesions produced by mechanical pressure (*10*) and radio-frequency heating have

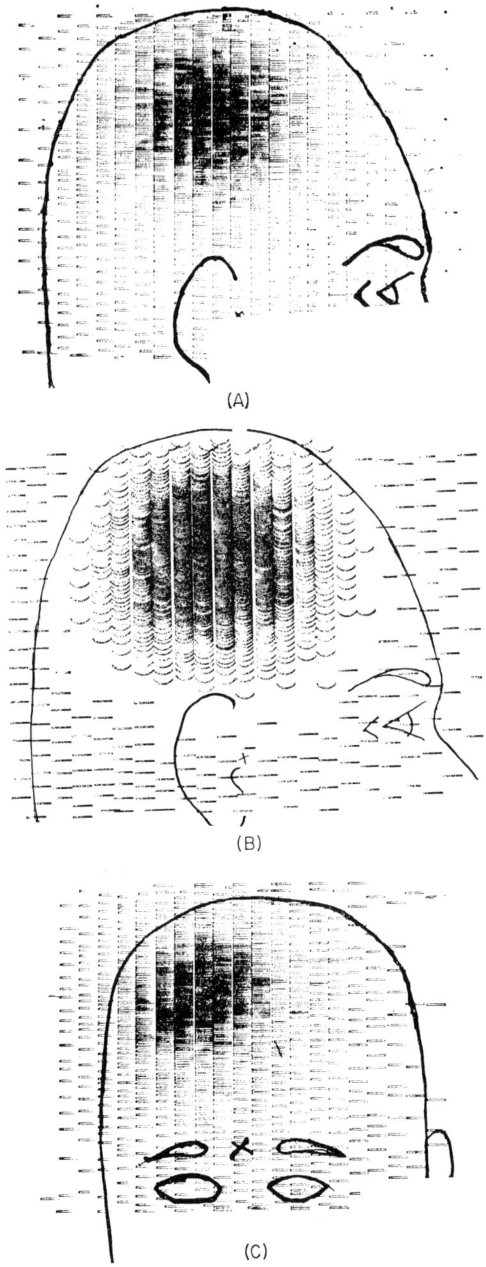

FIG. 12. ^{74}As positron scan of patient with meningioma. (A) Coincidence scan, lateral view showing marked frontal-parietal abnormality. (B) Unbalance scan, lateral view. Concentration of curved marks shows right unbalance. (C) Coincidence scan, A-P view with right superior abnormality.

shown that the tracer is taken up not only in the permanently damaged lesion proper but also in the surrounding tissue that was subjected to transient damage. A curious effect is that the uptake of arsenic continues to be high in the surrounding tissues that is histologically normal brain.

This extended uptake is useful for the localization of vascular lesions. Vascular disease may produce an ischemic region in the brain with transient or permanent damage. An analysis of the scans of such patients has shown that when the neurological deficit is transient, the scan tends to be normal, whereas with permanent neurological deficit, the scan is abnormal. For localizing these lesions arsenic is more effective than

TABLE III
CORRELATION OF SCANNING RESULTS AND CLINICAL DIAGNOSIS OF CONFIRMED TUMORS[a]

	Scan classification[b]				
	1	2	3	4	Total
Glioblastoma multiforme	186	28	8	3	255
Metastases	70	27	25	15	137
Meningioma	103	13	2	5	123
Astrocytoma	33	15	11	14	73
Oligodendroglioma	28	22	9	9	68
Recurrent	30	8	2	0	40
Miscellaneous (CNS)	81	51	45	39	216
Carcinoma (non-CNS)	25	16	23	23	87
Brain tumor suspects	78	83	69	79	309
	634	263	194	187	1278

[a] Period 1953–1963. Agent, ^{74}As-labeled arsenate.

[b] Classes: 1, definitely abnormal; 2, probably abnormal; 3, probably normal; 4, definitely normal.

copper or RISA (*12*). In general, scans of vascular lesions look different from those of tumors. They tend to be less dense, to be more diffuse, and to have less well-defined margins.

Scanning results in a number of other diseases (*2*) are summarized in Table IV. Some of these which, either metabolically or mechanically, produce focal regions of abnormal brain tissue yield positive scans. On the other hand, functional disorders, such as many epilepsies, appear negative.

In a significant number of instances false abnormal scans have been recorded with no demonstrable focal lesion. Since the patients had disease, and in several cases succumbed to it, clearly some phenomenon was occurring metabolically to cause increased tracer uptake.

Reading and interpreting of scans requires a certain amount of practice. Since the picture depends upon the trace materials used, the amount of data processing applied, and the metabolic and anatomical characteristics of the particular patient, all the information available on a scan will not be immediately obvious. As in any other pattern recognition problem, training and understanding of the purpose and peculiarities of the technique will aid greatly in making full use of this diagnostic method.

TABLE IV
CORRELATION OF SCANNING RESULTS AND CLINICAL DIAGNOSIS OF NONNEOPLASTIC DISEASE[a]

	Scan classification[b]				
	1	2	3	4	Total
Cerebrovascular disease	82	81	75	73	311
CVD Suspect	10	14	23	34	81
Convulsive disorders	32	74	130	198	434
Infections	30	34	27	38	129
Trauma	25	40	32	55	152
Degenerative disease	22	32	68	83	205
Headache	7	31	44	97	179
Miscellaneous	63	138	150	252	603
No diagnosis	83	121	133	187	524
	354	565	682	1017	2618

[a] Period 1953–1963. Agent, ^{74}As-labeled arsenate.
[b] Classes same as in Table III.

REFERENCES

1. Anger, H. O., and Gottschalk, A., Localization of brain tumors with the positron scintillation camera. *J. Nucl. Med.* **4**, 326 (1963).
2. Aronow, S., Brownell, G. L., Lovo, S. L., and Sweet, W. H., Analysis of 8 years' experience in positron scanning for brain tumor localization. *J. Nucl. Med.* **3**, 198 (1962).
3. Askenasy, H. M., Anbar, M., Laor, Y., Lewitus, Z., Kosary, I. Z., and Guttmann, S., The localization of intracranial space-occupying lesions by fluoroborate ions labelled with F^{18}. *Am. J. Roentgenol., Radium Therapy Nucl. Med.* **88**, 350 (1962).
4. Bagnall, H. J., Benda, P., Brownell, G. L., and Sweet, W. H., Positron-scanning with copper-64 in the diagnosis of intracranial lesions: partition of copper-64 versenate in, and excretion from, the body. *J. Neurosurg.* **15**, 411 (1958).
5. Bell, R. E., Graham, R. L., and Petch, H. E., Design and use of a coincidence circuit of short resolving time. *Can. J. Phys.* **30**, 35 (1952).

6. DiChiro, G., RISA encephalography and conventional neuroradiographic methods. A comparative study. *Acta Radiol.* Suppl. **201,** 101 (1961).
7. Draper, J. E., and Fleischer, A. A., Fast coincidence circuit for slow pulses. *Rev. Sci. Instr.* **31,** 49 (1960).
8. Evans, R. D., "The Atomic Nucleus." McGraw-Hill, New York, 1955.
9. Gruhle, W., Impuls-Zeitformer für schnelle Koinzidenzstufen. *Nucl. Instr. Methods* **4,** 112 (1959).
10. Hacker, H., Aronow, S., and Soloway, A. H., Differential concentration of arsenic-74 and copper-64 in experimental lesions in cat brain. *Neurochirurgia* **7,** 100 (1964).
11. Mealey, J., Jr., Brownell, G. L., and Sweet, W. H., Radioarsenic in plasma, urine, normal tissue, and intracranial neoplasms. *AMA Arch. Neurol. Psychiat.* **81,** 310 (1959).
12. Ojemann, R. G., Aronow, S., and Sweet, W. H., Scanning with positron-emitting radioisotopes: Occlusive cerebral-vascular disease. *Arch. Neurol.* **10,** 218 (1964).
13. Shealy, C. N., Aronow, S., and Brownell, G. L., Gallium-68 as a scanning agent for intracranial lesions. *J. Nucl. Med.* **5,** 161 (1964).
14. Wrenn, F. W., Jr., Good, M. L., and Handler, P., The use of positron-emitting radioisotopes for the localization of brain tumors. *Science* **113,** 525 (1951).

CHAPTER 19

RADIOISOTOPE CAMERAS

HAL O. ANGER

DONNER LABORATORY OF MEDICAL PHYSICS AND BIOPHYSICS
UNIVERSITY OF CALIFORNIA
BERKELEY, CALIFORNIA

I. STATIONARY DEVICES FOR TRANSLATING RADIOISOTOPE DISTRIBUTION INTO VISUAL IMAGES

Radioisotope cameras are relatively new instruments for imaging the distribution of radioisotopes *in vivo*. Instead of scanning the subject point-by-point, they view all parts of the field continuously. Recently, scintillation cameras have emerged from the research laboratory into practical use. At the end of 1966, about 60 commercially made cameras were in routine use in hospitals and research laboratories.

The main advantage of γ-ray cameras over radioisotope scanners is that they can take pictures of isotope distribution in a much shorter time. There are two reasons for this higher speed. First, currently available cameras are about 10 times as sensitive as conventional scanners and therefore gather the same information in 1/10 the time. Second, the picture-taking speed of cameras is not limited by mechanical factors. They view the entire picture area continuously, and when a subject contains enough radioactivity, they can take pictures at the rate of one per second or faster. The picture-taking speed of scanners is limited by how fast their probes can scan the picture area, and they require at least several minutes to scan most organs.

Shorter exposure times have important clinical advantages. First, rapid sequences of still pictures and motion pictures can be taken to determine the dynamic functions of organs. Second, multiple views of an organ from various angles can be obtained in a short period of time. This improves the visibility of lesions and other abnormalities. Third, more patients can be studied per day with one instrument, an important economic advantage.

In addition, continuous sensitivity to all parts of the field allows numerical counting data to be obtained from any part of the field as a function of time for dynamic processes.

Gamma-ray cameras that employ parallel multichannel collimators have a greater depth of focus, or ability to see sharply at all depths, compared to scanners with focused collimators. This is an advantage when viewing thick organs like the liver and brain.

Radioisotope cameras can be constructed to allow considerable flexibility in the positioning of patients. The camera can be positioned to obtain frontal, lateral, or oblique views while the patient is lying down, sitting, or standing. If a memory oscilloscope is employed, the picture of an organ under examination can be seen building up as the exposure proceeds, thus verifying early during the exposure that the final picture will be satisfactory.

Positron cameras are a special form of radioisotope camera that employ coincidence techniques to image positron emitters. Some chemical elements have no suitable γ-ray emitting isotopes but have positron emitters which in turn emit 0.51 MeV γ-ray pairs. Positron coincidence cameras offer high sensitivity and resolution for these isotopes. They also offer tomographic operation, in which activity lying on planes deep within the subject is sharply imaged while activity lying on other planes is blurred. Furthermore, any number of images, each showing a different plane sharply resolved, can be produced by suitable electronic circuitry during a single exposure.

In this section, a brief survey of different approaches to stationary imaging devices is presented.

A. Contact Methods

When a radioactive subject is very thin, the simplest method of imaging the distribution of radioactivity is to place X-ray film in contact with the subject, expose for a length of time, and then develop the film. This is the well-known method used to obtain autoradiographs of tissue sections.

Although the contact method of imaging "sees" the whole picture area during the entire exposure time, the overall sensitivity is low because many γ rays or β particles must strike a given area on the film before visible blackening results. Therefore, exposure times are long.

This method provides good resolution only when the distance separating the subject and film is very small. For two point sources to be resolved in the image, they should be roughly no farther from the film than they are from each other. Therefore, the contact method is not useful even for imaging the thyroid gland, which is only 2 to 3 cm below the surface. It is limited to the skin and accessible parts of the alimentary tract (*47*).

B. Camera-Type Devices with Direct Radiographic Recording

Of the various particles and rays emitted by radioactive isotopes, only X rays and γ rays have enough penetrating power to reach the surface of the body from deep-lying organs. Furthermore, these rays are always emitted isotropically and they cannot be focused or scattered predictably. However, satisfactory images of the deeper organs of the body can be obtained by selective interference, a method of blocking out or absorbing all but a small fraction of the rays with image-producing collimators. The remaining rays travel on to form an image of the subject at the exit side of the collimator. Two such collimators are the pinhole collimator, consisting usually of a single hole in a conical lead shield (Section III,A) and the multichannel collimator, consisting of hundreds or thousands of channels in an absorber plate (Section III,C). By either means, a γ-ray image of an object located deep within the body can be produced at a plane on the opposite side of the collimator. If a radiographic film or other detection means is located at this plane, an image of the subject can be obtained.

This method of producing images has been applied in the following ways. Roentgen in 1896 used a pinhole aperture and photographic film to obtain an image of the X-ray-emitting anode of one of his first tubes. In 1949 Copeland and Benjamin (*24*) used a γ-ray pinhole camera and X-ray film to obtain pictures of radium needles. In 1952 the author (*2*) used a γ-ray pinhole camera, a solid, thallium-activated, sodium iodide intensifying screen, and blue-sensitive photographic film to obtain pictures *in vivo* of a metastatic thyroid lesion containing a therapeutic quantity of ^{131}I. An activity concentration of 1 mCi/cm^2 and 1-hr exposure were necessary to obtain detectable blackening of the film.

In 1953, Johansson and Skanse (*38*) reported the use of a multichannel collimator, solid sodium iodide crystal, and blue-sensitive film to obtain *in vivo* pictures of the thyroid gland and metastatic lesions. In 1955 Kellershohn and Pellerin (*39*) used a multichannel collimator, a mosaic of sodium iodide crystals, and mercury vapor–sensitized film to obtain a further increase in sensitivity. In this case, each element of the crystal mosaic was lined up with a channel in the collimator. Yasukochi (*58*) has reported using a multichannel collimator and radiographic film to obtain images of phantom sources containing ^{125}I.

However, none of the above methods of obtaining images is sensitive enough for clinical diagnostic use.

C. Scintillator Mosaic with Image Amplifier

An obvious method of improving the sensitivity of the methods described in the previous section was to convert the γ-ray image into a light image by means of a scintillator, and then amplify the light with image intensifiers. In Fig. 1 a mosaic of 241 sodium iodide crystals, each contained in a separate cell in an aluminum holder, is shown in contact with the input of a Philips single-stage image amplifier (*3, 46*). The tube was identical to the type intended for X-ray image amplification except that the X-ray-sensitive phosphor was absent and the 5-inch photocathode was deposited directly on the inside of the glass envelope. A pinhole aperture projected a γ-ray image of the subject on the crystal mosaic. When a γ ray interacted with an element of the mosaic, light was produced, which caused electrons to be emitted from a small area of the image-amplifier photocathode. These electrons were accelerated within the tube and focused by an electron lens onto an output phosphor.

The intensified image appearing at the output screen was either viewed directly or recorded on photographic film.

With this instrument, an image of a therapeutic quantity of ^{131}I in the stomach of a patient with metastatic thyroid disease was observed visually. Movements of the patient's stomach were readily visible, thus indicating the value of camera-type instruments for dynamic studies. However, the sensitivity was still too low for diagnostic use. Because of field emission in the image amplifier, the background was equivalent to 10 $\mu Ci/cm^2$ when photographic recording was used, and because of the low gain of the image amplifier, an activity concentration of 200 $\mu Ci/cm^2$ of ^{131}I was necessary for visual observation. Despite the low sensitivity,

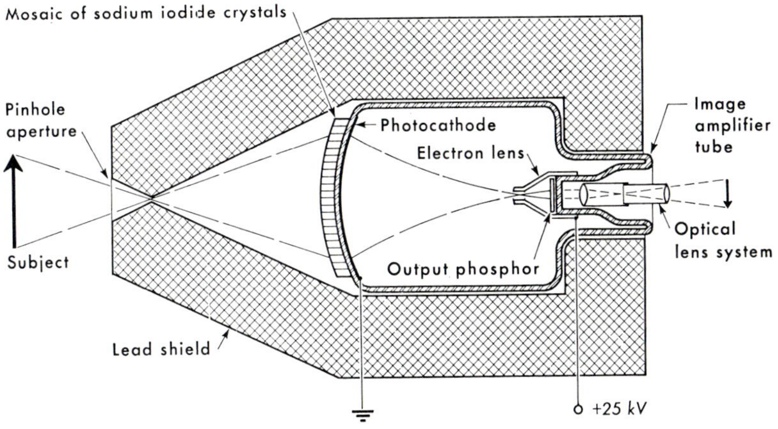

FIG. 1. Early version of γ-ray camera employing mosaic of sodium iodide crystals and image amplifier (*46*).

this instrument clearly demonstrated the potential usefulness of camera-type imaging devices.

D. The Scintillation Camera: Position-Sensing Multiplier Phototube Array with Solid Sodium Iodide Crystal

A new approach to a sensitive camera-type instrument was taken by the author in 1956 (*4, 5*). The result is the scintillation camera, which employs a solid sodium iodide scintillation crystal viewed by an array of multiplier phototubes, as shown in Fig. 2. A computing circuit, used in combination with the phototube array, senses the position of scintillations in the crystal and sends signals to an image-readout oscilloscope that reproduces the scintillations as point flashes of light. When a scintillation occurs at an intermediate point between phototubes, its position is still determined because of the proportionate division of light among the tubes. The accuracy of determining the position of scintillations in cameras, which employ larger crystals and more multiplier phototubes, allows 1000 picture elements to be resolved at medium γ-ray energies.

The signals from the multiplier phototubes are summed and pulse-height selection is employed to eliminate scintillations not falling within the photopeak of the γ-ray spectrum, thus reducing background by the

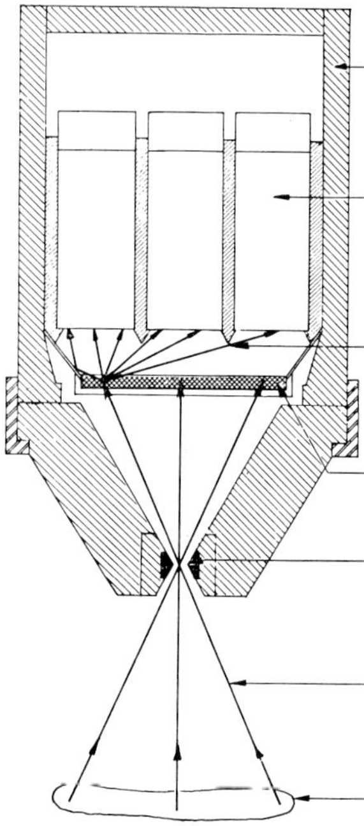

FIG. 2. Scintillation camera with 4-inch diameter solid sodium iodide crystal and seven multiplier phototubes (*4, 5*).

same method used in conventional radioisotope scanners. Excellent pulse-height resolution results from the efficient collection of light from the sodium iodide crystal.

A time exposure of the oscilloscope screen is taken with a Polaroid camera, and an image of the active areas of the subject results. Pinhole and multichannel collimators are used to image γ-ray emitters (Section III), and coincidence collimation of annihilation radiation is used for positron emitters (Section IV).

Recent models, including one that is commercially available,* employ 11-inch diameter crystals viewed by an array of 19 multiplier phototubes (*8, 9*). With the 11-inch camera, pictures of nearly all organs of

* Nuclear-Chicago Corp.

the body can be taken in a fraction of the time required by conventional radioisotope scanners. Brain tumor pictures have been taken in 10 sec, and stop-motion pictures have been taken of ^{99m}Tc going through the heart and kidneys at the rate of one picture per second (*14*).

By the use of the multiplier phototube array, many of the limitations of image amplifiers are avoided. High gain is readily obtained, tube background is negligible, and there is convenient remote reproduction of the images. Coincidence and dot-shifting techniques are easily used in conjunction with positron emitters. Also, there is no practical limit to the size of the camera except for limitations in the manufacture of the sodium iodide crystal.

The useful γ-ray energy range of phototube-array scintillation cameras is about 0.07 to 0.7 MeV. The upper limit is set by the inherent difficulties of collimating and detecting high-energy γ rays. The lower limit is a result of statistical phenomena discussed in Section II,C,2.

Because of the use of a solid homogeneous scintillator, rather than a mosaic, the images have no distracting patterns superimposed. Multichannel collimators with the most efficient hole spacing can be used without Moire effects. Furthermore, the ½-inch thick scintillator permits, without excessive resolution loss, the use of collimators in which γ rays travel at oblique angles. Also, resolution loss due to γ-ray scattering within the scintillator is minimized, as discussed in Section II,C,1.

By the use of analog-to-digital converters, the image information can be stored in digital form. Magnetic core memory systems with 1024 or 4096 elements are employed. Numerical data can be obtained from any desired picture area by digital computer techniques (Section V,C).

A more detailed description of the phototube-array scintillation camera is given in Section II.

E. Autofluoroscope

In 1962, Bender and Blau (*16, 17*) reported construction of a γ-ray imaging instrument called the autofluoroscope. It employed a mosaic of 293 sodium iodide crystals, each ⅜ inch in diameter by 2 inches long, viewed by a position-sensing multiplier phototube array. The electronic circuit and image readout system was the same as that employed for the scintillation camera (Section II,A,1). Collimation was achieved with a multichannel collimator having 293 tapered holes, one corresponding to each mosaic element. Television contrast enhancement was used in the display of the final image (*18*).

The authors reported taking static pictures of brain tumors and liver tumors with ⅕ to ⅒ the exposure time usually required with a conventional scanner. Also dynamic studies were made of Hippuran-^{131}I going through a kidney and ^{137m}Ba going through the heart *(18)*. Numerical data from organ compartments as a function of time were obtained by counting dots within prescribed areas in a sequence of pictures.

The purpose of the thick mosaic scintillator was to obtain high detection efficiency for medium- and high-energy γ rays. However, the sensitivity of the radioisotope cameras depends as much on the efficiency of the collimator as on the efficiency of the scintillator. Calculations indicate the collimator used with the autofluoroscope was relatively inefficient compared to other multichannel collimators. The net sensitivity, in terms of the number of γ rays detected per minute per microcurie of activity in the subject, was not reported. γ-Ray scattering and subsequent loss of resolution occur in thick sodium iodide crystals, as discussed in Section II,C,1.

The same authors have recently described a new rank-and-file coincidence method for determining which crystal in a mosaic detects a γ ray, and a system of recording the counts from each mosaic element in digital form in a magnetic core memory system* *(18, 19)*. Each of 300 crystals in the 9×6 inch mosaic is optically connected by two Lucite light pipes to one of 15 rank multiplier phototubes and one of 20 file multiplier phototubes. Simultaneous pulses from the two phototubes uniquely identify the mosaic element in which a scintillation occurs. The summed signal from the 15 rank phototubes is fed to a pulse-height selector, and the output provides a pulse that allows the magnetic core memory system to store the event. An anticoincidence system eliminates γ rays scattered between mosaic elements. Scintillations caused by both the original γ ray and the scattered γ ray are eliminated by this technique, since there is no method for distinguishing the original event.

The digital nature of the rank-and-file system lends itself to direct magnetic core storage of the data. Subsequently the data can be read out as a mosaic image on a cathode-ray tube. Any desired amount of background erase can be obtained nondestructively. Numerical data can be obtained from three picture areas by digital computer techniques (Section V,C).

F. Image-Converter γ-Ray Camera

In 1963 Ter-Pogossian described the camera shown in Fig. 3 for use with low-energy γ-ray emitters *(51)*. It employed an 8-inch diameter image-amplifier tube originally designed for use as an X-ray image intensifier. This type of tube has a thin X-ray-sensitive phosphor inside a glass envelope. When an X ray interacts with the phosphor, light is emitted

* Baird-Atomic, Inc.

which in turn causes electrons to be emitted from a photocathode deposited on the phosphor. These electrons are accelerated and focused by an electron lens onto an output screen. Each X ray that interacts with the input phosphor produces several thousand light photons at the output screen. The amplified flashes are recorded on fast Polaroid film.

This instrument was first used with the 27-keV X rays from ^{125}I. A multichannel collimator was employed to project an image of the subject on the input phosphor. Approximately 26% of the X rays that impinged on the glass envelope interacted with the input phosphor and produced a visible dot in the image. Pictures of phantoms containing as

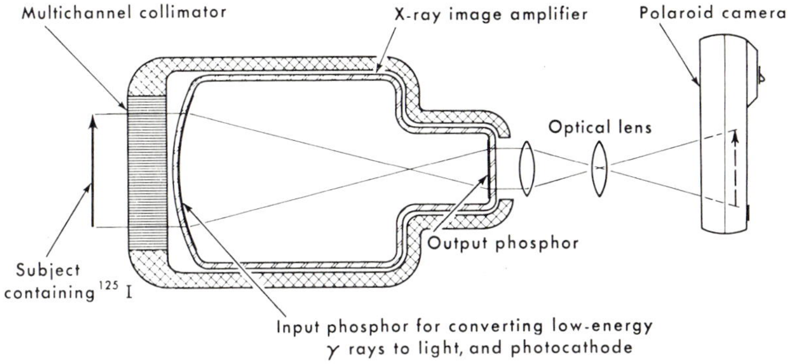

FIG. 3. γ-Ray camera employing X-ray image amplifier with internal input phosphor. This camera is for use with low-energy γ-ray emitters such as ^{125}I (*51*).

little as 25 μCi of ^{125}I were taken in 3 min. However, the first instrument was not applied clinically, because the large diameter of the image amplifier did not allow getting the instrument close enough to the thyroid gland of a patient. Also the input phosphor was located an appreciable distance inside the glass envelope of the image-amplifier tube, thus reducing the resolution of the X-ray image obtained from the multichannel collimator.

With specially constructed image-intensifier tubes, this type of instrument should provide good results with low-energy photon emitters. It has the advantages of simplicity and good detection efficiency for X rays and low-energy γ rays, and it promises good resolution when modified image-amplifier tubes become available (*52*).

Its disadvantages include low detection efficiency for medium-energy γ rays, and a lack of pulse-height selection to reduce background from scattered rays. Furthermore, X-ray emitters and low-energy γ-ray emitters have inherent disadvantages for imaging deep-lying organs. More

Compton scattering occurs in tissue at these energies and fewer of the scattered rays can be removed by pulse-height selection even if it is provided (*49*) (Section II,D,2). The net effect is a higher background of scattered dots in the images.

A similar instrument was reported by Kellershohn and Pellerin (*40*) in 1955. However, low-energy γ-ray emitters were not in use at that time and image amplifiers had higher backgrounds, so satisfactory sensitivity for clinical purposes could not be obtained.

G. Array of γ-Ray Counters

In 1955, Fucks and Knipping (*27*) reported constructing an instrument called the Gamma-Retina. It employed a fixed array of 39 Geiger–Müller counters and a collimator consisting of a lead plate with 39 holes, one corresponding to each counter. Whenever a γ ray was detected by a counter, a flash appeared in an array of glow lamps at a point corresponding to the position of the counter. The flashes were photographed with a motion picture camera to record the movement of tracer compounds. In 1964, an improved model was described that employed 100 scintillation counters in a 17×17 cm array (*28*). An intensity-modulated cathode-ray oscilloscope was used to display the detected γ rays. This instrument was built primarily to study heart function and to detect heart shunts *in vivo* by means of isotope angiocardiography. For preliminary studies with large dogs, 50 mCi of 7-day ^{177}Lu were injected and pictures were taken at a rate that showed the isotope traveling through the chambers of the heart.

The construction of a similar instrument built primarily for kinetic studies of tracer compounds in the brain has been reported (*35*). This instrument employs two 6×8 inch arrays of 63 scintillation counters each. A small focused collimator was provided for each counter. The counts from each counter were stored in a magnetic-core memory system. Numerical readout was by means of punched tape or typewriter, and images with any degree of background erase could be displayed on an oscilloscope.

Although simple in concept, these instruments are complex in construction and maintenance, and their resolution is limited to the center-to-center distance between counters in the array.

H. Spark-Chamber γ-Ray Camera

A new and very simple low-energy γ-ray camera employing a spark chamber as the detector was described in 1964 by Kellershohn (*41*). The 8-inch diameter chamber is filled with argon or xenon gas, and a potential of several kilovolts is maintained between a disk-shaped cathode and two grids. When X rays or γ rays produce recoil electrons in the gas between cathode and first grid, the potential difference causes additional free electrons and ions to be produced by collisions until an avalanche follows. The charged particles travel to the second part of the chamber, where they form the path for a visible spark. The sparks are photographed through a glass end of the chamber by an optical camera (*26*).

At the time of reporting, the detection efficiency of the spark chamber for the 27-keV X rays from ^{125}I was $\sim 10\%$ with xenon-filled chambers. Higher efficiencies can probably be obtained in the future by increasing the pressure of the gas.

I. Solid State Devices

During the past few years, a new method of detecting γ rays has been under development, namely, the use of solid state semiconductor detectors (Chapter 5). A mosaic of such detectors connected to a suitable image readout device and used with conventional pinhole or multichannel collimators offers an alternative method of producing a γ-ray camera.

At present the gross detection efficiency of the largest available germanium solid state detectors is limited to about 30% for 0.3-MeV γ rays, and the photopeak detection efficiency is about 5% for the same γ rays (*50*). The low detection efficiency compared with sodium iodide scintillators results because they are made from low-atomic-number material, and their sensitive volume is less than 1 cm thick.

Solid state detectors offer the potential advantage of much better pulse-height resolution than scintillation detectors, and thus more scattered γ rays could be rejected if these detectors could be employed. Mosaics with 100 or more elements are presently very expensive. Also, for best pulse-height resolution they must be operated at liquid nitrogen temperatures. Practical cameras using these detectors have yet to be developed.

II. DESCRIPTION OF SCINTILLATION CAMERA

A. Principle of Operation

The operation and performance of the multiplier phototube-array scintillation camera, discussed briefly in Section I,D, will be described in detail in this section. A commercial version of this instrument (Fig. 4A), employing an 11-inch diameter scintillator and 19 multiplier phototubes, is the most widely used clinical radioisotope camera at the time this chapter is being written.

The principle of operation of the phototube-array scintillation camera is illustrated in the drawing of the early model shown in Fig. 2. It employed a 4-inch diameter by ¼-inch thick sodium iodide crystal viewed by seven 1.5-inch diameter multiplier phototubes, arranged in a hexagonal array with six of the tubes at the points of a hexagon and the

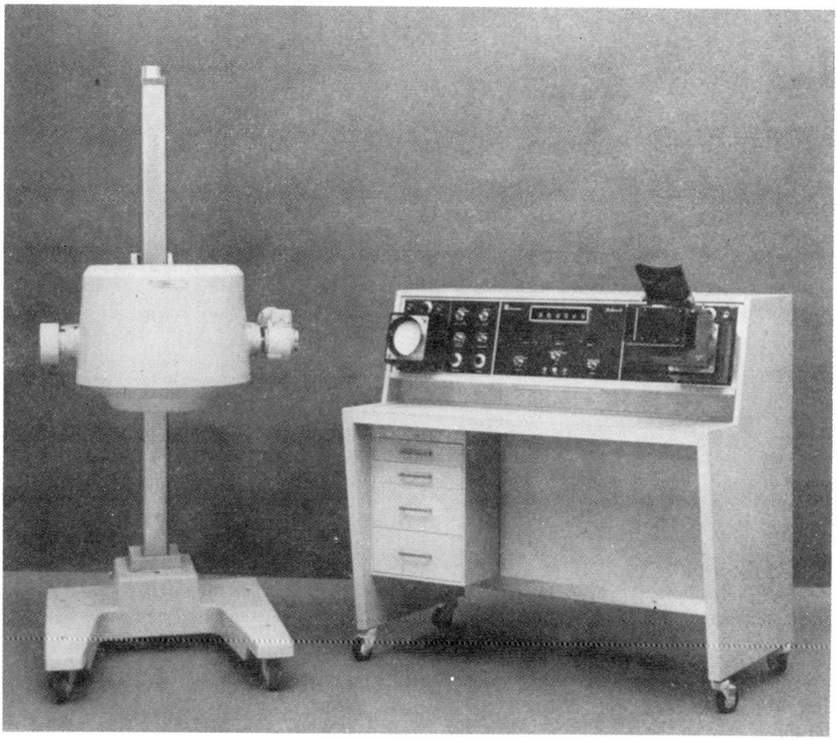

FIG. 4A. Commercially-manufactured scintillation camera (Pho/Gamma III, Nuclear-Chicago Corp.) employs an 11-inch diameter scintillator and 19 multiplier phototubes.

seventh at the center. The central plane of the crystal was about 1 inch from the photocathodes, thus allowing light from each scintillation to divide among the tubes.

The circuit for computing the location of scintillations and displaying them on the image-readout oscilloscope is shown in Fig. 4B. Pulse signals from the phototubes are fed through small capacitors to four output leads called the X^+, X^-, Y^+, and Y^- leads. The amount of signal transferred to each output lead is proportional to the capacitance value in picofarads given in the diagram. For instance, phototube No. 1 has a 30-pF capacitance to the X^+ lead, 10 pF to the X^- lead, 40 pF to the Y^+

lead, and zero capacitance to the Y^- lead. Therefore this phototube transfers most of its signal to the X^+ and Y^+ leads. Tube No. 7 in the center of the array has 20 pF to each lead, and therefore sends equal signals to the four leads.

Suppose a scintillation occurs directly under phototube No. 2. The light is emitted isotropically. Most of it is collected by phototube No. 2

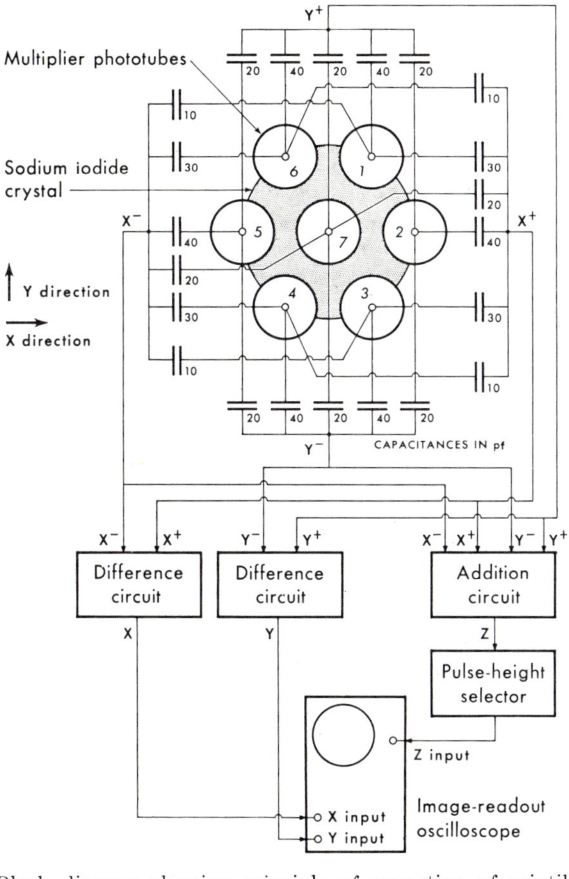

FIG. 4B. Block diagram showing principle of operation of scintillation camera using seven multiplier phototubes (5).

because this tube is closest and subtends a large solid angle. Smaller amounts are collected by tubes Nos. 1, 3, and 7, and still smaller amounts by tubes Nos. 4, 5, and 6. A large X^+ signal is generated by this scintillation because tube No. 2 is connected by a large capacitance to the X^+ lead. A small X^- signal is generated, and moderate but equal Y^+ and Y^- signals are generated.

These four signals are applied to analog computer elements and three new signals are produced that indicate the position and brightness of the scintillation. Signals approximately proportional to the X and Y coordinates of the scintillation are obtained as follows:

$$X = X^{+} - X^{-}$$
$$Y = Y^{+} - Y^{-}$$

The origin of the coordinate system is located at the center of the crystal. These equations assume that all scintillations are of equal brightness. For reasons given below, the only scintillations displayed on the readout oscilloscope are those nearly equal in brightness (photopeak scintillations) so the above condition is met approximately. The X and Y signals are applied directly to the X and Y inputs of the image-readout oscilloscope.

A third signal which is proportional only to the brightness of the scintillation without regard to its location in the crystal is called the Z signal. It is obtained as follows:

$$Z = X^{+} + X^{-} + Y^{+} + Y^{-}$$

This signal is applied to the input of a single-channel pulse-height selector. The window of the pulse-height selector is adjusted to accept only the photopeak of the γ-ray spectrum. Most scattered γ rays and many due to natural background are eliminated because they do not meet the pulse-height requirement.

To return to the description of what happens when a scintillation occurs under tube No. 2: when the X^{+}, X^{-}, Y^{+}, and Y^{-} signals are applied to the difference circuits, the X circuit puts out a large positive signal because the amplitude of the X^{+} signal is large, and the Y circuit puts out a signal of zero amplitude because the Y^{+} and Y^{-} signals are equal.

Normally, the beam of the image-readout oscilloscope is directed to the center of the screen and is cut off by a negative voltage on the control grid of the cathode-ray tube. When the X and Y signals are applied, the beam is deflected to a point on the right-hand side of the screen for a period of 1 μsec. At the same time, the X^{+}, X^{-}, Y^{+}, and Y^{-} signals have been summed in the addition circuit and the resulting Z signal applied to the input of the pulse-height selector. If the Z signal has the prescribed amplitude, the pulse-height selector produces an output pulse that turns on the beam of the image-readout oscilloscope for 0.5 μsec. The scintillation is reproduced as a point flash of light on the right-hand side of the oscilloscope screen.

Therefore, the cathode-ray tube presents a continuous readout of photopeak scintillations occurring in the crystal. The flashes are photo-

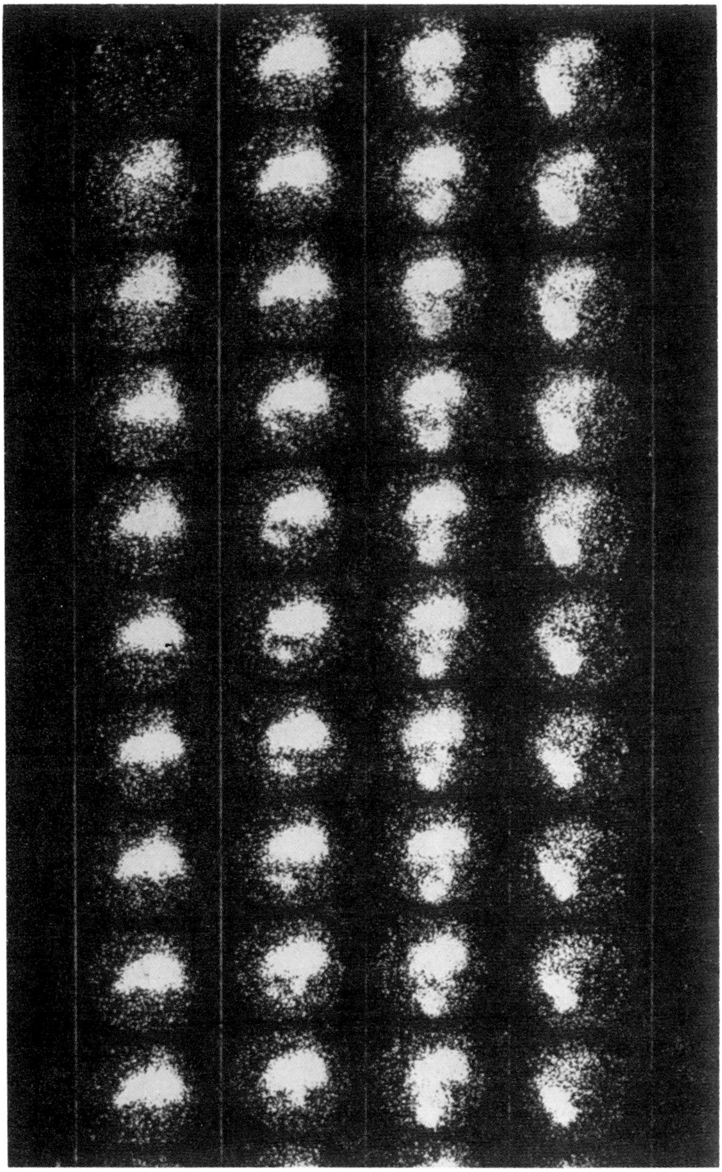

FIG. 5. Frames from "isotope movies" taken in 1960 showing 50 μCi of rose bengal-^{131}I taken up and excreted by the liver of a rat. Scintillation camera with pinhole collimation was used, and pictures were taken at one frame per minute.

graphed over a period of time with an optical scope camera, and the resulting picture shows the distribution of activity in the subject. Exposure times last from a second to a few minutes or more, and usually 1,000 to 100,000 or more dots are recorded on each picture.

Although only seven phototubes are used in this model of the scintillation camera, hundreds of picture elements can be resolved, because the scintillations are reproduced in approximately correct locations even when they occur at points intermediate between the phototubes. How accurately the position of the flashes on the readout oscilloscope corresponds to the original scintillations can easily be demonstrated by test pictures. Examples are shown for a larger instrument in Section II,C.

In the early scintillation cameras, a pinhole collimator was usually used to project a γ-ray image of the subject onto the crystal. Apertures from $\frac{1}{8}$ to $\frac{5}{16}$ inch in diameter were employed. In clinical practice these small instruments were used mostly for visualization of the human thyroid gland with ^{131}I.

They were also used to show the distribution of γ-ray-emitting isotopes in small animals. The first "isotope motion pictures" showing the movement of a tracer compound *in vivo* were taken in 1960. A series of still pictures from this film is shown in Fig. 5. They show 50 μCi of rose bengal-^{131}I being taken up by the liver and excreted into the duodenum of a rat. Pictures were taken at the rate of one frame per minute.

B. Scintillation Camera with 11-Inch-Diameter Crystal

With the availability of larger sodium iodide crystals, scintillation cameras with higher sensitivity and improved overall resolution were constructed (*8, 9, 14*) (Fig. 4A).

An outline drawing of the γ-ray-detecting head of a camera employing an 11.5-inch diameter crystal is shown in Fig. 6. The scintillator is viewed by a hexagonal array of nineteen 3-inch diameter multiplier phototubes. The phototubes are spaced about 1.5 inch from the central plane of the scintillator and are optically coupled to the scintillator by means of a Lucite light pipe or a mineral oil bath to maintain a high-refractive-index path between the crystal and the phototubes. The crystal is rough on all sides to reduce piping of the light to the edges of the crystal by repeated internal reflection. It is contained in a hermetically sealed can with a glass window and aluminum oxide reflector. A light deflector adjacent to the phototubes, shown in cross section in Fig. 6, reflects light that would normally fall between the tubes. This important component has been found empirically to improve the resolution and linearity of the pictures. The combination of elements including the scintillator crystal, multiplier phototube array, optical coupler, and the capacitor network is called an image detector.

A block diagram of the electronic circuit is shown in Fig. 7. The extra components used for coincidence collimation of annihilation radiation from positron emitters are also shown. The basic principle of operation of this large camera is the same as for the small camera described in Section II,A. The capacitor network is more complicated because of the larger number of phototubes employed. Details are given in another publication (*9*).

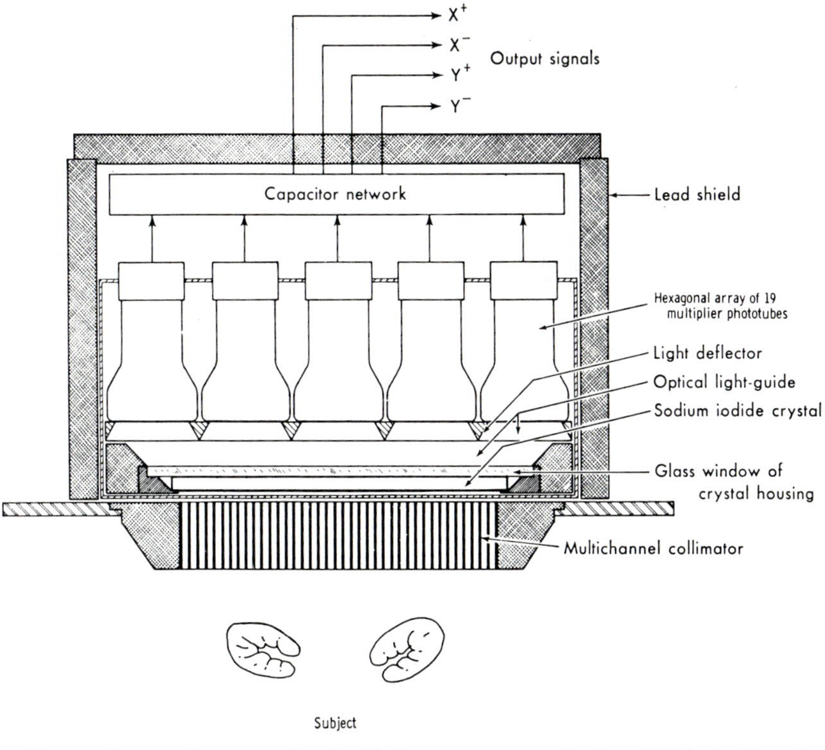

FIG. 6. Image detector of scintillation camera employing 11.5-inch diameter, 0.5-inch thick solid sodium iodide crystal and 19 multiplier phototubes (*8, 9*). Multichannel collimator is shown between crystal and subject.

Recently the difference circuits have been replaced by ratio circuits that perform the function

$$X = (X^+ - X^-)/Z \qquad \text{and} \qquad Y = (Y^+ - Y^-)/Z$$

With these circuits, the positions of flashes on the image-readout oscilloscope are independent of the brightness of the scintillation. Therefore, wide pulse-height selector windows can be used without the slight loss of position resolution that occurred at the edges of the pictures when difference circuits were used.

The γ-ray energy selector shown at the top of Fig. 7 is a variable attenuator that permits setting the pulse-height window of the scintillation camera to an isotope of given γ-ray energy while the voltages on the phototubes are kept constant. The method of adjusting the phototube voltages so that all have equal gain has been described (*9*). It is

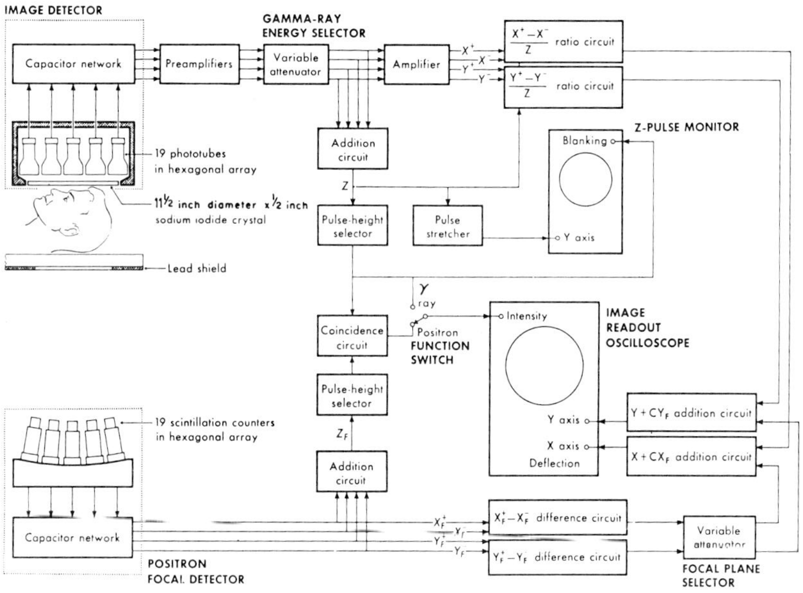

FIG. 7. Block diagram of γ-ray and positron scintillation camera employing image detector shown in Fig. 6 (*8, 9*).

easily accomplished with a collimated γ-ray source and the *Z*-pulse monitor oscilloscope described in the next paragraphs.

The *Z*-pulse monitor oscilloscope, shown at upper right of Fig. 7, gives the operator a means of quickly adjusting the pulse-height selector window to the photopeak of the isotope in use (*37*). The width of the window and the photopeak, and their relation to each other, can be observed visually. In this type of display, the width of the photopeak is represented by the vertical width of the bright line shown in Fig. 8A. The window is represented by the small superimposed dark area shown in Fig. 8B. The vertical width of the dark area is proportional to the width of the window. A properly adjusted window is shown in Fig. 8D.

This type of display is especially valuable when double isotope studies are performed, because the two photopeaks produce two bright lines and the window can be adjusted to coincide with either one of them very quickly as shown in Fig. 8G and 8H. Unsymmetrical adjustments can also be easily made when necessary in double isotope studies, or in cases where it is desirable to reduce acceptance of scattered γ rays to a minimum (*49*).

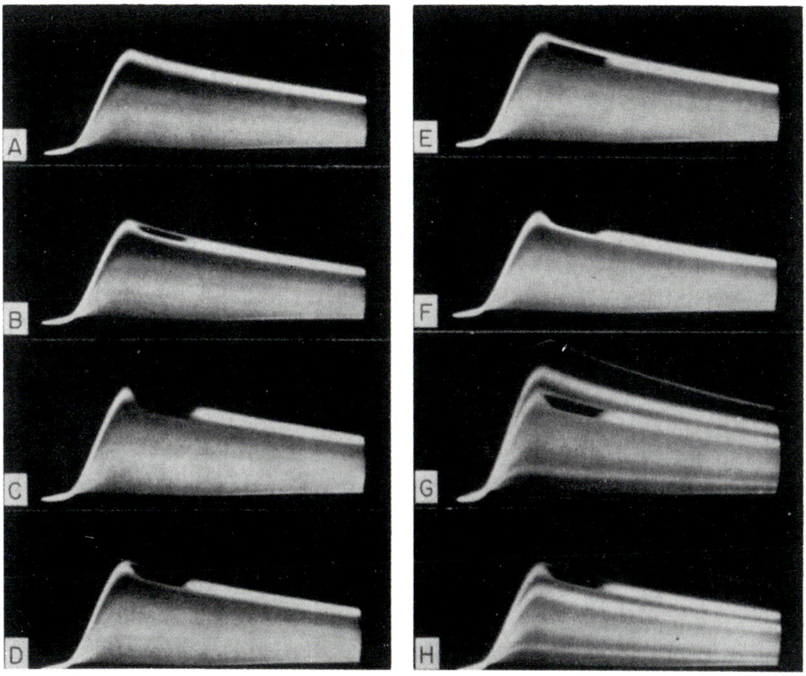

FIG. 8. Display seen in *Z*-pulse monitor scope. (A) Narrow white line at top is photopeak of ^{68}Ga. (B) Window of pulse-height selector centered on photopeak, but window too narrow to accept full photopeak. (C) Window wider than necessary. (D) Window width and height in proper adjustment. (E, F) Window not centered on photopeak. (G) Display shown in double isotope study with ^{203}Hg and ^{131}I. Window centered on 0.28-MeV ^{203}Hg photopeak. (H) Same double isotope study with window adjusted to 0.36-MeV ^{131}I photopeak.

The pulse-height resolution obtained with the image detector described here is equal to that of a good scintillation counter. This is due to the efficient light collection from the solid crystal and the direct coupling to the phototubes. The full width of the photopeak at half maximum is typically 8.7% for ^{137}Cs and 13.8% for ^{203}Hg when the entire scintillator is irradiated with γ rays. Good pulse-height resolution has the important advantage that a narrow pulse-height selector window can be used, providing maximum rejection of γ rays scattered by the subject and collimator. Maximum reduction of background due to cosmic rays and stray radioactivity is also obtained.

C. Factors Affecting Resolution and Sensitivity

The overall sensitivity of the scintillation camera is determined by two factors, namely the geometric efficiency of the collimator and the photopeak detection efficiency of the scintillator. The former is defined as the fraction of γ rays emitted from the subject that pass through the channels of the collimator, and the latter is defined as the fraction of γ rays impinging on the crystal that produce photopeak scintillations. Both factors are subject to approximate mathematical analysis.

The overall resolution is determined by three factors, the resolution of the γ-ray image produced by the collimator, the translation of this γ-ray image into a light image by the scintillator, and the accuracy of reproduction of the image in the scintillator on the image-readout oscilloscope.

The resolution and efficiency of γ-ray collimators is considered mathematically in Section III. The resolution and efficiency of positron coincidence collimation is considered in Section IV. The inherent position resolution obtainable from solid sodium iodide crystals, and the accuracy of reproduction of the image on the readout oscilloscope, are considered in the remainder of this section. In other types of imaging systems, additional factors may be important, such as the resolution of image amplifiers, the size of mosaic elements, and so forth, but these factors are not relevant here.

1. Inherent Detection Efficiency and Position Resolution of Sodium Iodide Scintillators

In the normal operation of the scintillation camera, each photopeak event that occurs in the image detector crystal is recorded as a visible dot on the picture. Photopeak events can result either from simple photoelectric interactions between the γ ray and the crystal or from multiple Compton-photoelectric interactions. The resolution of the image is decreased by the multiple interactions for reasons outlined below. Monte Carlo calculations have been performed to determine the image-resolution loss and the theoretical photopeak detection efficiency in sodium iodide as a function of γ-ray energy and scintillator thickness (*10*). Before the results of the calculation are presented, a detailed description is given of the types of interactions that occur.

Primary photoelectric interactions. In this kind of event, the original γ ray disappears and a photoelectron absorbs all of its energy. Light is emitted along the path of the electron, but its path length is very short. For instance, the range of a 0.36-MeV photoelectron in sodium iodide is 0.25 mm (*48*). In the image-resolution calculations all the light is assumed to come from the point where the interaction occurred. At low

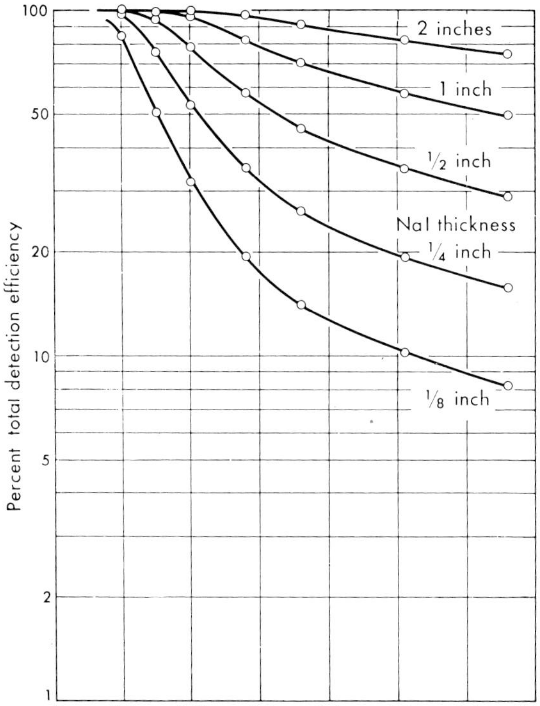

FIG. 9. Calculated gross (Compton plus photoelectric) detection efficiency for sodium iodide as a function of γ-ray energy and crystal thickness. Gross detection efficiency is defined as the fraction of γ rays striking the crystal that produce scintillations by either the Compton or photoelectric process (*10*).

γ-ray energies, primary photoelectric interactions are the main contributors to the photopeak in sodium iodide.

One or more Compton interactions followed by escape of a secondary γ ray from the scintillator. In this kind of event, part of the energy of the original γ ray is transferred to a Compton electron, and the remaining energy is carried away by a secondary γ ray. If the secondary γ ray escapes the scintillator, the interaction does not contribute to the photopeak of the pulse-height spectrum, because the Compton electron produces a relatively weak scintillation. The effect of these events on the photopeak detection efficiency and image resolution is not considered in the calculations because it was assumed they are rejected by the pulse-height selector.

One or more Compton interactions within the scintillator followed by photoelectric interaction of a secondary photon. These events contribute

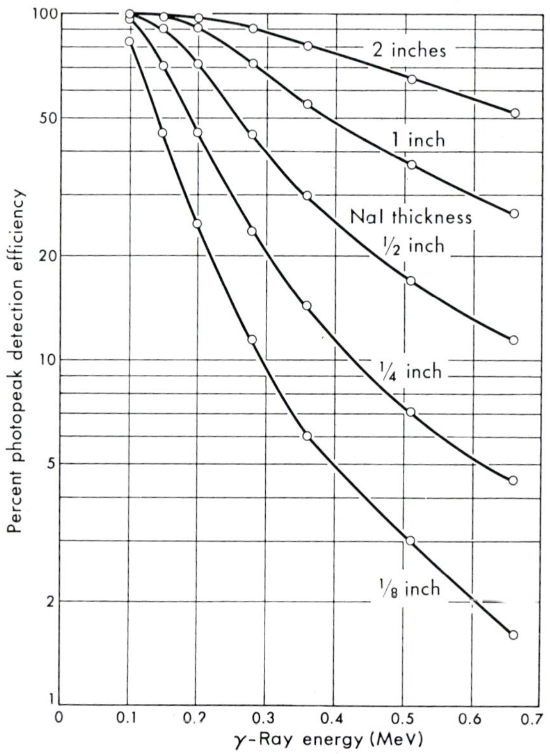

FIG. 10. Calculated photopeak detection efficiency for sodium iodide. Photopeak detection efficiency is defined as the fraction of γ rays striking the crystal that produce either a direct photoelectric interaction or a multiple Compton-photoelectric interaction (*10*).

to the photopeak, since all the energy of the original γ ray is absorbed in the scintillator. The scintillation from the first Compton electron is correctly positioned on the path of the primary γ ray, but the secondary scintillations are located a distance away. The computing circuit of the scintillation camera places a single flash on the oscilloscope at a point corresponding to the center of luminous intensity of the scintillations.

The probability of this kind of event as a function of the perpendicular distance from the primary γ ray to the center of intensity was calculated. These multiple Compton-photoelectric events are the main contributors to the photopeak at the higher γ-ray energies.

The gross detection efficiencies as a function of γ-ray energy for $\frac{1}{8}$-inch to 2-inch thick crystals of sodium iodide, as determined by analytic calculation, are shown in Fig. 9. Gross detection efficiency is the

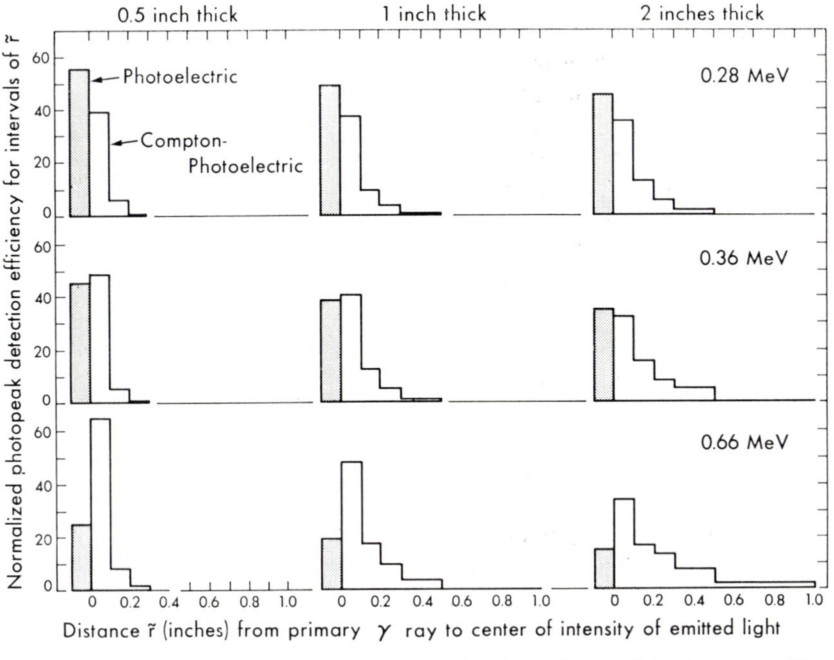

FIG. 11. Calculated loss of position resolution in sodium iodide due to multiple Compton-photoelectric interactions. The curves show the relative number of events occurring within intervals of $\tilde{r}$, where $\tilde{r}$ is the distance from the incident γ ray to the center of intensity of the light produced. Curves for 0.5-, 1-, and 2-inch thick crystals at three γ-ray energies are shown (*10*).

probability of producing any kind of scintillation, either Compton or photoelectric. The photopeak detection efficiency for the same crystals, as determined by the Monte Carlo calculation, are shown in Fig. 10. For a $\frac{1}{2}$-inch thick crystal, photopeak detection efficiencies are 90% for 0.15-MeV, 44% for 0.28-MeV, 29% for 0.36-MeV, and 17% for 0.51-MeV γ rays.

The theoretical loss of image resolution due to multiple Compton-photoelectric events in the scintillator is shown in Fig. 11. The numbers of primary photoelectric events are shown in the shaded columns, and the remaining portions of the curves show the number of Compton-photoelectric events as a function of $\tilde{r}$, where $\tilde{r}$ is the perpendicular distance from the primary γ ray to the center of intensity of the light produced. All curves are normalized to equal counting efficiency, since their purpose is to show only the image resolution. For a ½-inch thick crystal, $\tilde{r}$ is within the interval 0 to 0.1 inch for more than 90% of the photopeak events at the three γ-ray energies 0.28 MeV, 0.36 MeV, and 0.66 MeV. For a 2-inch thick crystal, a considerable number are outside this interval, particularly at the higher energies.

Conclusions reached from Figs. 10 and 11 are that good position resolution can be obtained from ½-inch thick crystals at all γ-ray energies, but high detection efficiency can be obtained only at the lower energies. For thick crystals, high detection efficiency can be obtained at high energies, but the position resolution is appreciably reduced by multiple scattering.

The results of these calculations are applicable to mosaics of sodium iodide crystals when no γ-ray shielding is employed between elements. When shielding is employed, many of the photopeak events will be reduced to ordinary Compton events as far as light output is concerned. If anticoincidence circuitry is employed to reject Compton-photoelectric events that produce scintillations in two different elements of the mosaic, the effective detection efficiency will be reduced by elimination of these events. Furthermore, the smaller the area of the mosaic elements, the lower the effective detection efficiency will become.

The photopeak detection efficiency has been measured experimentally for a solid 0.46-inch thick, 11.5-inch diameter, sodium iodide crystal by counting calibrated sources of ^{139}Ce, ^{203}Hg, ^{131}I, ^{68}Ge, and ^{137}Cs at known geometry. The pulse-height selector was set to accept nearly all the photopeak as shown in Fig. 8D. The results, together with calculated efficiencies for a 0.46-inch thick crystal, are shown in Table I. The

TABLE I
CALCULATED AND MEASURED PHOTOPEAK DETECTION EFFICIENCY FOR 0.46-INCH THICK SODIUM IODIDE CRYSTAL (10)

Isotope	γ-Ray energy (MeV)	Calculated photopeak detection efficiency (%)	Measured photopeak detection efficiency (%)
^{139}Ce	0.166	89	75
^{203}Hg	0.28	39	34
^{131}I	0.36	26	22
^{68}Ga	0.51	15	13
^{137}Cs	0.66	10.4	10

measured counting efficiency is smaller than the calculated efficiency, probably because photopeak pulses at the upper and lower limits of amplitude were not accepted by the pulse-height selector window. A small loss was also caused by escape of recoil electrons from the surface of the scintillator.

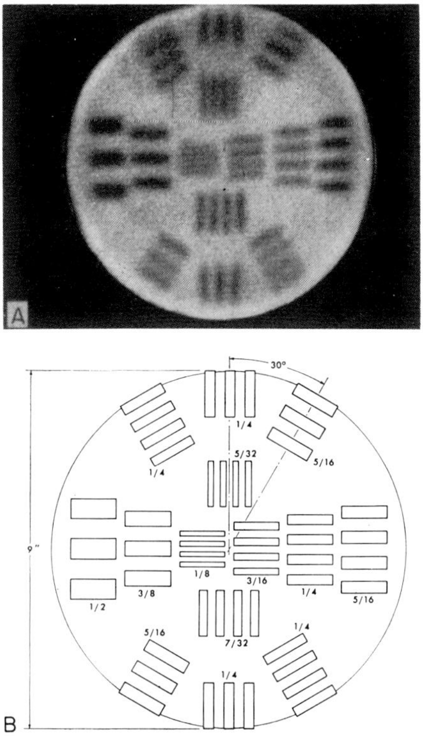

FIG. 12. (A) γ-Ray shadow picture of absorber bar pattern, demonstrating inherent resolution of 19-multiplier phototube image detector with 11.5-inch diameter, 0.5-inch thick scintillator. (B) Width of bars, equal to space between them, is shown on diagram in inches (*9*).

2. ACCURACY OF REPRODUCTION OF THE SCINTILLATOR IMAGE ON THE READOUT OSCILLOSCOPE

A test picture showing the inherent resolution obtained at 364 keV with the present 19-multiplier phototube image detector is shown in Fig. 12A. The phototubes had conventional S-11 photocathodes. An array of tungsten bars was placed 0.5 inch from the image detector. The size and spacing of the bars are shown in Fig. 12B. A point source of 364-keV

γ rays was located a few feet distant on the axis of the detector. Near the center of the picture, the $\frac{3}{16}$-inch bars are clearly resolved and the $\frac{5}{32}$-inch bars are barely resolved. The $\frac{1}{4}$-inch bars are also clearly resolved in the more difficult area at the edge of the picture. Further tests show that the $\frac{1}{4}$-inch bars can be resolved in the central area at 160 keV.

The accuracy with which multiplier phototube-array cameras can determine the position of scintillations in the crystal is limited by the statistics of electron production in the phototubes. The loss of resolution from this cause is inversely proportional to the square root of the brightness of the scintillation. This is the reason that the phototube-array scintillation camera cannot be used for very low-energy γ rays. A 27-keV γ ray from ^{125}I, for instance, releases only about 27 electrons from the photocathodes of all the phototubes combined when conventional tubes are used. When this small number of electrons is divided among the nearby multiplier phototubes, large statistical variations result, and positioning accuracy is poor. However, at medium γ-ray energies the inherent resolution is equal to or better than the resolution obtained from most γ-ray collimators.

The use of multiplier phototubes with higher quantum efficiency improves the inherent resolution of phototube-array scintillation cameras. Quantum efficiency is defined as the probability of release of a photoelectron from a photocathode by a single incident light photon. Phototubes with bialkali photocathodes have 1.5 to 2 times the quantum efficiency of the conventional tubes with S-11 photocathodes. These new tubes, recently available for the first time, provide a worthwhile improvement in the inherent resolution of the image detector. If the inherent resolution distance, R_i, is known for a given quantum efficiency, Q, and γ-ray energy, E_γ, the resolution distance, R_i', for a new γ-ray energy, E_γ', or quantum efficiency, Q', can be calculated by

$$R_i' = R_i[(E_\gamma/E_\gamma')(Q/Q')]^{1/2}$$

This equation is valid at low γ-ray energies where resolution loss due to multiple scattering of γ rays in the scintillator is not an appreciable factor (Section II,C,1).

The inherent resolution distance of the image detector and readout system can be accurately measured by the following method. A thin (0.05-inch wide) beam of γ rays from a slit collimator is directed at the scintillator and an exposure is taken. The source is then shifted a known distance, and a second exposure is taken on the same sheet of film. When a barely distinguishable double line appears in the resulting picture, the inherent resolution distance is just equal to the distance the source has been moved (*22*). The resolution distance of the 11-inch image detector with 19 bialkali-photocathode multiplier phototubes, when measured by this method, is 0.25 inch at 364 keV and 0.37 inch at 160 keV (*15*).

The second cause of inaccuracy in reproduction of the image is fixed in nature, rather than random, and appears as a spatial distortion, especially of scintillations located near the edges of the crystal. It is caused by the finite extent of the crystal and phototube array and by reflection of light at the edge of the high-refractive index sodium iodide crystal.

Mallard and Myers (*43*) have calculated the theoretical light collection of a seven-phototube array and showed that a nearly linear relationship exists between the position of each scintillation and the X and Y coordinate signals obtained from the difference circuits. However, the calculations were based on a simplified model, because it is difficult to take into account the effect of light reflections from the diffuse white surfaces that surround the crystal and the multiplier phototubes and the effect of multiple internal light reflections in the crystal.

No method has yet been described to accurately calculate the optimum parameters of the image detector. These parameters include the distance between multiplier phototubes and crystal, the shape of the light deflector, the surface treatment of the crystal, and so forth. The methods used to develop the present image detectors were empirical.

The linearity of image reproduction achieved with the 19-tube image detector is shown qualitatively in Fig. 13. These pictures were made by placing a radioactive "line source" at various positions under the camera and making multiple exposures. The line source consisted of a straight metal tube 12 inches long and ¼ inch in diameter filled with a solution of positron-emitting ^{68}Ge-^{68}Ga. Positron coincidence collimation was used and the source was 3 inches from the image detector housing in Fig. 13A and 1 inch away in Fig. 13B. The source was placed at 2-inch intervals to obtain the picture shown in Fig. 13B. Good linearity is achieved within an area 9 to 10 inches in diameter. The lines are reproduced reasonably straight and evenly spaced. Outside this area distortion is produced by reflection of light at the crystal edge. However, no difficulty results in the interpretation of the images if this edge distortion, called "edge packing," is recognized.

D. Factors Affecting Background

In radioisotope cameras and scanners, background dots are caused by (a) cosmic rays, (b) radioactive materials and X-ray equipment in the vicinity of the instrument, (c) radioactivity in the internal parts of the detector, (d) γ rays from the patient that pass through the detector shielding and the walls of the collimator, and (e) scattering of γ rays in the subject.

1. Stray Radiation

Causes (a), (b), and (d) above are minimized by adequate detector shielding and by the use of pulse-height selection. When tuned to 280-

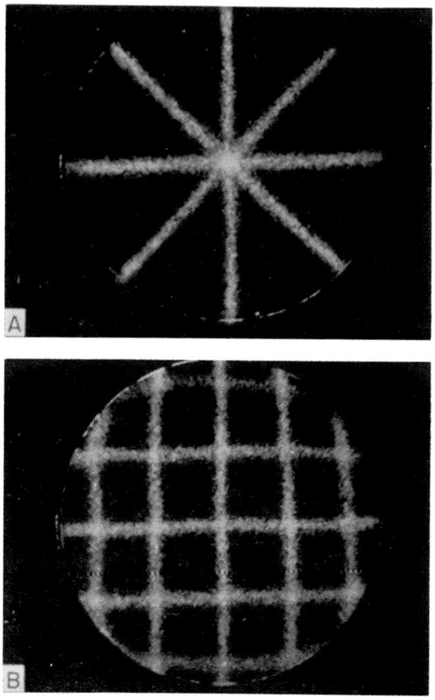

FIG. 13. Test patterns showing linearity of 11.5-inch scintillation camera using line sources and positron coincidence collimation. See text for explanation.

keV γ rays, the scintillation camera described in Section II,B has a background of about 100 dots per minute under normal conditions. Massive shielding cannot reduce the background much below this value, because presently available multiplier phototubes contain radioactive elements (^{40}K and radium) in the glass and other parts. Also some cosmic rays pass through any practical amount of shielding.

2. Scattered γ Rays and Their Rejection by Pulse-Height Selection

When the image detector is well shielded and the amount of radioactive material administered to the patient is adequate, the main cause of background dots is Compton scattering of the γ rays in surrounding tissue. When scattering occurs in the subject, any resulting dot in the picture is located at a position corresponding to the point of scattering, rather than to the point of origin of the primary γ ray. Medium-energy γ rays average 2 to 3 inches' travel in soft tissue before being scattered. Therefore, γ-ray scattering in soft tissue produces a diffuse halo of dots around the active parts of the subject.

Compton scattering occurs in roentgenography, but in this case most of the secondary radiation is absorbed by slit filters aligned parallel to the primary X-ray beam (Potter–Bucky filter). Also the number of scattered X rays is minimized by limiting the width of the X-ray beam to the area to be imaged. However, these techniques cannot be used for imaging the distribution of γ-ray emitting isotopes. The only useful method for reducing the number of these scattered γ rays is pulse-height selection. This technique has been used in radioisotope scanners for many years (*1*).

Not all scattered γ rays can be eliminated by pulse-height selection, because when a γ ray is scattered through a very small angle, the energy of the secondary γ ray is nearly equal to the original. The pulse-height selector window must have a finite width in order to accept most of the photopeak, so an appreciable change in energy must occur to cause rejection of the secondary γ rays. The situation is worse at low γ-ray energies because the secondary γ rays retain more of the original energy, and at the same time a wider pulse-height selector window must be used because the pulse-height resolution of scintillation detectors decreases at low energies. Also, more Compton scattering occurs at lower energies.

The energy retained by Compton-scattered γ rays can be easily calculated (*25*). Also, the angular distribution of the secondary γ rays can be determined from the Klein–Nishina formulas (*25*). Because multiple scattering occurs, an accurate calculation of the fraction of scattered γ rays removed by pulse-height selection at different primary γ-ray energies requires computer calculations using Monte Carlo methods. However, a rough indication of the fraction of scattered γ rays removed by pulse-height selection can be obtained from single-hit calculations, the results of which are shown in Fig. 14. These calculations assume a radioactive source 3 inches below the surface of soft tissue and a pulse-height selector window whose lower edge is set according to the pulse-height resolution expected at various energies. It was 9% below the primary γ-ray energy at 0.66 MeV and 20% below at 0.10 MeV. Intermediate values were based on assumption of a linear relationship between the lower edge and $(1/E_\gamma)^{1/2}$, where E_γ is the primary energy of the γ ray.

The curves in Fig. 14 show that at 0.36 MeV, 43% of the γ rays escape the subject without scattering or absorption (curve A) and 57%

are Compton scattered (curve B). All the latter will be shown on the picture if pulse-height selection is not used. If pulse-height selection is used, no more than 6% of the original γ rays will be Compton-scattered through small enough angles to get through the window and be shown on the picture (curve D). None of the γ rays is totally absorbed in the subject at this energy (curve C).

Thus, the usefulness of pulse-height selection at this medium γ-ray energy is apparent, because there is at least a factor-of-10 reduction in scattered γ-ray background. At lower energies, pulse-height selection is

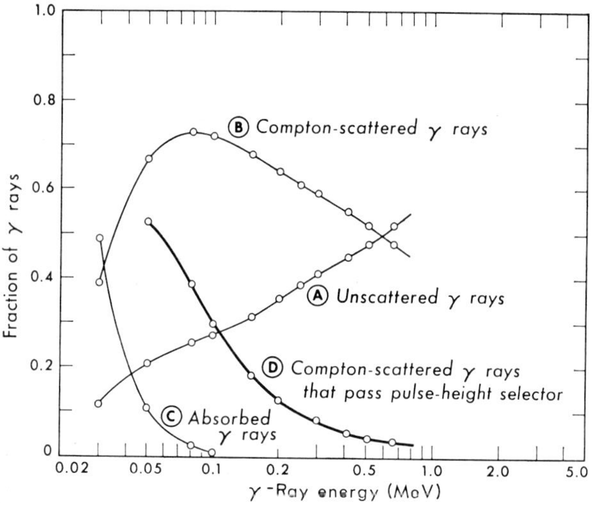

FIG. 14. Calculated fraction of γ rays from source 3 inches below tissue surface that (A) escape unscattered and unabsorbed, (B) escape but have been Compton scattered, (C) are absorbed and do not escape the surface of the tissue, and (D) are Compton scattered but not removed by pulse-height selector as described in text. Calculations assume only single hits, and therefore represent maximum values for curve D.

of less value, as the curves show. More scattering occurs, and pulse-height selection is less able to remove it. However, if multiple scattering were taken into account in the calculations, more improvement would be shown, especially at the lower energies.

III. IMAGE-PRODUCING COLLIMATORS FOR USE WITH γ-RAY EMITTERS

Three different methods of collimation can be used to project images of radioactive subjects onto a scintillator. They are pinhole collimation and multichannel collimation for γ-ray emitters, and coincidence collimation of annihilation radiation for positron emitters. The first two methods are discussed in this section and the third is discussed in Section IV.

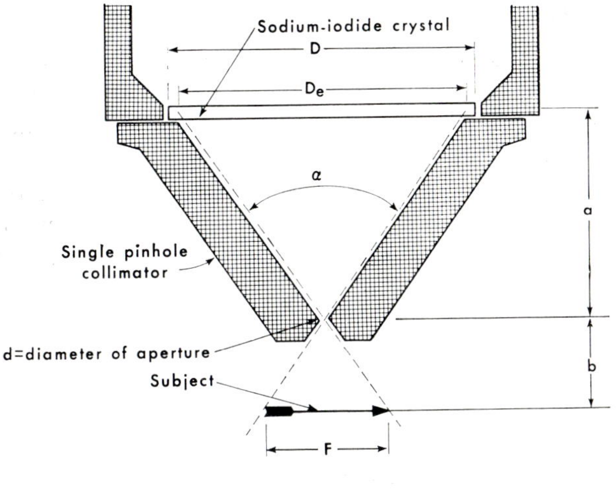

(A)

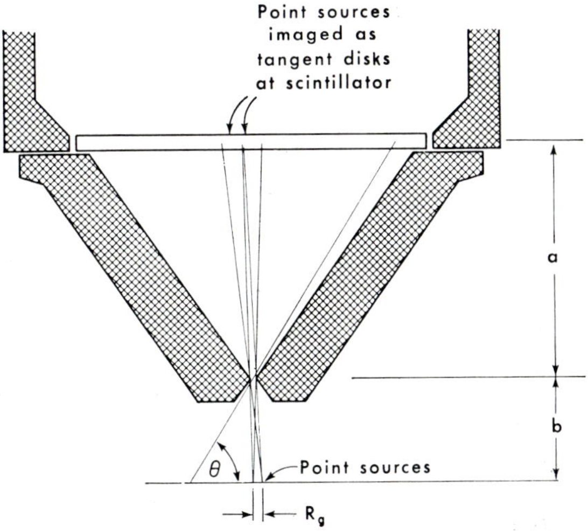

(B)

FIG. 15. (A) Single pinhole parameters relating to subject size and magnification. (B) Single pinhole parameters relating to resolution when resolution distance is defined as the distance between two point sources imaged as tangent disks at scintillator.

A. Pinhole Collimators

A pinhole collimator consists of a shallow aperture at the end of a lead shield, as shown in Fig. 15A. When γ rays enter the aperture, they continue traveling in straight lines to form an inverted image of the subject at the scintillator.

The geometric resolution and efficiency of single-aperture pinhole collimators have been discussed in previous publications (*6, 43, 46*). Briefly, the *geometric resolution distance*, R_g, of a pinhole collimator is given by

$$R_g = (a + b)d_e/a$$

where a is the distance from the aperture to the scintillator, b is the distance from the subject to the aperture, and d_e is the effective diameter of the aperture (Table II). As shown in Fig. 15B, the resolution distance, R_g, is defined as the distance between two point sources in the subject that are imaged as two disks that are tangent at the scintillator. The above equation does not take into account any resolution subsequently lost in the translation of the γ-ray image into a picture.

The *overall resolution distance*, R_0, is given by

$$R_0 = \left[R_g^2 + \left(\frac{b}{a} R_i\right)^2\right]^{1/2}$$

or

$$R_0 = \left[\frac{(a + b)^2 d_e^2 + b^2 R_i^2}{a^2}\right]^{1/2}$$

where R_i is the inherent resolution distance of the image detector and display system. R_i is 0.25 inch for 0.36-MeV γ rays and 0.38 inch for 0.14 MeV in the image detector described in Section II,B. When b is small with respect to a (when small subjects are being imaged), the magnitude of R_i has only a small effect on the overall resolution, because a magnified view of the subject is projected onto the scintillator. The term $[(b/a)R_i]^2$ is usually small compared to R_g^2.

The *effective diameter*, d_e, of a pinhole aperture is somewhat larger than the actual diameter d, owing to penetration of the edges of the aperture by γ rays. To reduce scattering of the γ rays, the apertures are usually made of tungsten, platinum, or other high-density material.

The effective diameter, d_e, of a pinhole aperture is given by

$$d_e = [d(d + 2\mu^{-1} \tan \alpha/2)]^{1/2}$$

where α is defined in Fig. 15A and values of μ^{-1}, the linear absorption coefficient in the aperture material, are given in Table II. Table III gives

TABLE II
VALUES OF μ^{-1}, MEAN FREE PATH OF γ RAYS IN COLLIMATOR MATERIAL[a]

Mean free path	Material	γ-Ray energy (MeV) 0.14	0.20	0.28	0.36	0.41	0.51	0.66
μ^{-1} (inches)	Pb	0.015	0.037	0.080	0.127	0.165	0.234	0.331
	Tungsten alloy	0.011	0.028	0.059	0.095	0.120	0.165	0.215
μ^{-1} (cm)	Pb	0.038	0.094	0.22	0.32	0.42	0.59	0.84
	Tungsten alloy	0.029	0.071	0.15	0.24	0.30	0.42	0.55

[a] Density of Pb = 11.4 gm/cm³; density of tungsten alloy = 18.5 gm/cm³. Values of μ interpolated from reference (*34*).

TABLE III
EFFECTIVE DIAMETER d_e (INCHES) FOR PINHOLE APERTURES WITH 70° ANGLE OF VIEW[a]

Actual diameter, d (inches)	Aperture material	γ-Ray energy (MeV) 0.14	0.20	0.28	0.36	0.41	0.51	0.66
0.125	Pb	0.135	0.149	0.172	0.195	0.211	0.238	0.272
	W	0.133	0.144	0.161	0.180	0.191	0.211	0.231
	Pt	0.132	0.140	0.154	0.171	0.183	0.197	0.219
0.187	Pb	0.197	0.212	0.237	0.262	0.280	0.311	0.350
	W	0.195	0.206	0.225	0.245	0.258	0.280	0.303
	Pt	0.193	0.197	0.211	0.228	0.238	0.257	0.281
0.250	Pb	0.260	0.275	0.301	0.327	0.347	0.380	0.422
	W	0.258	0.269	0.288	0.310	0.323	0.347	0.372
	Pt	0.256	0.265	0.280	0.299	0.309	0.330	0.356

[a] Calculated from the equation for d_e on p. 516.

the effective diameters of typical apertures in lead, tungsten, and platinum for several γ-ray energies.

For points on the central axis of a pinhole collimator, the *geometric efficiency* is given by

$$g = d_e^2/16b^2$$

where g is defined as the fraction of γ rays emitted by the subject that pass through the aperture. For points off the central axes, the geometric efficiency, g, is given by (*43*)

$$g = d_e^2 \sin^3 \theta/16b^2$$

where θ is the angle shown in Fig. 15B. When $\theta = 60°$, the geometric efficiency falls to 0.65 times the on-axis value. At the higher γ-ray energies this is partially offset by an increase in photopeak detection efficiency, because of the oblique path of the γ ray through the scintillator. The decrease in efficiency near the edge of the picture causes no particular problem in visual interpretation of the pictures. It should be taken into account if numerical data are to be obtained.

The *sensitivity, S,* in terms of the number of dots per minute recorded on the picture per microcurie of activity in the subject, with absorption in the subject neglected, is given by

$$S = 2.2 \times 10^6 \epsilon\eta(d_e^2/16b^2)$$

where ϵ is the photopeak detection efficiency of the scintillator and η is the abundance factor of the γ ray, or the average number of γ rays of a given energy emitted per disintegration.

For a given field size, pinhole collimators designed with a large acceptance angle, α, provide the best sensitivity and resolution. However, if α is too large, the working distance from subject to collimator becomes unconveniently small, there is excessive loss of resolution and sensitivity at the edge of the field, more scattering occurs in the aperture material, and foreshortening of the subject becomes excessive. Foreshortening refers to apparent magnification of the nearer parts of the subject. This is something that occurs with any type of camera using a wide-angle lens. An acceptance angle of 70° provides a good compromise among all these factors for most clinical purposes.

Pinhole collimators provides the best combination of sensitivity and resolution for small subjects that are positioned a short distance from the aperture. They can also be used to take pictures of very large subjects, such as an entire lung field or a grossly enlarged liver, by positioning the subject a large distance from the aperture. The aperture size can be easily changed to provide the best compromise between sensitivity and resolution. Also, pinhole collimators produce images that have no distorting patterns superimposed, because each point in the subject is imaged as a small circular area on the scintillator.

B. Pinhole Collimators with More than One Aperture

For some purposes, pinhole collimators with more than one aperture can be effectively used (*8, 14*). For the thyroid gland, three apertures provide three different views of the gland simultaneously, when the apertures are suitably positioned and when they are used with a large image detector. A section drawing of this collimator is shown in Fig. 16A. The central aperture projects a conventional view of the entire thyroid gland on the central portion of the scintillator. At the same time, the left aperture projects an enlarged oblique view of the left lobe on the left portion of the scintillator. The view is enlarged because the left aperture is closer to the subject than the central aperture. The right aperture projects a similar view of the right lobe on the right portion of the scintillator. As shown in Fig. 16B, three complete γ-ray images of the thyroid are produced by the three apertures, but the scintillator, represented by the circle, intercepts only one half of the two side images. The triple pinhole arrangement provides increased chances of seeing a nodule in or near the thyroid because each lobe is viewed from two different

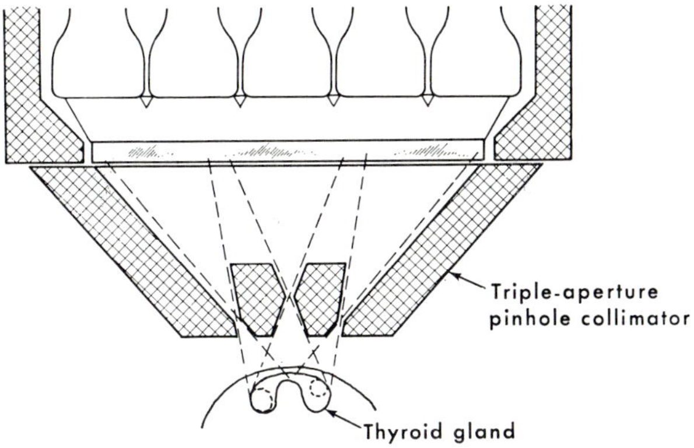

FIG. 16(A).

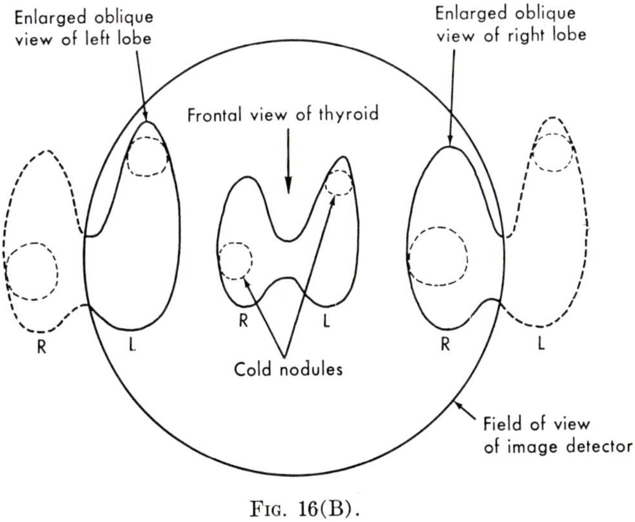

FIG. 16(B).

FIG. 16. (A) Section view of triple-aperture pinhole collimator used for imaging the thyroid gland. (B) Three complete γ-ray images of the gland are projected, but the image detector crystal intercepts only half of the two side views (*8*).

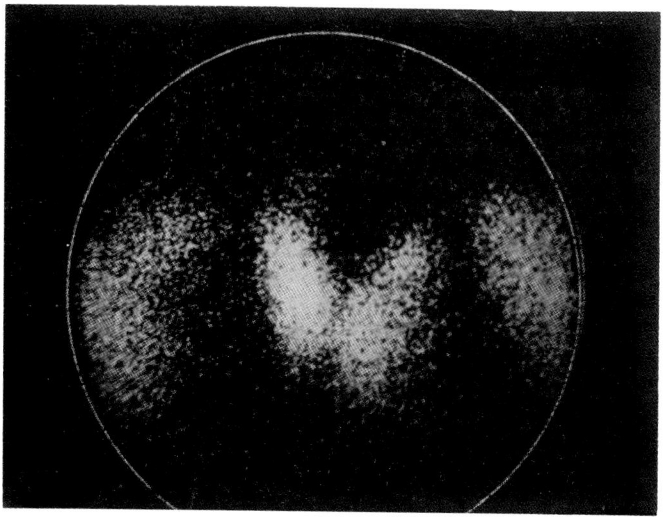

FIG. 16. (C) Triple aperture pinhole picture of thyroid gland. Cold nodule on posterior surface is clearly demonstrated in left oblique view. Gland contained 7 μCi of ^{131}I and exposure time was 7 minutes.

angles. Also, increased resolution is obtained in the two enlarged views. Furthermore, it is possible to determine whether specific areas of tissue are anterior or posterior to the gland by observing a shift in relative position of the tissue in the different views.

A picture taken with the triple-aperture collimator is shown in Fig. 16C. Exposure times are typically 5 to 10 min with 5 to 10 μCi of ^{131}I in the gland.

C. Multichannel Collimators

A multichannel collimator consists of a plate made of γ-ray absorbing material with hundreds or thousands of channels through it. Each channel accepts γ rays from only a limited area, and a γ-ray image of the subject results at the exit side of the collimator (*11, 44*).

The scintillation camera image detector with a typical parallel-channel collimator is shown in Fig. 6. In normal use the subject is located as close as possible to the entrance side of the collimator. Compared to pinhole collimators, multichannel collimators provide the best combination of sensitivity and resolution for large organs such as the brain, liver, and heart.

Collimators with parallel channels have the following characteristics. The size of the image is independent of the distance from subject to collimator. This is an advantage when an organ lies at an unknown depth and its size is to be determined. There is substantially uniform "depth response" in air. In other words, the same count-rate is obtained whether the subject is close to the collimator or distant, as long as the subject is imaged completely within the boundaries of the scintillator. Of course the depth response in tissue is modified by absorption and scattering.

The resolution of parallel-channel collimators is best for the parts of the subject closest to the collimator, and the resolution decreases with increasing distance from the collimator. In comparison, the resolution of focused collimators used for scanning is best for the parts of the subject at the geometric focus, which is usually 3 inches from the collimator. Their depth of focus is limited, and planes closer and farther away are less sharply resolved (*21, 23*). However, parallel-channel collimators can be designed to have the same geometric resolution at a distance of 3 inches as the typical focused collimators used for scanning. Then the parallel-channel collimator has a greater depth of focus, because it sharply resolves all the closer planes, whereas the focused collimator does not. Because clinical subjects are always several inches thick, the depth of focus, over which a relatively sharp image is obtained, should be taken into account in evaluating any collimation method.

Design of multichannel collimators. Multichannel collimators can be made with many combinations of hole diameter, length, and septal thickness. The formulas given in the next paragraphs assist in designing parallel-hole straight-bore collimators that have maximum efficiency for a given resolution and maximum γ-ray energy (*11*).

The mathematical analysis of this type of collimator is simplified if the assumption is made that the collimator moves sideways in the manner of a Potter–Bucky filter during the exposure time. The formulas have been derived by (a) assuming that the collimator moves relative to the subject and image detector during the exposure time, (b) determining the fraction of the time that a point source in the subject is visible to each element in the image detector, (c) determining the solid angle from the source to each element, and (d) integrating to obtain the overall counting efficiency.

For example, consider a collimator consisting of a rectangular array of square holes as shown in Fig. 17. This section view shows a plane through the center of a row of holes. The width of the holes is d, the length is a, and the septal thickness is t. The distance from the radioactive subject to the entrance of the collimator is b, and the distance from the exit to the central plane of the scintillator is c.

If the collimator is stationary, the distribution of γ rays has the

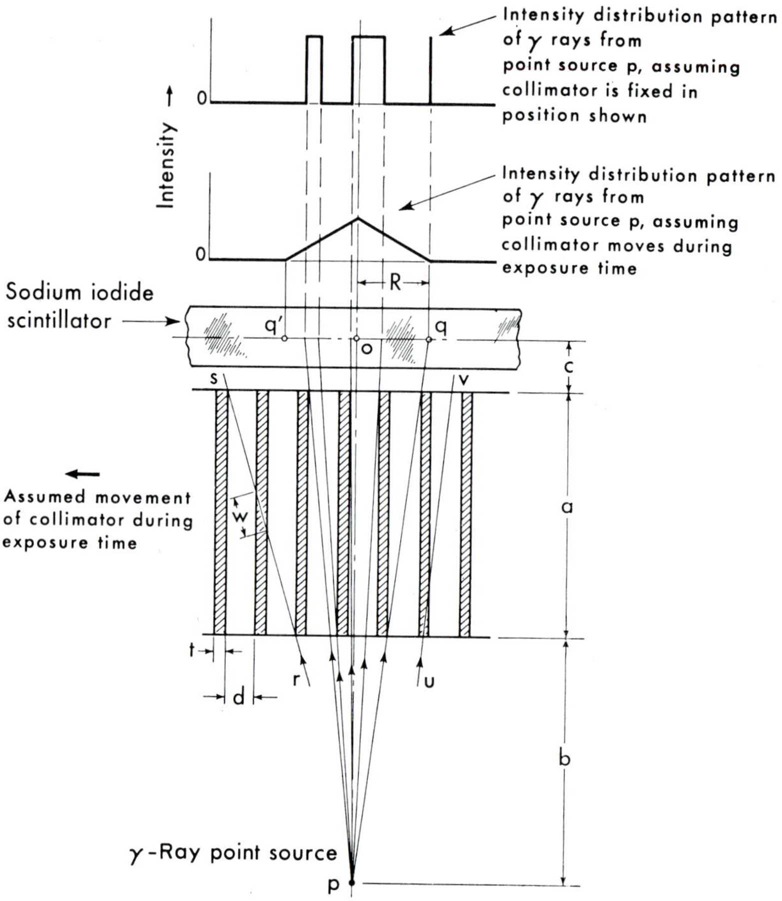

FIG. 17. Section view of multichannel collimator. γ-Ray pathways are shown at bottom, irradiated areas of scintillator when collimator is stationary are shown at top, and irradiated area if collimator moves during exposure time is indicated at center (*11*).

irregular shape shown at the top of Fig. 17, but if the collimator moves in the direction shown, the average distribution of γ rays that strike the scintillator has the triangular shape shown immediately above the scintillator. The intensity is a maximum at point o directly above the point source, and it falls linearly to zero, assuming opaque septa, at points q and q'.

The distance oq, which is equal to the full width of the triangular intensity curve at half maximum, is defined as the *geometric resolution distance*, R_g. From geometric considerations, it can be shown that

$$R_g = d(a_e + b + c)/a_e$$

As expected, the resolution distance R_g is smallest, or in other words the image is sharpest, when the distances b and c are small.

The effective length of the collimator is less than the geometric length because γ rays penetrate the edges of the collimator material, taking the path uv in Fig. 17. It has been shown (*45*) that the effective length of the collimator holes, a_e, is approximately given by

$$a_e = a - 2\mu^{-1}$$

where μ^{-1} is the mean free path of the γ ray in the material and μ is the total linear absorption coefficient (*25, 34*). Values of μ^{-1} in lead and tungsten are listed for several γ-ray energies in Table II.

The *geometric efficiency, g,* is given by

$$g = [Kd^2/a_e(d + t)]^2$$

where g is defined as the fraction of γ rays emitted by the subject that pass through the collimator channels. The γ rays that are scattered by the channel walls and any that travel through the septa are not included.

The value of the constant, K, depends on the shape of the holes and their distribution pattern. It has been determined mathematically and confirmed approximately by experiment that $K = 0.282$ for square holes in a rectangular array and $K = 0.238$ for round holes in a hexagonal array. Inspection of the above equation shows that g is independent of b, the distance between the subject and the collimator, provided the subject is completely imaged within the boundaries of the scintillator. Therefore, parallel-channel collimators should have uniform "depth response" in air, or in other words the count-rate of a subject in air should be independent of the distance from the collimator to the subject. This has been found by experiment to be approximately true.

The shortest distance a γ ray can travel through septal material when taking the unwanted path of minimum attenuation rs, shown in Fig. 17, is w. From experimental studies, acceptable images result when the narrow-beam (Compton plus photoelectric) attenuation of γ rays taking the path rs is 95% or more. Since $1 - (1/e)^3 = 0.95$, w should be equal to or greater than 3 times the mean free path of γ rays in the collimator material. With w known, the minimum permissible *septal thickness, t,* can be calculated for any hole diameter and length. From geometric considerations,

$$t = 2dw/(a - w)$$

The *sensitivity, S,* in terms of dots per minute recorded on the picture per microcurie of activity in the subject, neglecting absorption in the subject, is given by

$$S = 2.2 \times 10^6 \epsilon\eta \, [Kd^2/a_e^2(d + t)^2]$$

where ϵ is the photopeak detection efficiency of the scintillator, and η is the abundance factor or the average number of γ rays of a given energy emitted per disintegration. Values of ϵ are to be found in Table I. With the above equations, collimators can be designed that have optimum hole diameter, length, and septal thickness for a given subject-to-collimator distance, maximum γ-ray energy, and desired resolution.

The parameters of five multichannel collimators designed for maximum efficiency consistent with the stated geometric resolution distance and maximum γ-ray energy are given in Table IV. The material is lead, and all have hexagonal arrays of round holes. The calculated sensitivity in terms of dots per minute per microcurie takes into account the abundance factors of the principal γ rays. The Compton contribution of the high-energy components of ^{131}I was not included. The increase in resolution distance, R_g, and the increase in geometric efficiency because of γ rays penetrating the edge of the collimator material by the path *uv* in Fig. 17 were taken into account in the calculations. However, the increase in apparent efficiency by γ rays taking the paths *rs* was not included.

Other calculations indicate that higher sensitivity can be achieved if the collimators are made of tungsten alloy. The improvement results from having thinner septa and therefore more holes of the same diameter per unit area. The increase in sensitivity is 18% for collimators designed for 0.28 MeV maximum, 30% for those designed for 0.41 MeV, and 45% for those designed for 0.66 MeV γ-ray energies.

An example of a brain tumor picture taken with a multichannel collimator similar to No. 2 in Table IV and designed for 0.28 MeV maximum γ-ray energy is shown in Fig. 18A,B. The patient was given 700 μCi of Neohydrin-^{203}Hg and 4 hr later the pictures showing (A) left lateral and (B) back views were taken. The exposure time was 5 min each and 25,000 dots were recorded. A tumor is visible in the region at left of midline. Two small radioactive marker sources were placed at the corner of the eye and the bottom of the ear lobe for the lateral view, and at the ear canals in the back view. An outline of the head due to body background is also seen. The field of view of the camera is indicated by the circular line. The collimator used for this case had relatively high efficiency and moderate resolution.

Pictures of a brain tumor in another patient given 2 mCi of ^{99m}Tc as the pertechnetate ion are shown in Fig. 18C and 18D. Exposure times

TABLE IV

PARAMETERS OF FIVE MULTICHANNEL COLLIMATORS DESIGNED FOR MAXIMUM EFFICIENCY CONSISTENT WITH GEOMETRIC RESOLUTION DISTANCE AND MAXIMUM γ-RAY ENERGY

Collimator number:	1	2	3	4	5
Nominal maximum γ-ray energy (MeV):	0.20	0.28	0.28	0.36	0.41
Hole length, a (inches):	1.0	1.5	1.5	2.2	2.6
Hole diameter, d (inches):	0.111	0.225	0.150	0.193	0.213
Septum thickness, t (inches):	0.030	0.090	0.060	0.089	0.106
Number of holes in 10-inch diameter area:	4600	960	2090	1160	900
^{99m}Tc (0.14 MeV)					
Calculated dots/min-μCi	750	1080	490	336	282
Geometric resolution distance, R_g (inches)					
b = 1 inch:	0.28	0.47	0.30	0.32	0.34
b = 3 inches:	0.51	0.76	0.51	0.50	0.50
b = 5 inches:	0.74	1.07	0.71	0.68	0.67
^{203}Hg (0.28 MeV)					
Calculated dots/min-μCi	—	500	224	150	121
Geometric resolution distance, R_g (inches)					
b = 1 inch:	—	0.48	0.32	0.33	0.34
b = 3 inches:	—	0.82	0.54	0.52	0.52
b = 5 inches:	—	1.15	0.77	0.72	0.69
^{131}I (0.36 MeV)					
Calculated dots/min-μCi	—	—	—	101	80
Geometric resolution distance, R_g (inches)					
b = 1 inch:	—	—	—	0.34	0.35
b = 3 inches:	—	—	—	0.54	0.53
b = 5 inches:	—	—	—	0.75	0.72
^{198}Au (0.41 MeV)					
Calculated dots/min-μCi	—	—	—	—	85
Geometric resolution distance, R_g (inches)					
b = 1 inch:	—	—	—	—	0.35
b = 3 inches:	—	—	—	—	0.54
b = 5 inches:	—	—	—	—	0.73

NOTE: b is the distance from the source to the face of the collimator.

were 3 minutes each, and about 200,000 dots were recorded on each picture. Large amounts of ^{99m}Tc can be given without excessive radiation dosage to the patient because the half-life is short (6 hr) and no β particles are emitted (*36*). The energy of the emitted γ ray is 0.14 MeV. The ^{99m}Tc is obtained from a parent nuclide ^{99}Mo, which has a half-life of 2.8 days.

The collimator used for the study with ^{99m}Tc was specially designed for use with low-energy γ rays, and was made of lead foil and balsa wood. The balsa wood aided in fabrication of the array of 4000 square holes (*11*) and was left in place because it added strength and absorbed few γ rays. About 1000 dots per minute are obtained per microcurie of ^{99m}Tc, neglecting absorption in the subject. This high sensitivity is due partly to the high detection efficiency of the scintillator at 0.14 MeV and partly to the high geometric efficiency of the thin-septa collimator.

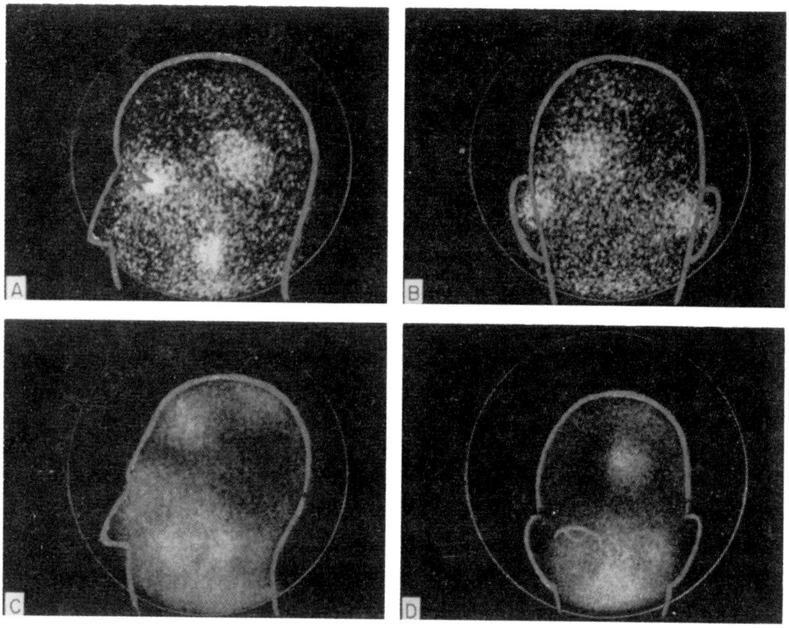

FIG. 18. (A) Left lateral and (B) posterior views of a brain lesion taken with Neohydrin-^{203}Hg and a multichannel collimator designed for nominal maximum γ-ray energy of 0.28 MeV. A prominent lesion and two small marker sources are seen in each view. (C) Left lateral and (D) frontal views of a brain lesion taken with ^{99m}Tc, a 0.14-MeV γ-ray emitter. A multichannel collimator designed for 0.20-MeV maximum γ-ray energy was used.

Dynamic studies with serial pictures to indicate organ function are shown in Fig. 19 (*30, 32, 33*). Two radioisotopes were employed in each study. Pulse-height selection was used to provide separate images of the two isotopes.

The first picture shows the renal parenchyma about 1 hr after injection of 50 μCi of Neohydrin-^{203}Hg. Exposure time was 5 min. The pulse-height selector was then changed to the 0.36-MeV γ rays from ^{131}I, making the camera insensitive to ^{203}Hg. Then, 100–200 μCi of Hippuran-

^{131}I was rapidly injected and series of 2-min exposures were taken. They show how rapidly Hippuran is cleared from the blood by the kidneys and whether any delay occurs in passage of urine from the pelvis of the kidney into the ureters and bladder. The second case (Fig. 19B) shows an abnormal left kidney with delayed clearance of Hippuran from the blood and holdup of urine in the kidney pelvis.

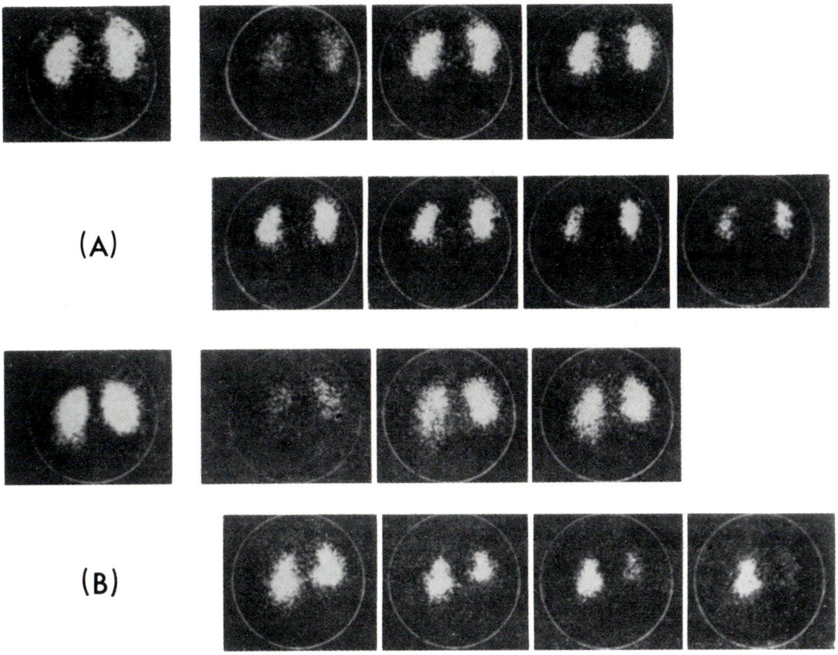

FIG. 19. Normal and abnormal dynamic kidney function studies. (A) First picture shows normal kidneys visualized with Neohydrin-^{203}Hg. Seven following pictures taken at 2-min intervals show clearance of Hippuran-^{131}I from blood after intravenous injection. (B) Same kind of study, but left kidney shows poor function.

IV. THE POSITRON CAMERA: COINCIDENCE COLLIMATION OF ANNIHILATION RADIATION FROM POSITRON EMITTERS

The instruments described in this section are special forms of radioisotope cameras for producing pictures of the distribution of positron-emitting nuclides (*6, 8, 12, 15*). Conventional image-producing collimators, such as pinhole or multichannel collimators, are not required. Whenever a positron is stopped by matter, it combines with a negative electron and produces two 0.51-MeV annihilation γ rays that travel away from their point of origin at 180° (Chapter 18). This property allows images to be formed with two detectors on opposite sides of the subject using coincidence circuitry and electronic computation techniques.

Positron cameras have several unique properties. When both detectors have position-sensing capabilities, high sensitivity can be obtained in combination with sharp resolution on organs deep within the subject. A "plane of best focus" exists that can be set to any desired level by adjustment of an attenuator in the electronic circuits. A tomographic effect can be obtained without movement of the patient or camera. One particular plane is shown in sharp focus while the other planes are superimposed but blurred. Furthermore, it is entirely feasible to have simultaneous readout of a number of focal planes during a single exposure. This can be accomplished by the use of two or more image readout oscilloscopes, each of which displays a different plane with sharp resolution. It can also be done by displaying a number of images in rapid succession at different locations on a single cathode-ray oscilloscope. At each location, a complete image of the subject can be shown with a different plane sharply resolved. Six or more planes can be read out simultaneously by this method.

Positron cameras have substantially uniform "depth response" in tissue, so that tumors deep within the body can be detected as easily as those on the surface. This is a unique property that cannot be obtained from instruments that detect single γ rays. The background count-rate in the absence of positron emitters is extremely low, only a few counts per hour. This permits taking long exposures of subjects containing very little activity.

Positron cameras have the following disadvantages and limitations. First, they are complex instruments employing many components. Second, there is a limit to the amount of radioactive material that can be used with them; overload can occur because of the very high count-rates, since there is no collimator between the image detector and the subject. However, the activity permitted before overload occurs in existing instruments allows pictures to be obtained with exposures as short as 1 min. Third, the availability of positron emitters is limited, as discussed in Section IV,F.

A. Types of Positron Cameras

Positron cameras can take several different forms, as described in the following paragraphs.

a. Unfocused Positron Cameras. In this relatively simple instrument, the same image detector described in Section II is employed, the subject is placed as close to the scintillator as possible, and a scintillation counter with a large thick crystal is located a distance away on the opposite side of the subject, as shown in Fig. 20A. When a γ-ray pair causes coincident scintillations in the two detectors, the scintillation in the image detector is displayed on the image-readout oscilloscope. Scintillations occurring in the image detector that are not in time coincidence with a γ ray detected by the scintillation counter are not displayed.

The remote γ-ray counter is called a focal detector because all γ-ray pairs that form an image of the subject must impinge upon it, and

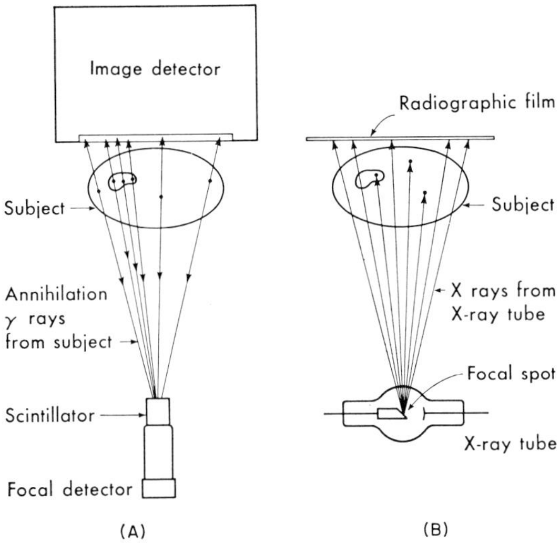

FIG. 20. (A) Positron camera with single remote γ-ray counter as focal detector. (B) Apparatus for taking X-ray radiograph of same subject. Geometry of image formation in the two cases is analogous.

therefore it is a focal point in the image geometry. The geometry of image formation is analogous to X-ray radiography, as shown in Fig. 20B. The focal spot of the X-ray machine is equivalent to the focal detector, and the X-ray film is equivalent to the image detector. In X-ray radiography, the radiation originates in the X-ray tube and a fraction of the rays are absorbed by the subject. In positron imaging, the radiation originates in certain areas of the subject, but since the radiation consists of γ-ray pairs traveling in opposite directions along straight lines and since all γ-ray pairs displayed on the image readout oscilloscope must pass through the focal detector, the geometry of image formation is the same. A slightly magnified image of the subject is projected on the image detector crystal.

Expressions for the resolution and sensitivity of this instrument are given in an earlier publication (*6*). The unfocused positron camera has been superseded by the more sensitive focused types described in the following sections.

b. Twin Image-Detector Focused Positron Camera. Another method of imaging positron emitters is to employ two identical image detectors located on opposite sides of the subject, as shown in Fig. 21A. Pulses

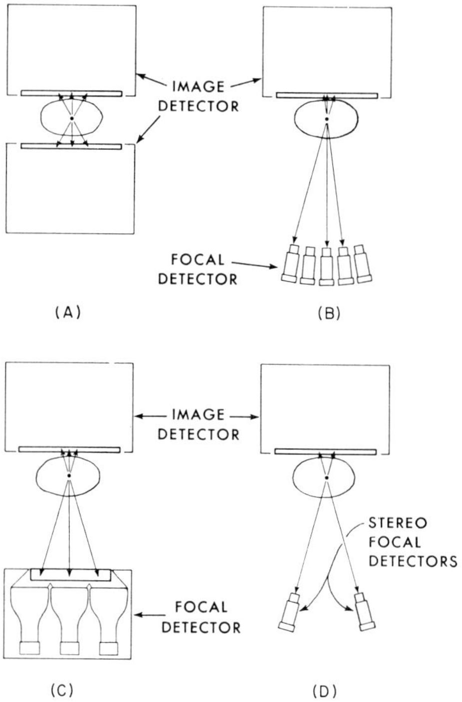

FIG. 21. (A) Focused positron camera employing two identical image detectors in close proximity to the subject. (B) Focused positron camera employing one image detector and a remote multiunit focal detector consisting of an array of scintillation counters. (C) Focused positron camera with remote solid-crystal focal detector. An array of multiplier phototubes determines the position of scintillations in the crystal. A relatively thick crystal is used to obtain high detection efficiency. (D) Stereo positron camera with two focal detectors.

from the two image detectors are sent to a coincidence circuit which responds only when simultaneous γ rays are detected. Activity lying on the central plane of the subject is shown with sharp resolution by taking a simple average of the x-coordinate signals from the two detectors and also an average of the y-coordinate signals. These new coordinate signals are sent to the deflection inputs of the image-readout oscilloscope, and the output of the coincidence circuit is sent to the intensity input. The beam of the cathode-ray tube is positioned by the averaged X and Y signals and is turned on momentarily when a coincidence occurs. The flashes are recorded by photographic time exposure, and an image of the positron distribution results. Other planes in the subject can be sharply resolved by taking weighted averages of the X and Y pulses from the two detectors (*6*).

Special properties of the twin-image detector camera include the following. Sensitivity can be quite high even though both scintillators are relatively thin, but it varies throughout the space between the detectors. Highest sensitivity is obtained for a point midway on the central axis between the two scintillators, because the solid angle of acceptable γ ray pairs is very high at this point. However, the sensitivity falls greatly near the outer edge of the field because of the smaller solid angle for producing coincident scintillations.

The depth of focus of the twin-image detector camera is relatively small. This is an advantage for tomographic operation where all planes are read out simultaneously, but it is a disadvantage in searching for lesions at unknown depth if only one image is produced per exposure. By means of suitable circuitry (*6*) the depth of focus can be made larger and the sensitivity more uniform, but then lower sensitivity results. The latter results partly because both detectors use relatively thin scintillators, and the overall sensitivity is proportional to the product of the photopeak detection efficiency of the two scintillators. The following types offer higher sensitivity for a given depth of focus.

c. Image Detector with Remote Multicounter Focal Detector. This type of positron camera uses a remote focal detector consisting of an array of scintillation counters with thick sodium iodide crystals, as shown in Fig. 21B. Good sensitivity is obtained because of the high detection efficiency of the focal detector. At the same time, high resolution is maintained on any given plane in the subject by means of an averaging, or dot-shifting technique, described in detail in Section IV,B.

d. Image Detector with Remote Imaging Focal Detector. The focal detector of this type of positron camera employs a large, thick solid sodium iodide crystal viewed by an array of 7 or 19 multiplier phototubes, as shown in Fig. 21C. The position of scintillations in the focal detector crystal is sensed by the same method employed in the image detector. Slightly higher resolution can be obtained with this type of camera than with the multiunit focal detector because of the higher resolution of the imaging focal detector. Additional information is given in Section IV,B.

e. Stereo Positron Camera. Simultaneous stereo views of positron emitters can be obtained with one image detector and two remote focal detectors, as shown in Fig. 21D. The two focal detectors are located a short distance apart so that a 6° to 10° angle is formed between the subject and the two detectors. When a γ-ray pair is detected by the left detector, the flash on the image readout oscilloscope is shifted to the left half of the cathode-ray tube screen by means of a pulse generator triggered by the signal from the left detector. When a γ-ray pair is detected by the right focal detector, the flash is deflected to the right side of the screen. Thus two separate adjacent images constituting a stereo pair are formed, each associated with one of the focal detectors. They are recorded by photographic time exposure and later viewed in a stereo viewer. The 6° to 10° difference in viewpoint of the two detectors provides the necessary stereo separation. The focal detectors can be single counters as shown in Fig. 21D or they can be the more efficient, position-sensing types shown in Fig. 21B and 21C.

B. Operation of Focal Detector and Computing Circuits

A block diagram of a positron scintillation camera is shown in Fig. 7. At the top left is the image detector, and located 20 to 30 inches below is the focal detector, consisting of 19 scintillation counters in a close-packed hexagonal array, each with a $1\frac{3}{4}$-inch diameter, 2-inch thick sodium iodide crystal. Pulse-height selectors adjusted to accept the 0.51-MeV photopeak are employed for both the image detector and focal detector.

The following analysis, though directed to the multiunit focal detector shown in Fig. 21B, also generally applies to the imaging focal detector shown in Fig. 21C. If a point source of positrons is located on a plane below the image detector, as shown in Fig. 22, each of the 19 scintillation counters images the source as a separate disk at the image detector. The diameter, d', of each disk is given by

$$d' = d(a/b)$$

where d is the diameter of each crystal in the focal detector, a is the distance from image detector to source, and b is the distance from the source to the focal detector. The distance, c', between centers of the disks is given by

$$c' = c(a/b)$$

where c is the center-to-center distance between crystals in the array.

Although the 19 disks are spread over a wide area on the image detector crystal, they are superimposed on the image-readout oscilloscope by means of the following dot-shifting technique. When a γ ray is detected by the center counter of the focal detector, the coincident scintillation in the image detector is shown on the image-readout oscilloscope without any shift from its normal location. However, when a γ ray is detected by any of the other 18 counters, a correction signal obtained from that counter shifts the position of the flash on the oscilloscope. The direction and magnitude of the correction signals are such that the 18 additional images of the point source are made to coincide with the image from the center counter. In other words, the point source is

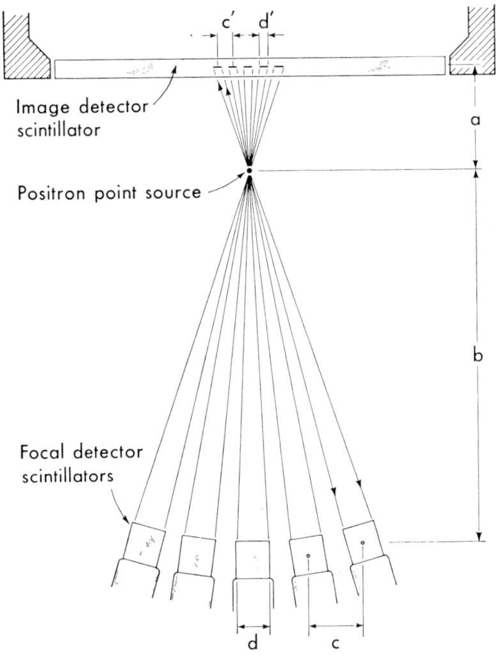

Fig. 22. Geometry of image formation in positron camera with multiunit focal detector. The five images of the point source shown on this diagram are superimposed by means of a dot-shifting technique when they are displayed on the image-readout oscilloscope (*8, 12, 15*).

brought into focus. All other points lying on the same plane are also brought into focus by correction signals from the focal detector.

The plane for which the correction signals are exact is called the plane of best focus. This plane can be set to any desired level in the subject by means of the focal plane selector, an attenuator shown in Fig. 7 that varies the strength of the correction signals. Since the electronic circuits are unable to sense the plane from which a γ-ray pair originates, the selection of the plane of best focus must be made by the operator. In a practical situation, the depth of an organ or tumor is often known, so the plane of best focus is set to that level. The resolu-

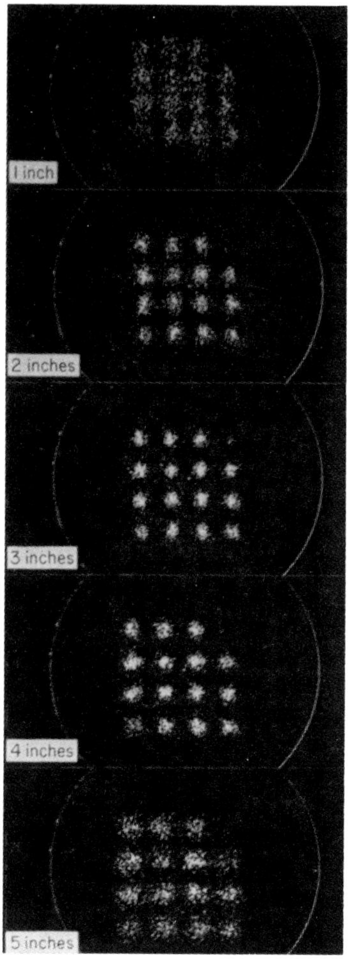

FIG. 23. Depth of focus of positron camera shown in Fig. 7. Plane of best focus was fixed at 3 inches and test source was located at 1, 2, 3, 4, and 5 inches. A slight enlargement of the image is apparent at 5 inches. This accounts for the better resolution of the sources compared to that at 1 inch.

tion of nearby planes is improved by the same correction signals even though the correction is not exact. In other words, a certain depth of focus is obtained, just as with an optical camera.

An illustration of the depth of focus obtained is shown in Fig. 23. The subject was a rectangular array of 14 point sources of a positron emitter with 1-inch center-to-center distance. The plane of best focus was set at 3 inches and pictures were taken with the test subject at several distances. Best resolution is obtained with the subject located 3 inches below the image detector, but almost equally good resolution is obtained with the subject located at 2 or 4 inches, even though the plane of best focus remains at 3 inches. In a brain tumor phantom study, small "tumors" were found to be almost equally visible as long as they were within 2.5 inches of the plane of best focus (*29*). Therefore, for clinical purposes, the depth of focus extends over 5 inches when the distance b is in the order of 20 inches.

C. Factors Affecting Resolution of Positron Cameras

Several factors affect the resolution of positron cameras.

a. Geometry of Image Formation. The geometric resolution distance, R_g, for positron cameras can be defined as the distance between two point sources located on the plane of best focus that are imaged as two tangent disks on the image detector. Then, referring to Fig. 22, it is apparent that

$$R_g = ad/b$$

For the multiunit focal detector shown in Fig. 21B and Fig. 22, $R_g = 0.27$ inch (7 mm) when $a = 4$ inches, $b = 22$ inches, and the diameter of the crystals in the focal detector is $d = 1.75$ inches.

When the solid-crystal focal detector of Fig. 21C is used, the geometric resolution is better. Preliminary tests indicate that the inherent resolution distance of this focal detector is about 0.5 inch. Therefore the geometric resolution distance $R_g = 0.08$ inch (2 mm) under the above conditions. However, the limitation in inherent resolution distance of the present image detector prevents this high resolution from being realized in practice. A very large number of dots would also be required in the images to overcome the statistical limitation of image formation.

b. Resolution of the Image Detector at High Count-Rates. The inherent position resolution of the image detector has been discussed in Section II,C. At 0.51 MeV, the present image detector resolution is about 0.25 inch. This resolution capability is maintained at count-rates up to about 10^7 scintillations per minute. When the integral count-rate from the image detector exceeds this rate, resolution begins to decrease. With no collimator between the subject and the image detector, the count-rate can reach this value with 20 to 50 μCi of positron emitter located a few inches from the image detector. However, the sensitivity is such that with this amount of activity excellent pictures can be taken in a few minutes.

High count-rate capability in the image detector and associated circuits is important in positron coincidence operation, because only about one scintillation per thousand is coincident with a count in the focal detector. Although some improvement can probably be obtained in the future by the use of faster, more complex, electronic circuits, the limitation in count-rate is due mostly to the time (~ 1 μsec) required for all the light to be emitted by the sodium iodide scintillator. Any large increase in count-rate capability will require a new scintillator material combining faster light emission with good detection efficiency for 0.51 MeV γ rays.

c. Range of Positrons in the Subject. When a positron is emitted in tissue it travels a few millimeters before it comes to rest and combines with a negative electron. Since the γ-ray pair is produced at the end of the path, there is a loss of resolution. The loss is not peculiar to the positron camera, however, since all instruments that detect γ rays from positron emitters suffer from the same effect.

The maximum range of positrons in tissue is nearly the same as for β particles of the same energy and thus can be in the order of a centimeter or more. However, the average effective range is a small fraction of the maximum. First, each particle undergoes scattering along its path and the net distance traveled from the point of origin is but a fraction of the total distance traveled (*20*). Second, the average energy of positrons emitted in radioactive disintegrations is usually 0.4 to 0.5 times the maximum energy (*42*). Third, the average distance traveled perpendicular to the line of sight of the positron camera is a fraction of the net distance. The latter follows since the positrons are emitted isotropically and only the lateral travel causes a loss of resolution. As a result of all these factors the net average perpendicular distance traveled by positrons is about $\frac{1}{4}$ of their maximum range. The resolution loss in soft tissue for 1-MeV positrons, for example, is about 2 mm.

d. Variation of Annihilation γ-Ray Directions from 180°. When a positron is annihilated, the two γ rays travel away from their point of origin at almost, but not exactly, 180°. The variation from 180° is due to the fact that the velocity of the positrons is not quite zero when they combine with an electron. They are slowed only to thermal velocity in tissue and the remaining momentum is transferred to the γ-ray pair. The resulting mean variation from antiparallelism is approximately $\frac{1}{137}$ radian or 0.4°. The effect on resolution can be calculated by simple geometry. For example, the loss is only about $\frac{1}{2}$ mm for a point source 4 inches from the image detector and 22 inches from the focal detector.

D. Sensitivity and Depth Response of Positron Cameras

The sensitivity, S, of the positron camera shown in Fig. 7 can be calculated from

$$S = 4.44 \times 10^6 f_a \epsilon_I \epsilon_F f_t(nd^2/16b^2)$$

where S is the sensitivity in terms of the number of dots per minute produced on the picture per microcurie of positron emitter in the field of view of the camera, f_a is the abundance factor of the positron, ϵ_I and ϵ_F are the photopeak detection efficiencies of the image detector and focal detector, f_t is the total tissue absorption factor for both γ rays, d is the diameter of the focal detector crystals, n is the number of counters in the focal detector, and b is the distance from subject to focal detector.

When a subject is imaged completely within the boundaries of the image detector, the sensitivity is inversely proportional to the distance between subject and focal detector. Because this distance is usually large, the sensitivity is nearly constant when the subject is within a few inches of the image detector. This is the normal condition, since best resolution is then obtained.

The calculated sensitivity of a positron camera with an 11.5-inch diameter, 0.5-inch thick sodium iodide crystal and a focal detector employing 19 separate counters with 1¾-inch diameter, 2-inch thick crystals is 1800 dots per minute per microcurie of 100% abundant positron emitter in air when the distance between image detector and focal detector is 22 inches. This agrees well with actual measurements using calibrated sources.

The measured half-absorption thickness of 0.51-MeV γ rays in tissue is 3.6 inches. A subject 6 inches thick has an absorption factor of 0.31. Therefore, the net sensitivity of the above instrument is about 560 dots per minute per microcurie of 100% abundant positron emitter in subjects 6 inches thick.

The depth response in tissue of positron cameras is unique when compared with instruments that detect single γ rays. When the subject has a constant thickness, the response is largely independent of depth. This follows because both γ rays of a pair must be detected to produce a dot, and the total path length of the γ rays through tissue is constant. The total tissue absorption factor, f_t, is the same whether the γ-ray pair originates from the center of the subject or from the top or bottom surface. It should be noted, however, that with subjects that vary in total thickness, the sensitivity is greater for the thinner parts of the subject because the total absorption of the two γ rays is less. This partly accounts for the brightness of the image at the edge of the patient's head in positron pictures taken of brain tumor patients.

E. Background of Positron Cameras

a. Stray Radiation. In the positron mode of operation, the background caused by cosmic rays and stray radioactivity is only a few counts per hour. This results from the stringent requirements for pulse height and time coincidence in the two detectors. Therefore, long exposures of objects containing very little activity produce quite satisfactory pictures. However, background dots are produced by other causes, as discussed below.

b. Accidental Coincidences. At the high count-rates often encountered in the image and focal detectors, the chance of accidental coincidences becomes appreciable. This results in dots at completely random locations on the pictures. The accidental rate, N_A, is given by

$$N_A = N_I N_F T$$

where N_I and N_F are the count-rates in counts per second for the image and focal detectors at the output of the pulse-height selectors and T is the coincidence gate width in seconds.

The present instrument operates satisfactorily at a gross count-rate of 10^7 cpm in the image detector. The coincidence gate width is 0.25 μsec, and the accidental coincidence rate at this gross count-rate is about 200 per minute. The true coincidence rate from γ-ray pairs is about 24,000 per minute under the same conditions. The accidental rate is minimized by shielding both detectors from active parts of the subject outside the field of view of the camera, as shown in Fig. 7.

c. Coincidences between Positron and γ Rays. Some radioisotopes emit one or more γ rays in coincidence with a positron. When these γ rays produce scintillations that pass the pulse-height selector, spurious dots result. A random background is produced, because there is no correlation between the directions of the γ-ray pair and the other γ rays. However, many positron emitters emit no coincident γ rays. Furthermore, all γ rays of less than 0.51 MeV are removed by pulse-height selection, and those with enough energy to pass the pulse-height selector usually produce a relatively small increase in background compared with the other causes listed here.

d. Small-Angle Compton Scattering. The third and major cause of background dots, particularly in thick subjects, is small-angle scattering of the 0.51-MeV γ rays. This subject has been discussed in general terms in Section II,D,2.

To illustrate the magnitude of the effect in thick positron-emitting subjects, the following case is considered. For a 6-inch thick subject, as calculated from the Compton-scattering coefficients for soft tissue, about 77% of the γ-ray pairs will undergo Compton scattering before they escape from the subject. Less than 1% are stopped by photoelectric interactions, and 23% escape unscattered. At 0.51 MeV, the pulse-height resolution is typically 10% and the lower edge of the pulse-height selector window is usually set about 5% below the center of the photopeak. The upper edge of the window is set high enough to include the entire upper portion of the peak.

From the Compton scattering formula, a 0.51-MeV γ ray must be scattered 18.8° to lose 5% of its energy. From the Klein–Nishina distribution, 8.7% of Compton-scattered γ rays are deflected 18.8° or less. Therefore 6.7% of the original γ-ray pairs are scattered through small angles and are still capable of passing the pulse-height selector. The result is that 78% of the dots shown on the picture are correctly located, since they are produced from unscattered γ-ray pairs. The rest are mislocated by varying amounts depending upon the scattering angle and the distance from the point of scattering to the image detector. The scattered dots produce a diffuse halo around the active areas of a thick subject. The effect can be partially removed by background-subtraction techniques, described in Section V.

F. Positron-Emitting Radioisotopes

A list of positron-emitting isotopes is given in Table V. Most positron emitters must be made in cyclotrons, because they require positive charged particle or energetic neutron bombardment for their production. Exceptions are ^{18}F and ^{64}Cu, which are easily produced in large amounts in neutron reactors. Other important exceptions are ^{68}Ga and ^{44}Sc, which are short-lived positron emitters easily obtained from long half-lived parents (*57*). Some positron emitters with considerable potential for medical research, such as ^{11}C and ^{15}O, have half-lives in the order of a few minutes, and therefore must be made near the site where they are used. The availability of these radioisotopes will no doubt improve in the future as small cyclotrons for the medical production of isotopes come into use (*52a*).

Positron emitters already in use with the positron camera include ^{18}F (*55*), ^{52}Fe (*12, 53, 54, 56*), ^{64}Cu, and ^{68}Ga (*7, 31*). In Fig. 24, frontal and right lateral views of a patient with a brain tumor are shown. The tracer compound was 700 μCi of EDTA-^{68}Ga, a positron emitter with a 68-min half-life obtained from a long-lived parent. In the lateral view, marker sources were placed at the corner of the patient's eye and the

TABLE V
LIST OF POSITRON-EMITTING RADIOISOTOPES

Element	Radioisotope	Half-life	Maximum β^+ energy (MeV)	Positron abundance (%)
Aluminum	^{26}Al	8×10^5 years	1.17	84
Arsenic	^{70}As	52 min	1.35	100
Arsenic	^{71}As	2.6 days	0.81	40
Arsenic	^{72}As	1.1 days	3.3	30
Arsenic	^{74}As	17.5 days	1.53	29
Bromine	^{75}Br	1.6 hr	1.70	~20
Bromine	^{76}Br	17.2 hr	3.57	~60
Bromine	^{77}Br	2.4 days	0.34	1
Carbon	^{11}C	20 min	0.97	99
Cesium	^{127}Cs	6.3 hr	0.68	3
Chlorine	^{34m}Cl	32 min	4.5	50
Chromium	^{49}Cr	42 min	1.54	100
Cobalt	^{55}Co	18.2 hr	1.50	~60
Cobalt	^{56}Co	77.3 days	1.5	20
Cobalt	^{58}Co	71 days	0.47	15
Copper	^{64}Cu	12.8 hr	0.66	19
Fluorine	^{18}F	1.9 hr	0.65	97
Gallium	^{66}Ga	9.5 hr	4.1	66
Gallium	^{68}Ga	1.1 hr	1.9	85
Germanium	^{69}Ge	1.7 days	1.2	33
Gold	^{194}Au	1.7 days	1.2	~3
Indium	^{109}In	4.3 hr	0.8	6
Iodine	^{121}I	2.0 hr	1.2	100
Iodine	^{124}I	4.5 days	2.20	~30
Iodine	^{126}I	13.3 days	1.11	1.3
Iridium	^{190}Ir	3.2 hr	2.0	10
Iron	^{52}Fe	8.3 hr	0.8	~57
Krypton	^{77}Kr	1.1 hr	1.86	~80
Krypton	^{79}Kr	1.4 days	0.60	5
Manganese	^{51}Mn	0.75 hr	2.16	100
Manganese	^{52}Mn	5.6 days	0.58	35
Molybdenum	^{90}Mo	5.7 hr	1.2	33
Nickel	^{57}Ni	1.5 days	0.85	50
Nitrogen	^{13}N	0.17 hr	1.19	100
Oxygen	^{15}O	2.0 min	1.68	100
Phosphorus	^{30}P	2.5 min	3.3	99
Palladium	^{101}Pd	8.5 hr	0.58	4
Praseodymium	^{139}Pr	4.5 hr	1.0	~6
Rhodium	^{102}Rh	210 days	1.24	~7.5
Rubidium	^{81}Rb	4.7 hr	0.33	13
Rubidium	^{84}Rb	33 days	1.6	19
Scandium	^{43}Sc	3.9 hr	1.2	100
Scandium	^{44}Sc	2.4 days	1.46	94

TABLE V (*Continued*)

Element	Radioisotope	Half-life	Maximum β^+ energy (MeV)	Positron abundance (%)
Selenium	^{73}Se	7.1 hr	1.7	63
Sodium	^{22}Na	2.6 yr	0.54	89
Technetium	^{93}Tc	2.7 hr	0.8	12
Technetium	^{94}Tc	0.9 hr	2.41	~75
Tin	^{111}Sn	0.6 hr	1.51	29
Titanium	^{45}Ti	3.1 hr	1.0	83
Vanadium	^{47}V	0.52 hr	1.89	100
Vanadium	^{48}V	16 days	0.69	56
Zinc	^{62}Zn	9.3 hr	0.66	~10
Zinc	^{65}Zn	254 days	0.32	2
Zirconium	^{89}Zr	3.3 days	0.91	25

bottom of the ear lobe. In the frontal view, markers were placed at the ear canals. A small tumor is visible in both views. The bright outline of the patient's head is caused by uptake of EDTA in the extracellular fluid space of skin and diploe.

V. RECORDING METHODS

A. Image Recording and Viewing

Because most radioisotope cameras display individual γ rays as momentary point flashes of light on a readout screen, some method must be employed to record this information and form a time-integrated visual image. For maximum usefulness, the image should be available for viewing shortly after the exposure is finished or, even better, it should be visible during the exposure time as it builds up.

The recording method should avoid any permanent loss of data due to saturation effects or lower-level cutoff. Saturation causes loss of information in the more intense parts of the image. It can result when two flashes occur at the same point if the recording method does not permit the double event to be displayed as a more intense dot. Lower-level cutoff causes loss of information in the less intense parts of the image and can occur if the recording method requires two or more flashes at the same point before a visible response results. Though a lower-level cutoff is useful in minimizing the effects of background, it should normally be avoided in the initial recording, because loss of picture information can occur if it is set to the wrong level.

Another requirement is that the dots be recorded and displayed in such a way that the observer can best comprehend the image represented by them. Proper dot size is important. If the dots are small and there is much open space between them, it is difficult for the observer to perceive small differences in dot density. If the dots are too large, resolution is lost. A method of modifying dot size by means of diffusion is described in Section V,A,2.

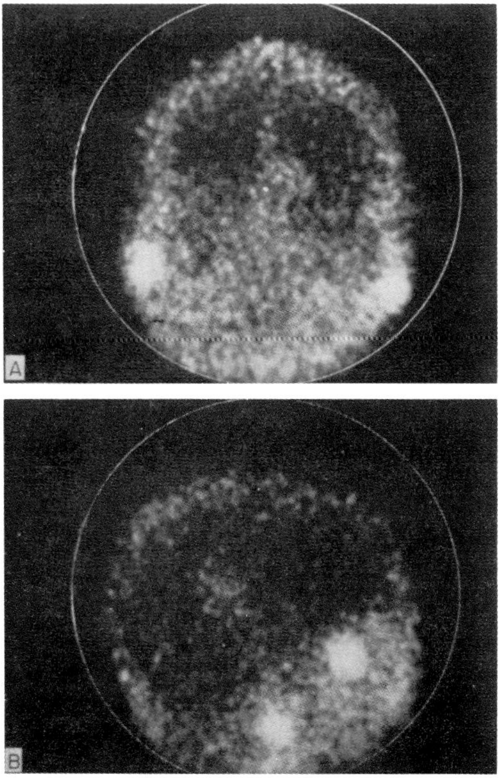

FIG. 24. (A) Frontal and (B) lateral views showing brain tumor. Positron coincidence collimation was used with EDTA-^{68}Ga as tracer compound (7).

In displaying the pictures, a compromise should be made between contrast and gradation. Gradation refers to the number of gray tones visible owing to increments in concentration of activity in the subject. Since amplifying contrast necessarily decreases gradation, contrast enhancement should be kept to the minimum necessary to show significant variations in the image. Contrast should not be amplified far beyond the point at which statistical variations become visible. When gradation is retained, images with large numbers of dots have depth and transparency. They display more significant information than high-contrast images. The latter look like silhouettes of an organ while the former may show internal parts as well.

1. SINGLE-LENS OR MULTILENS OSCILLOSCOPE CAMERA AND PHOTOGRAPHIC FILM

One method of recording images is to photograph the flashes appearing on the oscilloscope screen over a period of time with an optical camera and photographic film. If a single-lens oscilloscope camera and low-contrast film are used, proper exposure is easily obtained. Contrast enhancement and background suppression can be obtained by viewing the picture on closed-circuit television (*17, 18*).

If medium- or high-contrast film is used for the initial recording, contrast enhancement is obtained directly when the dots are numerous enough to overlap, but there is less exposure latitude, and proper exposure is difficult to achieve.

If the dots are not large and numerous enough to pile up, no contrast enhancement results from the use of moderate- or high-contrast film. However, when pictures are composed of only a small number of dots, the statistical variations in dot density are relatively great, and contrast enhancement has little or no value. A useful technique for some viewers is to record such pictures with sharply focused dots and view them through a diffusion filter as described in the following section.

Of all the types of photographic film available, Polaroid self-developing film is most convenient, because the image can be seen a few seconds after the exposure is made. This film normally yields medium-contrast positive prints. In the density-versus-exposure characteristic, there is a threshold that must be exceeded before the film responds. The print remains black even though the film has been exposed to a certain amount of light, and then with more exposure it turns gray, and with still more exposure, white. If the dots are numerous enough to pile up in parts of the image, the contrast characteristic provides moderate contrast enhancement and a lower-level cutoff.

The exposure problem with medium- and high-contrast films is easily solved by the multilens oscilloscope camera (*8, 13*) shown in Fig. 25. This optical camera has several small lenses with graded apertures mounted on a single lens board. Several small images of the cathode-ray tube screen are produced simultaneously on one sheet of film. Each lens allows a different amount of light to reach the film, and a range of over- to underexposure is achieved, with at least one satisfactory image assured. Subjects with considerable variation in amount of activity are rendered with no loss of information, because the most active parts of the subject receive proper exposure in one image and the less active parts in another. Furthermore, a wide range of exposure times can be used with no adjustment of the equipment. With long exposures, the slower lenses give satisfactory images, while with short exposures the faster lenses yield properly exposed images. Thus, the multilens camera gives a series of images with graded lower-level cutoff.

A six-lens picture of a rat 1.5 hr after injection of ^{18}F as the fluoride is shown in Fig. 26. Positron coincidence collimation was employed. All of the images were of course produced simultaneously. The first

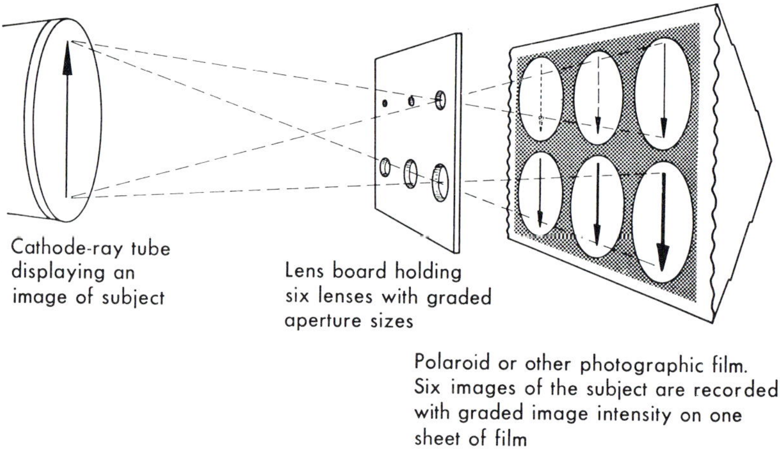

FIG. 25. Drawing of multilens oscilloscope camera, showing how images with graded intensity are formed (*13*).

shows a diffuse outline of the rat and background dots. The third image shows a clearer outline of the rat and indicates that ^{18}F is present in all the gross soft tissues. The fourth and fifth images begin to show the skeleton, where much of the ^{18}F concentrates. The sixth picture shows only the parts of the skeleton having the highest concentration of ^{18}F, the bladder, and one hydronephrotic kidney.

2. GAUSSIAN DOT DIFFUSION

Viewing the pictures through a diffusion filter transforms variations in dot density into different shades of gray (*13, 14*). Little or no contrast enhancement is then necessary, because the human eye is quite sensitive to small differences in gray tones when the picture is adequately illuminated. Diffusion has the effect of suppressing background because isolated dots are defocused and blend into the background, where they become less noticeable. At the same time, parts of the picture with large numbers of dots per unit area are highlighted, since the defocused dots add together to form a prominent bright area.

A satisfactory diffusion filter consists of a sheet of glass with a very finely pebbled surface, such as Tru-Site Picture Framing Glass.* With this filter the amount of diffusion obtained is directly proportional to the distance between the glass and the picture.

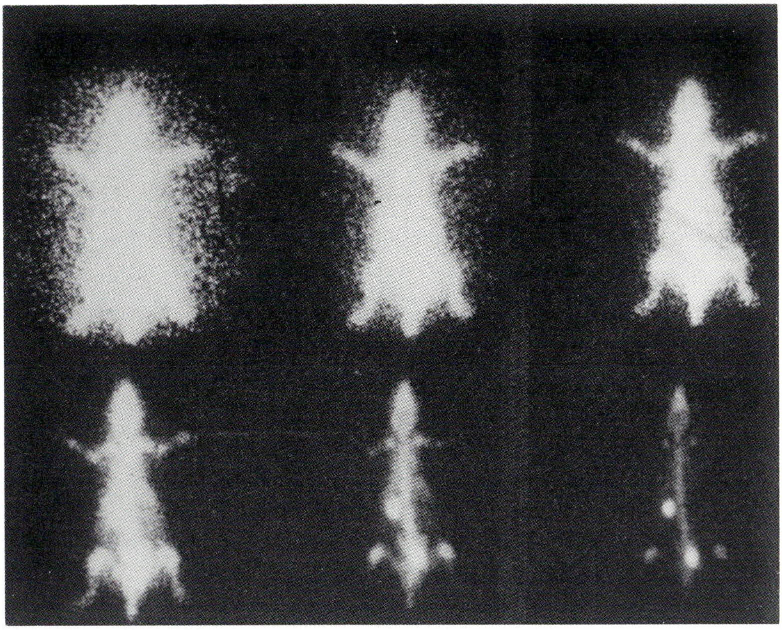

FIG. 26. Example of picture taken with six-lens camera, showing distribution of ^{18}F in a 200-gm rat *in vivo.* Twenty microcuries were administered intravenously, and 1.5 hr later a single 10-min exposure was made, simultaneously producing six images with graded intensity.

An example of the effect of diffusion is shown in Fig. 27. These pictures show the distribution of erythropoetic marrow in the shoulder area of a human subject. The tracer was 8.2-hr positron-emitting ^{52}Fe, and coincidence collimation was used. In the sharply focused original, Fig. 27A, marrow is shown in the humerus, the clavicle, and the scapula. In the diffused copy, Fig. 27B, it is also easily seen in the ribs, the oblique lines at the lower left. It is easy to overlook the ribs in the original picture, although they can be seen if the observer looks for them. In the diffused copy they are less likely to be missed.

A variation of the technique of viewing the sharply focused pictures through the diffusion filter is to record the picture initially with diffused dots. This can be done by placing the diffusion filter an inch or more in

* Dearborn Glass Co., Bedford Park, Illinois.

front of the cathode-ray tube. Alternatively it can be done by defocusing the cathode-ray beam with its focus control or by placing a defocusing lens in front of the scope camera. The use of the diffusion filter has the advantage that the light from each dot is spread into a nearly Gaussian pattern instead of a sharp-edged disk. The subjective effect of Gaussian diffusion is better than the other methods of defocusing. Furthermore, with the filter the diffusion is equal over the entire picture area, it is easy

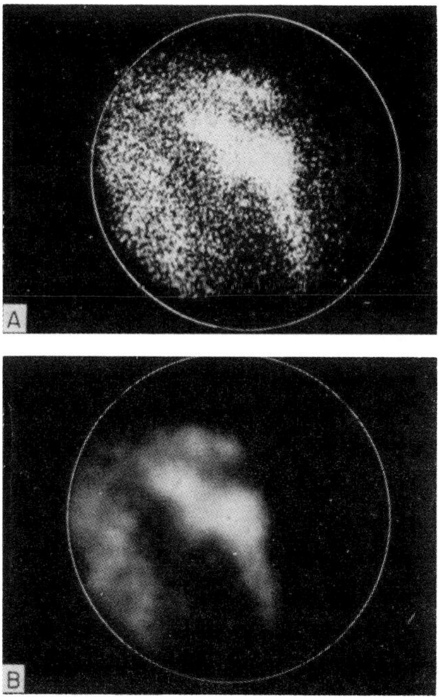

FIG. 27. Effect of diffusion filter on picture originally recorded with sharply focused dots. (A) Sharply focused original picture of distribution of erythropoietic bone marrow in shoulder area. (B) Same picture as it appears when viewed through diffusion filter. Isolated background dots are eliminated, and areas where there is a slight increase in the concentration of dots, such as the ribs (diagonal lines at lower left), become more apparent (*13, 14*).

to vary the amount, and it does not vary if the *f* stop of the oscilloscope camera lens is changed, as it does if a defocusing lens is used.

3. MEMORY-TYPE CATHODE-RAY TUBE

Mallard and Myers (*43*) reported constructing a γ-ray scintillation camera with a memory-type cathode-ray tube for readout and storage of the image. This is advantageous because the image is visible as it builds up. Thus, patients can be quickly positioned for the best possible view. Furthermore, the storage tube they used has a variable background suppression. After adjustment, the screen can be photographed to obtain a permanent record. Only significant pictures need be recorded.

The memory-type cathode-ray tube has a nonconducting storage mesh between a conventional electron gun and fluorescent screen. The electron gun deposits a charge on the storage screen at points corresponding to each dot in the image. This permits electrons from an electron "flood gun" to pass through and continuously illuminate a dot on the fluorescent screen. The image can be erased at any time by pressing a button that brings the potential of the storage mesh back to cutoff.

The requirements of a good storage tube are linear gray tone display, variable lower-level cutoff, adequate writing speed, and complete erasure of the previous image without residual effect on the following picture. Less ideal tubes can be used if their function is only to aid in aligning patients.

B. Motion Pictures

The movement of tracer compounds through organs can be shown either by taking motion pictures or by taking sequences of still pictures. Both show the dynamics of an organ, as well as its size and shape, and will probably become increasingly valuable in medical diagnosis and research.

Two methods can be used for recording and displaying motion pictures. The first is to record the flashes from the oscilloscope with a motion picture camera. Usually the action is speeded up by exposing each frame for a few seconds or more and then projecting the developed film at the regular speed of 16 or 24 frames per second. A process that may take many minutes in the patient is compressed to a few seconds of viewing time.

A second method of displaying motion is to record the x- and y-position signals for each dot in the image on magnetic tape and to play back the tape on a cathode-ray-tube monitor. By recording at slow tape speed and playing back at high speed, the action can be accelerated by factors of up to 100. The tape recording has the advantage that immediate playback is possible without the processing necessary for motion picture film. It also lends itself to obtaining numerical data, as described in Section V,C.

One of the problems in viewing motion pictures of dynamic processes is to present the pictures to the observer so he can visualize the information contained in them. Each frame of a motion picture film is composed of a small number of dots. When these flash onto the screen for only a small fraction of a second, it is often difficult to visualize what they show.

One answer to the problem is the use of image-persistence techniques. The purpose of the latter is to make each dot remain on the screen long enough to make a suitable impression on the observer. Image persistence can be obtained with closed-circuit television apparatus using a memory-type television camera tube called a Permachon (*18*). This special camera tube views the image-readout oscilloscope or a projected motion picture, and the persistent image is viewed on a television monitor.

Image persistence can also be obtained by projecting an image from a motion picture projector onto a light-sensitive long-persistence phosphor and viewing the phosphorescent image. A third method is to reprint motion picture film by a "slip-frame" technique so that each frame on the original is printed on several frames of the copy. A fourth method is to view a magnetic-tape recording on a cathode-ray tube having a long-persistent phosphor.

C. Numerical Data Recording and Readout

Several methods can be used to obtain numerical count-rate data from specific areas of a picture.

a. Direct Electronic Methods. A relatively simple method is to divide the image into halves, quarters, and so on, and electronically count the signals that produce dots within each area. For instance, to count flashes appearing on the right-hand half of the picture, a circuit that counts positive X signals but does not count negative X signals is used. Another circuit, sensitive only to negative X signals, counts flashes appearing on the left-hand side of the picture. By sending the outputs of these two circuits to ratemeters and a dual recorder, curves of the count-rate versus time in the two halves of the image detector are obtained.

The above arrangement is used for kidney-function studies with Hippuran-^{131}I. The curves are comparable to conventional renograms.

b. Visual Dot Counting. This technique consists of recording flashes from an image-readout oscilloscope on motion picture film, then visually counting dots within specified areas on each frame of the developed film (*18*). The number of counts per minute in the area is plotted as a function of time. This method is very flexible, since areas of any size or shape can be chosen, but it is laborious when large numbers of dots must be counted.

c. Magnetic Tape Recording with Numerical Readout. Numerical counts as a function of time can be obtained from a picture area of any size or shape by the following semiautomatic technique. First, the position and time of occurrence of all detected γ rays are recorded on magnetic tape. With the scintillation camera, this is done by recording all the X, Y, and Z pulses on a three-channel recorder. At the same time a picture of the organ under study is obtained from the readout oscilloscope with an optical camera.

By reference to the picture just obtained, a mask is made that blocks out all the picture except the area from which numerical counts are wanted. This mask is placed before the image-readout oscilloscope. Then the magnetic tape is played back and the flashes within the desired area are counted by a phototube. The counts are sent to a ratemeter and recorded as a function of time on a chart recorder. Additional areas may be treated in the same fashion by making new masks and replaying the tape.

This method is very flexible because the position and time of all detected γ rays are recorded on the tape and numerical data from any area can be read out at any time in the future. It also offers the advantage that motion pictures or additional still pictures can be printed out by replaying the tape.

d. Magnetic Core Memory. Another method of obtaining numerical data from specific areas of a subject, consists of dividing the picture electronically into a rectangular mosaic of picture elements and storing the counts that occur within each element in a magnetic core memory. The memory systems used in multiparameter analyzers are suitable. These devices can also display the stored data as intensity-modulated mosaic pictures on a cathode-ray tube with any desired amount of contrast amplification or background suppression. In addition, isocount contours can be shown by displaying all picture elements having a certain range of stored counts, while all elements with more or less counts are blanked out. Also, the data can be shown as an isometric display of a three-dimensional plot, where the third dimension represents the number of counts stored in each channel.

To obtain numerical data from a specific picture area, the picture elements within that area are selected and the counts within those channels are totaled. If dynamic processes are being followed, the data in the memory are periodically transferred to another memory device, because the magnetic core memory alone does not record the time at which the counts in a particular channel were received. Then by the use of conventional computer techniques the numerical counts in the selected area are plotted as a function of time.

ACKNOWLEDGMENTS

Most of the research reported in this chapter was done under the auspices of the U.S. Atomic Energy Commission. Additional support came from California

State Cancer funds. The author gratefully acknowledges the long-term support of Dr. John H. Lawrence, Director of the Donner Laboratory, and Dr. C. A. Tobias, Vice Chairman in Charge, Division of Medical Physics, University of California. The following physicians were instrumental in applying the scintillation camera to clinical use: Dr. Donald C. Van Dyke, Dr. Alexander Gottschalk, Dr. Leonard Schaer, Dr. Malcolm Powell, Dr. Saul Winchell, Dr. Rashid Fawwaz, and Dr. Carol Shkurkin. Mr. Yukio Yano did the chemistry on the special isotopes used. Thanks is extended also to Dr. William G. Myers, Biophysics Research Professor at Ohio State University, for his many stimulating discussions.

REFERENCES

1. Allen, H. C., Jr., and Risser, J. R., Simplified apparatus for brain tumor surveys. *Nucleonics* **13,** No. 1, 28 (1955).
2. Anger, H. O., Use of a gamma-ray pinhole camera for *in-vivo* studies. *Nature* **170,** 200 (1952).
3. Anger, H. O., Mortimer, R. K., and Tobias, C. A., Visualization of gamma-ray emitting isotopes in the human body. *Proc. 1st Intern. Conf. Peaceful Uses At. Energy, Geneva, 1955* Vol. 14, p. 204. United Nations, New York, 1956.
4. Anger, H. O., A new instrument for mapping gamma-ray emitters. Biology and Medicine Quarterly Rept. UCRL-3653 (1957).
5. Anger, H. O., Scintillation camera. *Rev. Sci. Instr.* **29,** 27 (1958).
6. Anger, H. O., and Rosenthal, D. J., Scintillation camera and positron camera. *Proc. Seminar Med. Radioisotope Scanning, Vienna, 1959* p. 59. Intern. At. Energy Agency, Vienna, 1959.
7. Anger, H. O., and Gottschalk, A., Localization of brain tumors with the positron scintillation camera. *J. Nucl. Med.* **4,** 326 (1963).
8. Anger, H. O., Gamma-ray and positron scintillation camera. *Nucleonics* **21,** No. 10, 56 (1963).
9. Anger, H. O., Scintillation camera with 11-inch crystal. Donner Laboratory Semiannual Rept. UCRL-11184, p. 69, 1963.
10. Anger, H. O., and Davis, D. H., Gamma-ray detection efficiency and image resolution in sodium iodide. *Rev. Sci. Instr.* **35,** 693 (1964).
11. Anger, H. O., Scintillation camera with multichannel collimators. *J. Nucl. Med.* **5,** 515 (1964).
12. Anger, H. O., and Van Dyke, D. C., Human bone marrow distribution shown *in vivo* by iron-52 and the positron scintillation camera. *Science* **144,** 1587 (1964).
13. Anger, H. O., Scintillation camera image recording. Lawrence Radiation Laboratory Rept. UCRL-11336 (1964).
14. Anger, H. O., Van Dyke, D. C., Gottschalk, A., Yano, Y., and Schaer, L. R., The scintillation camera in diagnosis and research. *Nucleonics* **23,** No. 1, 57 (1965).
15. Anger, H. O., Sensitivity, resolution, and linearity of the scintillation camera, Tenth Scintillation Counter Symposium, *IEEE Trans. Nucl. Sci.* **13,** No. 3, 380, 1966.
16. Bender, M. A., and Blau, M., The clinical use of the autofluoroscope (abstract). *J. Nucl. Med.* **3,** 202 (1962).
17. Bender, M. A., and Blau, M., The autofluoroscope. *In* "Progress in Medical Radioisotope Scanning" (R. M. Kniseley, G. A. Andrews, and C. C. Harris, eds.), TID-7673, p. 151. U.S. At. Energy Comm., Washington, D.C., 1963.

18. Bender, M. A., and Blau, M., The autofluoroscope. *Nucleonics* **21,** No. 10, 52 (1963).
19. Bender, M. A., The digital autofluoroscope. *Proc. Symp. Med. Radioisotope Scanning, Athens, 1964* Vol. 1, p. 391. Intern. At. Energy, Vienna, 1964.
20. Berger, M. J., Monte Carlo calculation of the penetration and diffusion of fast charged particles. *In* "Methods in Computational Physics" (B. Alder, S. Fernbach, and M. Rotenberg, eds.) Vol. 1, p. 135. Academic Press, New York, 1963.
21. Brownell, G. L., Theory of radioisotope scanning. *Intern. J. Appl. Radiation Isotopes* **3,** 181 (1958).
22. Brownell, G. L., Resolution of gamma imaging devices. Picker Scintillator 9, No. 2-C (1965).
23. Brucer, M., "Radioisotope Scanning. An Introduction to the Use of the Area Scan in Medical Diagnosis." Oak Ridge Institute of Nuclear Studies, Oak Ridge, Tennessee, 1958.
24. Copeland, D. E., and Benjamin, E. W., Pinhole camera for gamma-ray sources. *Nucleonics* **5,** No. 2, 44 (1949).
25. Davisson, C. M., and Evans, R. D., Gamma-ray absorption coefficients. *Rev. Mod. Phys.* **24,** 79 (1952).
26. Forsaith, A. L., Horwitz, N. H., and Lofstrom, J. E., The resolution of a spark imaging camera (Spintharicon) with parallel channel collimators. *Phys. Med. Biol.* **11,** 411 (1966).
27. Fucks, W., and Knipping, H. W., Eine Gamma-Retina. *Naturwissenschaften* **42,** 493 (1955).
28. Fucks, W., Knipping, H. W., Liese, E., and Schumacher, G., Zur diagnostischen Verwendung von Isotopen am Krankenbett, insbesondere in der Herz- und Krebsklinik. *Atomkern Energie* **9,** 271 (1964).
29. Gottschalk, A., and Anger, H. O., Sensitivity of the positron scintillation camera for detecting simulated brain tumors. *Am. J. Roentgenol., Radium Therapy Nucl. Med.* **92,** 174 (1964).
30. Gottschalk, A., and Anger, H. O., Renal scintiphotography with the gamma ray scintillation camera and Hg^{203} Neohydrin. *Radiology* **84,** 861 (1965).
31. Gottschalk, A., McCormack, K. R., Adams, J. E., and Anger, H. O., A comparison of results of brain scanning using Ga^{68}-EDTA and the positron scintillation camera, with Hg^{203}-Neohydrin and the conventional focused collimator scanner. *Radiology* **84,** 502 (1965).
32. Gottschalk, A., and Anger, H. O., Use of the scintillation camera to reduce scanning time. *J. Am. Med. Assoc.* **192,** 448 (1965).
33. Gottschalk, A., and Anger, H. O., Progress in radioisotope scanning: Clinical application of scintillation cameras and short lived isotopes. *In* "Progress in Atomic Medicine" (J. H. Lawrence, ed.), p. 78. Grune & Stratton, New York, 1965.
34. Grodstein, G. W., X-ray attenuation coefficients from 10 keV to 100 MeV. *Natl. Bur. Std. (U.S.) Circ.* **583** (1957).
35. Gross, W., Schlesinger, E. B., and de Boves, S., A scintillation camera for kinetic studies of the distribution of radioactive nuclides in the brain. *Proc. Symp. Med. Radioisotope Scanning, Athens, 1964* Vol. 1, p. 401. Intern. At. Energy Agency, Vienna, 1964.
36. Harper, P. V., Beck, R. N., Charleston, D., and Lathrop, K. A., Optimization of a scanning method using Tc^{99m}. *Nucleonics* **22,** No. 1, 50 (1964).
37. Harris, C. C., Eason, H. O., Francis, J. E., Jr., and Bell, P. R., An oscilloscope monitor for scintillation spectrometers. *J. Nucl. Med.* **1,** 280 (1960).

38. Johansson, S. A. E., and Skanse, B., A photographic method of determining the distribution of radioactive material *in vivo*. *Acta Radiol.* **39,** 317 (1953).
39. Kellershohn, C., and Pellerin, P., Scintillator grid localizes gamma emitters photographically. *Nucleonics* **13,** No. 12, 34 (1955).
40. Kellershohn, C., and Pellerin, P., "Sur la possibilité d'utiliser un tube amplificateur d'image pour mettre en évidence la localisation et la distribution d'un corps radioactif". *Compt. Rend. Soc. Biol.* **149,** 533 (1955).
41. Kellershohn, C., Desgrez, A., and Lansiart, A., Deux nouveaux types, de détecteur pour camera a rayons X ou γ. *Proc. Symp. Med. Radioisotope Scanning, Athens,* Vol. 1, p. 333. Intern. At. Energy Agency, Vienna (1964).
42. Loevinger, R., Japha, E. M., and Brownell, G. L., Discrete radioisotope sources. *In* "Radiation Dosimetry" (G. J. Hine and G. L. Brownell, eds.), p. 693. Academic Press, New York, 1956.
43. Mallard, J. R., and Myers, M. J., The performance of a gamma camera for the visualization of radioactive isotopes *in vivo*. *Phys. Med. Biol.* **8,** 165 (1963).
44. Mallard, J. R., and Myers, M. J., Clinical application of a gamma camera. *Phys. Med. Biol.* **8,** 183 (1963).
45. Mather, R. L., Gamma-ray collimator penetration and scattering effects. *J. Appl. Phys.* **28,** 1200 (1957).
46. Mortimer, R. K., Anger, H. O., and Tobias, C. A., The gamma-ray pinhole camera with image amplifier. *Conv. Record I.R.E. 1954* Pt. 9, pp. 2–5 (1954).
47. Rabinowitz, J. L., Shockman, A. T., and Bogash, M., The *in vivo* autoradiography of human prostate—a preliminary communication. *J. Nucl. Med.* **5,** 72 (1964).
48. Ramm, W. J., Scintillation detectors. *In* "Radiation Dosimetry" (G. J. Hine and G. L. Brownell, eds.), p. 278. Academic Press, New York, 1956.
49. Ross, D. A., Harris, C. C., Satterfield, M. M., Bell, P. R., and Jordan, J. C., Low-energy gamma emitters in scanning and other clinical applications. *In* "Radioaktive Isotope in Klinik und Forschung" (K. Fellinger and R. Höfer, eds.), Vol. 6, p. 108. Urban & Schwarzenberg, Berlin, 1965.
50. Shirley, D. A., Applications of germanium gamma-ray detectors. *Nucleonics* **23,** No. 3, 62 (1965).
51. Ter-Pogossian, M. M., Kastner, J., and Vest, T. B., Autofluorography of the thyroid gland by means of image amplification. *Radiology* **81,** 984 (1963).
52. Ter-Pogossian, M. M., and Eichling, J. O., Autofluorography with an X-ray image amplifier. *Proc. Symp. Med. Radioisotope Scanning, Athens, 1964* Vol. 1, p. 411. Intern. At. Energy Agency, Vienna, 1964.
52a. Ter-Pogossian, M. M., and Wagner, H. N., Jr., A new look at the cyclotron for making short-lived isotopes. *Nucleonics* **24,** No. 10, 50 (1966).
53. Van Dyke, D., Anger, H. O., and Pollycove, M., Effect of erythropoietic stimulation on marrow distribution in man, rabbit, and rat as shown with Fe^{59} and Fe^{52}. *Blood* **24,** 356 (1964).
54. Van Dyke, D. C., and Anger, H. O., Patterns of marrow hypertrophy and atrophy in man. *J. Nucl. Med.* **6,** 109 (1965).
55. Van Dyke, D., Anger, H. O., Yano, Y., and Bozzini, C., Bone blood flow shown with F^{18} and the positron camera. *Am. J. Physiol.* **209,** 65 (1965).
56. Yano, Y., and Anger, H. O., Production and chemical processing of iron-52 for medical use. *Intern. J. Appl. Radiation Isotopes* **16,** 153 (1965).
57. Yano, Y., and Anger, H. O., A gallium-68 positron cow for medical use. *J. Nucl. Med.* **5,** 484 (1964).
58. Yasukochi, H., Study of the scintillation camera. *Nippon Acta Radiol.* **2,** 246 (1964).

CHAPTER 20

SINGLE AND MULTIPLE DETECTOR SYSTEMS FOR WHOLE-BODY COUNTING

JOHANNES G. MEHL*

DIVISION OF HEALTH, SAFETY, AND WASTE DISPOSAL

INTERNATIONAL ATOMIC ENERGY AGENCY

VIENNA, AUSTRIA

The purpose of whole-body counting is the determination of the total radioactivity in human bodies. From this the quantities of radioactive elements or radioactive compounds present in the body at the time of measurement can be assessed. Such data yield valuable information in physiological and toxicological radioisotope research, medical radioisotope diagnosis and therapy, and diagnosis and treatment of radioactive poisoning.

Periodic whole-body radioactivity measurements permit the determination of the retention and excretion of radioactive substances in a subject and may replace radioactivity analysis in urine and (or) feces

*Present address: Gesellschaft für Kernforschung m.b.H., Karlsruhe, Federal Republic of Germany.

samples. If these are combined with simultaneous measurements of the radioactivity in blood, tissues, or organs, valuable information can be obtained concerning the metabolism of radioactive tracers (7).

I. PRINCIPLES OF WHOLE-BODY COUNTING

Whole-body counting consists of the measurement of photons radiated from the body by detector systems external to the subject. It is therefore confined to measurements of radioisotopes which emit photons capable of penetrating the body tissues and other absorbing media positioned between the radioactive deposit in the body and the radiation-sensitive detector volume. It does not matter whether the photons are emitted directly (γ radiation) or indirectly (annihilation radiation, Bremsstrahlung) by the radioisotope in question, but for purposes of counter design and for quantitative measurements the number of photons emitted per disintegration and their energy or energy distribution must be known.

For whole-body radioactivity measurements a detector-to-body geometry must be chosen so that the response of the detector is not significantly affected by the distribution of the radioisotope within the body. This objective can be achieved in two ways.

(1) Large radiation detectors are positioned around the body in almost a 4π geometry, so that most photons emitted from the body during the measurement strike the detector.

(2) One or several small radiation detectors in fixed positions are placed around the body or are moved on fixed tracks along the body, so that the photons that strike the detector (or detectors) are a representative fraction of all the photons emitted from the body during the measurement.

Liquid and plastic organic scintillation detectors are now preferred for large detector systems, but high-pressure ionization chamber systems are still in use. Characteristics of large organic scintillators and their use for whole-body counting are described in Chapter 21.

In single and multiple detector systems G-M counters, proportional counters, and scintillation counters are used. However, for measurement of photons of medium and high energies, preference is given to thallium-activated sodium iodide crystal detectors because of their high counting efficiency per unit detector volume. They also permit discrimination between different photon energies, which makes them superior to organic scintillators. For photons of very low energy, in the case of high activity levels or if discrimination between different photon energies is not required, other detectors may be more suitable for technical or economic reasons.

In this chapter the design, performance, and calibration of single and multiple detector systems for whole-body radioactivity measurements are discussed. Detailed consideration is given to systems using NaI(Tl) crystal detectors.

Several problems in whole-body counting arise primarily from the fact that the heights and weights of persons vary over a wide range. Within the same person the distribution of the radioactivity may change with time. Furthermore, the range of activity levels is fairly wide.

A proper design of whole-body counters will help to minimize the problems of whole-body radioactivity measurements. A detector-to-body geometry should be chosen aiming for a response of the counter to photons emitted from the body independent of body build and the distribution of the radioactivity within the body. The detection limit of the counter should be adequate for the measurement of the expected photon emission rates. This implies that reasonable counting statistics are obtained within a counting time suitable for the persons to be measured and also that overloading of the counting equipment at high count-rates is prevented. Finally, it should be possible to assess the contribution to the count-rate from radiation originating outside the body and from other radioisotopes within the body with a sufficient accuracy in order to permit appropriate correction for their interference.

II. DESIGN OF SINGLE AND MULTIPLE NaI(Tl) DETECTOR SYSTEMS

A. Fundamental Data

The design of NaI(Tl) crystal whole-body counters depends largely upon the expected photon emission rate from the body, the maximum counting time, and the accuracy with which the total radioactivity of the body must be determined.

1. PHOTON EMISSION RATE

The photon emission rate, P, of the body can be assessed from the formula

$$P = 2.22 \times 10^6 A\eta\alpha \quad \text{(photons per minute)} \tag{1}$$

where A is the activity of the radioisotope in microcuries, η the number of photons of energy E_γ emitted per disintegration, and α the body transparence for photons of energy E_γ.

Values for η are listed in the physics and nuclear medicine literature. The body transparence, α, for photons, measuring the photopeak only, has been observed to be nearly independent of the photon energy within an energy range from $E_\gamma = (0.2\text{–}2)$ MeV. A value of $\alpha = 2/3$ is a close approximation of experimental findings (*11*).

High photon emission rates are to be expected where γ-ray emitters such as ^{131}I or ^{198}Au are used for radioisotope therapy. Doses between about 10^3 and 10^5 μCi are administered. The total radioactivity of the respective isotopes in the body is to be measured over periods of several days up to weeks. If it is assumed that the detection of 1% of the administered dose would be sufficient for purposes of therapy control, the counter should be designed for measurement of activity levels between about 10 and 10^5 μCi corresponding to photon emission rates of about 10^7 and 10^{11} photons per minute.

Intermediate photon emission rates are to be measured in medical radioisotope diagnosis, where a large variety of γ-ray-emitting isotopes are administered at activity levels between 1 and 100 μCi. The total radioactivity of the body is to be measured over periods of days up to several weeks or even months. For the measurement of 1% of the administered radioactivity, the counter should be designed for activity levels between 10^{-2} and 100 μCi. In most cases counters designed for the measurement of photon emission rates between about 10^4 and 10^8 photons per minute will suffice. Such counters may also be used for the assessment of accidental high intakes of radioactive material.

Low photon emission rates are to be expected where natural radioactive deposits of ^{40}K, fallout deposits of ^{137}Cs, or body burdens at or below the maximum permissible values of radioisotopes of high radiotoxicity are to be measured. If, for purposes of medical diagnosis, radioisotopes of moderate radiotoxicity are applied, it is necessary to keep the administered radioactivity below the levels referred to above. Thus, also in medical radioisotope diagnosis, measurements of low photon emission rates may be required.

From the natural ^{40}K radioactivity of adults, which is about 0.1 μCi, a photon emission rate of 1.6×10^4 photons per minute can be expected. Average fallout ^{137}Cs deposits in adults (Germany, Karlsruhe-Landstuhl) rose from about 3×10^{-3} μCi (1961–1962) to 2×10^{-2} μCi (spring 1964). These values correspond to photon emission rates of 3.8×10^3 and 2.5×10^4 photons per minute, respectively.

Maximum permissible body burdens of radioisotopes of high radiotoxicity applicable to radiation workers are between 10^{-2} and 5 μCi. The corresponding values applicable to individual members of the public are, in general, taken as $1/10$ of these values for adults and $1/100$ of these values for children. Thus, for the measurement of individual members of the population total-body radioactivity levels as low as 10^{-4} μCi may be encountered. A body burden of 10^{-4} μCi would result in a photon emission rate of the body of 15 photons per minute, if it is assumed that the radioisotope in question emits 10 photons per 100 disintegrations.

2. COUNTING TIME

In medical radioisotope work, if the patient is in poor physical condition, or if children are to be measured, the counting time should not exceed a few minutes. In radioisotope diagnosis of less severe cases counting times of 10 to 15 min are normally accepted. If the radioactivity of persons is measured for purposes of surveillance in radiation protection a 20-min counting time is often routine. Frequently counting times of even 40 min are applied; in those cases special measures for the patient's welfare, such as music, television, and intercommunication systems between the measured individual and the operator, are found advantageous.

3. ACCURACY AND PRECISION

An accuracy of $\pm 25\%$ would be sufficient if the body radioactivity is assessed for purposes of radiation protection. In the case of an emergency, early measurements which permit only the assessment of the order of magnitude of the activity of the contaminants can also be of value.

Total-body radioactivity measurements performed for the control of radioisotope therapy would normally not require an accuracy better than $\pm 10\%$. For medical radioisotope diagnosis, in general, it is not necessary that the total radioactivity of the body be determined in absolute units, such as the microcurie. Only relative values of successive measurements are required. In many cases it would be desirable to obtain a precision of at least $\pm 5\%$.

B. Geometry

The fraction of the photons emitted by the body that strikes the crystal (or crystals) depends upon the detector-to-body geometry, Ω, which is defined by the formula

$$\Omega = (\phi_e/4\pi D_e^2) \tag{2}$$

where ϕ_e is the effective cross section of the detector system for photons emitted by the body, and D_e is the effective distance of the body from the detector system for crystals suspended with their axis perpendicular to the body axis. For purposes of design the effective cross section may be regarded as

$$\phi_e = \pi r^2 n \tag{3}$$

where r is the radius of the crystals, and n is the number of crystals.

The effective detector-to-body distance, D_e, depends on the positioning of the crystal (or crystals) with respect to the body. Various detector systems have been developed for achieving independence of the counter response from body build and distribution of the radioactivity within the body. These counting systems may be classified as stationary and moving systems.

1. Stationary Systems

In stationary systems the crystal (or crystals) and the body are in a fixed position during the measurements. The effective detector-to-body

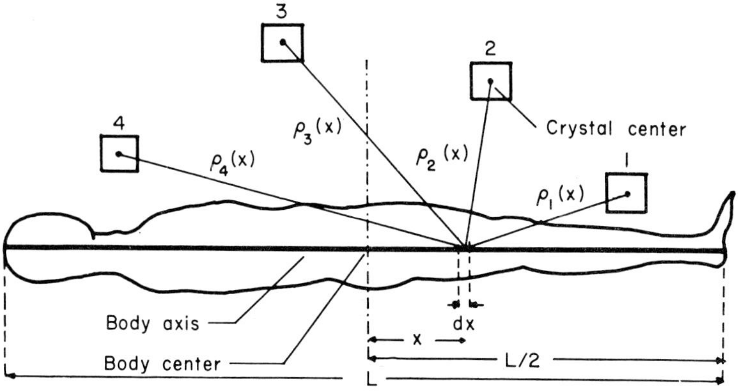

Fig. 1. Assessment of counter geometry for a line source representing the body of a subject.

distance, D_e, can be assessed to a first approximation from the response of the detector system to a line source of the length of the body and in a position corresponding to the long axis of the body (Fig. 1). The position of each crystal may be represented by its center. The response of a system of n detectors to the activity of a line element, dx, of the source can be assessed from the function

$$\frac{1}{\rho(x)^2} = \frac{1}{n}\sum_{i=1}^{n}\frac{1}{\rho_i(x)^2} \tag{4}$$

where $\rho(x)$ is the effective distance of the detector system as a whole and $\rho_i(x)$ is the distance of the ith detector from the line element dx. Both $\rho(x)$ and $\rho_i(x)$ depend on the position of dx defined by its distance x from the center of the line source. The uniformity of response of the detector system requires a minimum of variation of $1/\rho(x)^2$ for all values of x between $-L/2$ and $+L/2$, which is the full length of the line source.

The integral mean value of $1/\rho(x)^2$ for all values of x yields the effective distance, D_e, of the line source:

$$\frac{1}{D_e^2} = \frac{1}{L} \int_{-L/2}^{+L/2} \frac{dx}{\rho(x)^2} \tag{5}$$

In Table I formulas are given for the functions $1/\rho(x)^2$ and $1/D_e^2$ that apply to the geometrical data of various detector systems.

a. *Single-Crystal Systems.* Single crystals are used in a number of different geometries.

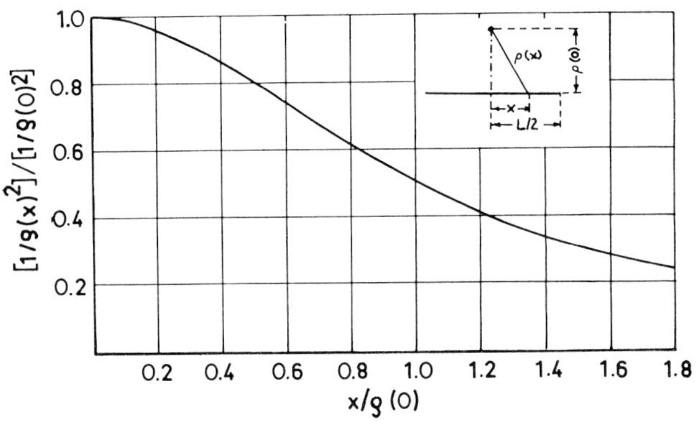

FIG. 2. Geometrical characteristics of single-crystal stretcher systems.

Single-crystal stretcher geometry: The design of an adequate counting geometry is simple for high photon emission rates (Section II,A,1). The detector-to-body distance can be made sufficiently large so that the detector response is nearly uniform for the full length of the body axis. The subject may lie on a stretcher close to the floor of the room. He may be measured in supine and, where necessary, also in prone position to permit averaging of differences in the self-absorption by body tissues. The crystal is normally suspended above the center of the body. For this case the function $1/\rho(x)^2$ is shown in Fig. 2. The ordinate is given in units of $1/\rho(0)^2$, where $\rho(0)$ is the detector-to-body (line source) distance. For a value of $\rho(0) = 250$ cm and a body length $L = 175$ cm, it can be seen from Fig. 2 that for elements at both ends of the line source ($x = 87.5$ and $x/\rho(0) = 0.35$) $1/\rho(x)^2$ is reduced to only 89% of its value at the center ($x = 0$). However, for a shorter distance, $\rho(0) = 50$ cm, the corresponding value of

$1/\rho(x)^2$ is reduced to 24%, so that significant errors may be expected when redistribution of the radioactive deposits occurs. In the two examples above the effective crystal-to-body distances are $D_e = 225$ cm and $D_e = 65$ cm, respectively (from formula given in Table I for $1/D_e^2$ of stationary single-crystal stretcher geometry).

TABLE I

System	Type	Definition	$1/\rho(x)^2$	$1/D_e^2$
Stationary	Single crystal			
	Arc	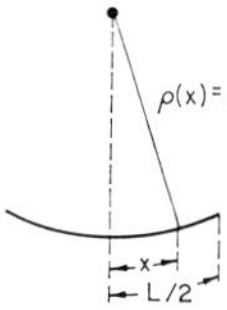	$1/\rho^2$	$1/\rho^2$
	Stretcher	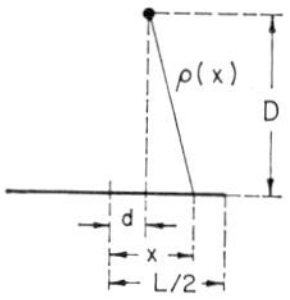	$\dfrac{1}{(x-d)^2+D^2}$	$\dfrac{1}{LD}\left(\tan^{-1}\dfrac{\frac{L}{2}-d}{D}+\tan^{-1}\dfrac{\frac{L}{2}+d}{D}\right)$
	Chair	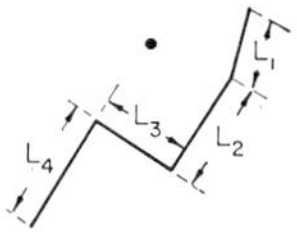 $L = L_1 + L_2 + L_3 + L_4$	For each part L_1, $L_2, \ldots L_n$ of the line source L as for single crystal stretcher system	$\dfrac{1}{L}\left(L_1/D_{e1}^2 + L_2/D_{e2}^2 + \cdots + L_n/D_{en}^2\right)$
	Multicrystal			
	Stretcher	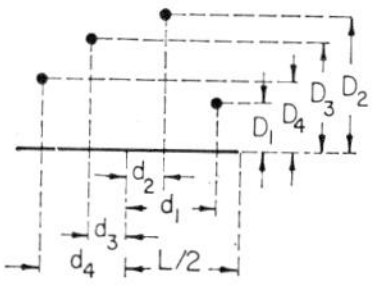	$\dfrac{1}{n}\sum_{\nu=1}^{n}\dfrac{1}{(x-d_\nu)^2+D_\nu^2}$	$\dfrac{1}{n}\sum_{\nu=1}^{n}\dfrac{1}{LD_\nu}\left(\tan^{-1}\dfrac{\frac{L}{2}-d_\nu}{D_\nu}+\tan^{-1}\dfrac{\frac{L}{2}+d_\nu}{D_\nu}\right)$
Moving	Single crystal			
	Constant speed	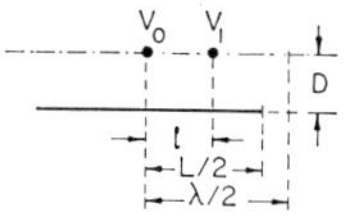 $V_0/V_t = 1$	$\dfrac{1}{\lambda D}\left(\tan^{-1}\dfrac{\frac{\lambda}{2}-x}{D}+\tan^{-1}\dfrac{\frac{\lambda}{2}+x}{D}\right)$	$\dfrac{2}{\lambda L}\left(\dfrac{\lambda+L}{2D}\tan^{-1}\dfrac{\lambda+L}{2D}-\dfrac{\lambda-L}{2D}\tan^{-1}\dfrac{\lambda-L}{2D}+\dfrac{1}{2}\ln\dfrac{4D^2+(\lambda-L)^2}{4D^2+(\lambda+L)^2}\right)$
	Variable speed	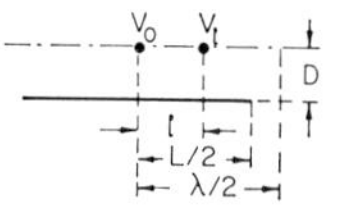 $V_0/V_t = 1 + kt$	$\dfrac{1}{\rho(x)^2}=\dfrac{1}{\lambda}\left[\dfrac{1+kx}{D}\left(\tan^{-1}\dfrac{\frac{\lambda}{2}-x}{D}+\tan^{-1}\dfrac{x}{D}\right)+\dfrac{1-kx}{D}\left(\tan^{-1}\dfrac{\frac{\lambda}{2}+x}{D}-\tan^{-1}\dfrac{x}{D}\right)+\dfrac{k}{2}\ln\dfrac{(\frac{\lambda}{2}-x)^2+D^2}{x^2+D^2}\cdot\dfrac{(\frac{\lambda}{2}+x)^2+D^2}{x^2+D^2}\right]$	

Single-crystal arc geometry: The effective detector-to-body distance of single-crystal systems can be reduced without losing the desirable characteristics of the large distance counting geometry. The subject is positioned on an arc and the crystal is suspended at the center of that arc (Table I). This keeps $1/\rho(x)^2$ constant for the entire length of the source. However, there is a limit for reducing the detector-to-body distance. If the radius of the arc is kept below 1.5 meter, the subject is not positioned comfortably, and measurements in the prone position become difficult.

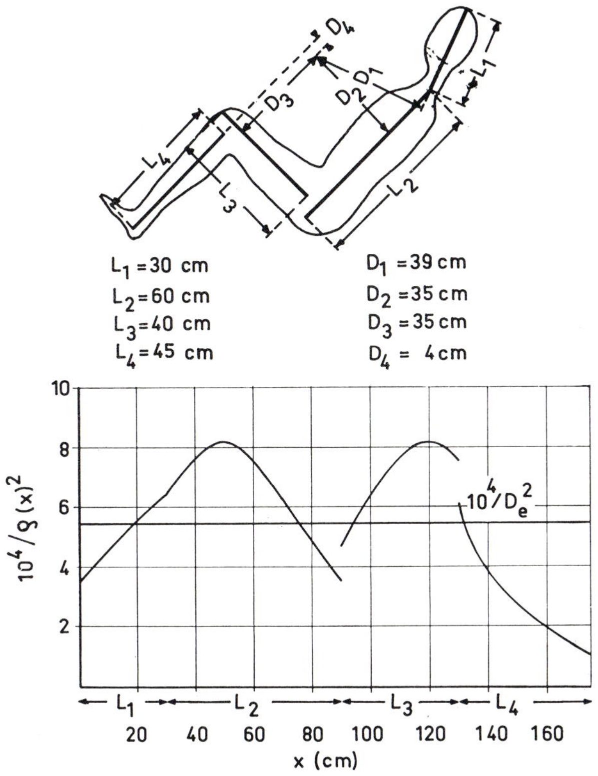

FIG. 3. Geometrical characteristics of a single-crystal chair system. See text.

Single-crystal chair geometry: Patients may be positioned in a chair more comfortably than on a stretcher or in an arc geometry. If the crystal is suspended at about 45 cm from the back and seat of the chair, it is then about at the center of an arc formed by the trunk and the thighs of the subject. However, if checked by the formulas given in Table I it becomes obvious that the detector response to elements of the four line sources (Fig. 3) taken to represent the body is not very uniform. The effective detector-to-body distance of the sources is $D_e = 43$ cm.

Though the single-crystal chair geometry does not fulfill very well the geometrical requirements of whole-body counters (Section I), it has found a fairly wide application. This is primarily due to the high sensitivity which is obtained by the small effective detector-to-body distance and to the ease of reproducing the geometrical conditions.

b. *Multiple-Crystal Systems.* Multiple crystals are used in a number of different geometries.

Two-crystal stretcher geometry: By using two crystals side by side either above or below a stretcher, it is possible to flatten the response of the detector system. If the crystals are close to the body, one at each end, it is obvious that the response to volume elements at the center of the body will be a minimum, and that to volume elements under each detector a maximum. If the detectors are placed closer to the body center, the minimum response becomes less pronounced and finally turns into a maximum.

For a line source of length L, it can be shown that the response to a source element at the center becomes equal to the response to source elements in the vicinity of each detector, if the distance of the crystals from the body center is $d = D/(3)^{1/2}$, where D is the distance of the crystals from the line source. For such a geometry, unless large values of D are used, the response of the system to elements at the ends of the line source is much lower than for elements at its central region. Therefore, in general, it is preferable to have the same reduced response to central elements as to line elements at each end of the source. It can be shown that this is the case if

$$d = [1/\sqrt{3}][D^2 + (L/2)^2]^{1/2}$$

In Fig. 4 $[1/\rho(x)^2]/[1/\rho(0)^2]$ is plotted as a function of x/L for various values of d. A flat response is achieved only for fairly large detector-to-body distances. When a 15% variation of the response is acceptable (Fig. 4, Curve 2) $d = 3L/8$ and $D = 8L/(11)^{1/2}$ can be used. Assuming a body length of $L = 175$ cm, these values correspond to $d = 66$ cm and $D = 73$ cm. The effective detector-to-body distance of that system would be $D_e = 95$ cm.

Four-crystal stretcher geometry: In Fig. 5 $[1/\rho(x)^2]/[1/\rho(0)^2]$ is plotted as a function of x for two four-crystal stretcher systems. Even for small detector-to-body distances the variation of the response of the detector system can be kept within 25% for about 140 cm of the body length. The effective detector-to-body distance for both cases is about

$D_e = 37$ cm. In stationary systems normally not more than four crystals are used. If the total crystal volume is divided into many small ones,

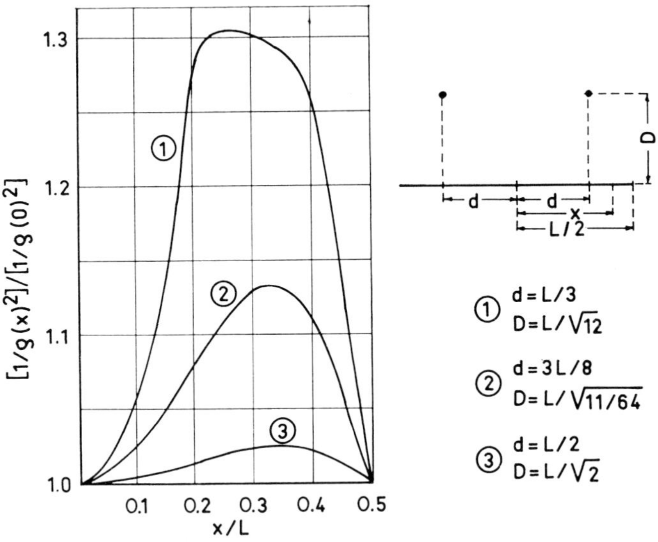

FIG. 4. Geometrical characteristics of two-crystal stretcher systems.

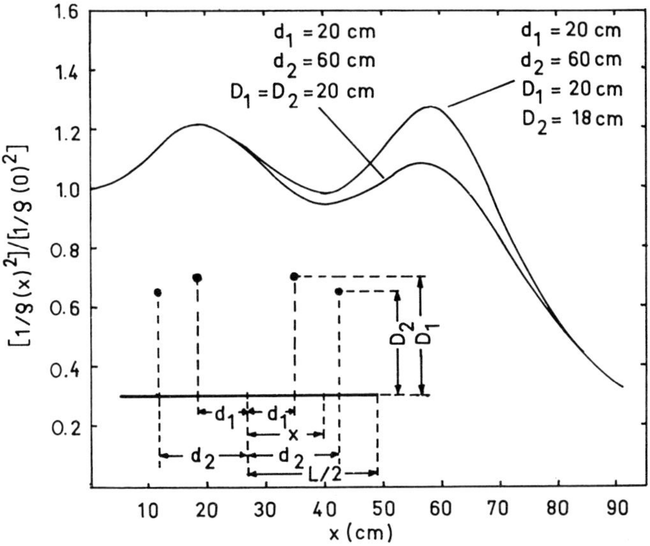

FIG. 5. Geometrical characteristics of four-crystal stretcher systems.

the poorer spectral response of small NaI(Tl) crystals and the problems of matching the various detectors for operation in a single counting system may become significant. Also the maintenance of the overall stability becomes more difficult. However, multiple detector systems, if equipped with collimating shields, are also useful for simultaneous measurements of partial body radioactivity at various body sites. If such measurements are contemplated, the number of detectors will be determined by the number of body sites for which simultaneous measurements are required.

2. MOVING SYSTEMS

The geometrical characteristics of a stationary n-crystal system can be achieved with only a single crystal when it is positioned subsequently at n different positions for $1/n$ of the total counting time at each. This would imply that the distribution of the radioactivity is not subject to significant changes during the counting time. Instead of this complex procedure it is easier to move the crystal continuously over the body and integrate the counts during a full movement.

a. *Single Crystal Systems.* Normally the subject is positioned alternately in prone and supine positions on a stretcher and the crystal is moved on a fixed track above the subject and parallel to the body axis. Of course it does not matter whether the crystal or the subject moves, or subject and crystal both move relative to each other. In fact, each of these systems is used. Movement of both crystal and subject is preferred if the space for moving the crystal beyond the stretcher ends is limited; movement of the subject is preferred where shadow shields (Section III,B) are applied.

Crystal movement at constant speed: In general, the crystal is moved at a constant speed. The counting geometry can be assessed from a line detector with a length equal to the crystal path. The formula for $1/\rho(x)^2$ and $1/D_e^2$ as a function of the length of the crystal path λ, its distance D from the line source of length L are given in Table I. In Fig. 6 $[1/\rho(x)^2]/[1/\rho(0)^2]$ is shown as a function of x/L for various values of D and λ. The response of the system to elements near the ends of the line source is flattened by increasing the length of the crystal path and by reducing the distance between the line source and the crystal. For a system with $\lambda = 235$ cm, $L = 175$ cm, and $D = 25$ cm the effective detector-to-body distance is $D_e = 47$ cm.

Crystal movement at variable speed: The decrease of $1/\rho(x)^2$ with increasing values of x can be compensated by lowering the speed of crystal movement with increasing values of l, the crystal position measured from the center of the path of crystal movement. The time interval during which the crystal sees the body from a position l is proportional to $1/v_l$ where v_l is the speed of crystal movement at l. In the formula for $1/\rho(x)^2$ given in Table I, it is assumed that the time interval is increased in proportion to l so that $(1/v_l) = (1/v_0)(1 + kl)$.

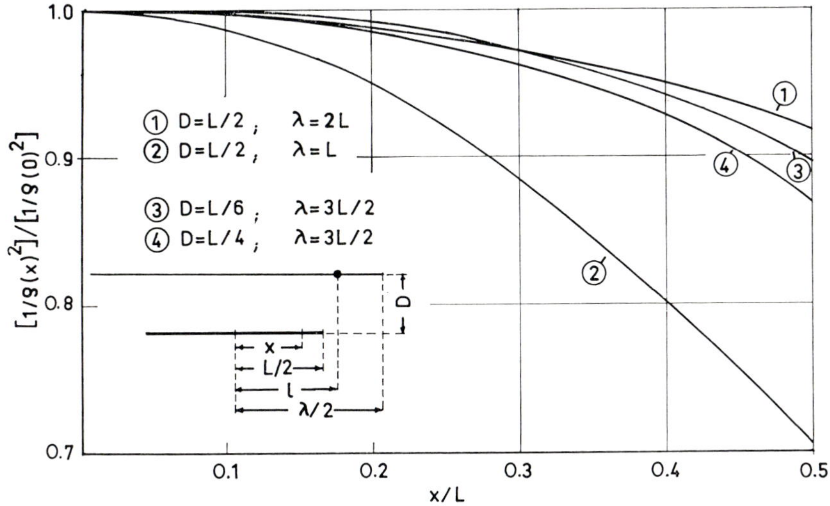

FIG. 6. Geometrical characteristics of single-crystal systems moving with constant speed.

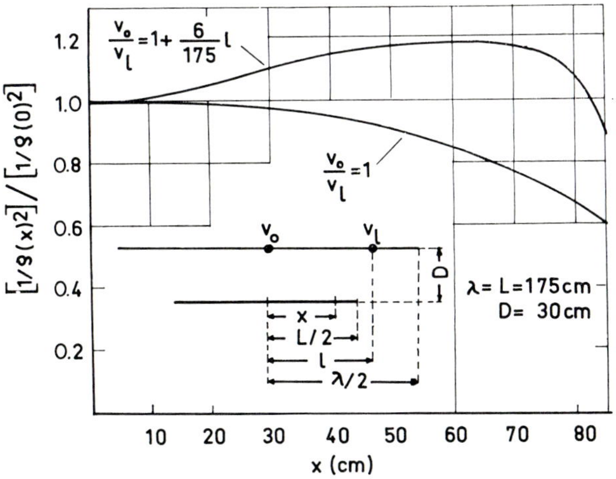

FIG. 7. Geometrical characteristics of a single-crystal system moving with variable speed.

The effect of variable speed of crystal movement on the function $[1/\rho(x)^2]/[1/\rho(0)^2]$ is shown in Fig. 7.

b. *Multiple Crystal Systems.* In order to prevent loss of time by repositioning of the subject for measurements in prone and supine positions, it is convenient to use two crystals, one below and one above the subject. Normally both crystals are moved simultaneously at constant speed. It appears that not much is gained by increasing the number of crystals further, though systems with four crystals are in use. The geometrical characteristics of multiple-crystal moving systems can be easily assessed from the formulas given for single-crystal moving systems.

C. Counting Statistics

1. Signal Count-Rate

With NaI(Tl) detectors quantitative measurements are usually based on the counts per unit time in the total absorption peak (photopeak) of

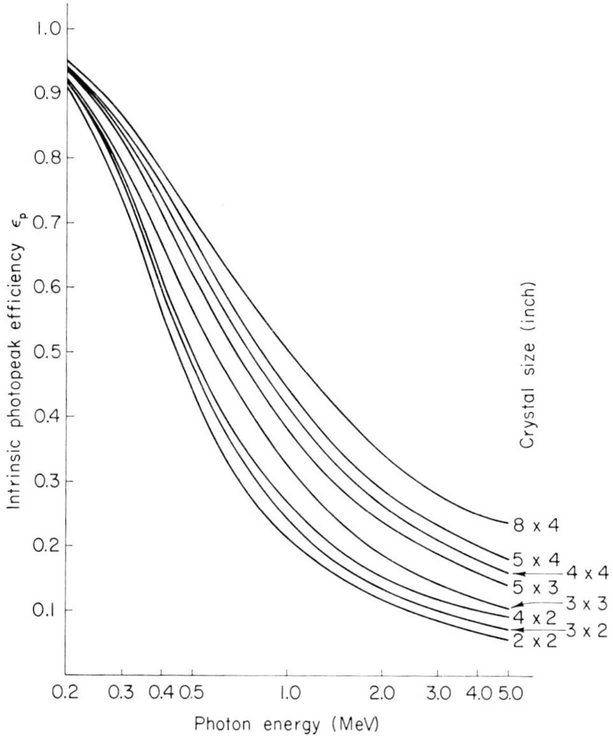

FIG. 8. Intrinsic photopeak efficiency (photofraction) of NaI(Tl) crystals as a function of photon energy for various crystal sizes (*20, 32*).

the γ radiation in question. Instead of the full width of the photopeak its central region may be used where the statistical precision is highest. Thus the counts (signal and background) are integrated in an energy interval ΔE usually symmetrical around the peak.

The signal count-rate, S, can be calculated as

$$S = P\Omega\epsilon_p F \quad \text{(counts per minute)} \tag{6}$$

where P is the photon emission rate of the body (Eq. 1), Ω is the fraction of the photons emitted from the body which strikes the crystal (or crystals) (counting geometry, Eq. 2), ϵ_p is the fraction of the photons striking the crystal (or crystals) that contributes to the photopeak (intrinsic photopeak efficiency), and F is the fraction of counts in the photopeak that is recorded in a preselected energy interval ΔE.

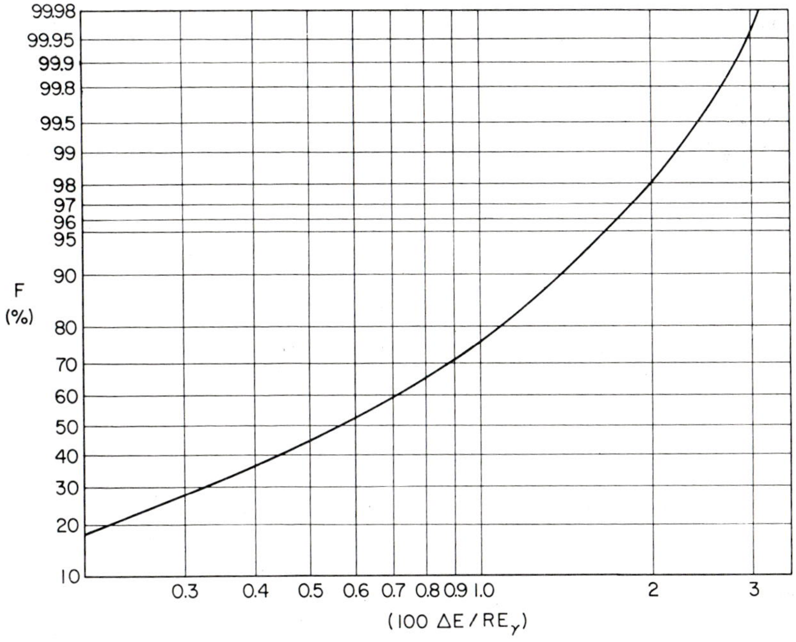

FIG. 9. Fraction, F, (percent) of the counts of the full energy photopeak that is within a preselected energy band ΔE. (E_γ is the energy of the photopeak, R its spectrometric resolution in percent.)

The intrinsic photopeak efficiencies, ϵ_p, of NaI(Tl) crystals obtained from interpolation of published data are plotted in Fig. 8 as a function of the γ-ray energy for crystal sizes between 2×2 inches and 8×4 inches.

The fraction, F, of the counts of the full energy peak, within a preselected energy interval, ΔE, symmetrical around the peak, can be easily assessed if the peak is assumed to be Gaussian in shape. Its shape can then be characterized by the line width or the spectrometric resolution, R, defined as the full width of the energy peak at half peak height in percentage of the peak energy, E_γ. In Fig. 9 F is plotted as a function of

$(100/R)(\Delta E/E_\gamma)$. It is noted that 95% of the counts of a photopeak are registered if $(100/R)(\Delta E/E_\gamma) = 1.65$. Therefore, it will be sufficient if the energy band ΔE is so selected that

$$\Delta E = 1.65 \times 10^{-2} R E_\gamma \tag{7}$$

The variation of the resolution, R, with the γ-ray energy can as a first approximation be assumed to be proportional to the inverse square root of the γ-ray energy (Chapter 6, Section IV,A). Average values of resolution data of NaI(Tl) for the ^{40}K ($E_\gamma = 1.46$ MeV) and the ^{137}Cs ($E_\gamma = 0.662$ MeV) γ rays as determined from values reported by 50 laboratories (*8*), are best represented by the following equation:

$$R = (3.35 \times 10^2)/(E_\gamma)^{1/2} \qquad \text{(percent)} \tag{8}$$

where the γ-ray energy, E_γ, is given in kiloelectron volts.

Using the above value for the resolution, R, the width of the energy interval, ΔE, follows as

$$\Delta E = 5.5(E_\gamma)^{1/2} \tag{9}$$

2. BACKGROUND COUNT-RATE

The count-rate due to radiation other than the photons of the radioisotope under consideration in the body is referred to as background count-rate. Background count-rate given for a wide energy interval (0.1 to 2.0 MeV) is designated $\overline{B}$. The background count-rate, B, within a narrow energy interval, ΔE, can be determined from $\overline{B}$ if the spectral distribution of the background pulses is known.

Two components contribute to the background count-rate. The first, B_c, is the counter background count-rate, which can be determined without a person or with a nonradioactive phantom in the counting position. It results from built-in contamination, cosmic and environmental radiation. The second, B_b, is the background count-rate due to radiation from other radioisotopes within the body besides the one under consideration.

The built-in contamination of counting equipment may differ considerably depending on the materials used, their history, and their origin. Spurious amounts of radioactivity may become significant, when low photon emission rates of the body are to be measured. A range of observed contributions to the background count-rate, $\overline{B}_c$, is given in Table II for selected low-radioactivity equipment.

Cosmic and environmental radiation constitutes the largest fraction of the background count-rate, $\overline{B}_c$, for an unshielded crystal. For the energy range of 0.1–2 MeV unshielded NaI(Tl) crystals in normal laboratory buildings have background count-rates of 10 to 50 cpm/cm^3 of crystal volume. Inside good shields the background can be reduced to

TABLE II
CONTRIBUTIONS TO THE TOTAL BACKGROUND COUNT-RATE (0.1–2 MEV) OF A 7 × 3.5 INCH NaI(Tl) CRYSTAL IN A 2-METER STEEL CUBICLE, 20 CM THICK AND LINED BY 3 MM LEAD (*8*, *12*)

Origin of radiation	Contribution to background count-rate (cpm)
Steel shield and lead lining	110–300
Multiplier phototube assembly	100–700
^{40}K in crystal	15–30
Support of crystal and patient	40–100
Radon in air	5–250[a]
Cosmic and environmental radiation	160

[a] Varies with time and weather.

0.2 to 1 cpm/cm^3 (*8*). The transmission of steel shields to photons from environmental and cosmic radiation is given in Fig. 10. The values are affected little by the size of the crystal (*16*, *27*). As shielding material, 10 cm of steel is equivalent to 5 cm of lead or 80 cm of water, if prefer-

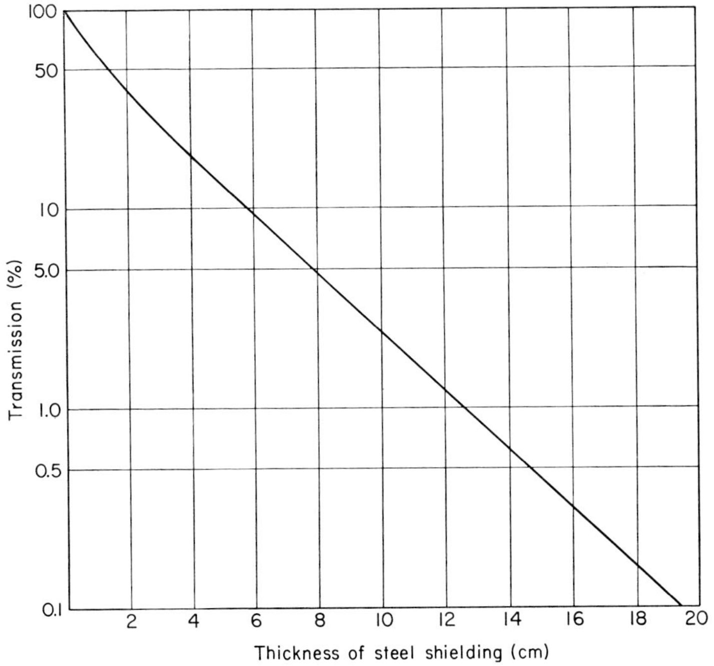

FIG. 10. Transmission of steel shields around NaI(Tl) crystals for photons of environmental and cosmic radiation within the 0.1–2 MeV energy range (*16*, *27*).

ence is given to these materials. A reduction of the background count-rate from cosmic and environmental radiation to levels comparable to those from built-in contamination requires shields with a transmission of less than 0.5%, which can be achieved by steel more than 15 cm thick.

The spectral distribution of the background radiation changes little

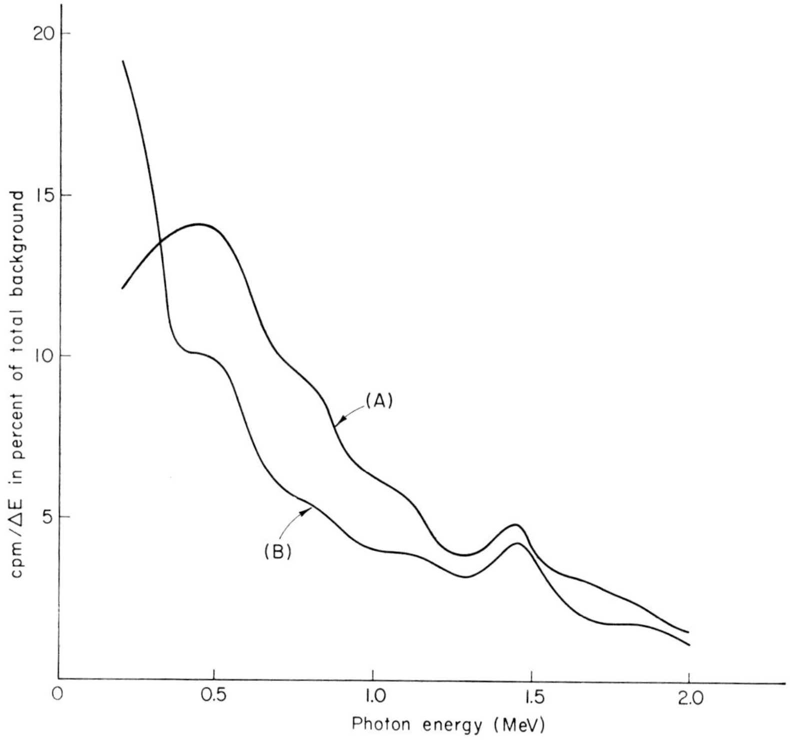

FIG. 11. Spectral distribution of the background count-rate, B_c, due to cosmic and environmental radiation and radiation from built-in contamination per energy interval $\Delta E = 5.5(E)^{1/2}$. (A) Moderate built-in contamination; background count-rate, 0.5 cpm per cubic centimeter of crystal volume. (B) Low built-in contamination and shield grading; background count-rate, 0.2 cpm per cubic centimeter of crystal volume.

with the thickness of the shield (*16*). Furthermore, it is nearly independent of the crystal size, at least below 1.3 MeV. In order to reduce the Compton scattered radiation within the shielded enclosure, its internal surfaces are lined with lead of 3 mm thickness. This reduces the intensity of the background spectrum at low energies. Figure 11 shows typical background spectra observed in steel rooms with 8-inch thick walls (*8*). Curve A refers to counters with moderate built-in contamination and Curve B refers to counters with low built-in contamination and reduced Compton scattered radiation (3 mm lead lining).

Of radioisotopes normally present in the body only ^{40}K and ^{137}Cs (Section II,A,1) contribute significantly to the photon emission. Their contribution B_b to the total background count-rate, B, in the energy interval ΔE could be assessed again from the total background count-rate to be expected within the 0.1–2 MeV energy interval and its spectral distribution. However, it is more convenient that the spectral distribution of each radioisotope is given in percentage of the count-rate of the photopeak which can be assessed from Eq. 6.

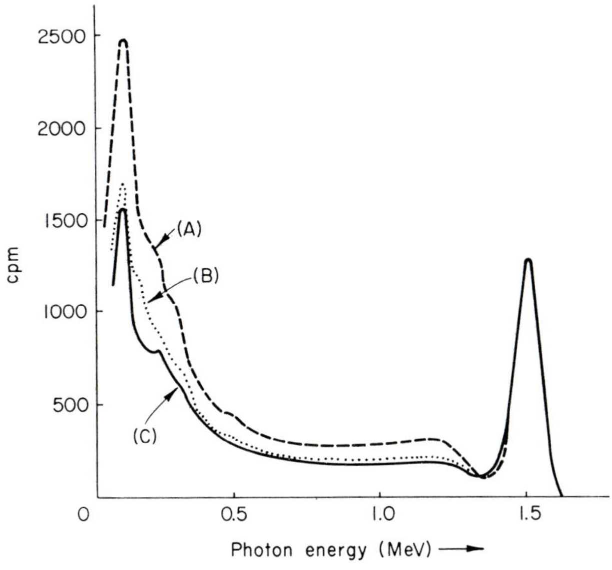

FIG. 12. Potassium-42 spectra obtained from measurements of the same patient with NaI(Tl) crystals of different sizes (*18*). (A) 4 inches in diameter, 4 inches high; (B) 9 inches in diameter, 4 inches high; (C) 11.5 inches in diameter, 4 inches high.

While the spectral distribution of the background is nearly independent of the crystal dimensions, this is not the case for spectra from radioisotopes. In Fig. 12 the net ^{42}K spectra are shown for the same patient measured with sodium iodide crystals of different diameters. The three spectra are normalized to the same area in the photopeak. The relative number of counts in the Compton region increases significantly with smaller crystals. Therefore, where crystals smaller than 8×4 inches are used, the contribution to the background count from ^{40}K and ^{137}Cs is higher at lower energies than for the large crystal, where most of the photons are completely absorbed. The contribution to the background counts from 140 gm potassium and ^{137}Cs burdens between 2.5 and 20 nCi as measured with an 8×4 inch crystal are given in Fig. 13. It was

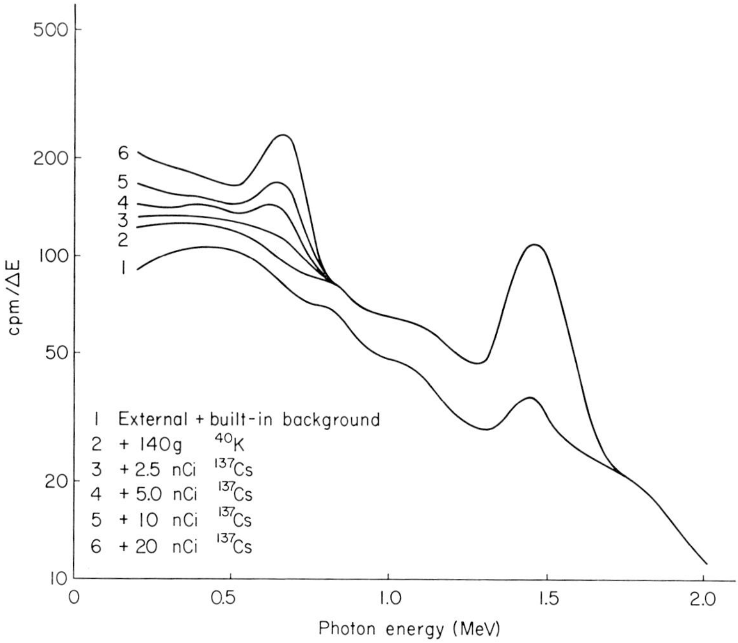

FIG. 13. Contribution to the background count-rate of an 8×4 inch NaI(Tl) crystal from cosmic and environmental radiation, radiation from built-in contamination, 140 gm potassium and ^{137}Cs burdens between 0.25 and 20 nCi [$\Delta E = 5.5(E)^{1/2}$].

assumed that the counter background (0.1–2 MeV) was 760 cpm, that its spectral distribution is that given in curve B of Fig. 11, and that the effective crystal-to-subject distance is about 45 cm.

3. DETECTION LIMIT

In addition to the errors from limitations of the detector-to-body geometry, the statistical standard deviation, σ_S, of the signal count-rate, S, limits the precision of the measurements. The standard deviation of S is given by

$$\sigma_S = \pm(100/S)[(T/t_T) + (B/t_B)]^{1/2} \quad \text{(percent)} \tag{10}$$

where $T = B + S =$ total count-rate, B is the background count-rate, and t_T and t_B are the respective counting times.

The *minimum detectable activity* is derived from the following consideration (*23*). If the total counts are different from the background counts by more than three times the standard deviation of the background counts, an effect has been observed with a 99.7% confidence level.

The probability of its being due to background count fluctuations alone is only 0.3%. The minimum detectable activity can therefore be considered that amount of activity which results in a total count that differs from the background count by three times the standard deviation of the background count. The detection limit should refer to the statistical variation of the counts attributable to radioactivity distributed in the body. For that reason the assessment of detection limits is based on the standard deviation of the body background count-rate, B_b. The value of B_b is obtained by separate measurements of the total back-

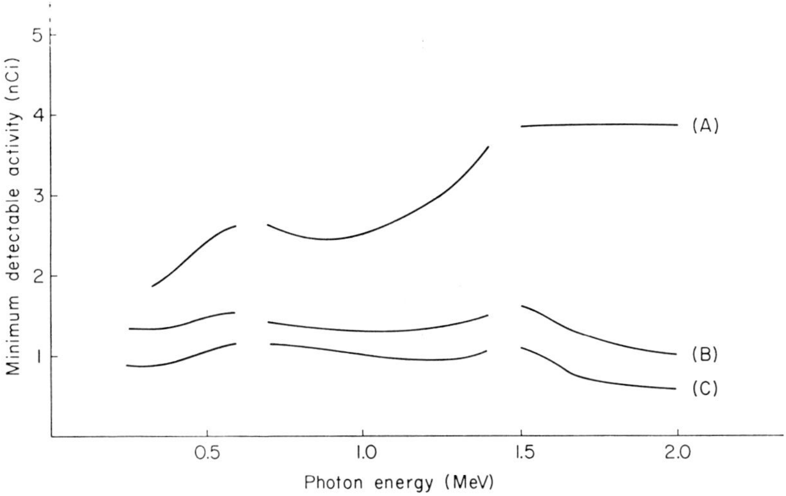

FIG. 14. Minimum detectable activity as a function of photon energy in the presence of 140 gm potassium and 10 nCi ^{137}Cs using a single NaI(Tl) crystal. The counting times are 20 min each (*14*).

(A) 4 × 4 inch crystal, $\overline{B}_c = 500$ cpm (0.1–2 MeV).
(B) 8 × 4 inch crystal, $\overline{B}_c = 2000$ cpm (0.1–2 MeV).
(C) 8 × 4 inch crystal, $\overline{B}_c = 900$ cpm (0.1–2 MeV).

ground count-rate, B, and the counter background count-rate, B_c. The standard deviation of B_b is

$$\sigma_{B_b} = [(B/t_B) + (B_c/t_c)]^{1/2} \quad \text{(cpm)} \tag{11a}$$

where t_B is the counting time of the total background (counter and body) and t_c is the counting time for the counter only. The detection limit, δ, follows then as

$$\delta = 3(A/S)[(B/t_B) + (B_c/t_c)]^{1/2} \quad (\mu\text{Ci}) \tag{11b}$$

where S/A is the signal count-rate per unit activity (counts per minute per microcurie), which is often referred to as the efficiency of the counting system.

Where low photon emission rates are to be measured t_B must be fairly long in order to achieve adequate counting statistics. In such cases it is not advisable to use significantly longer counting times for the measurement of B_c because of possible variations of B_c over extended periods. Therefore it appears reasonable that for purposes of design it is assumed that $t_B = t_c = t$, so that

$$\delta = 3(A/S)[(B_b + 2B_c)/t]^{1/2} \quad (\mu\text{Ci}) \tag{12}$$

If the characteristics of the background spectra (counter background and body background), the counting efficiency as a function of photon energy and the counting times are known, then the minimum detectable activity as a function of the photon energy can be assessed. The values given in Fig. 14 (*14*) apply to two crystal sizes (4 × 4 inches and 8 × 4 inches) under the following conditions:

(i) the radioisotope under consideration emits γ rays of one energy only;
(ii) one photon is emitted per disintegration of the radioisotope ($\eta = 1$);
(iii) apart from the radioisotope in question, the body contains 140 gm potassium and 10 nCi ^{137}Cs;
(iv) B and B_c are each measured for a period of 20 min ($t_B = t_c = t = 20$);
(v) the effective detector-to-body distance, D_e, is about 45 cm.

Because it is impossible to distinguish between an increased ^{137}Cs or potassium content and a small amount of a contaminant emitting photons of an energy close to 662 keV or 1.46 MeV, respectively, the curves have breaks at these energies. The effect of an increased background on the detection limit is small, as shown by the two lower curves. The advantage of large crystals over small ones is well demonstrated. The use of several small crystals reduces the detection limit by about $\sqrt{n}$, where n is the number of crystals.

III. PERFORMANCE OF SINGLE AND MULTIPLE NaI(Tl) DETECTOR SYSTEMS

It is advisable for technical as well as economic reasons that the range of photon emission rates which are to be measured by any one counter is limited to about four decades. Therefore different types of counters are designed for measurement of high, intermediate, and low photon emission rates.

A. High Photon Emission Rates

The design of an adequate counting system is a minor problem, where such high photon emission rates as defined in Section II,A,1 are to be measured. The detector-to-body distance can be made so large that the sensitivity is nearly uniform over the full length of the body. The patient may lie on a stretcher close to the floor and can be measured in supine and where necessary also in prone position. This permits averaging of differences in self-absorption by body tissue. In order to keep the background count-rate stable and within reasonable limits, moderate collimation of the detector is indicated. In addition, control of movement and use of large radiation sources in the environment during the measurements is necessary.

An illustration of a whole-body counter designed for purposes of radioisotope-therapy control is shown in Fig. 15. The detector-to-body

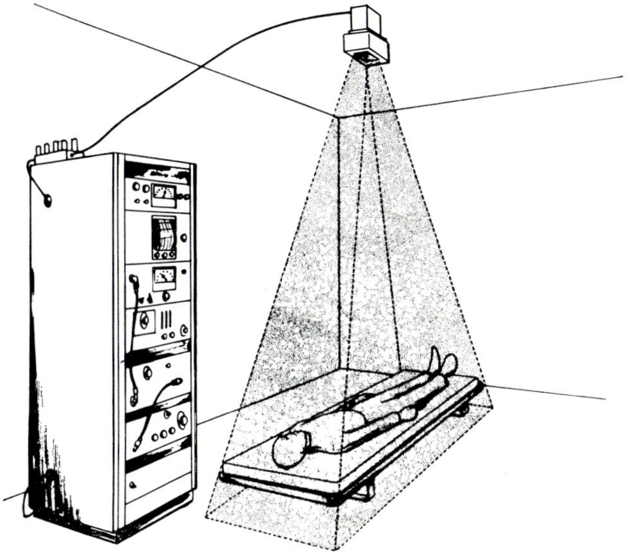

FIG. 15. Single-crystal stretcher geometry with moderate collimation for the measurement of high photon emission rates (*22*).

distance is about 2.5 meters. The detector is a 2×2 inch NaI(Tl) crystal mounted in a collimator viewing the bed. A curved lead attenuator, which passes only 10% of the 364-keV ^{131}I γ rays, is used when the count-rates become too high for the electronics system ($>$ 10 mCi). For ^{131}I within an activity range of about 50 μCi to 150 mCi a 1-min counting time is routine, while with a 10-min counting time reasonable counting statistics down to 10 μCi are obtained.

B. Intermediate Photon Emission Rates

With moderate room shielding and a larger crystal the geometry described above (Section III,A) could also be used for counting intermediate photon emission rates, as defined in Section II,A,1. However, a reduction of the detector-to-body distance is more economical. If instead of the 2.5 meter single-crystal stretcher geometry a 1-meter arc technique is applied, the sensitivity is increased by a factor of 6. This is insufficient where only small crystals are available. Therefore a chair geometry (Section II,B,1,a) is often used (Fig. 16). The effective de-

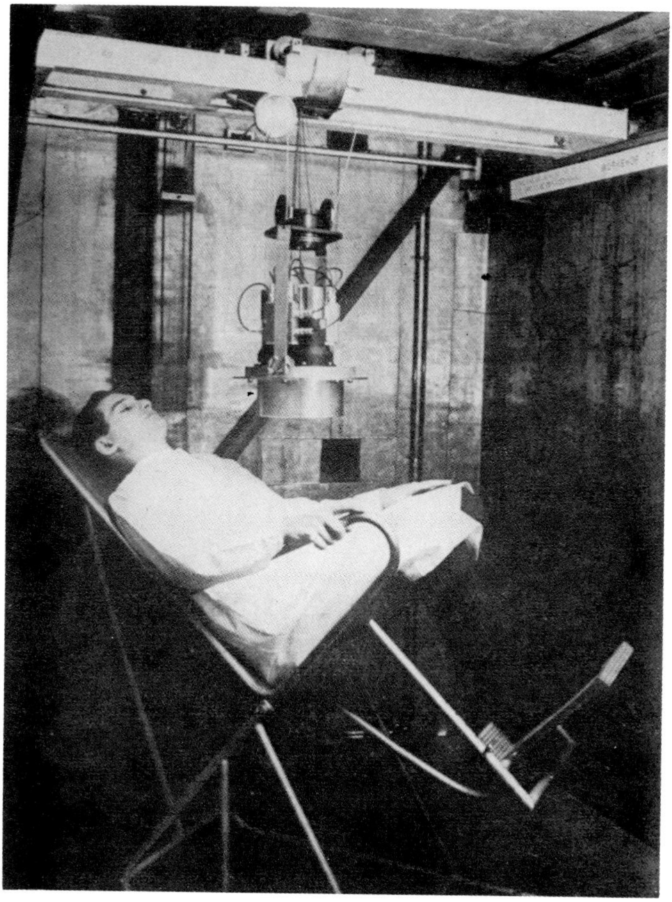

FIG. 16. Subject in tilted chair geometry. (Courtesy of International Atomic Energy Agency, Vienna)

tector-to-body distance is thereby reduced to about 45 cm, which increases the sensitivity of the 2.5-meter stretcher geometry by a factor of about 25. A serious disadvantage of chair geometries is their nonuniformity of response to radioactivity in different parts of the body (Fig. 3). Therefore, redistribution of radioactivity may cause serious errors in the interpretation of the results.

Recently multiple detector-stretcher geometries, and single-crystal moving systems have been preferred. A four-crystal stretcher geometry with a trough shielding is shown in Fig. 17. The crystals at the bottom of the lead trough view the entire length of the body through a radiolucent stretcher which can be wheeled over the shield-detector assembly. If equipped with four 3×3 inch crystals the system is more than a hundred times as sensitive as the high-level counter (Fig. 15). It operates most usefully in the 0.1- to 100-μCi range (*21*).

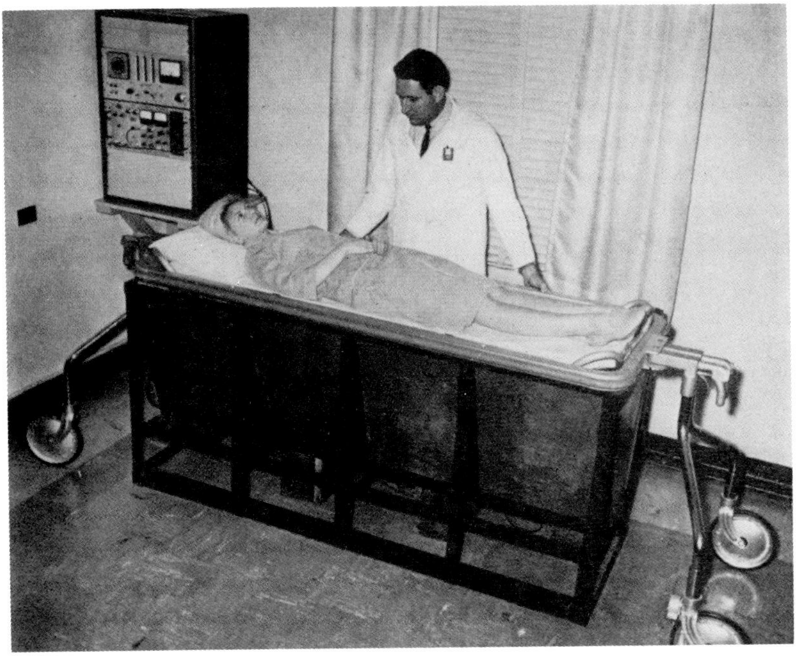

FIG. 17. Four-crystal stretcher geometry with lead trough shield for the measurement of intermediate photon emission rates (*21*).

A single-crystal moving system is shown in Fig. 18. Instead of a complete enclosure by room shielding, a *shadow shield* is used. It consists of a collimating shield placed around the detector and a large shield behind the subject, so shaped as to cast a shadow over the area viewed by the crystal. The background spectrum of a completely closed room shield of the same material and thickness is compared in Fig. 19 with the background spectrum obtained with the shadow shield of Fig. 18. For all practical purposes, they are identical.

C. Low Photon Emission Rates

Technical data and illustrations of whole-body counters for the measurement of low photon emission rates have been compiled recently (*8*).

Low-level whole-body counters differ from those designed for intermediate photon emission rates by larger crystals and heavier shielding.

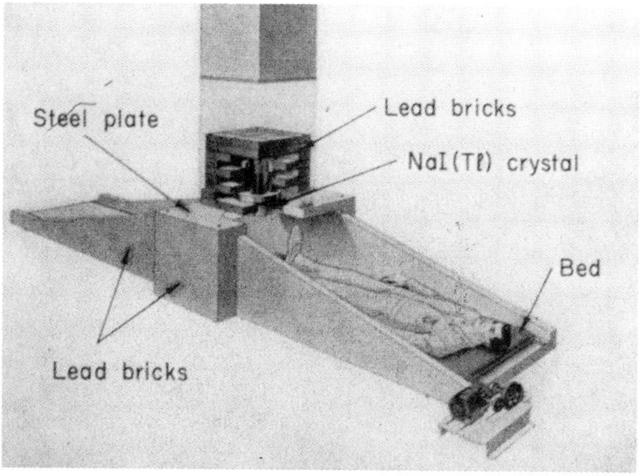

FIG. 18. Single-crystal moving system with shadow shield (*25*).

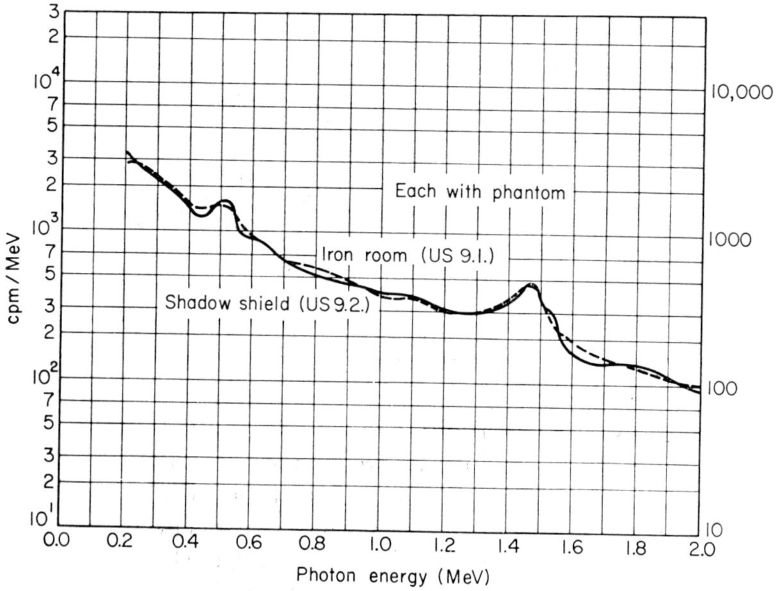

FIG. 19. Comparison of background spectra of a 9⅜ × 4 inch crystal in a shadow shield and in a steel room with walls 25 cm thick (*8*).

Most are equipped with a single 8 × 4 inch crystal, though up to six crystals and a total crystal volume of 10^4 cm^3 are used. The geometries are the same as those for the measurement of intermediate photon emission rates. The present trend of development is toward single- and multiple-detector moving systems (*7*).

Massive room shielding is inevitable for the measurement of photon energies below 300 keV. Preference is given to steel and lead. Water is seldom used, mainly because laboratory space is normally limited. If possible pre-1945 steel is used. Otherwise premonitoring of steel samples is required for checking of contamination by ^{60}Co and fallout products. Surface contamination from fallout products must be removed before assembly. Since magnetic fields can affect the operation of multiplier phototubes, the steel must be kept away from strong magnetic fields such as used by magnetic cranes. A detailed description of the construction of a room made from steel sheets is given by Miller *et al.* (*19*). With steel walls 10 to 20 cm thick or lead walls 5 to 10 cm thick, background count-rates in the 0.1–2.0 MeV energy range have been reported between about 0.2 and 1 cpm per cubic centimeter of crystal volume, with most of the values below 0.5 cpm per cubic centimeter (*8*).

Special consideration must be given to the ventilation of low-background enclosures. Frequently forced ventilation with 5–30 changes per hour is used. This provides fresh air for the occupant and also reduces the accumulation of radon daughter products which can significantly contribute to the background. In general, the air is filtered by absolute filters, to reduce contamination by particulate airborne radioactivity, which includes radon daughter products on dust. Several counting rooms are equipped with aged air systems and (or) closed air circuits for use when gaseous radionuclides contribute significantly to the background radiation. The contribution of airborne radioactivity increases with the volume of the room, which is mostly in the range of 6–10 cubic meters.

IV. CALIBRATION OF SINGLE AND MULTIPLE NaI(Tl) DETECTOR SYSTEMS

The formulas given in Section II for the design of whole-body counters are based on a number of assumptions. The accuracies of the photon emission rates of the body, the counting efficiencies of the crystals, and the characteristics of the counting geometry of a particular system as calculated from these formulas are therefore limited. A more accurate determination of the detector response to the body radioactivity is obtained from calibration procedures.

A. Effects of Angle of Radiation Incidence

The effect of the angle of radiation incidence with respect to the crystal axis on the resolution and counting efficiency has been investigated with point sources of different γ-ray energies (0.12–1.3 MeV) and crystal sizes up to 8 × 4 inches (*3, 13, 24*). For angles between 0° and 45° the photopeak counting efficiency decreases by not more than 15% for 1.3-MeV photons and does not increase by more than 15% for 120 keV photons, provided that the crystal is uncollimated. For 0.6-MeV photons the photopeak efficiency varies very little with the angle of incidence and the spectrometric resolution changes by less than 10% with 5 × 4 inch crystals (*24*). These effects may be important where the counting geometry requires a wide solid angle, such as in stationary single-crystal geometries with small detector-to-body distances. In moving systems or multiple-crystal stationary systems the effect is less important.

B. Effect of Body Mass on the Counter Background

The background count-rate is affected by the mass of the body in the counting position. If no or only moderate shielding is applied the overall (0.1–2.0 MeV) background count-rate is reduced by the absorption of background radiation in the body. With heavy shielding an increase of the overall background count-rate may be observed from background radiation scattered by the body. The effect decreases with increasing detector-to-body distances and increases with body mass. The increase of the background count-rate (0.1–2.0 MeV) is normally less than 7%. In the energy interval between 100 and 150 keV an increase of up to 20% has been observed with a 5 × 4 inch crystal and up to 50% with a 4 × 0.2 inch crystal (*1, 9*).

Phantoms used for these investigations should be "nonradioactive" and the effective atomic number of the phantom should be similar to that of body tissue. Preference is given to sugar phantoms, though phantoms consisting of distilled water in a set of bottles such as described below are also used.

C. Effect of Body Mass on the Counting Efficiency

The counting efficiency is often defined as the ratio of the number of counts registered in the photopeak to the number of photons of energy E_γ emitted by an isotope in the body. The reciprocal value is, in general, referred to as the calibration factor of the system. The counting efficiency as a function of photon energy shows a maximum at about 200 keV. At lower energies the efficiency decreases because of absorption of photons in the body and crystal housing. At higher energies the photopeak efficiency decreases owing to Compton interactions of the photons in the crystal. The counting efficiency versus photon energy for a single 8 × 4 inch crystal chair geometry is given in Fig. 20. The values depend largely on the detector-to-subject geometry and cannot be generalized.

The effect of body weight and shape on the counting efficiency depends largely on the particular counting system. In most counting systems a decrease of the counting efficiency is observed with increasing body weight per unit body height. An increase may also be observed if the effective detector-to-body distance decreases significantly with increasing body weight per unit body height and if the photon energy is sufficiently high to minimize photon absorption.

Attempts have been made to correlate the variation of counting efficiency with a parameter often referred to as the *effective body thickness*. It is assessed from absorption measurements with point sources

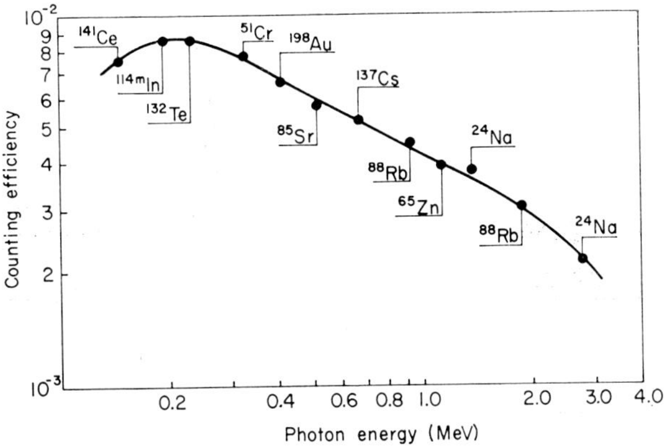

FIG. 20. Counting efficiency of a single-crystal chair system as a function of photon energy (*2*).

behind the subject at various positions such as shoulder, hip, and knees (*4, 6*). Another method is based on matching the shape of the spectrum from the *in vivo* measurement of the subject, with that of a point source at a position equivalent to the body center, by varying the thickness of phantom material in front of and behind the source (*17*). However, since these methods are laborious and time consuming, they are not very suitable for routine measurements of a large number of persons of different body build.

Correction factors for different body builds have been derived. It has been found (*15*) that the effective body thickness, t, can be calculated as

$$t = \text{const } (W/H)^{1/2}$$

where W is the body weight (kilograms) and H the body height (centimeters). Correction curves for the counting efficiency for different body weights and heights have been published for a single-crystal chair system (*15*), a four-crystal stretcher system (*30*), and single-crystal arc and chair systems, as well as single-crystal moving systems (*5*).

For a limited number of radioisotopes the counting efficiency of the system can be determined from *in vivo* measurements (Section IV,D); otherwise the use of phantoms is required. Such phantoms must be sufficiently realistic with respect to the particular counting geometry. If the detector-to-body distance exceeds about 45 cm, or, if the 4π geometry is applied, the phantoms may be composed of ordinary polythene bottles filled with solutions of the radioisotope (*26, 33*). More realistic phan-

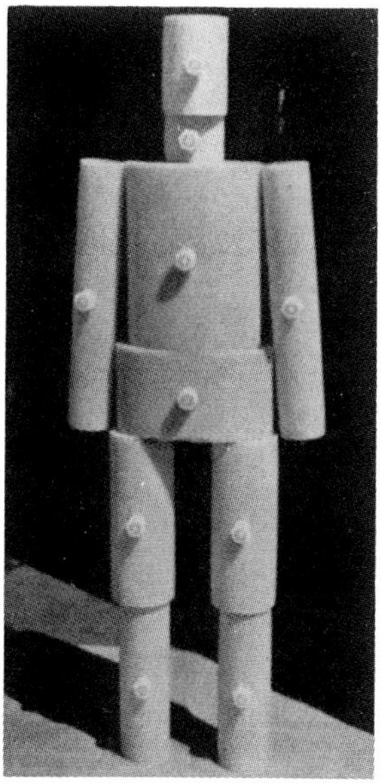

FIG. 21. Phantom of a 70-kg, 170-cm man composed of containers with elliptical and cylindrical cross section. (Grey and Marten Ltd.)

toms are used (Fig. 21) where shorter detector-to-body distances are applied (*28, 31*). A very realistic phantom of an adult (73.5 kg, 175 cm) is the "Remcal" manikin.* The plastic body shell contains hollow plastic models of the major organs, such as lungs, liver, stomach, heart, spleen, kidneys, urinary bladder, and so forth. Naturally, the costs of phantoms increase the more refined they are. In general, sufficiently accurate information can be obtained from phantoms which represent the major sections of the body, such as head, neck, chest, hip, arms, thighs, and legs.

* Alderson Research Laboratories Inc.

D. Effects of Distribution of the Body Radioactivity on the Counting Efficiency

Whole-body counters should be so designed as to minimize variations of the counting efficiency with changes of the distribution of the radioactivity. This cannot be achieved to such a degree that variations in distribution can be ignored. Count-rates measured after administration of a radioisotope and corrected for radioactive decay and excretion vary with time until the distribution of the radioactivity is rather stable. This is caused by changes of the photon emission rate and the photon spectrum, by differences in photon absorption and scattering, and by changes of the effective counting distance.

In order to prevent errors from redistribution effects, that time has been determined when an equilibrium distribution has been reached. This is done either by checking variations of the count-rate profile over the length of the body as a function of time (preferably by scanning with a slit collimator), or by observing any changes in the photon spectrum, such as variations of the peak-to-valley ratios.

The administration of a known amount of radioactivity to volunteers or patients for purposes of instrument calibration is of course restricted to radioisotopes of short physical and (or) biological half-life, so that the radiation dose to the subject is minimal. For natural potassium the *in vivo* calibration method would only be applicable if potassium suitably enriched with ^{40}K were available. The effective half-life of ^{137}Cs is too long to permit its application for *in vivo* calibrations. However, in these cases it is possible to use other radioisotopes of the respective elements with short effective half-lives, which emit photons of about the same energy as the radioisotope for which the calibration is required. For ^{40}K calibrations it is preferable to use ^{42}K ($E_\gamma = 1.51$ MeV, $T = 12.4$ hours) (*10, 18, 29*) and for ^{137}Cs calibrations, ^{132}Cs ($E_\gamma = 0.669$ MeV, $T = 6.2$ days) (*5, 30*).

The efficiency of counters as a function of radioactivity distribution has been determined with point sources in phantoms (*3, 5, 21, 28*). From the results of such measurements, the response of counter systems were computed for sources evenly distributed throughout distinct body compartments and the body as a whole.

A comparison of whole-body counter calibrations obtained from *in vivo* measurements, phantom measurements, and computer calculations have shown a remarkable agreement of the results (*5*). This verifies the reliability of whole-body counter measurements.

REFERENCES

1. Bengtsson, L. G., Human beta bremsstrahlung detection by means of thin and thick sodium iodide crystals. *Proc. Symp. Assessment Radioactivity Man, Heidelberg, 1964* Vol. I, p. 91. Intern. At. Energy Agency, Vienna, 1964.

2. Boulenger, R. R., Colard, J. F., and Henry, J., Compteur Humain total du CEN à Mol. *Proc. Symp. Whole-Body Counting, Vienna, 1961* p. 309. Intern. At. Energy Agency, Vienna, 1962.
3. Chabra, A. S., An improved whole-body counting geometry with a single NaI(Tl) detector (8 × 4 inches). *Radiology* **82,** 816 (1964).
4. Clark, S. D., Dudley, R. A., Kuchta, D. R., Shanahan, M. M., Tavla, M., and Visacci, F. I., Radium and mesothorium toxicity in human beings. *In* "Radium and Mesothorium Poisoning and Dosimetry and Instrumentation Techniques in Applied Radioactivity" (R. D. Evans, ed.), M.I.T. Ann. Progr. Rept. AECU-4285, p. 1 (1959).
5. Dudley, R. A., and Ben Haim, A., Calibration problems in whole-body counting with NaI(Tl) detectors. *Proc. Panel, Clin. Uses Whole-Body Counting, Vienna, 1965* p. 92. Intern. At. Energy Agency, Vienna, 1966.
6. Evans, R. D., Radium poisoning, II. Quantitative determination of radium content and radium elimination rate of living persons. *Am. J. Roentgenol. Radium Therapy* **37,** 368 (1937).
7. International Atomic Energy Agency, *Proc. Panel, Clin. Uses Whole-Body Counting, Vienna, 1965.* Intern. At. Energy Agency, Vienna, 1966.
8. International Atomic Energy Agency, "Directory of Whole-Body Radioactivity Monitors." Intern. At. Energy Agency, Vienna, 1964.
9. Lidén, K. V. H., and McCall, R. C., Low-energy-photon detectors for whole-body counting. *Proc. Symp. Whole-Body Counting, Vienna, 1961* p. 145. Intern. At. Energy Agency, Vienna, 1962.
10. McNeill, K. G., and Green, R. M., Measurements with a whole-body counter. *Can. J. Phys.* **37,** 683 (1959).
11. Malamos, B., Belcher, E. H., Binopoulos, D., and Constantinides, C., The use of whole-body counting techniques in clinical studies with ^{59}Fe, ^{22}Na, ^{82}Br, ^{58}Co-labelled vitamin B_{12} and ^{131}I-labelled albumin. *Proc. Symp. Whole-Body Counting, Vienna, 1961* p. 435. Intern. At. Energy Agency, Vienna, 1962.
12. Marinelli, L. D., Miller, C. E., May, H. A., and Rose, J. E., Low-level gamma-ray scintillation spectrometry: experimental requirements and biomedical applications. *Advan. Biol. Med. Phys.* **8,** 81 (1962).
13. May, H. A., Angular response of scintillation detectors. Argonne National Laboratory, Radiological Physics Division Semiannual Report, July through December, 1960. Rept. ANL-6297, p. 30 (1961).
14. Mehl, H. G., and Rundo, J., Preliminary results of a world survey of whole-body monitors. *Health Phys.* **9,** 607 (1963).
15. Meneely, G. R., Rolf, H. L., Weiland, R. L., Heyssel, R. M., and Lagemann, R. T., The use of computers in whole-body counter data processing. *Proc. Symp. Whole-Body Counting, Vienna, 1961* p. 379. Intern. At. Energy Agency, Vienna, 1962.
16. Miller, C. E., The human spectrometer. Argonne National Laboratory, Radiological Physics Division Semiannual Report July through December 1957. Rept. ANL-5829, p. 114 (1958).
17. Miller, C. E., Low-intensity spectrometry of gamma radiation emitted by human beings. *Proc. 2nd Intern. Conf. Peaceful Uses At. Energy, Geneva, 1958* Vol. 23, p. 113. United Nations, New York, 1958.
18. Miller, C. E., An experimental evaluation of multiple-crystal arrays and single-crystal techniques. *Proc. Symp. Whole-Body Counting, Vienna, 1961* p. 81. Intern. At. Energy Agency, Vienna, 1962.

19. Miller, C. E., Marinelli, L. D., Rowland, R. E., and Rose, J. E., Reduction of NaI background. *Nucleonics* **14,** No. 4, 40 (1956).
20. Miller, W. F., Reynolds, J., and Snow, W. J., Efficiencies and photofractions for gamma radiation on sodium iodide crystals. Argonne National Laboratory Rept. ANL-5902 (1958).
21. Morris, A. C., Jr., A diagnostic-level whole-body counter. *J. Nucl. Med.* **6,** 481 (1965).
22. Morris, A. C., Jr., Ross, D. A., and Travis, J. C., A high-level whole-body counter. *Intern. J. Appl. Radiation Isotopes* **15,** 391 (1964).
23. National Commission of Radiation Protection, A Manual of Radioactivity Procedures. Recommendations of the National Committee on Radiation Protection and Measurements. Report No. 28. *Natl. Bur. Std.* (*U.S.*) *Handbook* **80** (1961).
24. Naversten, Y., A two-crystal scanning-bed counter for accurate determination of whole-body activity. *Proc. Symp. Assessment Radioactivity Man, Heidelberg, 1964* Vol. I, p. 55. Intern. At. Energy Agency, Vienna, 1964.
25. Palmer, H. E., and Roesch, W. C., A shadow shield whole-body counter. *Health Phys.* **11,** 1213 (1965).
26. Percival, D. R., and Anderson, J. I., Whole-body counting. Idaho Operation Office, USAEC, Rept. IDO-12021, p. 39 (1962).
27. Rasmussen, N. C., Bulkley, J. B., Harman, G. J., and Beique, R. A., Low γ-ray background enclosure. *In* "Radium and Mesothorium Poisoning and Dosimetry and Instrumentation Techniques in Applied Radioactivity" (R. D. Evans, ed.), M.I.T. Ann. Progr. Rept. AECU-3504, p. 36 (1957).
28. Rundo, J., Body radioactivity measurements as an aid in assessing contamination by radionuclides. *Proc. 2nd. Intern. Conf. Peaceful Uses At. Energy, Geneva, 1958,* Vol. 23, p. 101. United Nations, New York, 1959.
29. Rundo, J., Some calibration problems of whole-body gamma-ray spectrometers. *Proc. Symp. Whole-Body Counting, Vienna, 1961* p. 121. Intern. At. Energy Agency, Vienna, 1962.
30. Rundo, J., and Taylor, B. T., The assessment of radioactive caesium in man. *Proc. Symp. Assessment Radioactivity Man, Heidelberg, 1964* Vol. II, p. 3. Intern. At. Energy Agency, Vienna, 1964.
31. Suguri, S., Measurements with a whole-body counter. *Proc. Symp. Whole-Body Counting, Vienna, 1961* p. 219. Intern. At. Energy Agency, Vienna, 1962.
32. Vegors, S. H., Jr., Marsden, L. L., and Heath, R. L., Calculated efficiencies of cylindrical radiation detectors. Idaho Operation Office, USAEC, Rept. IDO-16370 (1958).
33. Woodward, K. T., Randolph, E. L., Jr., Van Hock, R., Hartgering, J. B., Claypool, H. A., Manskey, A. A., Jr., and Noble, J. J., The Walter Reed whole-body counter facility. U.S. Army Medical Research and Development Command, Washington, D.C., 1960.

CHAPTER 21

LARGE ORGANIC SCINTILLATION DETECTORS

MARVIN A. VAN DILLA, ERNEST C. ANDERSON,
CHESTER R. RICHMOND
LOS ALAMOS SCIENTIFIC LABORATORY
UNIVERSITY OF CALIFORNIA
LOS ALAMOS, NEW MEXICO
AND
ROBERT L. SCHUCH
UNIVERSITY OF CALIFORNIA AT SAN DIEGO
LA JOLLA, CALIFORNIA

I. LIQUID AND PLASTIC SCINTILLATORS

Large counters using liquid and plastic scintillators include three sizes: (1) counters for human adult subjects; (2) intermediate counters for dogs and babies; and (3) small animal counters for rats, mice, and biological samples. Only (1) and (3) will be discussed, and examples will be chosen largely from the liquid scintillation counters developed at Los Alamos. Much of the discussion is directly applicable to any organic scintillator, including those for cattle and food samples. The organic scintillators (Chapter 9) differ from the inorganic scintillators (Chapter 6) in that their density is close to unity and their average atomic number is low, about 6. They are available in much larger sizes and a very wide variety of shapes. Thus, for large samples, the organic scintillator offers the advantages of much higher counting efficiency and of a considerable degree of independence of sample size, shape, and position at the cost of some, but not all, of the energy resolution of the sodium iodide crystal. The organic scintillator is, therefore, the method of choice when the γ-ray spectrum of the sample is comparatively simple and a high degree of counting precision is desired, or when large numbers of very low-level samples must be measured in minimum time. The sodium iodide system is indicated when complex spectra are to be analyzed or when the location of the activity within the sample is to be accurately determined.

A quantitative example of the advantage of high counting efficiency is the measurement of natural potassium (^{40}K) in people by means of its 1.46-MeV γ-ray emission. This can be done at our laboratory with two counters: a liquid scintillator (Humco II, described in Section III) and a 9×6 inch sodium iodide spectrometer. The efficiency, background, and counting time necessary for 2.3% statistical precision on a 70-kg subject containing 150 gm potassium are shown in Table I. With the liquid scintillator, only one-tenth the counting time is needed, clearly a substantial advantage.

TABLE I

NATURAL POTASSIUM MEASUREMENTS WITH TWO TYPES OF WHOLE-BODY COUNTERS

	Cpm per 150 gm K	Background (cpm)	Time for $\sigma = 2.3\%$ (min)
Humco II	5400	22,000	$3\frac{1}{3}$
9×6 inch NaI(Tl)	180	210	35

Liquid and plastic scintillators have practically the same density, average atomic number, and quantum efficiency. Actual counter design, however, depends on which is used. The size of plastic blocks is limited to the order of a cubic foot, whereas much larger liquid scintillators are practical. The cost of liquid scintillators is lower, although containment problems lessen the difference. Containers for liquids have to be leakproof; this is a soluble engineering problem but it is easier for plastics. Reflectors with maximum reflectivity (such as MgO powder) can be used around plastics; less efficient reflectors are used with liquids because of their high index of refraction. Liquid scintillators are more transparent to their own fluorescence. With currently used liquid scintillators or plastics, no fire hazard exists while early solvents like toluene were highly inflammable.

Human counters using liquid scintillators tend to be 2π or 4π systems viewed by an array of large-area multiplier phototubes (*20*). They subtend a solid angle of 2π or 4π steradians about the subject corresponding to 50 or 100% geometrical efficiency, respectively. The same instrument made with plastic scintillators tends to be a collection of blocks arranged about the subject in 2π geometry or less (*3*).

The world distribution of both types of human counters is given in Table II. Details of performance for most of these counters have not yet been published. Counting efficiency would be expected to drop with decreasing geometry. This seems to be the case for the Leeds counter and the Japan Atomic Energy Research Institute counter. Both have somewhat less than 2π geometry. Their responses are 1200 and 960 cpm, respectively, for an adult containing 150 gm K, in contrast to 5400 cpm for Humco II with almost 4π geometry. Energy resolution should be about the same for all of these counters, and is in the range 25 to 35% for the Los Alamos and Leeds counters for ^{40}K γ rays.

II. γ-RAY ABSORPTION IN LOW-Z DETECTORS

The energy deposition spectrum of organic scintillators is largely determined by the Compton process (*9*). If the detector is small (linear dimensions of the order of centimeters), a scattered γ ray escapes and a continuous spectrum of secondary electrons is produced. If the detector is large (of the order of 1 meter), multiple scatter followed by eventual photoelectric absorption of the degraded photons occurs, giving rise to a line spectrum.

The exact calculation of the interactions of γ rays with a large absorbing mass is very difficult because of the complex series of events which occurs and because an analytic expression cannot be written for the spectrum following multiple scattering. Satisfactory solutions can be obtained on large electronic computers using a technique known as the Monte Carlo method (*20, 22*). This method makes use of the laws of chance to select typical scattering events in the proper proportion. A large number (of the order of thousands) of such events are calculated, and the average of the calculations is the theoretical prediction for a physical experiment. The accuracy of the method is determined by the precision with which the fundamental events are mirrored in the calculation model and the number of calculations that it is feasible to perform. The results of such a Monte Carlo calculation (histogram) for the case of ^{137}Cs γ rays incident on a small (volume about 1 cm^3) xylene scintillator are compared in Fig. 1 with the Klein–Nishina analytic function (smooth curve), which is applicable in this case since more than one scattering event is improbable in such a small volume.

TABLE II

HUMAN COUNTERS USING ORGANIC SCINTILLATORS (1964)

Location	Type	Builder[a]	Scintillator[b]	Shield
Los Alamos Sci. Lab., New Mexico	4π Liquid	LASL	1800 Liters TS-28 with PPO + POPOP	Steel room (7-inch armor plate)
Army Med. Res. Unit Europe, Landstuhl, Germany	2π Liquid	LASL	280 Liters TEB with ϕ_3 + POPOP	3-Inch lead baffle
Walter Reed Army Inst. of Res., Washington, D. C.	4π Liquid	D	600 Liters HF with ϕ_3 + POPOP	5-Inch steel cylinder
Purdue Univ., Lafayette, Indiana	4π Liquid	M, P	560 Liters HF with PPO + POPOP	6-Inch steel room
Cornell Univ., Ithaca, New York	2π Liquid	M	280 Liters TS-28 with PPO + POPOP	6-Inch steel room
Univ. Rochester, New York (for babies)	4π Plastic	M	167 Liters	5- to 8-Inch lead shot
Univ. Illinois, Urbana, Illinois	4π Liquid	M	560 Liters TS-28 with PPO + POPOP	5-Inch mild steel
Univ. Hamburg, Hamburg, Germany	4π Liquid (modular)	P	1600 Liters HF with ϕ_3 + POPOP	5-Inch steel room
Univ. Leeds, Leeds, England	3 Plastic blocks	Univ. Leeds	NE-101	Steel room (five $\frac{1}{2}$-inch steel plates)
Dept. National Health and Welfare, Ottawa, Canada	4 Plastic blocks	NE	NE-102	Steel room (8 inches thick)
Japan Atomic Energy Res. Inst., Tokai-Mura, Japan	9 Plastic blocks	—	—	Steel room (8 inches + 3-mm lead)
Natl. Inst. Rad. Sci., Chiba, Japan	8 Plastic blocks	MAPI	National Scinti-light, MEW	Steel room (6-inch iron + 3-mm lead + 3-mm Lucite)
Natl. Inst. Health, Bethesda, Maryland	18 Plastic blocks	RCL, D	Plastic	Steel room ($6\frac{1}{4}$ inches thick)

NOTE: See footnotes on facing page.

[a] Builders:

D	=	Dixie Mfg. Company, Baltimore, Maryland.
LASL	=	Los Alamos Scientific Laboratory, Los Alamos, New Mexico.
M	=	Metrix, Inc., Deerfield, Illinois.
NE	=	Nuclear Enterprises, Edinburgh.
P	=	Packard Instrument Company, Downers Grove, Ill.
RCL	=	Radiation Counter Laboratories, Skokie, Illinois.
MAPI	=	Mitsubishi Atomic Power Industries, Inc., Tokyo, Japan.

[b] Scintillators:

ϕ_3	=	terphenyl.
PPO	=	diphenyloxazole.
αNPO	=	α-naphthylphenyloxazole.
POPOP	=	phenylenebis(phenyloxazole).
TEB	=	triethylbenzene.
TS-28	=	Shell Oil commercial paint solvent.
HF	=	Arapahoe commercial scintillation solvent.
NE-101, 102	=	Nuclear Enterprises commercial plastic scintillators.
Pilot-B	=	Pilot Chemicals commercial plastic scintillator.
MEW	=	Matsushita Electric Works, Ltd., Osaka, Japan.

The agreement is excellent. It is interesting that the code indicates that in about 1% of the cases multiple scatter will occur, giving rise to pulses with energy greater than the maximum for single scattering.

As the scintillation detector is made larger, multiple scattering becomes more probable, and the spectrum becomes more complicated. Figure 2 shows the results of the Monte Carlo calculation for a test tank detector 15.5 inches in diameter and 11 inches thick in comparison with experimental results. There is a great deal of single and double scattering as evidenced by the double peak in the computed Compton spectrum. The energy of the first peak corresponds to 478 keV, the maximum energy that can be transferred in a single collision of the incident 662-keV γ rays. The scattered γ ray from this interaction has an energy of 184 keV so that the maximum energy transfer in a second backscatter is 77 keV, giving a total maximum of 545 keV for the double scattering maximum. This corresponds closely to the energy of the second peak.

A small amount of photoelectric absorption, amounting to about 3.3% of the total interactions, occurs in a detector of this size. In order to compare this calculated energy spectrum with that observed experimentally, it is necessary to broaden the computed spectrum to allow for statistical effects. These include fluctuations in number of scintillation photons produced per million electron volts deposited and in the number of photoelectrons and the multiplication factor in the multiplier phototube, variations in photocathode sensitivity, variations in light collection efficiency from various parts of the scintillator, and nonlinearity of

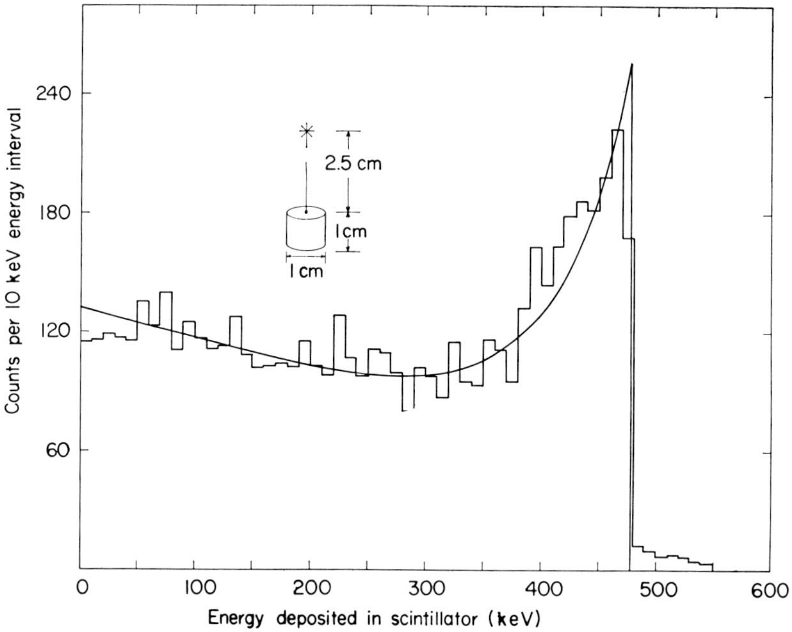

FIG. 1. Spectrum produced by 0.66-MeV ^{137}Cs γ rays incident on small liquid scintillator of about 1-cm^3 volume. Histogram, Zerby–Moran code prediction unbroadened; smooth curve; Klein–Nishina formula.

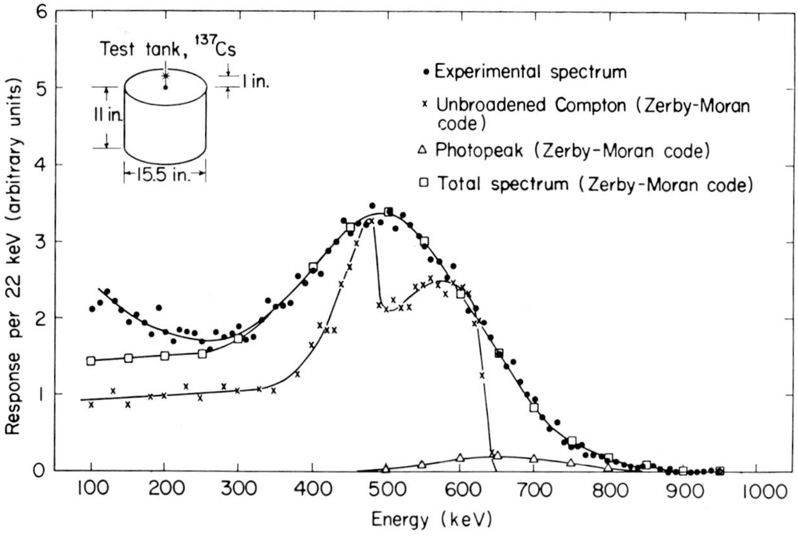

FIG. 2. Spectrum produced by 0.66-MeV γ rays incident on test tank; experimental result compared with Zerby–Moran code prediction.

scintillator (light output not strictly proportional to energy but depending on the details of energy deposition). While the broadening cannot be predicted in detail, it is assumed proportional to the square root of the energy of the event, that is, statistical effects are assumed to be dominant. The energy deposition spectrum was, therefore, broadened by means of a Gaussian function applied to the information in each channel with the standard deviation of the Gaussian set proportional to $E^{1/2}$, where E is the energy of the channel.

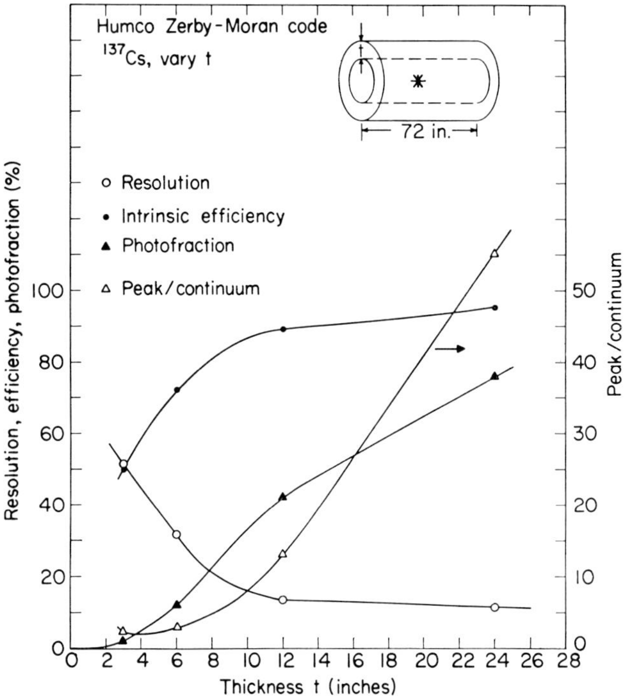

FIG. 3. Theoretical performance of counters of the Humco II type as function of scintillator thickness for 0.66-MeV γ rays; Zerby–Moran code predictions for optimum optics.

The solid points in Fig. 2 are the experimental results for the test tank, and the squares give the corresponding calculation using a broadening factor chosen to fit the experimental results best. Agreement is excellent, except in the lowest energy region, where the experimental results are higher than the theoretical. This may be due to γ rays scattered by the environment or to optical imperfections, or both.

The escape of backscattered γ rays cannot be eliminated by increasing the thickness of detectors in this geometry, and hence this design yields an inherently broad peak. With an interior source (that is, well-type geometry), γ rays backscattered from one side of the counter reenter the scintillator after recrossing the well and are subject to further absorption. Figure 3 shows the theoretical performance curves for a series of counters with a 72-inch long, 18-inch diameter sample well surrounded by a layer of liquid scintillator of varying thickness. Note that for a 12-inch thickness a resolution of 14% and an efficiency of 90% are predicted (optimum optics) with little gain for greater thick-

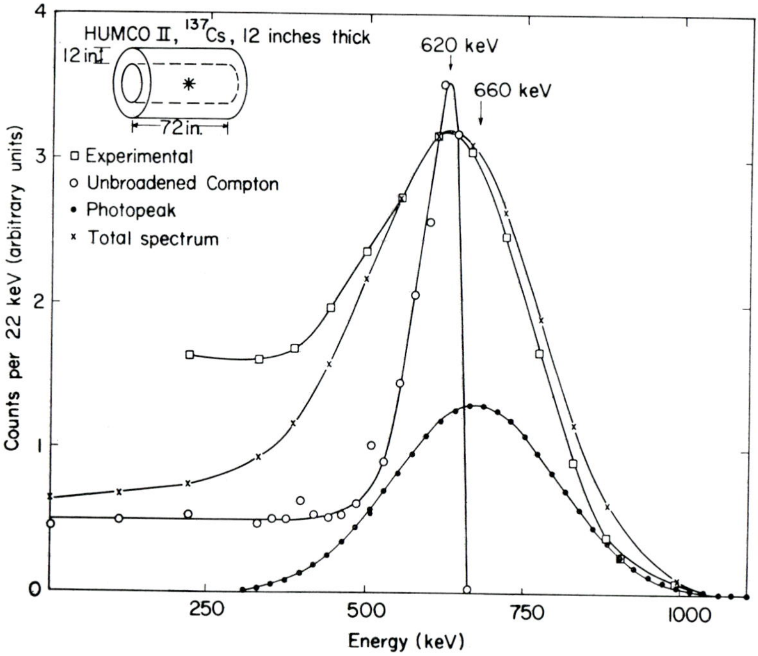

FIG. 4. Spectrum produced by 0.66-MeV γ rays incident on Humco II; experimental result compared with Zerby–Moran code predictions.

nesses, although photofraction and peak-to-continuum ratio continue to improve.

The model with 12 inches of scintillator thickness corresponds closely to Humco II, the large human counter (Section III). A comparison of theoretical and experimental resolution for this counter is given in Fig. 4 for ^{137}Cs γ rays. The unbroadened energy deposition spectrum calculated for multiple Compton scattering is a narrow peak at 620 keV. Total absorption now accounts for 42.5% of the interactions. Proper selection of the broadening factor produces good agreement with the experimental spectrum except at lower energies. A considerable improvement in peak-to-continuum ratio has been obtained recently by more careful selection of multiplier phototubes, better balancing of their individual gains, and an improved pulse amplifier. This results in better agreement between the experimental and computed spectra.

The theoretical analysis of γ-ray absorption shows the principle of design of a large organic γ-ray counter with energy resolution approaching that of sodium iodide crystals and an efficiency approaching 100%. Comparison with actual results so far attained shows that the theoretical performance has not yet been approached, however. The difficulties appear to lie in the problems of complete collection of the scintillation light and its conversion into the electrical signal. Light collection independent of the location of the scintillation in the detector is very difficult to attain. Use of total internal reflection (*5*) or materials of maximum reflectivity like MgO or Al_2O_3 powder is impractical for liquid scintillators. Transparency of the scintillator must be very high because of the very long (meters) path of the scintillation light between emission and collection. Finally, nonuniformities in the efficiency of the photocathodes of the multiplier phototubes introduce additional dispersions.

III. THE LOS ALAMOS LIQUID HUMAN COUNTER

A. Description of Counter

The present discussion is based on Humco II, the instrument currently in use at Los Alamos Scientific Laboratory. Many of the operating characteristics are similar for the other counters listed in Table I; however, counting efficiency and resolution are better for Humco II than can be attained for smaller detectors (Section II).

Humco II is a 72-inch long steel tank, hexagonal in outer cross section, with an 18-inch diameter well made of 0.030-inch thick stainless steel passing down the axis to accommodate the subject (Fig. 5). The layer of liquid scintillator around the well has a minimum thickness of 12 inches and consists of about 400 gallons of a solution of 4 gm/liter PPO and 0.04 gm/liter POPOP in TS-28 (a commercial hydrocarbon paint solvent). Scintillation light is collected by 24 16-inch multiplier phototubes (DuMont K-1628). The anodes are connected directly in parallel, and the summed signal is fed into a single charge-sensitive preamplifier (to eliminate capacitance loading). Tubes are balanced for equal overall gain by adjusting the high voltage applied to each with a potentiometer in series with the bleeder resistors. The single high-voltage supply (rated at 3000 V, 15 mA) has a stability of 0.005% per hour drift, according to the manufacturer. The charge-sensitive preamplifier feeds the scintillation pulses to a transistorized amplifier with maximum gain of 1000. This, in turn, feeds a bank of six single-channel pulse-height analyzers set to cover the range from 0.1 to 2.7 MeV. Six scalers collect the data for a preset time, usually 100 sec, and automatically operate an IBM card punch. A multichannel analyzer is used for energy calibration and alignment of the system and for occasional identification of simple spectra.

The counter tank is contained in a steel room with 7-inch thick walls to minimize interference by outside sources of radiation. The subject is introduced into the counting volume by means of a canvas sling moving in a steel trough passing through the wall of the steel

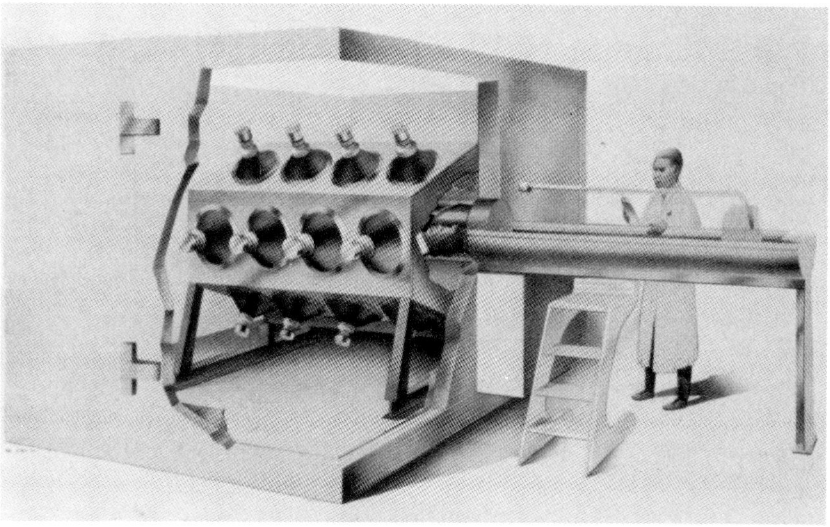

FIG. 5. The Los Alamos Human Counter (Humco II), showing scintillator tank and multiplier phototube arrangement.

room. The opening in the shield is sealed by a steel plug which rides in the trough at the end of the sling. The subject well is ventilated, illuminated, and supplied with a communications system, as well as with recorded music or radio. The subject has complete control over the transport mechanism and can bring himself out of the counter at any time by pressing a switch. Claustrophobia has not been a problem.

The energy resolution obtained is illustrated in Fig. 6, which shows spectra obtained from point sources of ^{40}K, ^{65}Zn, ^{54}Mn, ^{137}Cs, and ^{131}I. Pairs of γ rays as close together as ^{54}Mn (842 keV) and ^{65}Zn (1.12 MeV) or ^{65}Zn and ^{40}K (1.46 MeV) can be determined simultaneously, but these represent the practical resolution limits of the counter. Resolution (full width at half maximum) ranges from 30% for ^{40}K to 50% for ^{137}Cs.

Since the efficiency of the counter is very high (roughly 80%), γ rays which are emitted simultaneously (in cascade) produce appreciable sum peaks. This is illustrated in Fig. 7 for ^{60}Co and ^{22}Na. The two ^{60}Co γ rays (1.17 and 1.33 MeV) are not resolved but produce a single line at 1.1 MeV. Detection of both γ rays produces the sum peak at 2.2 MeV. In the case of ^{22}Na, three γ rays are involved: two annihilation quanta of 0.51 MeV each and the 1.28-MeV γ ray. The sum of one annihilation

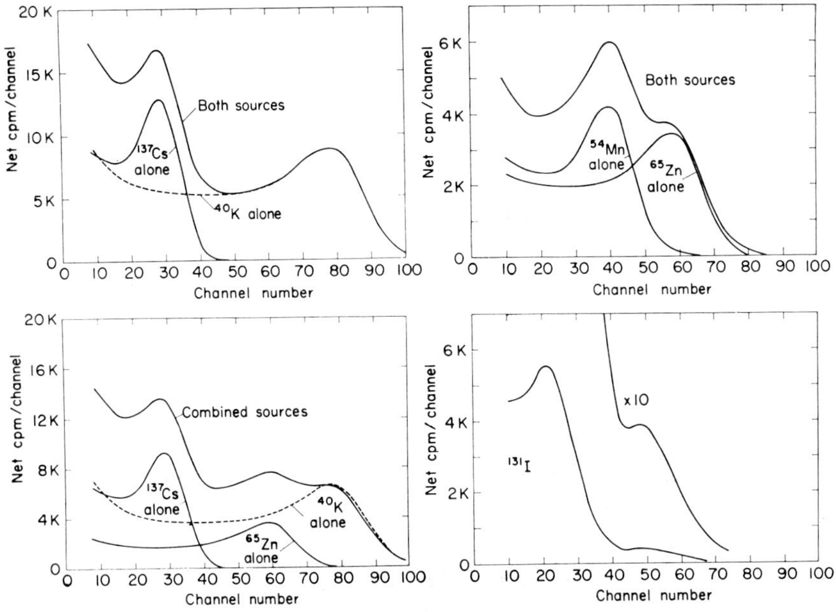

FIG. 6. Spectra produced by several important radionuclides in Humco II.

quantum and the γ ray should produce a peak at 1.56 MeV, while a triple sum would give peaks at 1.73 to 1.85 MeV, depending on the multiplicity of scattering. These sum peaks can be extremely useful, since they lie in a spectral region comparatively free from interferences. For example, the ^{24}Na sum peak at 3.9 MeV facilitates the diagnosis of whole-body neutron exposure in the presence of fission product contamination. The ^{60}Co sum peak permits its use as a double tracer, with ^{59}Fe (Chapter 12, Section I,4).

Two other spectra of interest are those from ^{228}Th and ^{226}Ra shown in Fig. 8. These are quite different from the more familiar ones obtained with low-geometry systems because here sum peaks predominate. In the case of radium, the 1.1-MeV peak is due to the 0.607-0.77 MeV cascade, and the 1.6-MeV peak is due to the 0.607-1.12 MeV cascade in RaC′. In

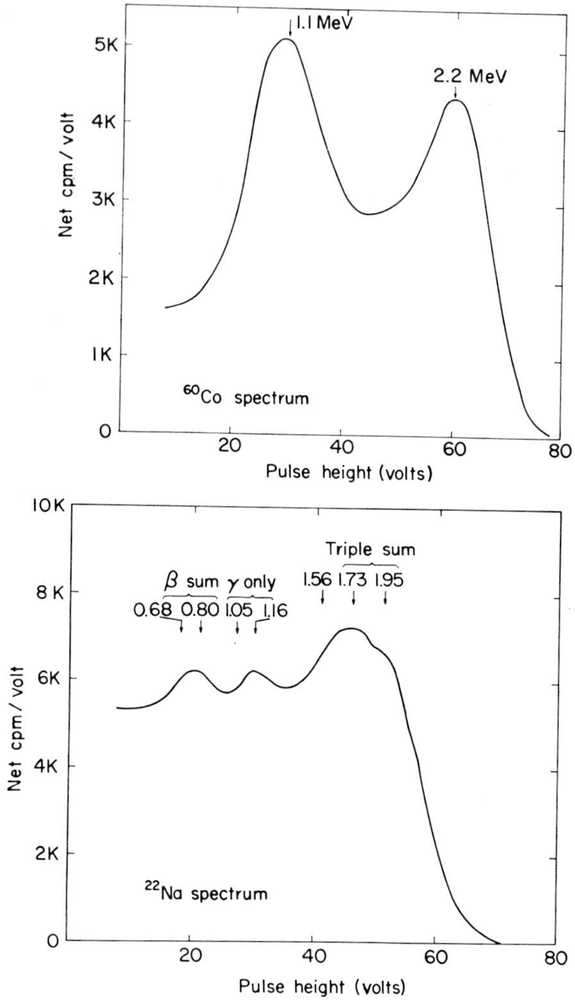

FIG. 7. Spectra produced by ^{60}Co and ^{22}Na in Humco II; sum peaks are prominent.

the case of thorium, the 3.0-MeV peak is due to the 2.61-0.58 MeV cascade in ThC″.

The energy calibration of Humco II is shown in Fig. 9. Peak pulse height is proportional to energy deposited when the latter is taken as the maximum for double Compton scatter.

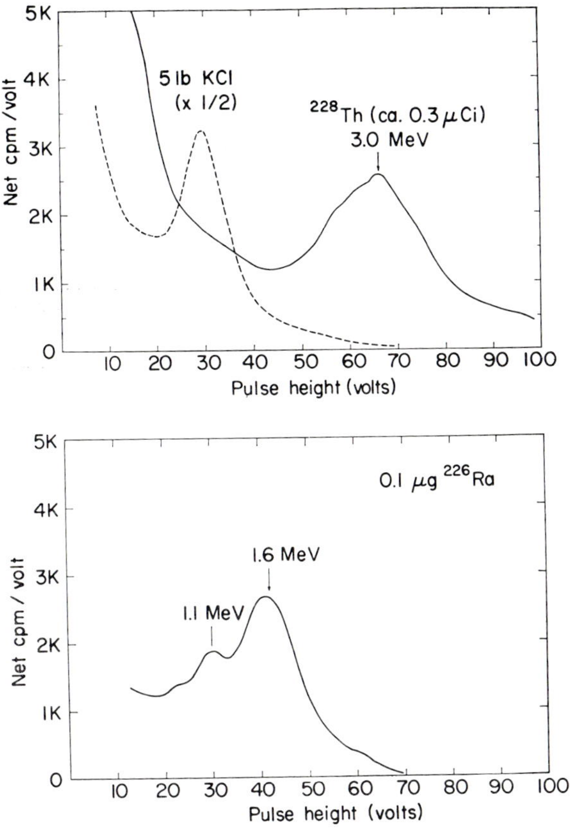

FIG. 8. Spectra produced by ^{228}Th and ^{226}Ra in Humco II.

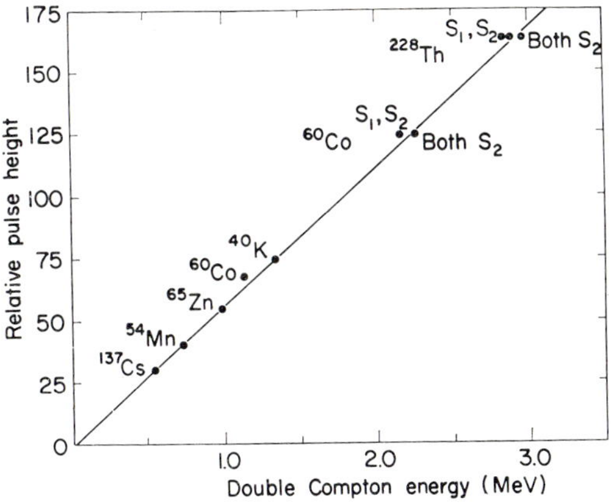

FIG. 9. Energy calibration of Humco II with toluene filling; S_1 refers to single scatter, S_2 to double scatter, and either or both to a cascade γ-ray pair.

The capability of the counter for multiple tracer experiments is summarized in Table III. Any nuclide listed can be determined simultaneously with any other nuclide from a different group, provided the amounts are not too disparate. Members of adjacent subgroups can be resolved only with difficulty.

TABLE III
RESOLUTION CAPABILITY OF HUMCO II

Group	Nuclide	Full energy of γ ray(s) (MeV)	Double-Compton energy
1	^{32}P	Bremsstrahlung	—
	^{90}Sr		
2	^{214}Pb (RaB)	0.24–0.35	0.16[a]
	^{203}Hg	0.28	0.19
	^{51}Cr	0.32	0.23
	^{131}I	0.36	0.27
3a	^{198}Au	0.41	0.31
	^{85}Sr	0.51	0.40
3b	^{137}Cs	0.66	0.55
	^{54}Mn	0.84	0.73
4	^{64}Cu	1.02 (β + annihilation)	0.80
	^{86}Rb	1.08	0.96
	^{65}Zn	1.12	1.00
	^{59}Fe	1.20 (1.10 and 1.29)	1.08
5a	^{40}K	1.46	1.34
	^{42}K	1.53	1.41
5b	^{214}Bi (RaC)	1.73 (sum)	1.60[a]
	^{22}Na	2.30 (sum)	1.80[a]
6	^{60}Co	2.50 (sum)	2.25
7	^{208}Tl (ThC″)	3.20 (sum)	3.00[a]
8	^{24}Na	4.12 (sum)	3.93

[a] Observed energy of a broad complex peak.

The differential background count-rate of Humco II is shown in Fig. 10.

B. Geometrical Sensitivity

The well-type design of Humco II was chosen to minimize changes in counting efficiency due to position of the radioactivity. The success of the design is indicated by Fig. 11, which shows the relative counting efficiency for a 2-kg KCl source moved along the axis of the counter compared with the effect calculated from geometrical end-losses only. Over the central 4 ft of the well, the variation in efficiency is only $\pm 5\%$. For a nuclide such as ^{131}I, which concentrates in the neck region, some care is necessary in calibrating and in positioning subjects. For most

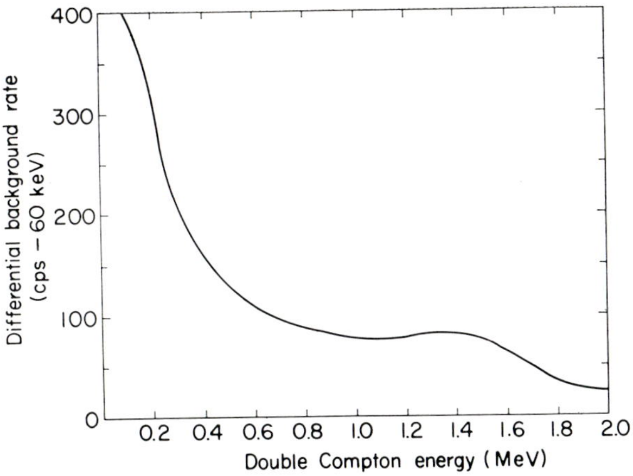

FIG. 10. Differential background count-rate of Humco II.

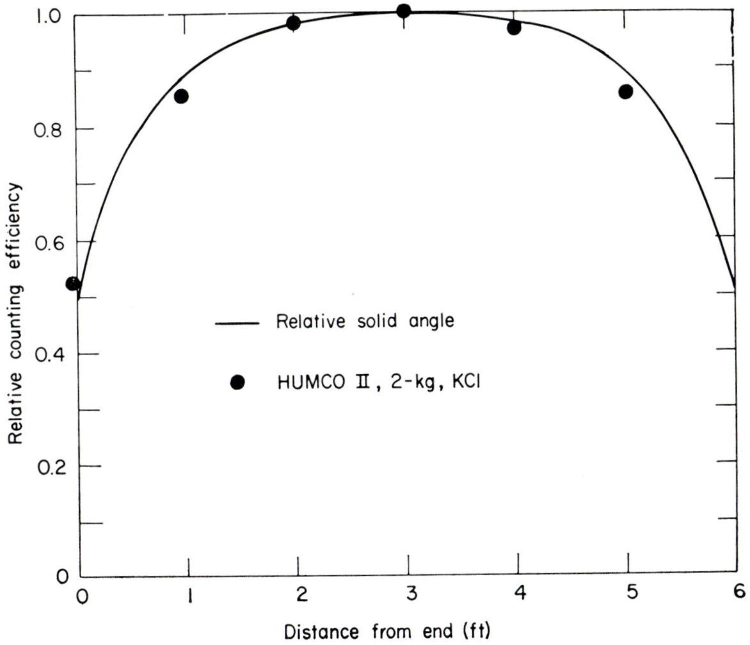

FIG. 11. Counting efficiency of Humco II relative to geometrical center for a 2-kg KCl source on axis.

nuclides, however, geometrical effects do not contribute significantly to the errors of measurement.

The radial sensitivity variation of Humco II is small. If a small ^{137}Cs source is moved from the geometrical center to the bottom of the well, equidistant from the ends of the counter, the count-rate in the ^{137}Cs channel increases only 1%.

C. Efficiency and Calibration

The self-absorption of the human body is of the order of 50% even for γ rays as energetic as those of ^{40}K. It is, therefore, necessary to calibrate the counter for each nuclide which is to be determined quantitatively. While the counter is relatively insensitive to the position of a point source within the well, different distributions of radioactivity in the human body can lead to significantly different self-absorption factors. It is, therefore, necessary that the calibration for counter efficiency be carried out *in vivo* with care and with close attention to the details of the mixing and distribution of the calibrating dose. Phantom measurements are of limited usefulness for accurate work, although they appear to be reliable to within a few percent for a nuclide such as ^{40}K with a comparatively simple, nearly uniform distribution.

Humco II has been accurately calibrated for ^{40}K and ^{137}Cs. The procedure is to administer intravenously accurately known doses (of the order of 0.1 to 1 μCi) to volunteer subjects chosen for a variety of weights and heights. In the first few hours, body radioactivity is measured frequently (the spacing depending on the mixing rate) until their count-rates no longer change with time. If this time is so long that appreciable excretion occurs, this must be collected and measured. Calibrations must be obtained for each nuclide in all channels below the peak, since a high-energy γ ray produces significant numbers of counts in the lower channels which must be taken into account in multiple tracer experiments.

Calibration curves for ^{40}K (obtained using ^{42}K for the administered activity) are shown in Fig. 12 and for ^{137}Cs (using ^{137}Cs or ^{132}Cs) in Fig. 13. These curves have proved to be very reproducible when repeated at intervals on different subjects. The background is 355 counts per second in the potassium channel and 560 counts per second in the ^{137}Cs channel. It is estimated that the absolute error resulting from the uncertainty in these curves is about 2% for ^{40}K determinations. Analysis of the residual variance of the data about the least-squares fit has failed to disclose any significant correlation with any parameter of bodily measurement. Within the range of shapes covered it is, therefore, concluded that gross body weight is the sole parameter determining the ^{40}K efficiency.

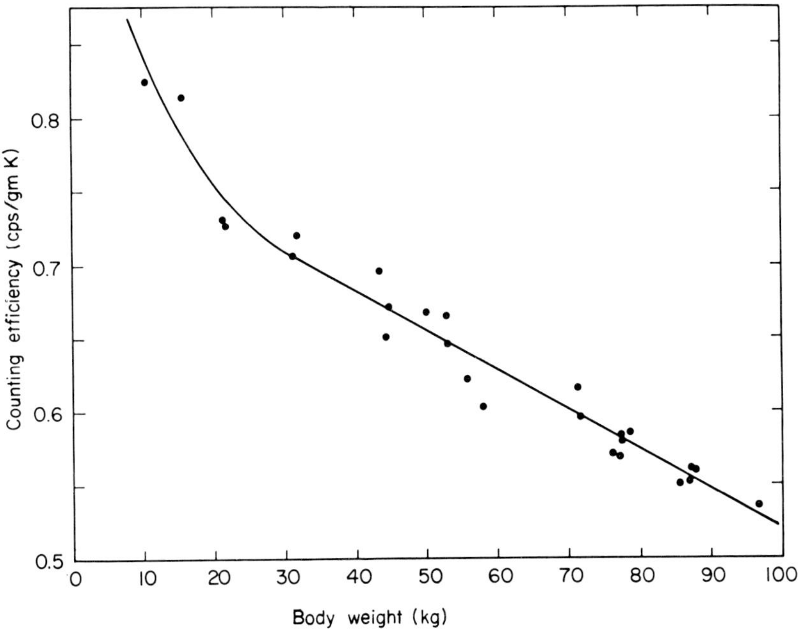

FIG. 12. Counting efficiency of Humco II for normal body potassium as a function of body weight.

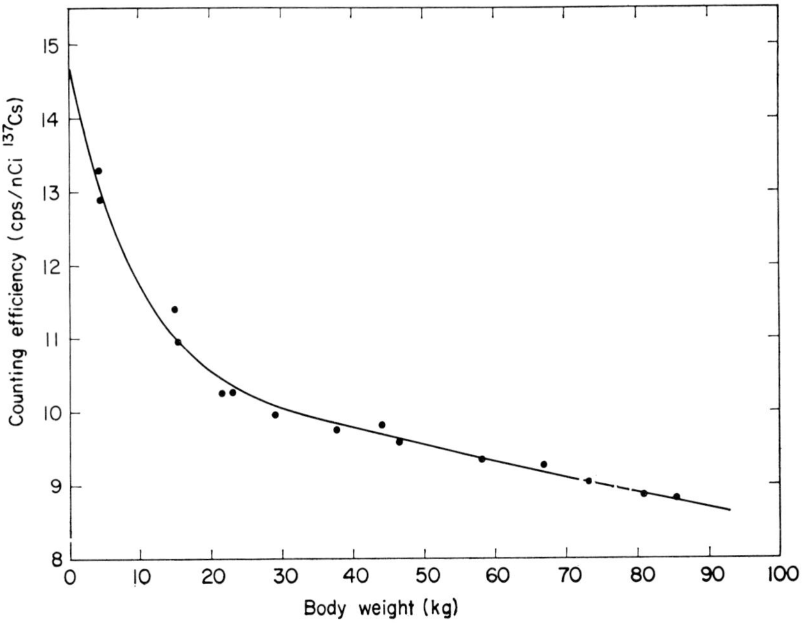

FIG. 13. Counting efficiency of Humco II for body ^{137}Cs as a function of body weight.

D. Metabolic Studies

1. Body Potassium

The results of the studies of total body potassium using whole-body counters are of general interest, since potassium is an important body component and natural ^{40}K constitutes an important background activity whose variations limit sensitivity and accuracy in the measurement of other nuclides. In addition, the studies which have been made of the precision and accuracy attainable in natural potassium measurements give a valuable indication of the long- and short-term instrumental stability, as well as of the practical limits on absolute calibration of the detector.

The total amount of potassium in the adult male body is quite variable, showing a standard deviation of $\pm 10\%$ for selected age groups, with the average ranging from 2.1 to 1.7 gm of K per kilogram for ages between 20 and 70 (*2*). Women average 15% less than men in these units. In terms of the natural ^{40}K radioactivity, this is of the order of 0.1 μCi, of which only 10% decays by γ-ray emission. The net count-rate of 5400 cpm from this amount of ^{40}K is considerably less than the background of 22,000 cpm for Humco II. As a result, the demands on counter stability are quite stringent. The counting statistics tend to be the parameter limiting the accuracy, and the errors are to a good approximation not percentage errors but rather absolute errors (for example, in grams of K) more or less independent of the amount of potassium present. This puts a high premium on the use of very large samples and makes the measurement of, for example, the potassium content of small children very difficult.

No human counters give absolute results, they must be calibrated. It is important here to distinguish between precision and accuracy. Precision can be evaluated from the reproducibility of a series of measurements. Accuracy, on the other hand, can be determined only if the true, absolute value is known; accuracy is the important parameter when one compares results obtained by different methods.

Extensive studies (*1*) have shown that the precision of the determination of the total potassium content of a sample or subject is given by the counting statistical error for counting times up to 30 min (Chapter 3, Section I,B). For a counting time of 3 min, the standard deviation is about ± 3 gm and for 30 min ± 1 gm for Humco II. Additional γ-ray activity can be detected with a similar precision provided the potassium background can be determined on the same subject. This corresponds to a sensitivity of 0.2 nCi total body burden (at 100% γ-ray abundance) for a 3-min counting time, assuming a self-absorption coefficient similar to that of potassium.

Proof of the absolute accuracy of a determination of total body potassium by 4π counting is not easy because of the lack of a completely satisfactory standard of comparison. Destructive chemical analysis of the human body is very difficult and rarely feasible. Isotopic dilution methods (*4*) are somewhat uncertain, principally because of the impossibility of proving the degree of mixing, and are technically difficult because of the short half-life of ^{42}K. Comparison with sodium iodide crystal spectrometry is unsatisfactory, since this method suffers from the same type of errors which affect the 4π counter and, in addition, is sensitive to the subject's shape.

The results of absolute potassium determinations by ^{40}K counting and by ^{42}K isotope dilution (*4*) show that ratios of exchangeable ^{42}K to total potassium measured on the same individuals range from 0.92 to 0.99, with a mean of 0.96 for five normal male subjects. Comparison (*1*) of the averages for two different population groups (same sex and age range) gave 1.012. Comparison with sodium iodide spectrometry of the same three subjects in four different laboratories gave a ratio of 0.98 (spectrometer to 4π counter), with a range of 0.90 to 1.03. Comparison with sodium iodide spectrometry for population averages gave an average ratio of 1.05, with a range of 0.92 to 1.16 for six groups from four laboratories. From these results, we conclude that the absolute accuracy of the 4π counter method for the determination of total body potassium is better than ± 6 gm and probably better than ± 3 gm.

Comparable studies of precision and accuracy have not been made for other nuclides. To the extent that electronic instability is limiting, similar conclusions will apply. However, potassium is a particularly favorable case; it combines a high γ-ray energy with nearly uniform distribution in the body, thus minimizing the variations that can be caused by the change in self-absorption associated with translocation. The magnitude of these effects remains to be established experimentally for other nuclides.

2. RADIOCESIUM METABOLISM

The study of radiocesium retention kinetics in man is of practical importance because ^{137}Cs is produced in high yield from both uranium and plutonium fission and hence is a by-product of nuclear reactors and nuclear weapon tests. The entry of fallout ^{137}Cs into the biosphere and man has prompted the measurement of biological parameters needed to estimate human radiation protection guides. Both 28-year ^{137}Cs and 6.6-day ^{132}Cs have been used; a recent study using ^{132}Cs illustrates the general technique and problems encountered (*18*).

Each of the four subjects was counted in Humco II prior to ^{132}Cs injection to establish the preexperimental γ-ray background. Then 1 ml of ^{132}Cs chloride containing about 0.65 μCi was injected into the antecubital vein, and measurements were carried out for 45 days. Standards of ^{137}Cs were used throughout this experiment, since both isotopes emit

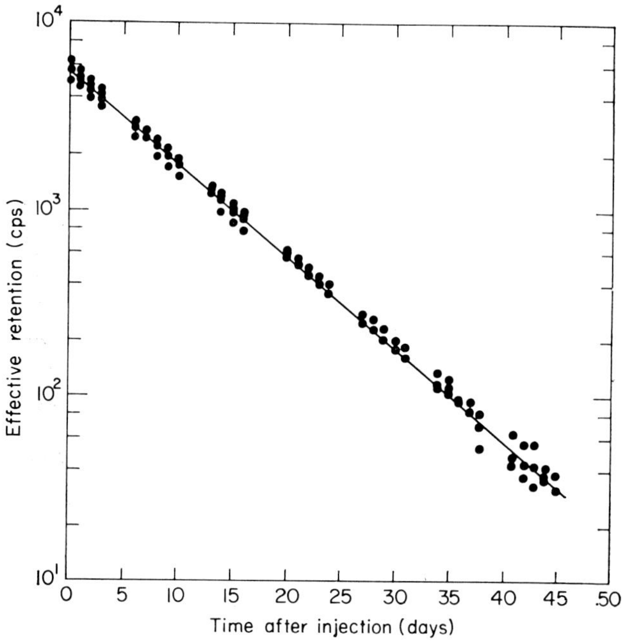

FIG. 14. Retention of ^{132}Cs in four subjects as a function of time after intravenous injection.

γ rays of almost identical energy and the almost negligible decay of the ^{137}Cs during the experiment is very convenient. An additional bonus is an independent estimation of the ^{132}Cs half-life.

The resulting data are shown in Fig. 14. This plot is part of the output of an IBM 7090 computer which has been programmed to fit a simple exponential function to the experimental data by a least-squares procedure (*14*). For the averaged data of the four subjects the effective half-life is 6.07 days. Using a physical half-life of 6.59 days obtained from the measurements of the ^{137}Cs and ^{132}Cs standards, an average biological half-life of 77.5 days is computed.

Several interesting points should be mentioned. First, the biological half-life of ^{137}Cs for normal adults is 100 to 135 days (*15, 19*); the low value obtained with ^{132}Cs is due to the large amount of stable cesium in the original material. Second, the biological half-life computed from the experimentally observed effective half-life is very sensitive to the value used for the physical half-life. Therefore, care must be used when the physical and effective half-lives are approximately equal. Third, the observed count-rate varied less than 2% between injection and the time of first excretion, some 3 to 4 hr later. This observation indicates the insensitivity of Humco II to early changes in bodily distribution of this radionuclide. Fourth, constancy of Humco II calibration was checked with an extended ^{137}Cs source (in a 5-gallon jug of water) whose spectrum resembled that of the subjects, not a point source.

3. ZINC METABOLISM

Zinc is an essential trace element that functions in certain enzymes concerned with proteolysis and cellular respiration. This element is also thought to participate in erythropoiesis and myelogenous bone marrow functioning and to be involved in skin metabolism. It is present in hair in concentrations of roughly 200 parts per million.

Little is known about the behavior of this element in the body. Large-volume whole-body counters afford a means of investigating zinc metabolism using ^{65}Zn. Figure 15 shows the whole-body biological retention of orally administered ^{65}Zn by two normal men (*17*). The kinetics of body retention are described by the linear sum of three exponential processes for roughly 1 year. Note the similarity of the rate constant of the last term in each retention equation. This term is presumed, on the basis of related studies, to represent turnover of skeletally bound ^{65}Zn.

Biological retention of orally administered ^{65}Zn by the same male subject with and without supplemental dietary zinc is shown in Fig. 16 (*11*). The gastrointestinal absorption was about a factor of 2 lower after the subject received 10 mg of zinc per day as zinc acetate for about 1 month.

IV. 2π MULTIPLE PLASTIC COUNTER

A large organic scintillation counter at the National Institutes of Health has a unique design, which combines the geometrical efficiency of a 2π system with some ability of localization (*3*). It consists of 18 blocks of plastic scintillator ($12 \times 12 \times 6$ inches each) arranged below a horizontal trough (Fig. 17). This trough has been marked with tape to indicate the positions of the detectors. The control console contains an array of push-button switches, which permit the selection of any com-

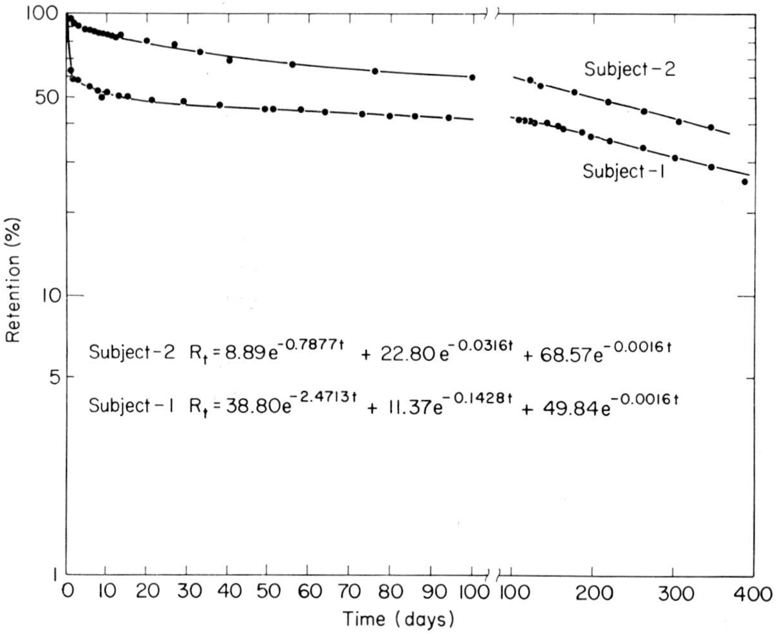

FIG. 15. Retention of ^{65}Zn in two subjects as a function of time after oral ingestion.

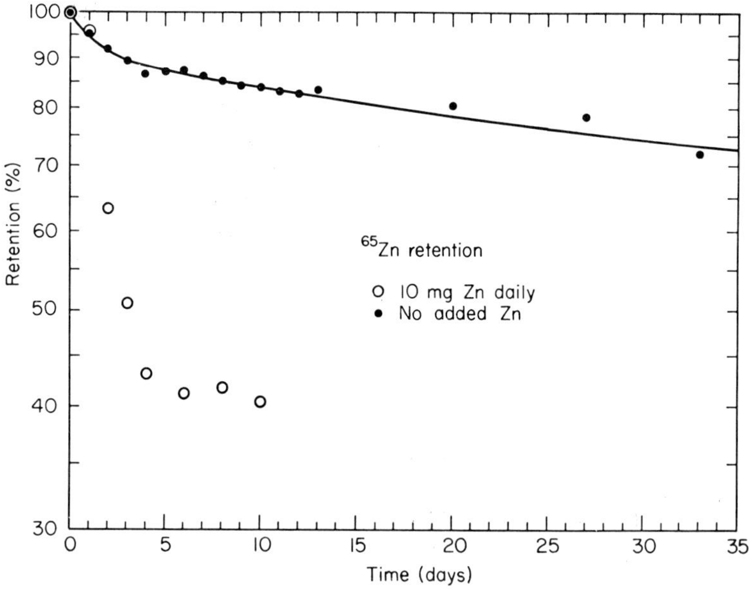

FIG. 16. Effect of supplemental zinc on ^{65}Zn retention in one subject.

bination of detector units, the summed outputs of which are recorded in each of four energy channels on separate scalers. With this system, the difference in organ burden, as between liver and spleen for example, can be determined, but not the distributions within an organ.

An important feature is the facility for transferring bed-ridden patients (osteoporosis) into the counter without trauma. One survey of

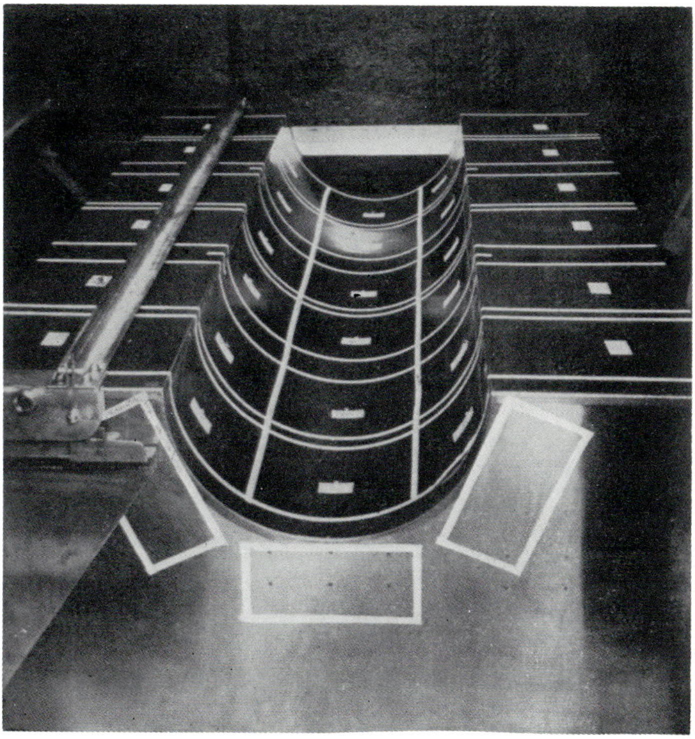

FIG. 17. Multiple plastic human counter at the National Institutes of Health, showing patient trough and metal shell. The positions of the 18 plastic scintillator blocks have been indicated by tape.

the applications of this counter is shown in Table IV. Most of the cases required multiple counts, sometimes over a period of several days.

The background in the channel containing the ^{40}K peak (0.75 to 1.7 MeV) is 50 cps. The potassium calibrations were made with arrays of 2-lb boxes of sugar, a KCl tube down the center of each one. The counting efficiency decreases with increasing weight; the ratio of the counting efficiency of a 50-kg sugar phantom to that of a 100-kg sugar phantom was determined as 1.25.

TABLE IV
MEDICAL APPLICATIONS OF THE NIH WHOLE-BODY COUNTER

Isotope	Purpose
^{40}K	Neuromuscular disorders
^{47}Ca	Mostly multiple myeloma
^{51}Cr	Refractory anemias
^{57}Co	Vitamin B_{12} studies
^{59}Fe	Incompletely diagnosed anemias
^{131}I	Study of macroglobulins

V. SMALL ANIMAL COUNTERS

A. Design and Performance

Although mice and rats may be counted in the larger detectors, accuracy and sensitivity are limited unnecessarily by the large background. A variety of systems (*6, 7, 8, 10, 16, 21*) has been designed especially to study biological phenomena in small animals, and now several models are available commercially (Section VI). It is convenient to have the long axis of the counter horizontal. This orientation is also advantageous for measuring liquid samples of large volume containing

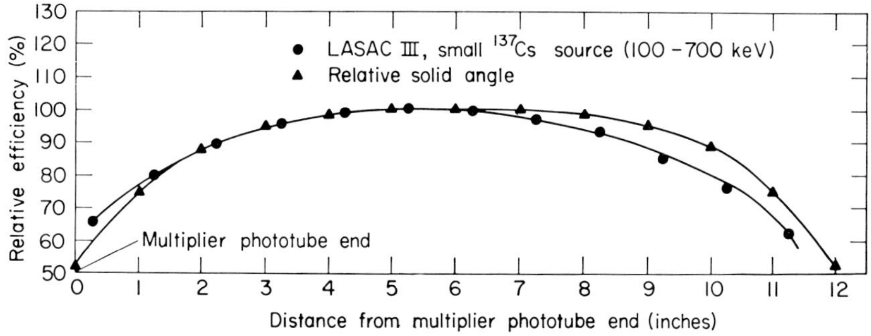

FIG. 18. Theoretical and observed response of LASAC III as a function of ^{137}Cs source position.

material which tends to settle out during the period of assay. Counting efficiency is less sensitive to radial displacement of the source than to axial displacement to the end of the counter. A counting chamber with both ends open is more sensitive to changes in sample positioning than is the well-type with one end of the counting chamber closed by scintillator solution. In the latter design, reproducible geometry and maximum efficiency are easily achieved by positioning the sample against the end wall of the counting chamber. Regardless of the detector tank design, the relation between sensitivity and source position along the counting chamber axis should correspond to that predicted by geometry (that is, solid angle subtended at source by scintillator). Good agreement means good light collection and hence good design (Fig. 18).

Many of the commercially available counters are based on a liquid scintillation counter for small animals (Fig. 19). This counter consists of a detector tank 12 inches in length and about 12 inches in diameter with a 4.25-inch diameter hole down the center to contain the sample.

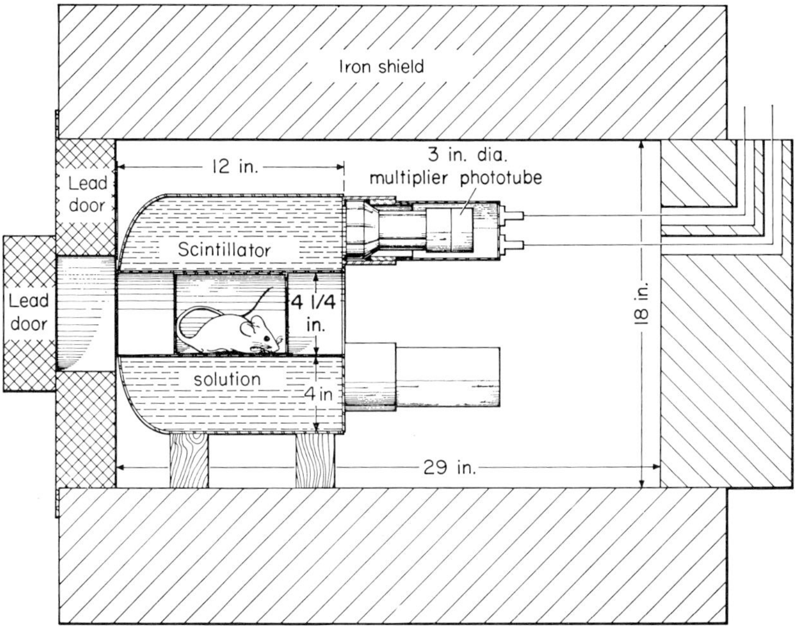

FIG. 19. Schematic diagram of detector and shield of the Los Alamos Small Animal Counter (LASAC III).

The sample is surrounded by a 4-inch thick annular ring of scintillator solution (4 gm terphenyl per liter plus 0.05 gm POPOP* per liter toluene). All inside surfaces of the detector tank are painted with a TiO_2-pigmented epoxy resin reflective coating. Seven 3-inch diameter multiplier phototubes are fitted on a flat plate at the rear end of the tank. The background shield is made of 7-inch thick steel plates. The hinged front of the shield is a stainless steel shell filled with lead and fitted with a sliding lead-filled door which, when moved laterally, per-

* 2,2′-*p*-Phenylenebis-(5-phenyloxazole).

mits access into the counting chamber. The multiplier phototubes are individually balanced for gain, and their signals are connected in parallel. The combined output of the tubes is fed into transistorized electronic circuitry that provides amplification and sorting of pulses into

TABLE V
LASAC III PERFORMANCE

^{137}Cs efficiency (75 to 600 keV)[a]	40%
Background (75 to 600 keV)	4000 cpm
^{137}Cs Half-resolution	20%
^{65}Zn efficiency (75 to 1100 keV)	40%
Background (75 to 1100 keV)	4700 cpm
^{65}Zn half-resolution	16%
Noise level	70 keV

[a] Energy calibration is based on the assumption that peaks in γ-ray spectra correspond to maximum energy deposition by single Compton scatter.

four energy bands. Output data are punched on paper tape in binary coded decimal form, and computer techniques are used to handle the large amount of data which accumulate (*14*). The performance of this

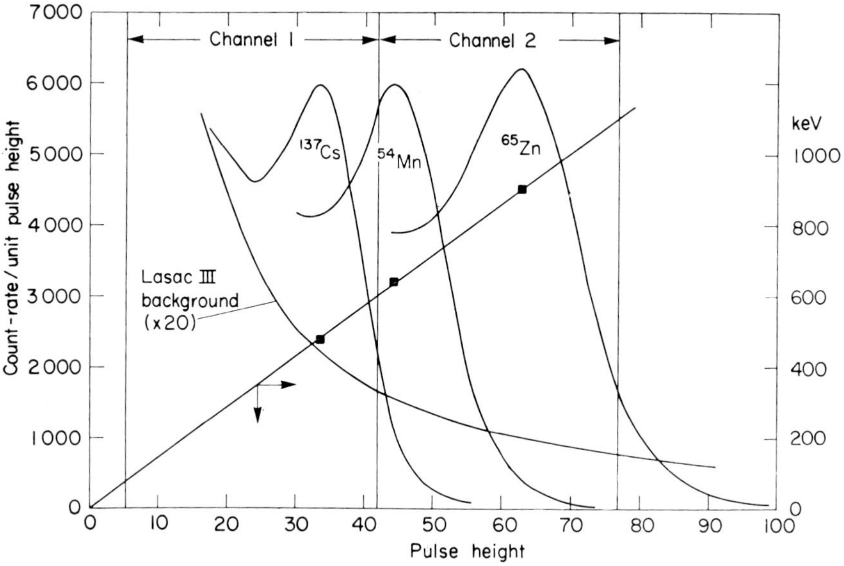

FIG. 20. Spectra produced by ^{137}Cs, ^{54}Mn, ^{65}Zn, and background in LASAC III.

counter is summarized in Table V. Minimum detectable activity of ^{137}Cs is of the order of 0.1 nCi for a 100-sec count of source and background (that is, standard deviation due to counting statistics for a weak source equals 0.1 nCi). The spectra of three radionuclides and background obtained with a multichannel analyzer are shown in Fig. 20.

B. Sodium Metabolism in Rats

A useful application of this small animal counter is a study of the effects of age, sodium depletion, and sodium repletion on the long-term retention pattern of ^{22}Na by rats (*13*). Twenty-four Sprague-Dawley rats received about 0.5 μCi of ^{22}NaCl intraperitoneally; half the animals were fed normally and half were on a low sodium diet. Forty days after injection, the low sodium group was fed normally and allowed to replete their sodium for the rest of the experiment. Of the animals fed the regular lab chow the younger rats lost ^{22}Na at a faster rate initially yet retained more at later times than the older rats. Data indicate that both age groups retain ^{22}Na tenaciously during sodium restriction. During this period, young rats retained more radiosodium than the older rats. Of the initially administered ^{22}Na, only 4 and 16%, respectively, was lost from young and older animals over the 40-day sodium depletion period. Immediately after sodium repletion, both age groups lost ^{22}Na at an accelerated rate. A salient feature is the large difference between the amounts of ^{22}Na retained by the normal and repleted groups at long times after administration. The computer-derived retention equation (0 to 163 days) for the biological retention of ^{22}Na for the rats on a normal diet is

$$R_t = 98.60e^{-0.16341t} + 1.19e^{-0.03511t} + 0.59e^{-0.00257t}$$

VI. ARM COUNTERS

Liquid scintillation detectors designed specifically to measure radioactivity in the human forearm are useful in clinical diagnosis. Determination of the amount of radioactivity in the blood is ordinarily accomplished by measuring the activity of blood samples withdrawn by venepuncture. An annular detector (Fig. 21) constructed to measure conveniently the human arm *in vivo* can be used in clinical diagnostic tests instead of or as an adjunct to tests requiring venepuncture. The counter measures the radioactivity both in blood and in other contiguous arm tissues. Measurement of the entire muscular blood-rich portion of the forearm requires less counting time for a given dose than measurements on samples of circulating blood. Hence, radioactivity levels can be followed in the patient for longer periods of time. Additional advantages include reproducible geometry and patient comfort through the reduction or elimination of repeated venepunctures, especially with sick patients and children. The assay is done while the patient is reclining in a comfortable chair (*12*).

TABLE VI

COMMERCIAL COUNTERS DESIGNED FOR ARM COUNTING AND/OR SMALL ANIMAL COUNTING[a]

	Packard Model 440 (ARMAC)	Metrix MX-15 (Bio-Met)	Electro-Fab
Sample well length (inches)	8	$17\frac{3}{8}$	16
Sample well diameter (inches)	$4\frac{1}{2}$	5	7
Scintillator thickness (inches)	4	4	3
Scintillator type	Liquid	Plastic	NE-102 plastic
Multiplier phototubes	Six 3-inch tubes	Eight 3-inch tubes	Eight Amperex XP-1031
Multiplier phototube location	Far end	Far end	Each end
Shielding	2 Inches lead	Lead shot + steel	2 Inches lead
Total weight (lb)	1600	—	2500
^{137}Cs half-resolution	Stated 25%	Stated 25%	Stated 21%
^{137}Cs counting	Integral efficiency stated about 50%	Sensitivity (10 min) stated 0.04 nCi	—
Counting application	Arm, small animal, small samples	Arm, small animal, small samples	Mainly small animal and small sample

[a] See Appendix, Section III.

Several commercially available counters are described in Table VI. Information on mechanical details and electronic design is not included but is obtainable from the manufacturer. The Bio-Met is also available with sodium iodide detectors. The Electro-Fab unit is designed mainly for small animals and other samples of similar size.

Certain diagnostic tests can be made by measuring the disappearance of a labeled dye from the systemic circulation; an example is the liver

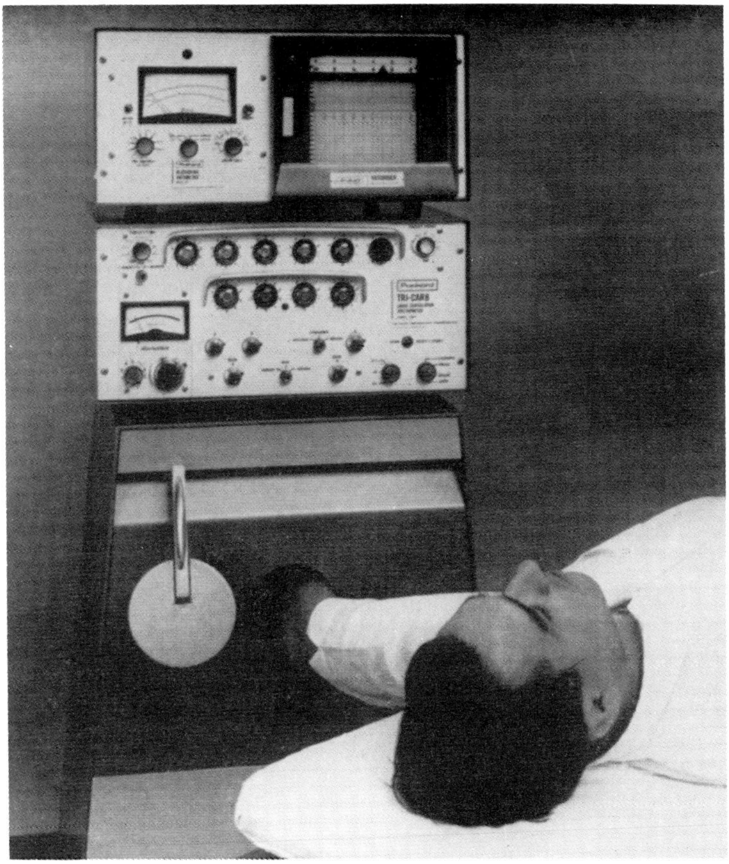

FIG. 21. ARMAC (Packard Instrument Comp.) for arm counting and small animal counting.

function test (*12*). Ten microcuries of ^{131}I-labeled rose bengal dye is injected intravenously into one arm while the other is positioned in the detector. Changes in the circulating radioactivity are recorded continuously. Figure 22 shows the arm activity as a function of time for healthy persons and others with inflammatory hepatitis. At 1 hr, three times more dye remained in the arms of patients with hepatitis.

In essence, this type of diagnostic test indirectly measures the rate of uptake of a labeled material by a specific tissue or organ. The technique obviates the problem of crystal positioning relative to the organ,

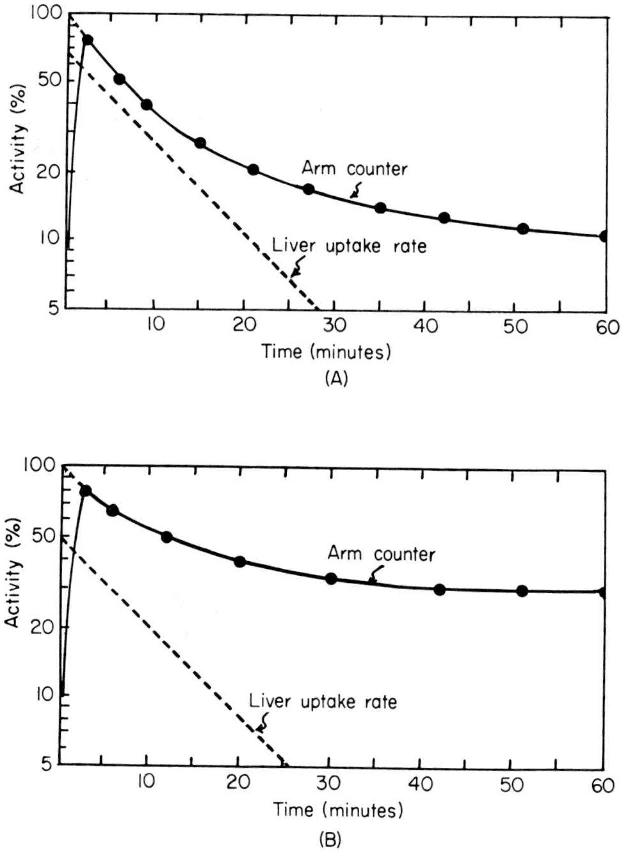

FIG. 22. Arm activity as a function of time after intravenous injection of ^{131}I-labeled rose bengal dye for (A) normal subjects and (B) patients with inflammatory hepatitis.

which is inherent to external probe techniques. However, other problems such as tracer recycling and deposition in other arm tissues arise.

Diagnostic tests possible with arm counting techniques are erythrocyte survival, plasma iron clearance, plasma protein survival, intestinal fat absorption, sodium retention, and blood volume. Also, studies on thyroid function, phagocytic activity, and vitamin B_{12} absorption appear promising. The application of the arm counter to diagnostic and clinical medicine has barely been exploited and represents a potential area for research.

REFERENCES

1. Anderson, E. C., Determination of body potassium by 4π gamma counting. *In* "Radioactivity in Man" (G. R. Meneely and S. M. Linde, eds.), p. 211. Thomas, Springfield, Illinois, 1965.
2. Anderson, E. C., and Langham, W. H., Average potassium concentration of the human body as a function of age. *Science* **130,** 713 (1959).
3. Andrews, H. L., Peterson, D. C., Murphy, R. E., and Myers, E. J., An organic plastic, localizing whole-body counter. *J. Nucl. Med.* **6,** 667 (1965).
4. Boling, E. A., Taylor, W. L., Entenman, C., and Behnke, A. R., Jr., Total exchangeable potassium and chloride and total body water in healthy men of varying fat content. *J. Clin. Invest.* **41,** 1840 (1962).
5. Brini, D., Peli, L., Rimondi, O., and Veronesi, P., On large scintillation counters. *Nuovo Cimento* [10] Suppl. II, 1048 (1955).
6. Brownell, G. L., Ellett, W. H., Rydin, R. A., and Hine, G. J., Large plastic scintillator for radioactivity measurement. *Health Phys.* **5,** 27 (1961).
7. Cook, J. D., and Valberg, L. S., Evaluation and use of a large plastic scintillator for gamma counting. *J. Lab. Clin. Med.* **61,** 317 (1963).
8. Dunavant, B. G., and Christian, J. E., A large-volume 4π liquid scintillation detector. *Intern. J. Appl. Radiation Isotopes* **8,** 223 (1960).
9. Evans, R. D., "The Atomic Nucleus," p. 677. McGraw-Hill, New York, 1955.
10. Forrester, R. H., Conrad, M. E., Jr., and Crosby, W. H., Measurement of total body iron^{59} in animals using whole-body liquid scintillation detectors. *Proc. Soc. Exptl. Biol. Med.* **111,** 115 (1962).
11. Furchner, J. E., and Richmond, C. R., Effect of dietary zinc on the absorption of orally administered Zn^{65}. *Health Phys.* **8,** 35 (1962).
12. Lushbaugh, C. C., and Schuch, R. L., Clinical use of the arm counter in blood clearance studies. *Advan. Tracer Methodol.* **1,** 314 (1963).
13. Richmond, C. R., Furchner, J. E., and Cummins, B. M., Effect of age, sodium depletion and sodium repletion on the retention of sodium^{22} by rats. *J. Nutr.* **76,** 210 (1962).
14. Richmond, C. R., Furchner, J. E., Dean, P. N., and McWilliams, P., Electronic processing and analysis of metabolic data. *Health Phys.* **10,** 3 (1963).
15. Richmond, C. R., Furchner, J. E., and Langham, W. H., Long-term retention of radiocesium by man. *Health Phys.* **8,** 201 (1962).
16. Richmond, C. R., Furchner, J. E., and Trafton, G. A., Comparison of predicted and measured equilibrium levels for chronically administered Cs^{137}. *Health Phys.* **7,** 219 (1962).
17. Richmond, C. R., Furchner, J. E., Trafton, G. A., and Langham, W. H., Comparative metabolism of radionuclides in mammals. I. Uptake and retention of orally administered Zn^{65} by four mammalian species. *Health Phys.* **8,** 481 (1962).
18. Richmond, C. R., London, J. E., Dean, P. N., and Furchner, J. E., Whole-body retention of intravenously administered ^{132}cesium by man. Los Alamos Scientific Laboratory Report LA-3132-MS. p. 49 (1964).
19. Taylor, M. P., Vennart, J., and Taylor, D. M., Retention and excretion of caesium-137 by man. *Phys. Med. Biol.* **7,** 157 (1962).

20. Van Dilla, M. A., and Anderson, E. C., Human counters using liquid scintillators. *Proc. Symp. Whole-Body Counting, Vienna, 1961* p. 41. Intern. At. Energy Agency, Vienna, 1962.
21. Woodward, K. T., Richmond, C. R., and Langham, W. H., Measurement of retention and excretion of radioisotopes of the alkali metals by mice and rats, using an annular liquid scintillation counter. *Proc. 1st Health Phys. Soc., 1956* p. 79 (1956).
22. Zerby, C. D., A calculation to predict the pulse-height response function from gamma-ray scintillation counters. *Proc. Total Absorption Gamma-Ray Spectrometry Symp., Gatlinburg, Tenn., 1960*. TID-7594, p. 80. U.S. At. Energy Comm., Washington, D.C., 1960.

APPENDIX

GERALD J. HINE AND ROBERT LOEVINGER
SECTION OF MEDICINE, DEPARTMENT OF RESEARCH AND ISOTOPES,
INTERNATIONAL ATOMIC ENERGY AGENCY, VIENNA

I. ELECTRON RANGE AND GAMMA-RAY ABSORPTION

TABLE I
PHYSICAL DATA FOR DETERMINATION OF γ-RAY TRANSMISSION[a]

Radioisotope	γ-Ray energy[b] (MeV)	Total γ-ray absorption coefficient (cm^{-1}): Water	Sodium iodide	Lead
^{125}I	0.033	0.30	—	—
^{197}Hg	0.077	0.18	8.07	—
^{99m}Tc	0.140	0.15	2.57	22.7
^{203}Hg	0.279	0.12	0.643	4.87
^{131}I	0.364	0.11	0.463	2.95
^{198}Au	0.412	0.105	0.404	2.42
Annihilation	0.511	0.096	0.338	1.7
^{137}Cs	0.662	0.085	0.272	1.2
^{60}Co	1.25	0.063	0.188	0.66

[a] Hubbell, J. H., and Berger, M. J., Nat. Bur. Std. (U.S.) Report 8681 (1965).
[b] The values of the γ-ray energy listed have been used for determining the absorption coefficients.

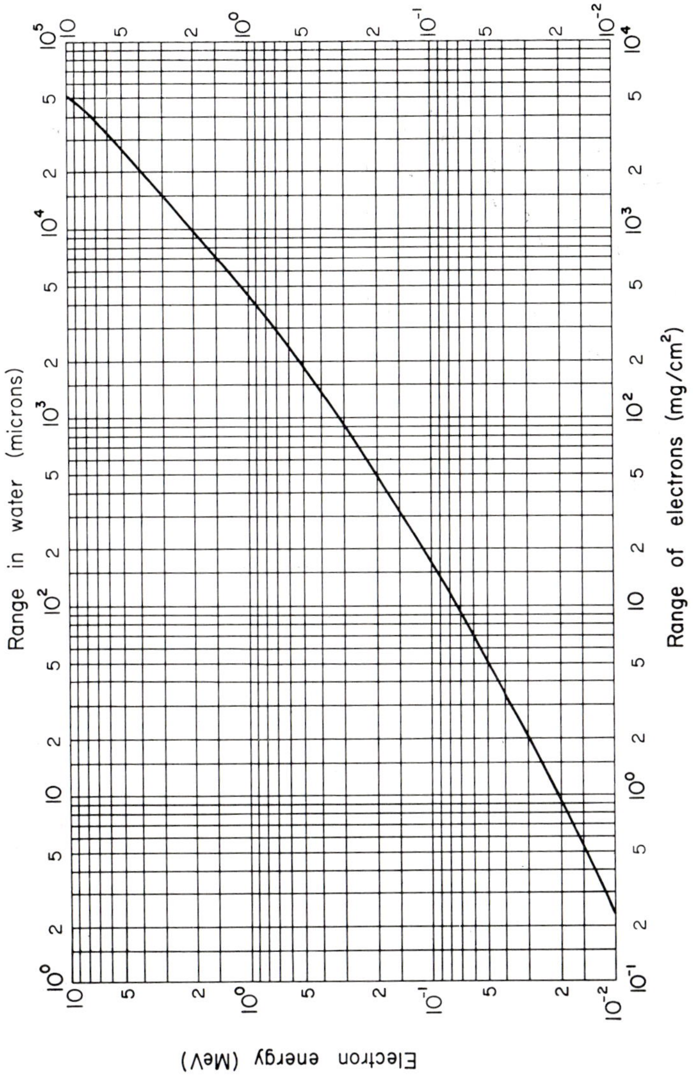

FIG. 1. Maximum range of electrons as a function of electron energy.

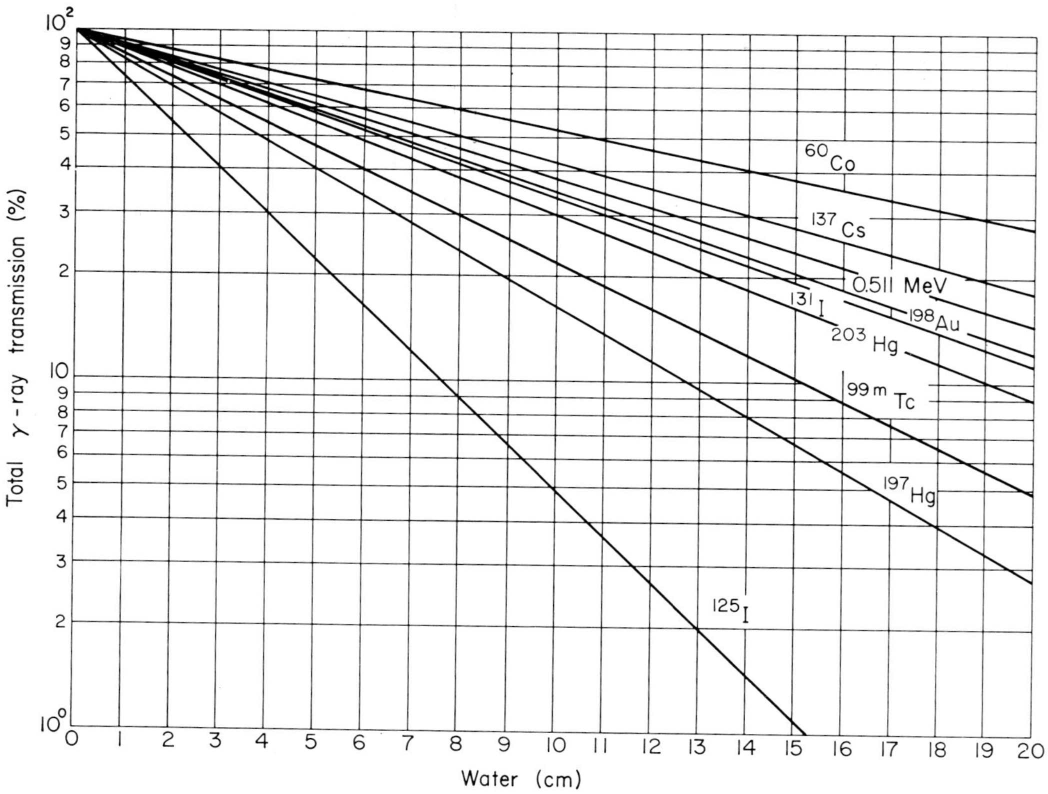

FIG. 2. Absorption (total) in water of the γ rays emitted from various radionuclides. The fraction absorbed equal one minus the fraction transmitted which is plotted in percent as a function of the thickness of the water absorber (Data plotted from Table I).

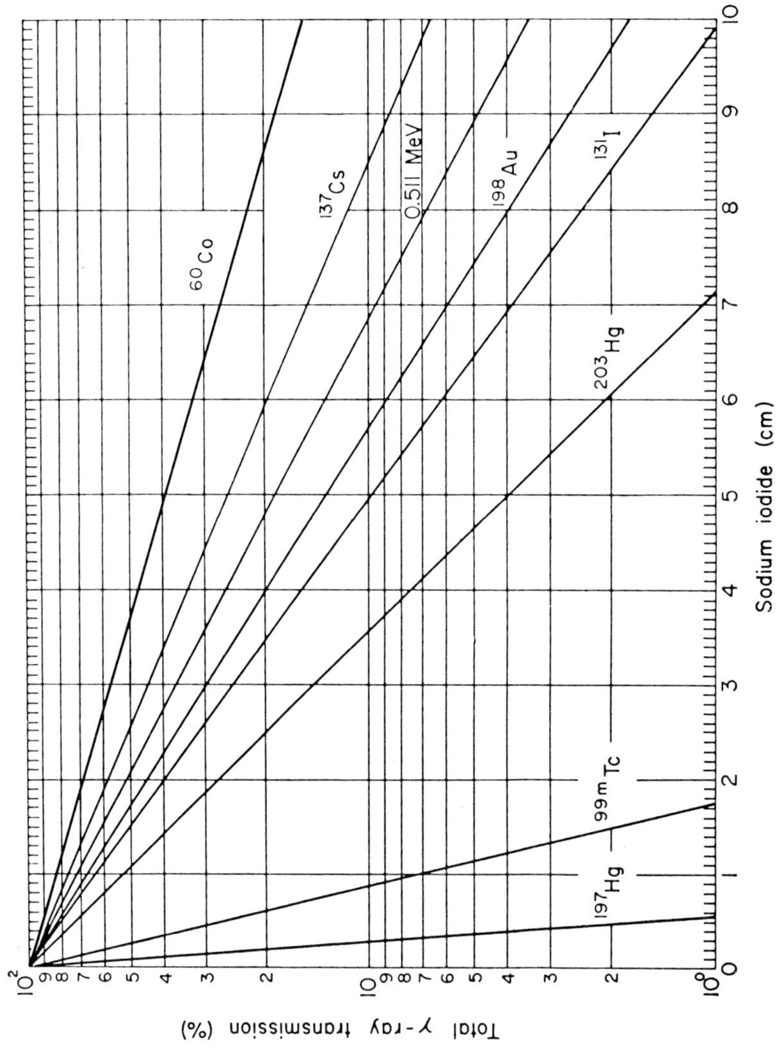

FIG. 3. Absorption (total) in sodium iodide of the γ rays emitted from various radionuclides. The fraction absorbed equals one minus the fraction transmitted which is plotted in percent as a function of the thickness of the sodium iodide absorber (Data plotted from Table I).

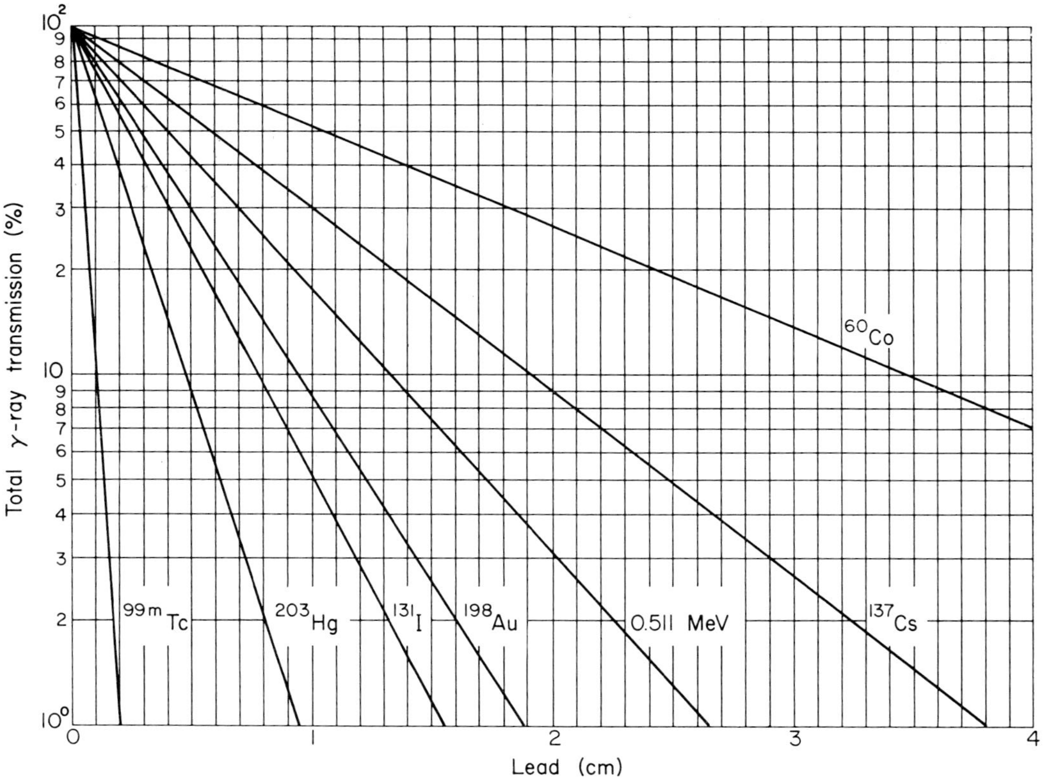

FIG. 4. Absorption (total) in lead of the γ rays emitted from various radionuclides. The fraction absorbed equals one minus the fraction transmitted which is plotted in percent as a function of the thickness of the lead absorber (Data plotted from Table I).

II. APPLICATION AND RADIATION DOSE OF RADIOISOTOPES IN MEDICINE

The figures and tables on the following pages deal with the total radiation dose received from administered radioisotopes.

TABLE II

Total Mean Radiation Dose to Standard Man from Some Administered Radioisotopes[a]

Organ or pool	Type of study	Radio-nuclide	Chemical form	Administration: Activity (μCi)	Administration: Route	Mean dose to standard man[b] (mrad per μCi administered): Whole body	Blood	Bone marrow	Kidney	Liver	Spleen	Thyroid
Thyroid gland	Uptake	^{131}I	Sodium iodide	1–25	oral	0.4						1500
		^{132}I	Sodium iodide	1–25	oral	0.1						40
	Scan	^{131}I	Sodium iodide	50–100	oral	0.4						1500
		^{125}I	Sodium iodide	50–100	oral	0.4						1000
		^{99m}Tc	Pertechnetate	1000	i.v.	0.01						0.3
Ferrokinetics	Iron absorption	^{59}Fe	Ferrous citrate	3–5	oral							
		^{59}Fe	Ferric chloride	3–5	oral	3					15	
	Plasma iron transport, degree and site of erythropoiesis	^{59}Fe	Ferrous citrate	3–10	i.v.							
		^{59}Fe	Ferric chloride	3–10	i.v.	20						
Circulatory system	Liver blood flow	^{198}Au	Colloidal gold	15	i.v.	2		4		40	40	
	Placental localization	^{131}I	Serum albumin	1–5	i.v.	2	20					1
		^{51}Cr	Tagged RBC	10	i.v.	0.3	2					
		^{99m}Tc	Albumin	1000	i.v.	0.02	0.05					
Blood	Plasma volume	^{131}I	Serum albumin	3–20	i.v.	2	20					1
		^{51}Cr	Serum albumin	25–100	i.v.	0.2	2					
	Red cell volume and survival	^{51}Cr	Tagged RBC	50	i.v.	0.3	2				40	
	Red cell survival	^{32}P	DFP	100–300	i.v.		100					
	Platlet survival	^{32}P	DFP	100	i.v.		50					
		^{14}C	Serotonin	4	i.v.		4					
Spleen	Scan	^{51}C	Tagged RBC	200–300	i.v.	0.3	2				40	
Body water	Total water	^{3}H	Tritiated water	1000–2000	i.v., oral	0.2						
Sodium space	Exchangeable sodium	^{22}Na	Sodium chloride	3–20	i.v.	20		120				
		^{24}Na	Sodium chloride	50–100	i.v.	2						

Skin, visible mucous membranes, cavity linings, eye.	Tumor diagnosis, localization	^{32}P	Disodium phosphate	100–500	i.v.	8		40		30	30	
Brain	Scan, tumor localization	^{203}Hg	Chlormerodrin	500–700	i.v.	0.4			80			
		^{197}Hg	Chlormerodrin	700–1500	i.v.	0.1			5			
		^{131}I	Serum albumin	300–1500	i.v.	2	20					
		^{131}I	PVP	300–500	i.v.	1	30					
		^{99m}Tc	Pertechnetate	10,000–15,000	i.v.	0.01						0.1 (thyroid blocked)
Liver	Scan, tumor localization, structure	^{131}I	Rose bengal	100–150	i.v.	0.4						
		^{198}Au	Colloidal gold	100–200	i.v.	2		4		40	40	
		^{131}I	Aggregated albumin	300–500	i.v.	0.1				0.6		
		^{99m}Tc	Colloidal sulfide	2000–10,000	i.v.	0.02		0.02		0.3	0.3	
	Function	^{131}I	Rose bengal	15	i.v.	0.4						
Kidney	Scan	^{203}Hg	Chlormerodrin	150	i.v.	0.4			80			
	Function	^{197}Hg	Chlormerodrin	150	i.v.	0.1			5			
		^{203}Hg	Chlormerodrin	10–50	i.v.	0.4			80			
		^{197}Hg	Chlormerodrin	10–50	i.v.	0.1			5			
		^{131}I	Hippuran	10–30	i.v.	0.03			0.6			
		^{125}I	Hippuran	10–50	i.v.	0.01			0.2			
Absorption studies	Vitamin B_{12}	^{57}Co	Vitamin B_{12}	0.5	oral	5				80		
		^{58}Co	Vitamin B_{12}	0.5	oral	20				400		
		^{60}Co	Vitamin B_{12}	0.5	oral	200				5000		
	Fat	^{131}I	Triolein or oleic acid	1–50	oral	0.6						
	Calcium	^{47}Ca	Calcium chloride	10	oral			20				
		^{45}Ca	Calcium chloride	5	oral			80				
Bone	Tumor localization	^{85}Sr	Strontium chloride	30	i.v.			10				

[a] The entries of the first six columns are based on tables given in the following reference: Silver, S., *Nucleonics* **23,** (8), 106 (1965).

[b] There is no general agreement on the biological assumptions that are the basis of internal dose computations and therefore the published dose values vary significantly. The mean radiation doses given in the last seven columns are based on the following references: Osborn, S. B., and Ellis, R. E. *In* "The Science of Ionizing Radiation" (E. E. Etter, ed.), Chap. 29, Charles C Thomas, Springfield, 1965. Seltzer, R. A., Kereiakes, J. G., and Saenger, E. L., *New England J. Med.* **271,** 84 (1964). Smith, E. M., *J. Nucl. Med.* **6,** 231 (1965).

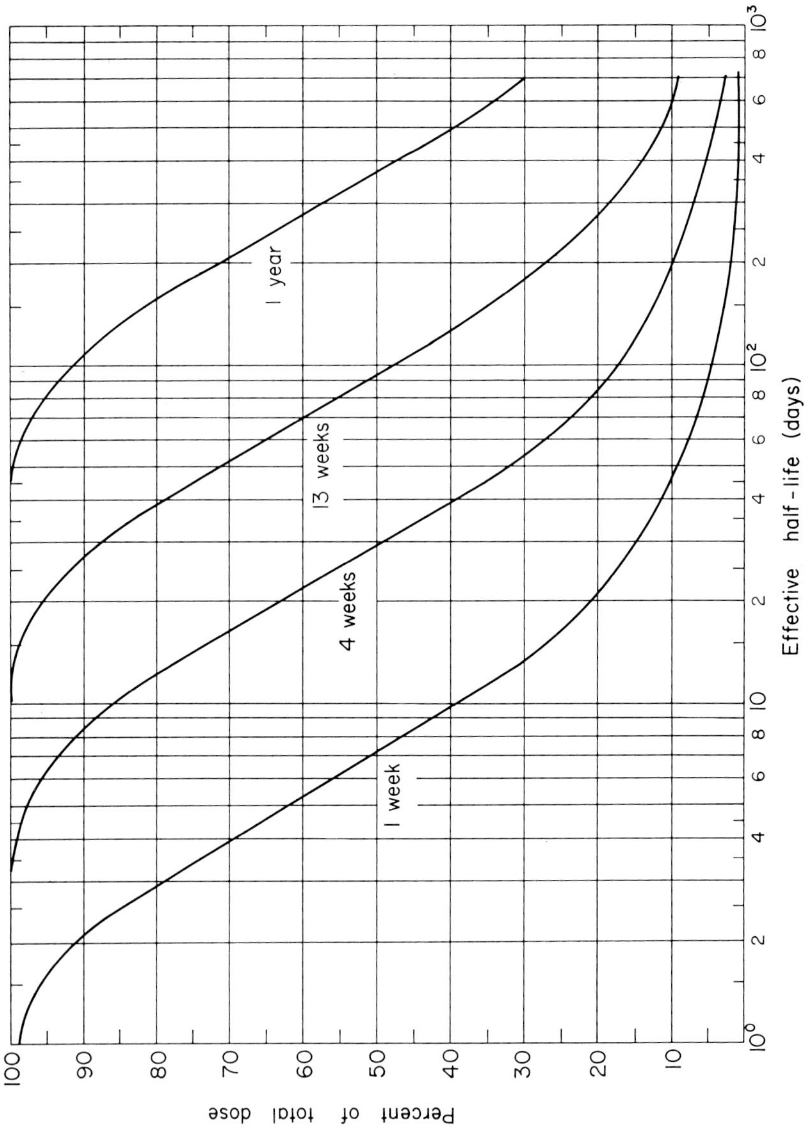

FIG. 5. See legend, opposite page.

TABLE III
TOTAL MEAN RADIATION DOSE FROM ADMINISTERED RADIOISOTOPES, FOR VARIOUS AGES, RELATIVE TO STANDARD MAN[a]

		Age group (years)				
Organ or pool	Std. man	15	10	5	1	New-born
Whole body, and organs except thyroid	1.00	1.0–1.3	1.6–2.0	2.6–3.4	4–6	7–25
Radioiodine in thyroid gland	1.00	1.3	2.3	3.3	8	25

[a] The table gives the radiation dose for each age group relative to the radiation dose for standard man listed in Table II. The data have been calculated from Tables III and IV of R. A. Seltzer, J. G. Kereiakes, and E. L. Saenger, *New Eng. J. Med.*, **271**, 84 (1964).

III. MANUFACTURERS OF NUCLEAR INSTRUMENTS AND THEIR PRODUCTS

The number of companies and their products which find applications in nuclear medicine is constantly increasing. Therefore only an approximate list of all companies and their products can be given. To indicate the product area of each company nineteen different categories were chosen somewhat arbitrarily, giving preference to items produced specifically for use in nuclear medicine. Some categories encompass a variety of instruments. For example, "counters" includes all sizes and types for widely different applications. Under "counting assemblies" complete counting units are listed including some with heavy lead shielding, sample holders, preamplifier, etc. However, some components, such as multiplier phototubes and scintillators, are listed separately, though they ordinarily are parts of counting assemblies and are not purchased as separate items. A list of such components might be of help to those engaged in developmental work.

Some types of instruments are not listed, for various reasons. High voltage power supplies are available from all manufacturers of scalers and ratemeters and are frequently an integral part of such instruments.

FIG. 5. Percent of total radiation dose delivered in various times, as a function of the effective half-life. The ordinate gives the radiation dose to an organ (or to the whole body) during 1 week, 4 weeks, 13 weeks, and 1 year, in percent of the total dose delivered during an infinitely-long time as listed in Table II. The abscissa gives the effective half-life in the organ (or whole body) in days. Example: during the first 4-week interval, 27% of the total dose is delivered to an organ by a radionuclide with a 2-month effective half-life. The graph is based on values given by J. Vennart, and M. Minski, *Brit. J. Rad.* **35**, 372 (1962).

Coincidence circuits, though used in liquid scintillation counting and low-level beta-ray measurements, cannot be regarded as instruments employed separately in nuclear medicine. While the contrary may be true for scintillation cameras in the near future, for the present compilation they are regarded as part of scanning instrumentation. Magnetic tape recorders for data storage, data readout instruments such as electronic recorders, data plotters, and paper punch tape are accessories generally used in many fields. They are mostly produced by companies outside the nuclear medicine field.

The companies with headquarters in the United States are listed separately from those located in other countries. This should not indicate any difference regarding the performance or usefulness of their products or otherwise. This division which results in two lists of about equal lengths, simplified their compilation and may enable the user to find the desired information faster.

The choice of companies to be included in this tabulation was difficult. It appeared unjustified to consider only the large companies which are in existence for many years because original and advanced instruments have become available from companies which were founded only recently. On the other hand, some of these companies have ceased to exist in some cases even after an initially successful start. Some companies produce scalers for industrial purposes which could be used in nuclear medicine; however, they were excluded to keep the list reasonably short. This also applies to companies producing health and safety instrumentation used mainly at reactor sites or other nonmedical installations.

The addresses of all listed companies are given and the reader is advised to obtain detailed information concerning their products from the companies themselves. The list of categories of products follows.

Categories of Products Applicable in Nuclear Medicine

1. Amplifiers
2. Chromatographic apparatus
3. Counters (G-M, prop., flow)
4. Counting assemblies (G-M, scintillation)
5. Dosimeters
6. Liquid scintillation counting assemblies
7. Low-background counting assemblies
8. Multichannel analyzers (100 channels or more)
9. Multiplier phototubes
10. Phantoms
11. Pulse-height analyzers (single, double)
12. Ratemeters
13. Sample changers (automatic)
14. Scalers
15. Scanners—Scintillation cameras
16. Scintillators (organic, inorganic)
17. Semiconductor detectors
18. Survey meters—Monitors
19. Whole-body counters

Names, Addresses, and Products of Nuclear Instrument Companies

(The italic numbers refer to categories of products applicable in nuclear medicine as listed on page 630.)

A. HEADQUARTERS IN THE UNITED STATES

Alderson Research Labs., Inc.
48–14 33rd Street
Long Island City 1, N.Y.
5, 10

Ames Atomium, Inc.
575 Middlesex Turnpike
Billerica, Mass. 01865
4, 12, 14

Amperex Electronic Corp.
230 Duffy Ave.
Hicksville L.I., N.Y. 11802
3, 9

ANS, Inc.
P.O. Box 241
Huntington, N.Y. 11744
6

AtoMation Inc.
Division of C. W. Reed Co., Inc.
5959 S. Hoover Street
Los Angeles, Calif.
4, 10, 14, 15, 19

Baird-Atomic, Inc.
33 University Road
Cambridge, Mass. 02138
1–5, 7, 8, 11–15, 18

Beckman Instruments, Inc.
2500 Harbor Blvd.
Fullerton, Calif. 92634
6, 7

Bradley Semiconductor Corp.
275 Welton Street
New Haven 11, Conn. 06506
17

Controls for Radiation, Inc.
130 Alewife Brook Parkway
Cambridge, Mass. 02140
5

Curtis Nuclear Corp.
1948 E. 46th Street
Los Angeles, Calif. 90058
4, 11, 12, 14, 15, 18

Eberline Instrument Corp.
805 Early Street
Santa Fe, New Mexico 87501
5, 14, 18

Edgerton, Germeshausen & Grier, Inc.
(EG&G)
130 Robin Hill Road
Goleta, Calif. 93017
5

Eldorado Electronics
601 Chalomar Road
Concord, Calif.
1, 11, 14

Electro-Fab
18034½ Ventura Blvd.
Encino, Calif.
4, 11, 12

Electro-Nuclear Laboratories, Inc.
(ENL)
115 Independence Drive
Menlo Park, Calif. 94025
1, 17

Eon Corporation
175 Pearl Street
Brooklyn, N.Y. 11201
3, 18

Fairchild, DuMont
Electron Tubes
750 Bloomfield Ave.
Clifton, New Jersey
9

Franklin Electronics, Inc.
East Fourth Street
Bridgeport, Penn. 19405
1, 11, 14

Gelman Instrument Co.
600 S. Wagner Road
Ann Arbor, Mich. 48106
5, 18

Hamner Electronics Co., Inc.
Subsidiary of Harshaw Chemical Co.
P.O. Box 531
Princeton, New Jersey 08540
1, 3, 4, 7, 11, 12, 14, 17

Harshaw Chemical Co.
1945 East 97th Street
Cleveland, Ohio 44106
3, 5, 16, 17

Hewlett Packard
1501 Page Mill Road
Palo Alto, Calif. 94304
4, 11, 14

Hughes Semiconductor Div.
500 Superior Ave.
Newport Beach, Calif.
17

Hunkar Instrument Development Laboratories, Inc.
2882 Wasson Road
Cincinnati, Ohio 45209
1, 4, 11, 13, 14

Interstate Electronics Corp.
707 East Vermont Ave.
Anaheim, Calif.
1, 4, 7, 11, 14

Isomet Corp.
433 Commercial Ave.
Palisades Park, New Jersey 07650
16

Isotopes, Inc.
123 Woodland Ave.
Westwood, New Jersey, 07675
3, 16, 17

Johnston Laboratories, Inc.
3617 Woodland Ave.
Baltimore, Md. 21215
7

Landsverk Electrometer Co.
641 Sonora Ave.
Glendale, Calif. 91201
5, 18

Leighton Labs, H.W.
250 Titus Ave.
Warrington, Penn.
3, 18

Lionel Electronic Laboratories, Inc.
Hoffman Place
Hillside, New Jersey 07205
3, 12, 14, 18

LND, Inc.
3230 Lawson Blvd.
Oceanside, N.Y. 11572
3

Madison Research & Development Labs., Inc.
7617 Donna Drive
Middleton, Wisc. 53562
5

Metrix, Inc.
P.O. Box 6222
Denver, Colorado 80206
4, 7, 19

Northern Scientific, Inc.
303 Price Place
Madison, Wisc. 53711
8

Nuclear-Chicago Corp.
333 East Howard Ave.
Des Plaines, Ill. 60018
1–8, 11–15, 18

Nuclear Corp. of America (Nucor)
2 Richwood Place
Denville, New Jersey
12, 14–16, 18

Nuclear Data, Inc.
114 West Golf Road
Palatine, Ill. 60067
3, 4, 7, 8, 11–14

Nuclear Development Lab., Inc.
P.O. Box 7034
Kansas City, Missouri 64113
3

Nuclear Diodes, Inc.
1640 Old Deerfield Road
Highland Park, Ill.
4, 16, 17

Nuclear Measurements Corp. (NMC)
2460 N. Arlington Ave.
Indianapolis, Indiana 46218
3, 4, 7, 11, 12, 14, 15, 18

Nuclear Research Corp.
Street Road at 2nd Street Pike
Southampton, Penn. 18966
3, 11, 13, 18

Nucleonic Corp. of America (NCA)
196 De Graw Street
Brooklyn, N.Y. 11231
3, 5, 11–14, 18

Numec Instrument & Controls Corp. (Numinco)
300 Seco Road
Monroeville, Penn. 15146
2, 3, 5, 14

Oak Ridge Technical Enterprises, Corp. (ORTEC)
111 Midland Road
Oak Ridge, Tenn. 37830
1, 11, 14, 17

Ohio Nuclear, Inc.
1725 Fall Ave.
Cleveland, Ohio 44113
4, 15

Packard Instrument Company, Inc.
2200 Warrenville Road
Downers Grove, Ill. 60515
2, 4, 6, 8, 11–14, 16, 19

Picker Nuclear
1275 Mamaroneck Ave.
White Plains, N.Y. 10605
1, 2, 4, 6, 7, 10–15, 18

Pilot Chemicals, Inc.
36 Pleasant Street
Watertown, Mass. 02172
16

Princeton Gamma-Tech, Inc.
P.O. Box 641
Princeton, New Jersey 08540
17

Quartz Products Corp.
698 Somerset Street
Plainfield, New Jersey
16

Radiation Counter Labs., Inc. (RCL)
5121 W. Grove Street
Skokie, Ill.
1, 3, 4, 8, 11–14, 18

RCA Electronic Components & Devices
415 S. 5th Street
Harrison, New Jersey 07029
9

Reuter-Stokes Electronic Components, Inc.
18530 S. Miles Parkway
Cleveland, Ohio 44128
3

Solid State Radiations, Inc.
2261 S. Carmelina Ave.
Los Angeles, Calif. 90064
17

Sturrup Nuclear
Div. Canberra Industries, Inc.
50 Silver Street
Middletown, Conn. 06458
1, 11, 12, 14

Technical Associates (TA)
140 W. Providencia Ave.
Burbank, Calif. 91502
3, 4, 7, 11–14, 18

Technical Measurement Corp. (TMC)
441 Washington Ave.
North Haven, Conn. 06473
2, 7, 8, 17

Tennelec Instrument Co., Inc.
140 E. Division Road
Oak Ridge, Tenn. 37830
1, 17

Tracerlab,
Div. of Laboratory for Electronics, Inc.
1601 Trapelo Road
Waltham, Mass. 02154
1–7, 11–14, 18

Victoreen Instrument Company
10101 Woodland Ave.
Cleveland, Ohio 44104
1, 3–5, 8, 11–14, 18

Wilkens Instrument and Research, Inc.
P.O. Box 313
Walnut Creek, Calif.
2

Wood Counter Lab. N., Inc.
1525 E. 53rd Street
Chicago, Ill. 60615
3

B. Companies with Headquarters Outside the United States

ACEC (Ateliers de Constructions Electriques de Charleroi)
Ave, E. Rousseau
Charleroi, Belgium
1, 3, 4, 11–14, 18

Dynatron Electronics
St. Peters Road, Furze Platt
Maidenhead, Birkshire, U.K.
1, 4, 11, 14

EKCO Electronics Ltd.
Southend-on-Sea, Essex, U.K.
1, 2, 4–6, 11–16, 18

Elliott Brothers Ltd.
Elstree Way
Borehamwood, Hertfordshire, U.K.
17

Elliott Nucleonics Ltd.
Century Works, Lewisham
London, S.E. 13, U.K.
11, 12, 14

Elron Electronics Industries Ltd.
88 Hagiborim Street
Haifa, Israel
1, 4, 11, 12, 14, 18

EMI Electronics Ltd.
Blyth Road
Hayes, Middlesex, U.K.
1, 4, 9, 11, 12, 14, 18

Ferranti Ltd.
Kern House 36, Kingsway
London, W.C. 2, U.K.
17

Finska Kabelfabriken Aktiebolag
P.O. Box 10419
Helsinki, Finland
8, 11

Fleming Instruments Ltd.
Caxton Way
Stevenage, Hertfordshire, U.K.
1, 11, 12, 14

Frieseke & Hoepfner GmbH
Tennenloher Str. 41
8520 Erlangen-Bruck, Germany
1–6, 11–15, 18

General Radiological
Bessemer Road
Welwyn Garden City, Hertfordshire, U.K.
1, 5, 12, 14, 18

Grey & Marten Ltd.
City Lead Works, Southwark Bridge
London, S.E.1., U.K.
10

Hilger & Watts Ltd.
98, St. Pancras Way
London, N.W.1, U.K.
16

Intertechnique, SA
B.P. 1
78 Plaisir (S.-et-O.), France
1, 4, 6–8, 11–15, 18

IDL (Isotope Development Ltd.)
Bath Road, Beenham
Reading, Berkshire, U.K.
1–7, 11–15, 18

Ital Elettronica S.P.A.
Via Ignazio Pettinengo 72
Roma, Italy
1, 3, 4, 11, 12, 14, 15, 18

Kobe Industries Corp.
5, Wadayama-dori, 1-Chome Hyogo-ku
Kobe, Japan
1, 3, 4, 6, 8, 11–14, 16, 18

Kyoto Electronics Mfg. Co. Ltd.
11, Kawa Higashi-Cho
Fushimi-ku
Kyoto, Japan
16

Laben (Laboratori Elettronici e Nucleari) S.p.a.
Via Edoardo Bassini 15
Milano, Italy
1, 8, 11, 12, 14, 18

Labgear Ltd.
Cromwell Road
Cambridge, U.K.
1, 3, 4, 7, 11–14, 18

Laboratoire Central de Telecommunications
46, Avenue de Breteuil
Paris 7e, France
3

Laboratoire Industriel d'Electrique Belin
296, Av. Napoléon Bonaparte
Rueil-Malmaison (S.-et-O.), France
1, 4, 6, 9, 11, 14, 16

Laboratorium Prof. Dr. Berthold
7547 Wildbad (Schwarzwald), Germany
1–4, 11–14, 18

Landis & Gyr, Inc.
Zug, Switzerland
1, 3–5, 11, 12, 14, 15, 18

La Physiotechnique
34 Av. Aristide Briand
Arcueil (Seine), France
5

La Radiotechnique
130, Avenue Ledru-Rollin
Paris 11e, France
3, 9, 16, 17

L'Electronique Appliquée
98, rue Maurice Arnoux
Montrouge (Seine), France
1, 4, 11, 12, 14

Massiot Philips
40, Avenue Hoche
Paris 8e, France
2–5, 7, 11, 13–15

MBLE (Manufacture Belge de Lampes et de Materiel electronique, S.A.)
80, rue des Deux-Gares
Bruxelles 7, Belgium
1–7, 11–14, 18

Mécaserto
126, Boulevard d'Alsace-Lorraine
Le Perraux (Seine), France
4, 13, 15, 17

Mesco
55, rue Benoit-Malon
Gentilly (Seine), France
1, 4, 5, 11, 12, 14, 18

Metrimpex
B.P. 202
Budapest 62, Hungary
1, 3–5, 8, 11, 12, 14–16, 18

Metronex
Al. Jerozolimskie 44
Warsaw, Poland
1, 3–5, 11, 12, 14, 16, 18

Mitsubishi Atomic Power Industries, Inc.
4, Ohtemachi 1-chome Chiyoda-ku
Tokyo, Japan
1, 3, 4, 7–9, 12–14, 18

Nash & Thompson
Hook Rise
Tolworth, Surrey, U.K.
16

Noratom A/S
Holmenveien 20, Vinderen
Oslo 3, Norway
4, 7, 12–14, 18

Nuclear Enterprises Ltd.
Sighthill
Edinburgh 11, U.K.
550 Berry Street
Winnipeg 21, Manitoba, Canada
1, 4, 6, 8, 11–19

Nuclear Research Application Ltd.
Emefco House, 107 Bell Street
Reigate, Surrey, U.K.
1–5, 7, 11–14, 16–18

Omnipol
Washingtonova 11
Praha 3, Czechoslovakia
1, 3–5, 8, 11, 12, 14, 18

Philips
Eindhoven, Holland
1–5, 7–9, 11–16, 18

Physikalisch-Technische Werkstätten
Lörracherstrasse 7
Freiburg im Breisgau, Germany
5

Quartz & Silice, S.A.
8, rue d'Anjou
Paris 8e, France
16, 17

RCA Victor Co. Ltd.
1001 Lenoir
Montreal 30, Canada
17

Reichert-Elektronik
Petrisberg
55 Trier, Germany
18

Research Electronics Ltd.
Bradford Road
Cleckheaton, Yorkshire, U.K.
1, 4, 11, 12, 14

SAIP (Soc. d'Applications Industrielles de la Physique)
38, rue Gabriel-Crie
Malakoff (Seine) France
1–5, 8, 11–14

SELO (Società Elettronica Lombarda)
Via G. D. Vittorio 307/28
Sesto San Giovanni
Milano, Italy
1, 3, 4, 7, 8, 11–15, 18, 19

Shimadzu Seisakusho Ltd.
18, Nishinokyo-Kuwabaracho
Nakagyo-ku, Kyoto, Japan
1, 3–5, 11, 12, 14, 15, 18

Siemens-Wernerwerk AG
Rheinbrückenstrasse 50
75 Karlsruhe-West Germany
1, 4, 5, 11–15, 18

Sierex Ltd.
15–18 Clipstone Street
London, W.1., U.K.
10

Simtec ltd.
3400 Metropolitan Blvd. East
Montreal 38, Canada
1, 17

SRAT (Soc. de Recherches et d'Applications Techniques)
41, rue Emeriau
Paris 15e, France
18

Stephen, R. A. & Co. Ltd.
Miles Road
Mitcham, Surrey, U.K.
5

Techniques Nucleaires
82, rue de Montigny
Argenteuil (S.-et-O.), France
1, 4, 11, 12, 14

Technopromexport
18,1 Ovchinnikovskaya nabersjnaya
Moscow, J-324, U.S.S.R
1, 3–5, 8, 9, 11, 12, 14, 18

Telefunken A.G.
Elisabethstrasse 3
7900 Ulm, Germany
2, 4, 5, 8, 11–14, 18

Toshiba
(Tokyo Shibaura Electric Co. Ltd.)
1-1 Uchisaiwa-cho, Chiyoda-ku
Tokyo, Japan
4, 5, 11, 12, 14, 18

Trombay Electronic Instruments
A.E.E.T.
Bombay 74, India
1, 4, 11, 12, 14, 18

Twentieth Century Electronics Ltd.
King Henry's Drive
New Addington, Croydon, Surrey, U.K.
3, 9, 17

Wallac Oy
Turku 5, Finland
1, 4, 5, 11–14, 18

AUTHOR INDEX

Numbers in parentheses are reference numbers and indicate that an author's work is referred to although his name is not cited in the text. Numbers in italic show the page on which the complete reference is listed.

C

D

N

O

P

S

Y

Z

SUBJECT INDEX

S

T

C 6
D 7
E 8
F 9
G 0
H 1
I 2
J 3